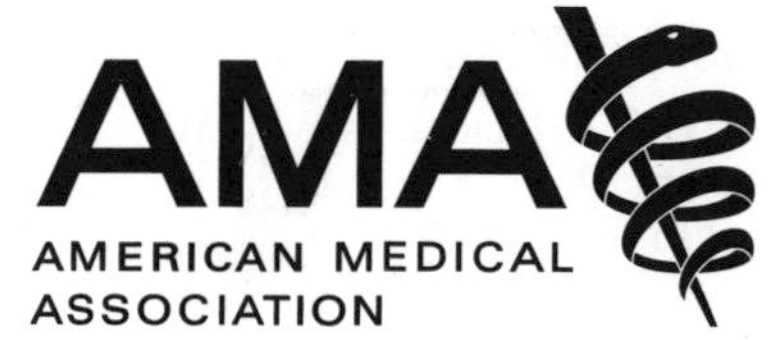

RISK ADJUSTMENT

DOCUMENTATION & CODING

SHERI POE BERNARD, CCS-P, CDEO, CPC, CRC

Risk Adjustment Documentation & Coding

Executive Vice President, Chief Executive Officer: James L. Madara, MD
Chief Operating Officer: Bernard L. Hengesbaugh
Senior Vice President, Health Solutions: Laurie A.S. McGraw
Vice President, Operations: Denise Foy
Manager, Book and Product Development and Production: Nancy Baker
Senior Developmental Editor: Lisa Chin-Johnson
Production Specialist: Mary Ann Albanese
Vice President, Sales: Lori Prestesater
Director, Channel Sales: Erin Kalitowski
Executive, Key Account Manager: Mark Daniels
Vice President, Marketing and Strategic Initiatives: Dave Sosnow
Product Manager, Print and Digital Products: Carol Brockman
Marketing Manager: Vanessa Prieto

Printed in the United States of America. 18 19 20 / TB-WE / 9 8 7 6 5 4 3 2 1

AMA publication and product updates, errata, and addenda can be found at amaproductupdates.org.

Internet address: www.ama-assn.org

To purchase additional copies of this book, contact the American Medical Association at 800 621-8335 or visit the AMA store at amastore.com. Refer to item number OP287018.

The AMA does not directly or indirectly practice medicine or dispense medical services. This publication does not replace the AMA's ICD-10-CM codebook or other appropriate coding authority. The coding information in this publication should be used only as a guide.

U.S. public laws and federal rules and regulations included in this publication are in the public domain. However, the arrangement, compilation, organization, and history of, and references to, such laws and regulations, along with all ICD-10-CM data and other materials are subject to the above copyright notice.

The Center for Medicare & Medicaid Services is responsible for the Medicare content contained in this publication and no endorsement by the AMA is intended or should be implied. Readers are encouraged to refer to the current official Medicare program provisions contained in relevant laws, regulations, and rulings. The Centers for Disease Control and Prevention is responsible for the ICD-10-CM content contained in this publication and no endorsement by the AMA is intended or should be implied. Readers are encouraged to refer to the current *ICD-10-CM Official Guidelines for Coding and Reporting* provisions contained in relevant guidelines for coding and reporting.

The American Medical Association ("AMA") and its authors and editors have consulted sources believed to be knowledgeable in their fields. However, neither the AMA nor its authors or editors warrant that the information is in every respect accurate and/or complete. The AMA, its authors, and editors assume no responsibility for use of the information contained in this publication. Neither the AMA nor its authors or editors shall be responsible for, and expressly disclaims liability for, damages of any kind arising out of the use of, reference to, or reliance on, the content of this publication. This publication is for informational purposes only. The AMA does not provide medical, legal, financial, or other professional advice and readers are encouraged to consult a professional advisor for such advice. The contents of this publication represent the views of the author[s] and should not be construed to be the views or policy of the AMA, or of the institution with which the author[s] may be affiliated, unless this is clearly specified.

Library of Congress Cataloging-in-Publication Data

Names: Bernard, Sheri Poe, author. | American Medical Association, issuing body.
Title: Risk adjustment documentation and coding / by Sheri P. Bernard.
Description: Chicago, IL: American Medical Association, [2018] | Includes bibliographical references and index.
Identifiers: LCCN 2017060194 | ISBN 9781622027330
Subjects: | MESH: International statistical classification of diseases and related health problems. 10th revision. Clinical modification. | Clinical Coding | Chronic Disease--economics | Documentation | Practice Management, Medical | Risk Adjustment | Severity of Illness Index
Classification: LCC RB115 | NLM W 80 | DDC 616.0076--dc23 LC record available at https://urldefense.proofpoint.com/v2/url?u=https-3A__lccn.loc.gov_2017060194&d=DwIFAg&c=iqeSLYkBTKTEV8nJYtdW_A&r=tWLRptOfAe8Swd0MiddLUysmHcNwwaujBy6V3K7jcZk&m=xYslcMdUwxRMTRK1Y3_5BCryyZ5CPXqJIVX7CeMNVz8&s=oNP0X7L7makSkEeHduYlvf0wtu9SNFW3X1xE2ff0ep8&e

ISBN 978-1-62202-733-0

OP287018:AC69:03/18

Contents

Foreword

As a general internist trained at the University of Tennessee in Memphis from 1976 to 1982, I believed that my professional success only required that I master medical science and work hard to bend the natural history of my patients' diseases to their favor.

It was not until the last year of my residency I learned there was a business side of medicine whereby Current Procedural Terminology (CPT®) coding was essential to my fee-for-service revenue cycle. It wasn't really that hard: five CPT codes for new outpatients, five CPT codes for established outpatients, several CPT codes for consultations and inpatient care, and certain CPT codes for the hospital and office procedures I performed. ICD-9-CM did not seem to matter, other than ensuring that certain CPT codes (eg, for ancillary services) would be paid. As such, I used the most generic ICD-9-CM codes I could remember to represent my patients' illnesses, such as 250.00 for diabetes, 496 for COPD, 401.1 for hypertension, and 780.79 for malaise and fatigue, given that these codes got all my lab tests covered, my patients were tired, and their doctor was tired!

Upon the second year of my hospital medical practice in 1984, CMS (then HCFA) introduced diagnosis-related groups (DRGs) that placed my county-owned community hospital on a budget for each admission. I had no clue that my inpatient documentation and its translation into ICD-9-CM (now ICD-10-CM/PCS) codes established these budgets. As such, I continued to document terms like "urosepsis," "non-cardiac chest pain," "altered mental status," "healthcare-acquired pneumonia," "poorly controlled diabetes," and similar terms, which, upon ICD-9-CM coding review, created skimpier DRG budgets than alterative language like "sepsis due to a urinary tract infection," "chest pain likely due to GERD," "metabolic encephalopathy," "pneumonia probably due to aspiration requiring clindamycin," "uncontrolled diabetes," and other coding descriptors that added revenue my hospital depended on.

It wasn't until 1999 that I learned coders could not clinically interpret the medical record to assign codes essential to inpatient DRG-based risk adjustment (RA). I thought the coders could just see the feathers, quacking, waddling, web feet, and the other clinical indicators in my patients' records and code "duck." Even though hospitals developed and deployed clinical documentation improvement (CDI) programs addressing our documentation habits, many physicians resisted, believing that these exercises only benefited the hospital, not the physicians' revenue cycles.

So how does this affect this book?

With the implementation of the Patient Protection and Affordable Care Act in 2011, whereby it was charged with modifying CPT-based fee-for-service reimbursement, CMS began holding physicians financially accountable for their cost efficiency with the value-based payment modifier (VBPM), which, much like hospital DRGs, was risk-adjusted based on the inpatient and outpatient codes physicians and hospitals reported, not a clinical abstraction of the conditions our patient populations experienced. No longer would my ICD-9-CM code of 250.00 work for complicated diabetes; I now had to state and code that the patient had diabetic nephropathy (250.70) along with chronic kidney disease, stage 4 (585.4), which added weight to my "expected cost" if I were to be deemed cost efficient and not be financially penalized. I had to learn to document and code "functional quadriplegia" for my bedridden patients with severe physical disabilities or frailty (an ICD-9-CM/ICD-10-CM administrative term that has no references in the world literature in http://www.pubmed.gov), drug or alcohol dependence (as opposed to drug or alcohol use or abuse), chronic hypoxemic respiratory failure (as opposed to dependence on supplemental oxygen), and systolic heart failure (instead of systolic heart dysfunction) to succeed with the VBPM.

Furthermore, with the enactment of the Medicare Access and CHIP Reauthorization Act of 2015

(MACRA), CMS increased physician accountability for risk-adjusted cost efficiency through either an alternative payment model (APM) or the merit-based incentive payment system (MIPS). Beginning in 2021, about a third of a 7% bonus or penalty (9% in 2022) will be based on how much is spent on my patient panel in comparison to how much it should have cost based on what is documented and coded in the record. While many APMs are now risk-adjusted, data collection for MIPS-based cost-efficiency models begins on January 1, 2019.

Now, not only must I know how to code better, I must also know how to document in an unfamiliar ICD-10-CM dialect to support the codes affecting risk adjustment (RA). If my documentation does not match the ICD-10-CM code I submit, my practice becomes vulnerable to second guessing by government-sponsored RA data validators (RADVs) or allegations by the Department of Justice of "upcoding," which could lead to criminal convictions, financial penalties, and even jail time.

Sadly, given that most physicians pick their own codes but have little knowledge of how the ICD-10-CM Alphabetic Index, Tabular List, Guidelines, or AHA's *Coding Clinic for ICD-10-CM* and *ICD-10-PCS* works, we are all vulnerable to these allegations of willful neglect or reckless disregard if we do not learn how physician RA works and what we must do to protect our practices. This text addresses how ICD-10-CM works and how we are to manage severity and risk adjustment essential to MACRA, APMs, and MIPS.

As a physician since 1979 and an AHIMA-certified coder since 2001, I attest that *Risk Adjustment Documentation & Coding*, will be more important than Harrison's *Textbook of Internal Medicine*, Sabiston's *Textbook of Surgery*, or other fundamental clinical texts as your practice navigates the treacherous waters of ICD-10-CM coding compliance. Sheri Poe Bernard, an accomplished writer and certified coder well versed in ICD-10-CM conventions, successfully outlines many of our documentation and ICD-10-CM coding risks and opportunities essential to the hierarchical condition categories (HCC) RA model CMS uses in judging our cost efficiency. She holds us accountable for how we define, diagnose, document, and deploy ICD-10-CM–based terminology in our medical records.

Using actual provider documentation examples, Ms. Bernard advocates workflows that compliantly identify, address, and report HCC-sensitive conditions like "functional quadriplegia," "acquired absence of small toe," "alcohol dependence in remission," "morbid obesity," "hypercoagulable states," "monoparesis," "stable angina," "systemic inflammatory response syndrome due to pancreatitis," and other conditions in lieu of less-specific alternatives. She encourages us to address old documentation habits, such as using the term "history of" when a patient actually has a condition (eg, instead of "history of breast cancer being treated with tamoxifen," documenting that the patient actually has breast cancer requiring adjuvant chemotherapy); not fully describing how we monitor, evaluate, address, or treat our documented and coded conditions; and assuring that whatever ICD-10-CM code we select is reflected in billing software is also reflected in our documentation. Ms. Bernard then alerts us to how RADVs or even the Department of Justice will view our documentation and ICD-10-CM coding practices to help us avoid fraud and abuse allegations or convictions.

I strongly urge you and your practice to embrace what Ms. Bernard has written and to develop documentation and coding policies, procedures, infrastructure, and practices implementing her suggestions. Not only will you have a better chance at avoiding an unintended penalty with the MACRA/MIPS/APM models, your practice will have better odds surviving an unwelcome RADV or Department of Justice inquiry into your billing workflow.

In addition, I hope this book will stimulate your interest and advocacy in addressing how ICD-10-CM coding conventions, guidelines, and advice are formulated by the ICD-10-CM Cooperating Parties (none of which is a physician group) and what role physician and/or specialty societies should play in amending these policies, especially since ICD-11 is slated to be released in 2018, albeit not for adoption in the United States. If physicians are not at the table in how ICD-11-CM will be formulated, we will be on the "menu."

I affirm Ms. Bernard in her work and congratulate the AMA in publishing the book on this important subject. With your help, feedback, and suggestions, I am sure the next edition will be even better than the first.

James S. Kennedy, MD, CCS, CCDS, CDIP
President
CDIMD – Physician Champions
A DBA of VP-MA Health Solutions, a Tennessee Corporation

Preface

Twenty-five years ago, hoping to change careers, I left my desk as a writer/editor at a daily newspaper for a job interview with a small medical publishing company. The interview was going well when the leader of the editorial team pulled out a copy of what could become my responsibility: a 14-lb treatise called *International Classification of Diseases, 9th Revision, Clinical Modification.*

"So," I said, flipping through the oversized paperback and eyeing the long lists of numbers and their associated descriptors, "this job is sort of like editing a phone book."

The editorial team erupted with good-natured laughter. By the end of the meeting, I had accepted the job.

Within months of exposure to my first ICD-9-CM code set files, I understood the joke. ICD-9-CM wasn't some dull list of inconsequential data, necessary only when one needed a plumber. Its annual updates revealed the agendas of our healthcare leaders, and provided a glimpse of new scientific discoveries. The classification of diagnoses was dynamic, and still is, reflecting our national health status.

As a lifelong learner, I have found the ICD to be a charismatic teacher. From the human papillomavirus epidemic to the adverse effects of terrorism, from homelessness to child sexual abuse, ICD codes speak of societal ills as well as physical ones. Code proposals are accompanied by health care data in support of code creation, offering up topical, short courses for issues such as newborn conditions related to Zika virus or anemia due to myelosuppressive antineoplastic chemotherapy. Medical science constantly brings new information to the table, and once a concept is accepted, the federal ICD managers codify it.

Unlike the obsolete phone book, ICD has strengthened over the years, albeit in an improved 10th revision. Accurate and complete diagnostic coding in the US health care industry is more important with each passing year. A synopsis of this importance can be seen in the timeline below, which represents both ICD-9-CM and ICD-10-CM as "ICD."

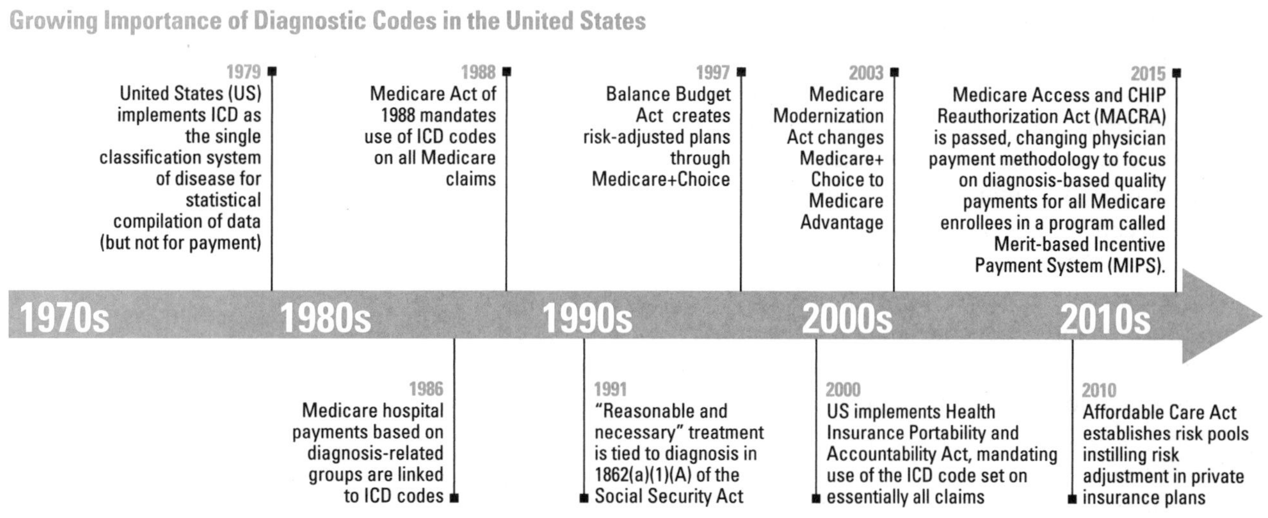

In risk adjustment, the severity of illness as represented by ICD-10-CM codes determines payment for insurance companies. In 2017, 19 million of 58 million Medicare enrollees participated in risk-adjusted Medicare Advantage plans, and 10.3 million were enrolled in private risk-adjustment pools under the Affordable Care Act. The Medicare Access and CHIP Reauthorization Act of 2015 became effective in 2017, and its Merit-based Incentive Payment System (MIPS) focuses on patient comorbidities as an increasingly important factor in physician payment for Medicare services. ICD-10-CM codes, naturally, are the method for conveying those comorbidities. Hospitals have been paid according to diagnoses since the 1980s; today, insurance companies and physicians are paid according to documented diagnoses, too.

In recent years, electronic adjudication of fee-for-service claims has become common. Insurers perform an automated review of electronic claims, looking for overbilling. This has led to a heightened awareness among physicians of a need for accuracy in CPT coding to ensure payments are not reduced or denied. Physicians and physician-based coders have been focused on the accuracy of documentation to capture *what* is performed, and they sometimes have taken shortcuts in documentation and coding to capture *why* it is performed. That "why" is conveyed through ICD-10-CM codes.

In the new reimbursement systems, severity of illness is a component of payment, reported with diagnosis codes. Physicians and coders must improve documentation and coding habits so that claims reflect the complexity of the diagnoses physicians treat and the work they do. *Risk Adjustment Documentation & Coding* helps physicians and coders improve the accuracy of coded diagnoses. Risk-adjustment (RA) coding and diagnostic coding in fee-for-service actually must follow the same guidance for coding, heretofore only routinely observed by hospital coders. The rules aren't new, but now that many physician and insurance payments are tied to outpatient diagnoses, the need for accurate diagnostic documentation and coding is urgent. As a result, *Risk Adjustment Documentation & Coding* is a perfect tool for physician office coders, insurance auditors, RA coders, educators, clinical documentation improvement specialists, and physicians, who need to know coding requirements in order to document sufficiently to capture the correct codes.

The guidance provided in this book comes directly from ICD-10-CM conventions and guidelines, the American Hospital Association's *Coding Clinic for ICD-10-CM and ICD-10-PCS,* and from the Centers for Medicare & Medicaid Services or other federal sources. This guidance is long-standing, and applies to everyone, not just RA coders. *Risk Adjustment Documentation & Coding* serves as an educational tool providing a foundation in proper code lookup and adherence to guidelines, and as an easy reference tool, with easy access to pertinent guidance and references. Appendix A and Appendix B are specific to RA. Appendix A reproduces the HCC and RxHCC tables for 2018 Medicare Advantage plans, and Appendix B provides a list of all ICD-10-CM codes that risk-adjust, their code descriptions, and the HCCs and RxHCCs specific to each code.

Appendix C provides the answers to questions at the end of each chapter, as well as exercises distributed throughout Chapter 4. Appendix D contains 12 teaching tools that may be reproduced and distributed to physicians and coders. One side of each tool contains documentation tips for a common chronic illness, and the other side contains code abstraction tips for the same chronic illness.

To enhance the active learning and/or training process, the following features have been added:

- **Abstract & Code It!** are clinical coding examples exercises provided throughout Chapter 4, which requires readers to abstract and code a clinical scenario, to test readers' understanding of the coding and documentation concepts covered for different topics.
- **Advice/Alert Note** highlights important information, exceptions to the rules, salient advice related to codes and diagnosis, such as federal guidance for coding and documentation from the *ICD-10-CM Official Guidelines for Coding and Reporting, Federal Register, 2008 CMS Risk Adjustment Data Validation Participant Guide*, or other federal regulatory guidance sources.
- **Chapter Opener** presents a general introduction and overview of the subject that may also cover some of the basic concepts and terminology necessary for understanding the topic. In most cases, the educational goals for the chapter are presented as well.
- **Clinical Coding Examples** illustrates a coding concept using a brief coding scenario or full

reproduction of the documentation related to a medical encounter, with coded results directly presented in the chapter.

- **Clinical Examples** demonstrates a clinical documentation concept using excerpts from a real medical record, with discussion of the critical deficits in content.
- **Coding Tip** provides practical advice, recommendations, and/or helpful information and reporting instructions about particular codes associated with a specific diagnosis, such as advice from the American Hospital Association's *Coding Clinic for ICD-10-CM and ICD-10-PCS*.
- **Definitions** of important and difficult terms are provided throughout the text at the bottom of the page in which the term appears, in order to negate the need for additional resources to learn the meaning of diagnostic, regulatory, or medical reimbursement terminology.
- **Documentation Tip** provides explanation of how ICD-10-CM classifies commonly documented phrases, as well as instructions on specificity requirements in coding, so that physicians can ensure the codes abstracted from their medical notes accurately reflect their patients' condition.
- **Example** provides samples to further demonstrate or highlight content and concepts covered in the chapter.
- **FYI** provides additional information that may help readers to better understand or provide additional background information regarding a topic or content such as documentation or coding issues, either by providing an illustration of a concept or by further defining terminology, diagnostic scoring systems, or code lists.
- **Sidebar** provides derivative story related to the main concepts covered in a particular section(s) of a chapter.
- **Evaluate Your Understanding** provides end-of-chapter exercises to allow students to evaluate their understanding of the concepts of each chapter using several types of exercises, such as:
  - **Answer questions**
  - **True/False statements**
  - **Internet-based** exercises provides links to online resources encourage readers to explore topics related to chapter concepts. Such exercises reinforce the need to keep abreast of the latest information in coding, documentation, RA, as well as the role technology plays in the current learning and teaching environment.
  - **Audit Exercises** are case study–based exercises that are provided in certain chapters as opportunities to practice abstracting and coding from the provided clinical scenarios.

Instructor or Training Resources

In addition to the features noted above, *Risk Adjustment Documentation & Coding* includes various resources to assist instructors and trainers in their course work and/or training. The following materials are part of the Instructor or Training Resources:

- PowerPoint Slides
- Two Course Exams (Theory and Practice)
- Test Bank (140 Questions [with answers and rationales])
- Mock Certification Exam (175 multiple choice questions [with answers and rationales] that can be used to assess students'/trainees' preparedness for certification and/or their overall understanding of RA, ICD-10-CM documentation and coding, HCCs, RxHCCs, how RA relates to medical financial matters, and clinical documentation improvement)

Download the Power Point slides at amaproductupdates.org. The rest of the instructor or training resources are only available to verified instructors. Please contact Amanda Brothers at amanda.brothers@ama-assn.org to receive access.

AMA Store offers complimentary review and instructor copies of books published by the American Medical Association to those schools purchasing directly from the AMA. Visit ama-assn.org/go/instructor-request to learn more about the program and submit your requests electronically. If you have questions regarding this title, please contact your AMA sales representative or account manager, or you may call 800 295-9895.

About the Author

Sheri Poe Bernard, CCS-P, CPC, CRC, CDEO, is one of the nation's leading developers of medical coding curricula and referential material. With more than 25 years of experience in coding and reimbursement, publishing, training, and test development, she is an expert communicator of coding concepts.

Bernard is a risk-adjustment consultant, as well as a freelance writer and educator. She is the author of the AMA's 2015 publication, *Netter's Atlas of Surgical Anatomy for CPT Coding* and the *2018 ICD-10-CM Chronic Disease Cards.* Previously, she was vice president of clinical coding content at American Academy of Professional Coders (AAPC). Prior to joining the AAPC as an employee, she served on its National Advisory Board for eight years and on the executive team of that board for four years. For 15 years, she created clinical coding products at Optum360® (Ingenix), where she developed a love for the International Classification of Disease. She is a frequent national speaker on topics involving CPT, ICD-9-CM, ICD-10-CM, and risk-adjustment coding.

About the Reviewers

The AMA and author sought input of multiple risk-adjustment and coding experts from across the nation to review for accuracy and completeness the contents of *Risk Adjustment Documentation & Coding*. The following reviewers provided feedback that was extremely helpful in finalizing the manuscript for *Risk Adjustment Documentation & Coding*. What follows is a description of the reviewers.

Suzan Hauptman, MPM; CPC; CEMC; CEDC; AAPC Fellow; Senior Principal at ACE Med Group

Suzan Hauptman has 25 years of experience in the medical insurance industry including coding management and clinical documentation improvement roles within regional hospital systems in Pennsylvania, auditing for consulting firms, and generating content for healthcare business publishers. She has a master's degree in public management with an emphasis in health, and is a regular contributor to numerous health business publications. She is a frequent speaker at local and national American Academy of Professional Coders (AAPC) events.

Mary A. Johnson, MBA/HM/HI©, CPC

Mary A. Johnson is currently the Medical Record Coding Program Director at Central Carolina Technical College. She has held this position since 2010. Her experience includes both on-campus and online teaching, as well as designing and implementing customized health information curricula. She also has been doing corporate training for over a decade. She is a frequent speaker, including the American Health Information Management Association (AHIMA) Assembly on Education; Health Professions Virtual Symposium; Allied Health Course Solutions; and AAPC local chapter meetings.

James S. Kennedy, MD, CCS, CDIP, CCDS

James S. Kennedy is the founder and President of CDIMD, a Nashville-based physician and facility advisory and consulting firm that advocates ICD-10-pertinent clinical documentation and coding integrity essential to healthcare revenue cycles and quality measurement. As a coding and clinical documentation integrity (CDI) expert with over 17 years of experience and as a frequent speaker to medical staff, Health Information Management (HIM) and CDI associations, Dr. Kennedy is nationally recognized for his subject matter expertise, communication skills, and problem-solving approach.

Debra Wheatley, CPC, CPMA

Debra Wheatley's healthcare career began as a chiropractic assistant who performed physiotherapy, billing, and radiology technologist duties. She began focusing more narrowly on medical coding and reimbursement after receiving her CPC in the healthcare division of Computer Sciences Corporation. She also coded for nephrology and neurosurgery specialties before joining DST Health Solutions, where she now specializes in risk adjustment and outpatient auditing. She became a Certified Professional Medical Auditor in 2012.

Acknowledgments

The culture of medical coders is one of generosity: busy people sharing their time and knowledge in the pursuit of education and accuracy. We are always learning, and always sharing what we learned. Every student I have met has shaped my understanding of the key concepts for accurate coding, and how best to teach these concepts. Many peers over the years have shared their resources, pointed me in the right direction, and corrected my misconceptions. I am indebted to all of you.

Writing this book was humbling. Only when I began to develop the manuscript did the many gaps in my knowledge surface. I am grateful to James S. Kennedy, MD, CCS, for filling in those gaps with eloquence and patience, and to the many coding friends I canvassed for federal citations and insight into risk-adjustment rules. Once the manuscript was written, my coding reviewers made astute edits that not only corrected mistakes, but noted when I had made errors of omission. I am very thankful to the many hours contributed by Mary A. Johnson, MBA/HM/HI©, CPC; Suzan Hauptman, MPM, CPC, CEMC, CEDC, AAPC Fellow; and Debra Wheatley, CPC, CPMA. These women know their business, and put quality first.

But no matter how fine-tuned the manuscript became, it would have been a disastrous performance without the orchestration provided by Lisa Chin-Johnson, AMA Senior Developmental Editor, who kept the team on schedule and brought many terrific ideas to the table. No one is as meticulous, as persuasive, or as supportive. I am also grateful to Richard Newman, former Director, Print and Digital Products, who was able to convince the AMA leadership of the importance of risk adjustment to physicians and their coders. The AMA as an organization is unequaled in the professionalism it brings to the medical coding publishing business. How lucky I count myself to be one of their published authors.

Finally, I am grateful foremost to my family, whose support and encouragement during the year I was writing this book was unflagging, in spite of all the time it took away from them. Michael, Charles, and Flora, you're the best!

At-a-Glance Review of the Features of *Risk Adjustment Documentation & Coding*

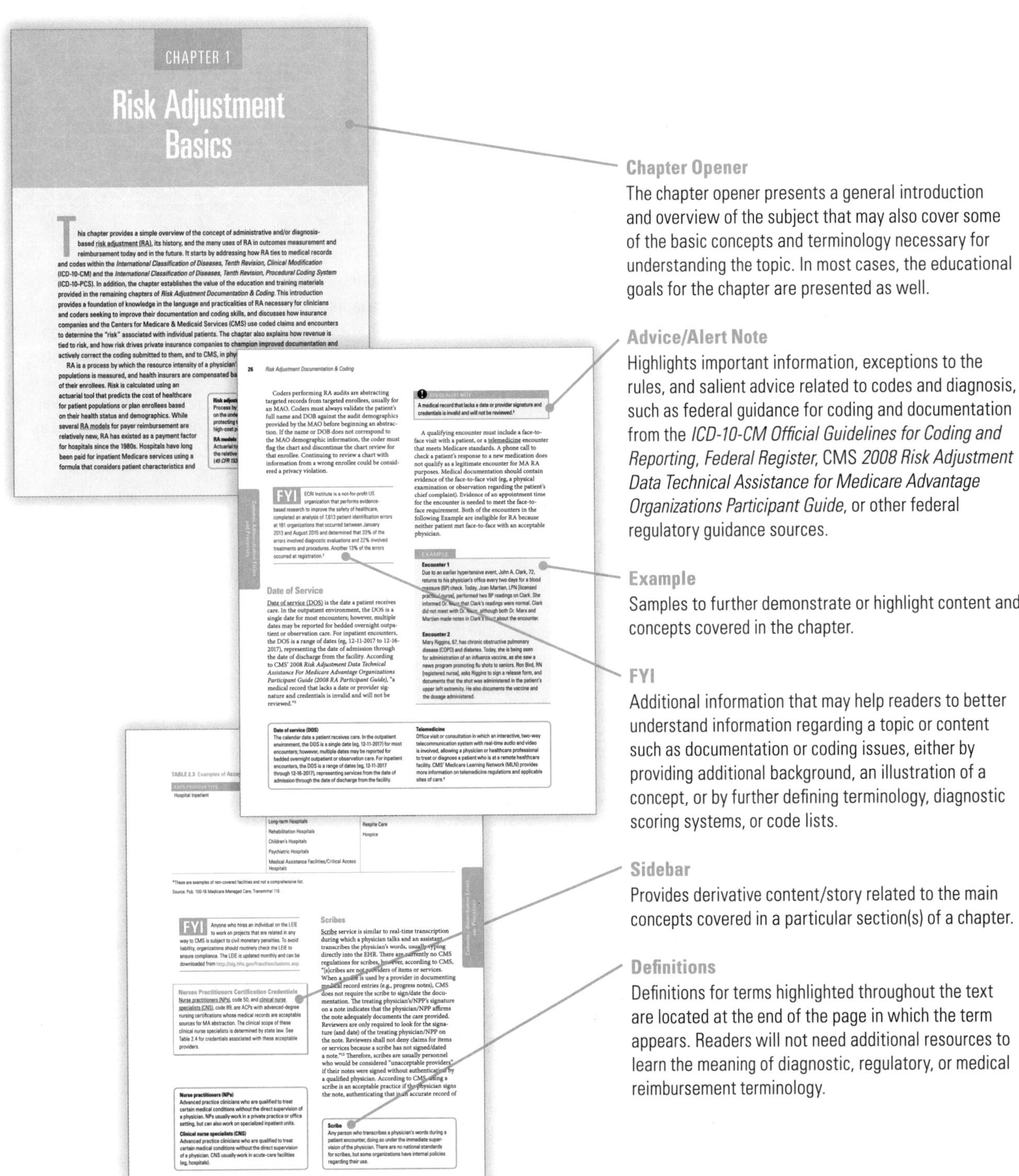

Chapter Opener

The chapter opener presents a general introduction and overview of the subject that may also cover some of the basic concepts and terminology necessary for understanding the topic. In most cases, the educational goals for the chapter are presented as well.

Advice/Alert Note

Highlights important information, exceptions to the rules, and salient advice related to codes and diagnosis, such as federal guidance for coding and documentation from the *ICD-10-CM Official Guidelines for Coding and Reporting*, *Federal Register*, CMS *2008 Risk Adjustment Data Technical Assistance for Medicare Advantage Organizations Participant Guide*, or other federal regulatory guidance sources.

Example

Samples to further demonstrate or highlight content and concepts covered in the chapter.

FYI

Additional information that may help readers to better understand information regarding a topic or content such as documentation or coding issues, either by providing additional background, an illustration of a concept, or by further defining terminology, diagnostic scoring systems, or code lists.

Sidebar

Provides derivative content/story related to the main concepts covered in a particular section(s) of a chapter.

Definitions

Definitions for terms highlighted throughout the text are located at the end of the page in which the term appears. Readers will not need additional resources to learn the meaning of diagnostic, regulatory, or medical reimbursement terminology.

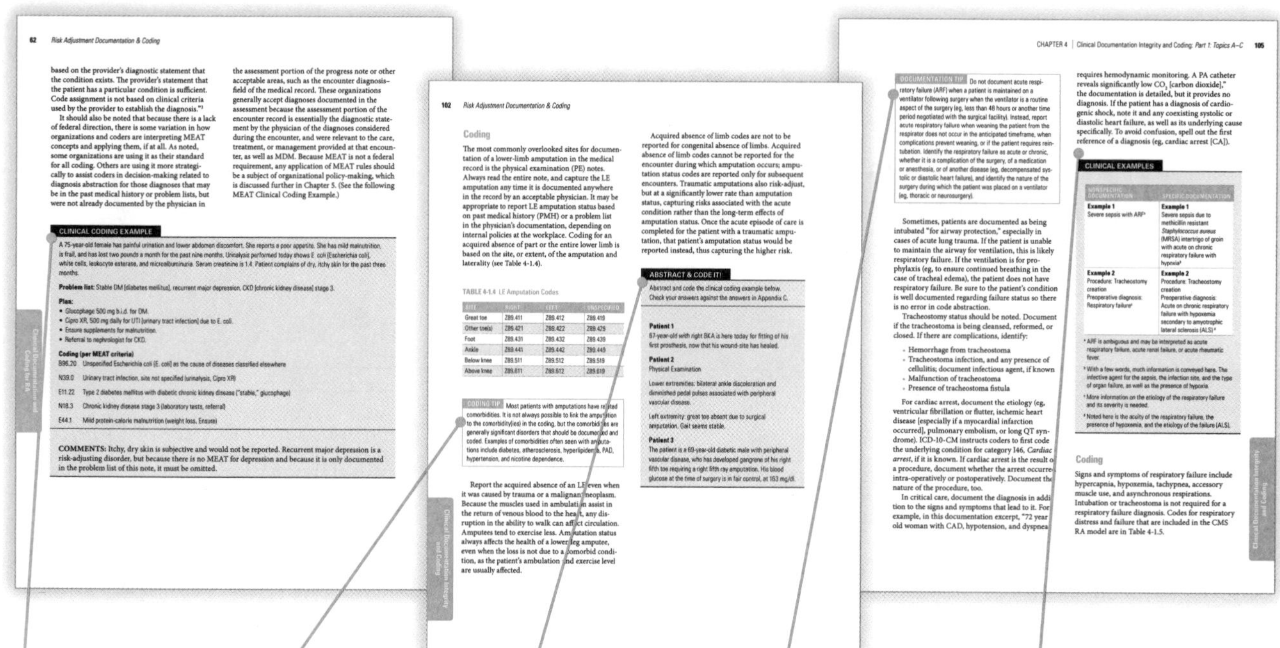

Clinical Coding Example
Illustration of a coding concept using a brief coding scenario or full reproduction of the documentation related to a medical encounter, with coded results directly presented in the chapter.

Coding Tip
Practical advice, recommendations, and/or helpful information and reporting instructions about particular codes associated with a specific diagnosis, such as advice from the American Hospital Association's *Coding Clinic for ICD-10-CM and ICD-10-PCS*.

Abstract & Code It!
Clinical coding examples exercises provided throughout Chapter 4 that requires readers to abstract and code a clinical scenario to test readers' understanding of the coding and documentation concepts covered for different topics.

Documentation Tip
Explanations of how ICD-10-CM classifies commonly documented phrases and instructions on specificity requirements in coding to help physicians ensure that the codes abstracted from their medical notes accurately reflect their patients' conditions.

Clinical Examples
Demonstration of a clinical documentation concept using excerpts from a real medical record, with discussion of the critical deficits in content.

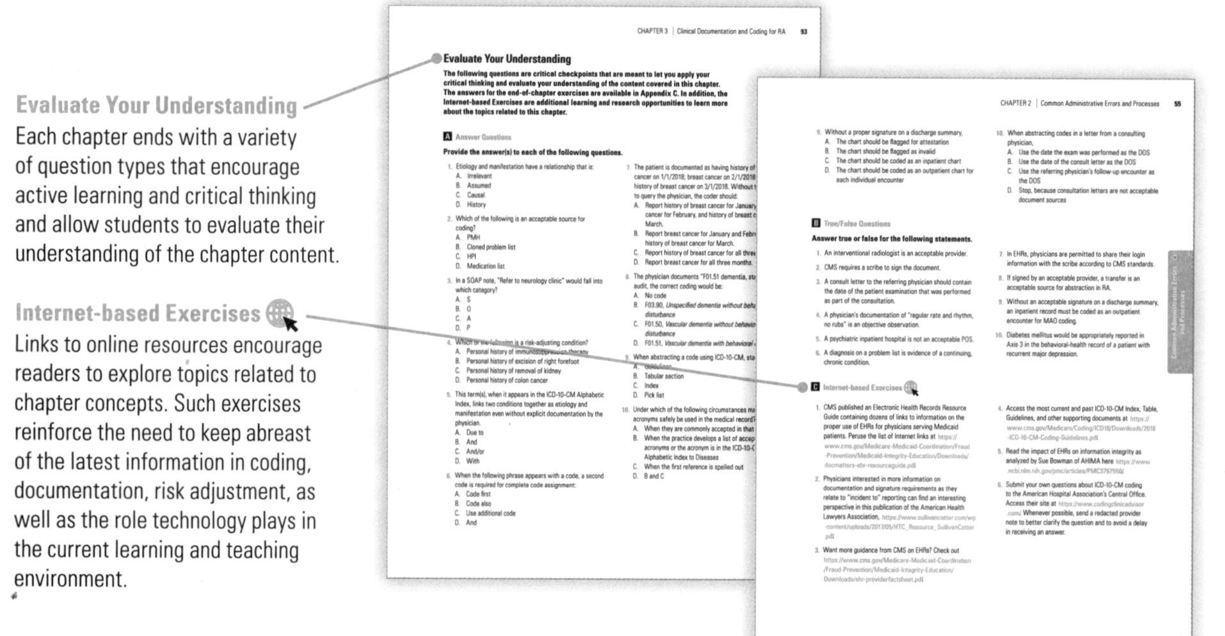

Evaluate Your Understanding
Each chapter ends with a variety of question types that encourage active learning and critical thinking and allow students to evaluate their understanding of the chapter content.

Internet-based Exercises
Links to online resources encourage readers to explore topics related to chapter concepts. Such exercises reinforce the need to keep abreast of the latest information in coding, documentation, risk adjustment, as well as the role technology plays in the current learning and teaching environment.

Introduction

Diagnoses are the cornerstone of medicine. Without a diagnosis, there is no treatment. Even an annual physical for a well patient is about screening for diagnoses. Even so, physician payment is based on the treatment or service performed, and these services are reported with Current Procedural Terminology (CPT®) codes. Because they are the "money codes," CPT codes have long been the focus of regulatory scrutiny and internal compliance plans. As a result, documentation and coding of diagnoses may not always be performed with the same level of meticulousness given to CPT documentation and coding.

Today, diagnoses have an increasing role in reimbursement. *Risk Adjustment Documentation & Coding* is directed toward a broad audience of virtually all treating physicians and other qualified healthcare providers, as well as all office staff involved in coding and billing. Participation in a risk-adjustment (RA) plan is not necessary to benefit from this book. Its goal is to improve diagnostic documentation and code abstraction so that the medical record is more complete, and claims data are more accurate. While this is essential for RA compliance, it should also be a goal of every physician and coder. The *OIG Compliance Program for Individual and Small Group Physician Practices* (*Federal Register* Vol. 65, No. 194, October 5, 2000, Notices, p. 59440) states, "One of the most important physician practice compliance issues is the appropriate documentation of diagnosis and treatment." Similarly, this is reinforced in the introduction to the 2018 *ICD-10-CM Official Guidelines for Coding and Reporting,* which states, "The importance of consistent, complete documentation in the medical record cannot be overemphasized. Without such documentation accurate coding cannot be achieved."

This Book's Mission

Risk Adjustment Documentation & Coding is not designed as a comprehensive guide to all RA issues. The complex calculations that determine the projected cost of a patient's disease burden for RA are briefly described in Chapter 1, but not to the depth that a RA plan would require in order to make these calculations. Localities, quality metrics, and a number of other factors that increase or decrease payments based on comorbidities are omitted from detailed discussion, because this book's mission is to promote clinical documentation improvement and coding excellence. Physicians and coders are not responsible for determining risk scores. They may want to understand which conditions risk-adjust to ensure these disorders are captured in the record appropriately, and this book will help them achieve that goal.

For the same reason, details on how to select and collect charts for RA audits, prepare for risk-adjustment validation audits (RADVs), and develop and manage an internal RA quality assurance and training program are omitted. The scope of this book is limited to documentation and coding, with a focus on those conditions that risk-adjust for the Medicare Advantage program under the Centers for Medicare & Medicaid Services (CMS). For this reason, the information included in the book addresses the hierarchical condition categories (HCCs) and prescription HCCs (RxHCCs) under Medicare Advantage, sometimes called CMS-HCCs. Another set of hierarchical condition categories called HHS-HCCs address risk-adjusted diagnoses in private risk pools under the Affordable Care Act. These are not discussed at length in this book, but for the most part, HHS-HCCs echo the Medicare Advantage HCCs and RxHCCs, with the exception of pediatrics and obstetrics.

Chapter by Chapter

An overview of the historic and current RA programs is provided in **Chapter 1, Risk Adjustment Basics,** along with an overview of how risk scores are calculated. Other federal initiatives that consider diagnoses in determining payment are also mentioned.

CMS requirements for signatures, encounter dates, and types of documentation appropriate for code abstraction are discussed in **Chapter 2, Common Administrative Errors and Processes.** The chapter concludes with an overview of chart formats for coders who may be unfamiliar with the variety of standardized formats available to physicians and other healthcare providers.

Chapter 3, Clinical Documentation and Coding for Risk Adjustment, offers guidance on what could and should be documented in the medical record in order to avoid any ambiguity or reversal in the event of an audit. These topics are general documentation and coding topics; for example, use of the phrase "history of," which could be applied to any diagnosis. Specific diagnoses are addressed in Chapter 4.

Most of the clinical documentation and coding advice and practices in Chapter 3 align exactly with excerpts from government documents offering federal guidance. In other cases, there are issues in which CMS and ICD-10-CM Guidelines have only provided general guidance and direction. For example, CMS requires a diagnosis to be "supported" in the medical record in order for it to be coded, but does not define "support." Chapter 3 discusses the spectrum of options and issues that organizations should consider as they determine their own coding and documentation policies.

Chapter 4, Clinical Documentation Integrity and Coding, by Topic, is divided into four parts by topics in alphabetical order. This chapter groups the HCCs and RxHCCs into topics for analysis (eg, all diabetes HCCs and RxHCCs are grouped together). A brief description of the diseases within the topic may include morbidity and mortality statistics and pathophysiology. Documentation guidance is addressed next, followed by a discussion of coding issues. These topics were separated so that a reader could focus on either or both disciplines of documentation and coding. Coding exercises accompany most topics in Chapter 4, and the answers are in Appendix C.

Chapter 5, Developing Risk-Adjustment Policies, applies to anyone developing ICD-10-CM coding policies, whether for RA or in private practice. There are many gray areas in coding in which there is no direction from the guidelines or from the American Hospital Association's (AHA's) *Coding Clinic for ICD-10-CM and ICD-10-PCS*. This chapter offers guidance on how to write, communicate, and maintain defensible coding policies. Keep in mind that the examples in this chapter are illustrative, and do not represent any endorsement from the American Medical Association (AMA) or the author that these sample coding policies would be accepted by CMS or other payers. It is every organization's responsibility to research and create its own coding policies.

Appendixes

Appendix A contains the tables for HCCs and RxHCCs under the Medicare Advantage programs for 2018. These are derived from the *Announcement of Calendar Year (CY) 2017 for Medicare Advantage (MA) Capitation Rates, Part C Payment Policies and Final Call Letter* and *Announcement of Calendar Year (CY) 2018 for Medicare Advantage (MA) Capitation Rates, Part D Payment Policies and Final Call Letter.* (There were no changes to RA factors (RAFs) for HCCs from 2017 to 2018, although there were changes to RxHCCs.) Included are reproductions of the HCC and RxHCC RAFs attachments from the announcements. These tables show the RAFs for each disorder based on patient demographics. There are also tables identifying HCC and RxHCC disease hierarchies with instructions for calculation, and HCC disease interactions calculations.

For more precise calculation of risk scores, a locality multiplier and understanding of the individual payer's quality scoring would be required. The intent of Appendix A is to provide physicians and coders with an understanding of the weight given to the diagnoses they are documenting/abstracting in order to illustrate the importance of accuracy and specificity.

Appendix B provides a very useful resource: a listing of all ICD-10-CM codes that map to HCCs or RxHCCs in code order, linked to the corresponding HCCs and/or RxHCCs. In some cases, a single ICD-10-CM code may link to more than one HCC or RxHCC. This provides a quick lookup for physicians or coders who wonder if a diagnosis risk-adjusts. Armed with the HCC or RxHCC, the reader can turn to Appendix A to determine the RAF of the diagnosis.

Appendix C provides answers to all end-of-chapter exercises, in addition to answers to Abstract & Code It! (clinical coding exercises) found throughout Chapter 4. Each answer includes a rationale of how the answer was derived.

Appendix D contains 12 training tools in which one is about general documentation and coding best practices and 11 are about documentation and coding for 11 common chronic diseases. For each disease covered, a page is dedicated to physician documentation and another to promote coding specificity and accuracy. These are available in PDF format and can be downloaded at amaproductupdates.org.

Quality Is the Key

As the tie between diagnoses and payment strengthens, physicians and coders risk exposure if the proper rules for diagnostic coding are not routinely followed in their offices. There are no losers in improving diagnosis coding and documentation, as these are essential to evidence-based medicine and improved outcomes. Complete documentation should not be considered an administrative burden; it is the foundation of all quality medical care. Compliant coding ensures that reported data accurately and consistently reflects the medical record—another worthy goal.

The guidance offered in *Risk Adjustment Documentation & Coding* is pertinent to all diagnostic documentation and to all diagnostic coding, regardless of payment methodology, place of service, or provider. It applies to everyone, not only RA participants. Diagnostic specificity and completeness are important. The correct ICD-10-CM codes convey the disease burden of a patient, necessary for care planning; the disease burden within a practice, necessary for resource management; and the disease burden throughout the country, critical to disease prevention and control. The entire spectrum of healthcare reimbursement is affected when diagnoses are not documented and reported with consistency and accuracy. Quality, as always, is the key.

CHAPTER 1

Risk Adjustment Basics

This chapter provides a simple overview of the concept of administrative and/or diagnosis-based risk adjustment (RA), its history, and the many uses of RA in outcomes measurement and reimbursement today and in the future. It starts by addressing how RA ties to medical records and codes within the *International Classification of Diseases, Tenth Revision, Clinical Modification* (ICD-10-CM) and the *International Classification of Diseases, Tenth Revision, Procedural Coding System* (ICD-10-PCS). In addition, the chapter establishes the value of the education and training materials provided in the remaining chapters of *Risk Adjustment Documentation & Coding*. This introduction provides a foundation of knowledge in the language and practicalities of RA necessary for clinicians and coders seeking to improve their documentation and coding skills, and discusses how insurance companies and the Centers for Medicare & Medicaid Services (CMS) use coded claims and encounters to determine the "risk" associated with individual patients. The chapter also explains how revenue is tied to risk, and how risk drives private insurance companies to champion improved documentation and actively correct the coding submitted to them, and to CMS, in physician and facility claims.

RA is a process by which the resource intensity of a physician's or group of physicians' patient populations is measured, and health insurers are compensated based on the underlying health status of their enrollees. Risk is calculated using an actuarial tool that predicts the cost of healthcare for patient populations or plan enrollees based on their health status and demographics. While several RA models for payer reimbursement are relatively new, RA has existed as a payment factor for hospitals since the 1980s. Hospitals have long been paid for inpatient Medicare services using a formula that considers patient characteristics and

Risk adjustment (RA)
Process by which health insurers are compensated based on the underlying health status of their enrollees, thereby protecting the insurers against losses due to high-risk, high-cost patients.

RA models
Actuarial tools used to predict healthcare costs based on the relative actuarial risk of enrollees in RA covered plans. (*45 CFR 153.20*)

procedures reported using the ICD-10-CM and ICD-10-PCS codes, which is currently embodied in the Medicare severity diagnosis-related group (MS-DRG) system. These MS-DRGs are based on ICD-10-CM and ICD-10-PCS codes derived from physician documentation, not the coder's clinical interpretation of the patient's circumstances, and are weighted or risk-adjusted based on coefficients assigned to each of these codes. Care provided to patients documented to be sicker is reimbursed at a higher rate than care to patients documented with less-serious illnesses. In MS-DRGs, it generally does not matter how many days the Medicare patient remains in the hospital or the cost of the care delivered by the hospital except for extreme circumstances. Payment is based solely on how sick the patient is, which is evidenced and based on the ICD-10-CM and ICD-10-PCS codes submitted by the facility. The advent of DRGs changed hospitals from a payment system based on payment for service provided to one that was based on the patient's condition.

Essentially, diagnosis-based RA models for payers are similar to the MS-DRG system, except the payment is made to the private insurance company over a specified period (eg, one year) rather than for an individual episode of care. Rather than assigning diagnostic codes to MS-DRGs, Medicare RA assigns codes to hierarchical condition categories (HCCs). Each HCC is assigned a value that contributes to an aggregated reimbursement that reflects the severity of the patient's illness, to pay for resources projected for patient care. For example, Patient A has uncomplicated diabetes (E11.9, HCC 19), which is assigned to one HCC. Patient B has diabetic ketoacidosis (DKA) (E10.10, HCC 17), assigned to a higher-valued HCC. Patient C has DKA (E10.10, HCC 17), diabetic polyneuropathy (E10.42, HCC 18 and 75), and a history of great toe amputation (Z89.419, HCC 189). Sicker patients will have more HCCs and/or higher-valued HCCs.

RA payment models for insurance plans were first mandated by the Balanced Budget Act of 1997 (BBA) and implemented by CMS for Medicare. The Medicare RA program allows CMS to pay private insurance plans for the known risks associated with insuring the Medicare beneficiaries they enroll. Risk scores measure individual enrollees' relative risks, and the scores are used to adjust payments that fund payments for each beneficiary's medical care.

RA expanded in 2014, when the Affordable Care Act (ACA) established an RA methodology to compensate insurance companies for insuring high-risk patients in affordable plans, which because of differing patient populations, uses different ICD-10-CM codes than that of Medicare. The ACA's program set up risk pools that would transfer premium revenue from plans with below-average actuarial risk to plans with above-average actuarial risk. Without an RA mechanism, a health plan gains a competitive advantage if it enrolls the healthy and avoids the sick. RA provides a safety net for insurers enrolling patients with pre-existing conditions.

Medicare Severity-Diagnosis Related Group (MS-DRG)
A classification system that categorizes diagnostic codes into groupings based on risk, for the purpose of reimbursement to hospitals for services provided to Medicare patients during an admission. Some private third-party payers have also adopted MS-DRGs.

Hierarchical condition categories (HCCs)
Classification mechanism in RA that groups ICD-10-CM codes into categories of risk for the purpose of projecting costs associated with care for health care plan enrollees. Diagnoses in each HCC have a similar risk for resource utilization, and each HCC is assigned a value associated with that risk.

Diagnosis-Based RA

In simplest terms, diagnosis-based RA is a methodology with a two-pronged goal: to ensure that patients' conditions are sufficiently diagnosed, documented, and coded in an effort to measure and monitor outcomes, and to accurately track the care needed through current and potential resources and reimburse accordingly. In more practical terms, RA widens the marketplace for health care insurers by compensating those insurers who enroll patients they would otherwise consider too risky to insure, ie, in order to inhibit the practice of what is known as "cherry picking" or "lemon dropping." This situation is defined as the practice of enrolling only the healthiest patients and discontinuing coverage for those with resource-intensive comorbidities. It also widens the marketplace of health care insurers for the enrollees, whose pre-existing conditions give rise to unaffordable medical premiums or total exclusion from insurance programs. Diagnosis-based RA is associated with insurance programs including Medicare Advantage (MA), Medicare prescription Part D coverage, Medicaid managed care plans, and the health insurance marketplace under the ACA. More than 75 million Americans are enrolled in risk-adjusting insurance plans, which is more than 20% of the insured population in the United States (US). Use of diagnosis-based RA approaches is now spreading to large employers that have a large pool of enrollees that include healthy as well as unhealthy employees in the commercial sector.

RA's effect goes far beyond the payer organizations and patients who participate. Risk is determined from the diagnoses in each patient's medical record, which are translated into ICD-10-CM codes. The diagnoses entered into the medical record by the physician must be specific, accurate, clinically valid, and written using ICD-10-CM's language if risk is to be captured accurately. Similarly, a lot rides on the correct abstraction of ICD-10-CM codes by physicians or coders in the inpatient or outpatient setting based on this documentation. RA, therefore, affects facilities, physician offices, medical coders, physicians, and payers—pretty much everyone in the health care documentation and coding continuum.

Diagnoses from physicians, other qualified health care providers, and hospitals are the source of most codes submitted for RA. RA rules for chart documentation and medical record abstraction are the same as the rules for physician or facility diagnostic coding, though the rules for physicians and inpatient facility coding differ. While hospitals and physician offices are expected to document and code according to the government's ICD-10-CM's conventions, guidelines, and official advice, enforcement of diagnostic coding guidelines in the outpatient arena has been lax for decades. This is due to several factors, such as:

- **Physician payment is based primarily on Current Procedural Terminology (CPT®) codes, so CPT code accuracy is the focus for outpatient coding.** Great care must be taken to document and code procedures and services accurately to ensure full payment and to prevent fraud or abuse. Coders in many physician offices ensure that ICD-10-CM codes abstracted from the record are valid only to the extent they support the medical necessity of the service provided. There is little oversight to ensure the diagnosis codes are as complete or precise as they could be and whether they conform to official ICD-10-CM conventions, guidelines, and advice, situations that could negatively affect RA. For example, a malignant neoplasm of the breast risk-adjusts, whereas a documented "history of breast cancer" does not, given that the first is coded with an actual malignant breast neoplasm code, while the second is coded with a personal history code. The official *ICD-10-CM Guidelines* stipulate that any malignancy undergoing active treatment (eg, toremifene for breast cancer) should be coded with the actual malignant neoplasm

Medicare Advantage (MA)
A type of health insurance for legal residents of the US who qualify for Medicare, administered by private insurance companies under contract with Medicare to provide coverage for hospitalization and physician care. Often, prescription drugs are included in the plans as well.

Medical record abstraction
Process in which a medical record is searched to identify data required for a secondary use; for example, for claims reporting, disease tracking, or resource utilization studies. For diagnoses, the narrative description of a disorder or disease is translated into an ICD-10-CM code and submitted with the claim for the encounter.

code, whereas the personal history code is applied only if the malignancy is not present or being actively treated. Either condition may justify a level 4 CPT evaluation and management office visit code to the oncologist, but the reported diagnosis may wrongly risk-adjust, or alternately, not risk-adjust when it should.

- **Physicians are not well trained in diagnostic coding.** Medical documentation may be the single most important obstacle to accurate RA coding. Many RA coders work remotely and cannot easily contact the physician for clarification of ambiguous documentation that does not mirror the terminology in the ICD-10-CM Alphabetic Index or Tabular List. Coders and auditors are often left with less than optimal notes from which to abstract codes. Beyond not fully understanding the documentation requirements of the ICD-10-CM, many physicians do not understand coding conventions and rules. With the advent of electronic health records (EHRs), physicians are increasingly selecting diagnosis and procedure codes from simple pull-down menus in the EHRs, and these diagnoses may not be supported by their documentation. These menus are often incomplete, and are usually not aligned with diagnostic coding guidelines required for compliant coding. In addition, physicians can create a subset of their code preferences within a drop-down list, thus limiting the broad spectrum of diagnosis codes available to code the encounter more accurately. Most physicians have received very little training in documentation as it relates to code abstraction for ICD-10-CM, or for the conventions and guidelines that govern code selection.
- **ICD-10-CM coding is complex and ever evolving.** Anyone abstracting ICD-10-CM codes is expected to follow the conventions, guidelines, as well as the official guidance provided in the American Hospital Association's (AHA's) *Coding Clinic for ICD-10-CM and ICD-10-PCS* (*Coding Clinic*), and other RA guidance and resources from CMS, which are sometimes found in nontraditional places. For example, most physicians have never heard of the AHA's *Coding Clinic*, much less used it. In another example, many RA auditing organizations continues to rely on CMS' *2008 Risk Adjustment Data Technical Assistance for Medicare Advantage Organizations Participant Guide* (*2008 RA Participant Guide*), even though the guide is updated annually. This is because CMS provided coding guidance in 2008 that has not been repeated in more recent participant guides. See the following Example from the often-cited 2008 *RA Participant Guide* (6.4.1, Co-Existing and Related Conditions) by RA audit firms even though it came from a 2008 guide. *(Note that this Example contains outdated* ***ICD-9-CM codes and HCCs**** *because the text is excerpted from a 2008 document.)*

EXAMPLE

Often cited by RA audit firms is this entry in the 2008 Guide, 6.4.1, *Co-Existing and Related Conditions.* Although the RA audit firms realize that the codes in this example are outdated ICD-9-CM codes, the message of the entry is that co-existing conditions should be reported even when they are not the chief complaint for medical encounters except those for minor presenting problems, hence they continue to use the guide:

> Co-existing conditions include chronic, ongoing conditions such as diabetes (250.XX HCCs 15-19*), congestive heart failure (428.0. HCC 80*), atrial fibrillation (427.31, HCC 92*), chronic obstructive and pulmonary disease (496, HCC 108*). These diseases are generally managed by ongoing medication and have the potential for acute exacerbations if not treated properly, particularly if the patient is experiencing other acute conditions. It is likely that these diagnoses would be part of a general overview of the patient's health when treating co-existing conditions for all but the most minor of medical encounters.
>
> Co-existing conditions also include ongoing conditions such as multiple sclerosis (340, HCC 72*), hemiplegia (342.9X, HCC 100*), rheumatoid arthritis (714.0, HCC 38*), and Parkinson's disease (332.0, HCC 73*). Although they may not impact every minor healthcare episode, it is likely that patients having these conditions would have their general health status evaluated within a data reporting period, and these diagnoses would be documented and reportable at that time.
>
> MA organizations must submit each required diagnosis at least once during a risk-adjustment reporting period. Therefore, these co-existing conditions should be documented by one of the allowable provider types at least once within the data reporting period.[1]

Another example is the narrative explanations provided by the National Center for Health Statistics (NCHS) when new ICD-10-CM codes are proposed. Sometimes, these narratives can gap-fill guidance on code usage. It is common for RA audit firms to use historic CMS documents.

EXAMPLE

This discussion, which was published in the September 22, 2015, meeting agenda of the ICD-10 Coordination and Maintenance Committee, indicates that coders may abstract diastolic/systolic heart failure based on documented ejection fraction, even when the physician does not document specifically systolic failure or diastolic failure.

> **Heart Failure with Reduced Ejection Fraction and with Normal Ejection Fraction**
>
> It is proposed to add inclusion terms related to ejection fraction for systolic heart failure, diastolic heart failure, and combined systolic and diastolic heart failure subcategories. The ejection fraction is a measure of the left ventricular function. In systolic heart failure, the ejection fraction is reduced. In diastolic heart failure, there is a normal ejection fraction or preserved ejection fraction. In combined systolic and diastolic heart failure, there is a reduced ejection fraction along with diastolic dysfunction.
>
> According to the 2013 American College of Cardiology Foundation/American Heart Association (ACCF/AHA) guidelines related to definitions of heart failure, the two principal forms of heart failure described are heart failure with reduced ejection fraction (HFrEF) and heart failure with preserved ejection fraction (HFpEF). The guidelines also note that "[b]ecause other techniques may indicate abnormalities in systolic function among patients with a preserved EF, it is preferable to use the terms preserved or reduced EF over preserved or reduced systolic function." It also notes that "[i]n most patients, abnormalities of systolic and diastolic dysfunction coexist, irrespective of EF." In addition, related to HFrEF, "those with LV systolic dysfunction commonly have elements of diastolic dysfunction as well."[2]

Inclusion notes now provide this information in the 2018 ICD-10-CM code set, however, before this change occurred, coders could cite those minutes when reporting heart failure based on ejection fraction. Minutes for the diagnostic coding portions of past ICD-10 Coordination and Maintenance Committee meetings can be accessed at www.cdc.gov/nchs/icd/icd10cm_maintenance.htm.

- **Time is the enemy.** With the advent of productivity standards for medical coders, and busy physicians coding from pull-down menus in EHRs, the accuracy of diagnostic coding has suffered. Correct diagnostic coding takes an investment in ICD-10-CM training, a commitment to time required to code properly, and vigilance to monitor the regulators for rule changes. When there are pressures to be more productive, it is usually the diagnostic coding that suffers.

EXAMPLE

Physician offices may sometimes document or code with less detail or accuracy than is optimal. For example:

- **Z00.00, Encounter for general adult medical examination without abnormal findings,** for the annual examination of a patient whose problem list includes hypertension and hypothyroidism. While Z00.00 is the reason for the visit, co-existing conditions should be reported secondarily; however, all too often, they are not reported because Z00.00 is sufficient to meet medical necessity requirements.
- **K70.30, Alcoholic cirrhosis of liver without ascites**, is documented and coded by the physician. While this is correct, guidance in the code set instructs coders to use an additional code to identify alcohol abuse or dependence. Although a patient's alcohol abuse or dependence risk-adjusts separately from any associated chronic liver condition, it often goes unreported in cases of alcoholic cirrhosis.

National Center for Health Statistics (NCHS)
Agency within the federal Centers for Disease Control principally responsible for updating and managing the ICD-10-CM coding system with a goal to provide data to guide US policies for health. NCHS co-chairs the ICD-10 Coordination and Maintenance Committee with CMS. Public meetings to discuss code changes are held twice yearly, usually in March and September. The meetings are held in Baltimore, but telecast live and also available as recordings.

Hospital diagnostic coding is usually more accurate than outpatient coding because hospital payment is tied to the diagnoses in MS-DRGs, and hospitals want to collect fair payment and avoid overpayment. Nevertheless, because hospital records can be hundreds of pages in length and hospital personnel have productivity requirements, secondary diagnoses that affect RA but do not affect the MS-DRG may be overlooked because of the volume of data. For example, a patient admitted with diabetes and end-stage renal disease (ESRD) with cardiovascular complications may also have a history of a below-knee amputation (BKA). BKA risk-adjusts; however, in this example, it may not be abstracted. The complexity of other illnesses in the patient's chart makes the amputation status seem insignificant; therefore, the BKA may not be documented, or if documented, it may not be abstracted.

The concepts of risk and RA are, at this point, ubiquitous. Like fee-for-service, pay-for-performance, and other payment methodologies that have shaped US health care reimbursement, RA has many applications. Risk is the basis of case mix in MS-DRGs. The concept of RA plans originated with Medicare, but models have also been developed for Medicaid and private insurance offered through the ACA.[3] Risk is also a calculation in the Value-Based Payment Modifier Program developed by CMS. Accountable care organizations (ACOs) are linking payments to quality and cost, and are using diagnoses as part of the metric for physician payments. Accurate documentation and coding for diagnoses is more important than ever.

Medicare and Medicare RA

Medicare is a federal program that provides health insurance to people who are 65 years or older, who have disabilities, or who rely on dialysis. Private insurance companies under contract to CMS administer Medicare programs. Most coverage rules are developed and enforced by CMS, with a few local exceptions. All US citizens who reach the age of 65, or who have ESRD, are eligible for Medicare Part A, hospitalization coverage. There is no charge for Part A. Citizens may opt to pay for Medicare Part B, outpatient coverage. Traditional Medicare coverage pays 80% of costs for eligible services under Parts A and B. The patient is responsible to pay 20% of eligible costs, considered co-insurance. Traditional Parts A and B coverage is administered by Medicare administrative contractors (MACs), which process claims and pay them with federal dollars.

Although Medicare provides a substantial safety net for enrollees, its coverage has limits. Medicare's expansion into diagnosis-based RA began as a result

Case mix
Actuarial analysis of a hospital's patient population based on risk associated with the diagnoses of the patient population for the purpose of allocating resources and reimbursement.

Value-Based Payment Modifier Program
Value modifiers enable differential payment to a physician or group of physicians under the Medicare Physician Fee Schedule (PFS) based upon the quality of care furnished compared to the cost of care during a performance period. The value modifier is an adjustment made to Medicare payments for items and services under the Medicare PFS. The diagnoses of the patient are a factor in determining the differential payment.[4]

Accountable care organizations (ACOs)
Groups of physicians or hospitals that come together voluntarily to share information and give coordinated high-quality care to their Medicare patients, linking payment to quality and cost.[5]

Medicare Part A
Medicare hospital facility coverage as well as hospice and skilled nursing facilities. There is no monthly charge to beneficiaries for this service, which pays 80% of covered hospitalization costs. Every US citizen over 65 years of age has Part A coverage (physician costs are not covered in Part A).

Medicare Part B
Medicare nonfacility coverage. Medicare beneficiaries must enroll in Part B, and pay a monthly fee, which is based on income level. This includes physician visits, preventive care, outpatient diagnostic tests, mental health care, and some home health services. Part B pays 80% of covered costs.

Medicare administrative contractor (MAC)
Private health insurer under contract with CMS to process and adjudicate Parts A and B medical claims for Medicare fee-for-service enrollees. There are 12 regional MACs across the country.

of the BBA of 1997,[6] which established Medicare Part C. Initially called Medicare+ Choice (now known as Medicare Advantage), Part C opened up Medicare programs to private insurers. The intent was to give consumers more options regarding their insurance coverage. Private insurers created plans that replaced the 20% liability with a maximum out-of-pocket (MOOP) and office-visit copays, offered vision services, health club memberships, or other benefits, and charged a small increase ($20 to $60) in the regular monthly Medicare premium. CMS oversaw the program. Medicare+ Choice plans were required to have features exceeding those of regular Medicare, to accept all eligible applicants, and to follow strict enrollment protocols.

Under Medicare+ Choice, insurers were paid a capitated rate for each Medicare-eligible enrollee in their program. From this capitated rate paid by CMS, the private insurers reimbursed Part A and Part B physicians for services to enrollees in their Medicare+ Choice program. However, providing insurance to a 65-year-old patient with simple hypertension has a different risk than providing services to a 65-year-old patient with hypertension, chronic kidney disease, congestive heart failure, and diabetic angiopathy. A capitated rate could lead to big losses for the insurer if too many patients had serious medical conditions, and Medicare enrollees usually consist of an older and less healthy population than the general population.

That is where RA entered the picture. Factors influencing the health of the enrollee (eg, age, economic status, and chronic disease) are evaluated and payment to the insurance plan covering the patient is *risk-adjusted*. In RA, a value is assigned to a group of chronic diseases (eg, chronic diabetic complications or metastatic cancers). Similar groups of chronic diseases were divided into HCCs. By reviewing the diagnostic codes assigned to the patient over the course of a year, a RA factor (RAF) could be calculated and payments recalibrated for each patient. A RAF is the total score of all risk factors for one patient for a total year. Each element of diagnostic or demographic data is assigned a value based on actuarial formulas. For Medicare Advantage, a RAF is used to predict future health care costs for health plan enrollees. The insurance company would receive significantly more reimbursement for covering the enrollee with multiple comorbidities than for the enrollee with simple hypertension, with the expectation that the cost of care for the enrollee with multiple comorbidities would be significantly higher.

FYI CMS maintains a Chronic Conditions Data Warehouse (CCW) that tracks certain diseases reported in claims among the Medicare and Medicaid populations. For Medicare in 2014, CCW determined these 10 comorbidities to have the highest incidence among Medicare patients: hypertension (57%); hyperlipidemia (46%); rheumatoid arthritis and osteoarthritis (31%); ischemic heart disease (28%); diabetes (28%); anemia (23%); chronic kidney disease (18%); chronic obstructive pulmonary disease (17%); depression (17%); and acquired hypothyroidism (15%). Federal spending for Medicare was $505 billion in 2014,[7] 14% of the total US budget.[8]

Medicare Part C
A combination of Parts A and B as offered by private insurance companies under MA plans. These plans may cost more, but offer more than traditional Parts A and B (eg, offering maximum out-of-pocket copays rather than a flat 20% fee, health club memberships, or vision care).

Capitated rate
A per-person fee, rather than a per-service fee, paid for providing coverage (eg, to an insurance company that has agreed to provide health insurance coverage to enrollees of a MA plan).

RA factor (RAF)
Total score of all risk factors for one patient for a total year. Each element of diagnostic or demographic data is assigned a value based on actuarial formulas. For Medicare, a RAF is used to predict future healthcare costs for health plan enrollees.

FYI

Medigap

Medigap programs are secondary insurance programs that cover what traditional Medicare does not. They are not RA programs. Medigap programs are usually more expensive than MA, and do not cover Part D. A patient with a Medigap policy will usually carry three insurance cards: one for Medicare, one for Part D coverage, and one for the Medigap plan. By contrast, an MA enrollee will usually have one card for all coverage. Traditional Medicare enrollees may have one card, or two, if they also subscribe to Part D. MA enrollees are excluded from Medigap plans. Medigap plans cover more of the costs not paid by Medicare.

RA was expanded to include drugs under the Medicare Prescription Drug, Improvement, and Modernization Act of 2003,[9] and at that time, Medicare+ Choice was renamed as Medicare Advantage (MA). Medicare Advantage organizations (MAOs) continue to grow, with one in three Medicare enrollees today choosing an MAO rather than traditional Medicare. Drug coverage, Medicare Part D, could be purchased separately with traditional Part B or with an MA program. During year-end open enrollment, Medicare enrollees can change their coverage plans, choosing traditional Medicare coverage or from among the variety of Part C and Part D plans.

Two separate HCC tables were created for Medicare RA: one for medical care under RA in Parts A and B—the HCCs that were previously mentioned; and the second for RA for outpatient pharmacy costs associated with the Medicare prescription benefit (Part D). This model is called the CMS prescription drug hierarchical condition categories (RxHCCs). (Table 1.2 provides a list of the 2018 RxHCCs, as covered in Part D.) Many disorders (eg, diabetes, heart failure, and cancers) risk-adjust in both HCC and RxHCC models. Patients with diabetes, heart failure, or cancer usually have more medical encounters and more prescribed medications and supplies. Some disorders risk-adjust only for HCCs. For example, pressure ulcers require medical care; however, medication is not routinely prescribed for patients with pressure ulcers. Some diagnoses risk-adjust for RxHCCs only (eg, hypothyroidism). Hypothyroidism is treated with daily synthetic thyroid replacement therapy, but does not usually increase the patient's need for medical encounters.

Note that for the most part, the RA discussion in this book will embrace both HCCs and RxHCCs without differentiating between the two systems in discussing coding and documentation. Regardless of whether it is HCCs or RxHCCs coding, or both, the requirements of compliant and complete documentation and coding are essential, and the focus of this book is improved documentation and coding for RA. When appropriate, specifics regarding RxHCCs or HCCs will be discussed, but keep in mind, the same set of documentation and coding rules apply to both HCCs and RxHCCs, all diagnosis-based RA models, and to all diagnostic coding. The only difference between RA coding and other diagnostic coding is that for RA, only a subset of diagnoses is addressed. Quick-reference tables are provided in Appendix B to identify diagnosis codes that map to MA HCCs and RxHCCs. Tables that show individual values associated with each HCC and RxHCC are presented in Appendix B.

Some HCCs/RxHCCs are grouped together when calculating risk scores. Only the most severe HCC is counted in the calculation. (See Appendix A and Table 1.3 for the RxHCC List of Disease Hierarchies.)

Medicare RA payments are prospective in nature, which means that diagnoses from claims filed the previous year are used to calculate the risk score of an enrollee for the current year for MAOs. (See Figure 1.1.) Conversely, RA payment under the ACA's health insurance marketplace is retrospective, also called concurrent. For these ACA risk pools, the claims data from a current period of time determine the payment for the current period.

ADVICE/ALERT NOTE

Medicare RA is prospective in nature, which means that diagnoses and encounters from the previous year are used to calculate the CMS payments for an enrollee for the current year to MAOs.

Medicare Part D

Prescription drug coverage through private health insurance companies offered to Medicare enrollees.

FIGURE 1.1 How Medicare RA Works

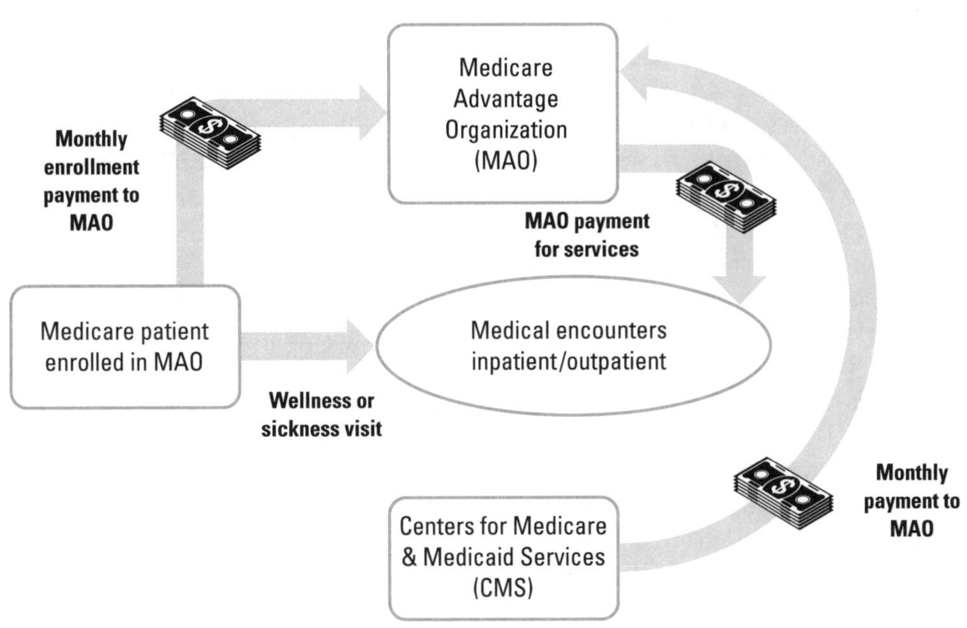

CMS' monthly payment to MAO is risk-adjusted based on the comorbidities of the enrollee rather than on the services provided. The base rate is capitated and risk-adjusted to reflect the chronic conditions of the patient.

Unintended Consequences

As with all major shifts in payment paradigms, diagnosis-based RA brought with it some unintended consequences. In particular, CMS did not predict how poor the accuracy of diagnosis coding in physician offices has been. For example, in a 2012 RA data validation (RADV) audit of PacifiCare for 2007, only 55 risk scores out of 100 beneficiaries were valid, according to a report from the Office of Inspector General (OIG). In a 2012 RADV audit of Paramount Care, Inc, for 2007, the OIG reported that only 56 of 100 beneficiaries had correct risk scores. In RA, the insurance company is held accountable for the accuracy of the diagnostic coding that is the basis for their payments from CMS. Historically, most insurers have had little or no direct authority over physician documentation or coding of diagnoses, but, according to the 2013 OIG Work Plan,[10] the MAOs are accountable for the ICD-10-CM codes submitted by physicians for RA:

> MA organizations are accountable for the performance of the entities with which they contract. MA organizations that delegate responsibilities under their contracts with CMS to other entities must specify in their contracts with those entities provisions that the entities must comply with all applicable Medicare laws, regulations, and CMS instructions. (*42 CFR § 422.504(i)(4)*).

In addition to inaccurate diagnostic coding, MAOs discovered that not all chronic conditions were being captured consistently. CMS requires that each HCC diagnosis be addressed at least once a year for the diagnosis to qualify for payment under RA. This provides incentive for the MAO to ensure each enrollee is receiving ongoing care for comorbidities, with a goal of improving the overall outcomes in the Medicare population. When people enrolled in MA plans skip preventive care, lifelong chronic diseases may disappear from risk scores and those diseases may worsen if unchecked.

EXAMPLE

Mary Tatum, 72, has had rheumatoid arthritis for 30 years, relies heavily on homeopathic medications, and refuses most traditional drug therapies. Last year, due to the discomfort of travel and her self-described stable condition, she canceled her annual physical. This year, she was hospitalized for six days with acute rheumatoid pericarditis. She is enrolled in an MA plan.

Because Tatum did not have contact with physicians in the previous year, no diagnosis of rheumatoid arthritis (or any other comorbidity) is associated with her risk score this year. Her capitated rate is the same as a healthy 72-year-old with no chronic conditions, but the MAO is still responsible for reimbursing all of the services she receives during her episode of care for pericarditis.

Many MAOs encourage physicians to perform outreach for members who are underutilizing the health care system. Had Tatum been encouraged to attend her annual examination or seek routine care, the pericarditis may have been diagnosed before hospitalization was required. At the very least, the MAO would have been compensated for the risks associated with her comorbidity(ies).

In addition to providing incentives to physicians who perform patient outreach, many MAOs also enlist clinical documentation improvement (CDI) trainers for physicians, in hopes this will boost HCC capture and reduce coding errors. Some MAOs require CDI as part of their contract agreements, and many MAOs hire auditors or have their own auditing departments review the coding of physicians seeing MA patients. Someone reading this course material would likely fall into one of these categories, as a current or prospective physician, coder, CDI specialist, contracted auditor, or MAO employee.

Medicare HCCs and RxHCCs

The determination of which diagnoses should risk-adjust has been distilled into several key points by CMS. The diagnoses considered for RA should be clinically meaningful; predictive of resource requirements; exclude extremely rare diseases; identify severity of disease; and be classifiable within ICD-10-CM. For MA, CMS has established a list of more than 9,000 diagnoses for chronic and acute conditions that map to about 80 HCCs and about 4,000 diagnoses that map to about 75 RxHCCs.

EXAMPLE

Diabetes mellitus falls into the following HCCs and RxHCCs:

HCC 17	Diabetes with acute complications
HCC 18	Diabetes with chronic complications
HCC 19	Diabetes without complication
HCC 122	Proliferative diabetic retinopathy with vitreous hemorrhage
RxHCC 30	Diabetes with complications
RxHCC 31	Diabetes without complications
RxHCC 241	Diabetic retinopathy

Each diabetes HCC and RxHCC has a specific value. HCC 19 (without complication) has a factor of 0.127, while HCC 18 (with chronic complications) has a factor of 0.371. Some codes will risk-adjust to more than one HCC/RxHCC. For example, diabetic polyneuropathy risk-adjusts to HCC 18 for the diabetes, HCC 75 for the neuropathy, and RxHCC 30 for the diabetes.

Clinical documentation improvement (CDI)
Betterment of the content of the medical record so that it accurately represents the author of the record, status of the patient's health, and diagnostic tests and treatments provided. CDI also endeavors to align the language of the medical record with the codes used in reporting diagnoses and services to have the secondary result of improved code abstraction.

The higher the RAF, the more resources are projected to be needed to manage the patient's health and the bigger the MAO RA payment. Risk factors are additive, ie, the risk scores for each chronic disease are tallied to determine the enrollee's final RAF score.

ADVICE/ALERT NOTE

Risk factors are additive, ie, the risk scores for each chronic disease are tallied to determine the enrollee's final RAF score.

Demographics contributing to a RAF include the enrollee's financial status, whether the enrollee lives independently or in an institution, age, and sex. RAFs undergo a final computation before payment is made, involving the enrollee's state and county to determine individual capitation rates. CMS uses these rates with the RAF to determine the final payment to the MAO for an enrollee. Some issues (eg, long-term institutional status and ESRD status) are considered for each month of the payment year. The details of the rules for determining RAF scores are more an accounting and actuarial function. However, it is beneficial for coders and physicians to be exposed to the weight given to the various HCCs and RxHCCs, and the process of determining a RAF, to heighten awareness of how proper documentation and coding affects RA scores and payments. For more information on RAF calculations and MAO payments, visit www.cms.gov/Medicare/Health-Plans/MedicareAdvtgSpecRateStats/Risk-Adjustors.html.

Proper documentation and effective coding communicate the severity of the patient's condition. The MAO wants to ensure that all available HCC-mapped diagnoses are captured and coded in the health record for appropriate charge capture. The MAO is equally motivated to ensure that diagnosis codes reported for a patient accurately reflect the patient's medical record, since CMS is vigilant in its audits of payments under the MA system, and will require reimbursement and may levy fines for overpayments. While no one should be expected to memorize all of the HCCs or codes that map to HCCs, it is relatively simple to become familiar with the categories of illness that risk-adjust and approach those categories of illness with care in documentation and abstraction.

HCCs/RxHCCs and their values are updated annually, as are the ICD-10-CM codes that map to them. Tables 1.1 and 1.2 are snapshots of the HCCs and RxHCCs for MA reporting during 2018, during which 2017 dates of service were processed to determine MAO payments. Included is the community RAF for an enrollee who is aged but not disabled or eligible for Medicaid. The complete tables are provided in Appendix A.

Medicaid
Healthcare program jointly funded with state and federal dollars that assists low-income US citizens or legal residents who otherwise could not obtain healthcare coverage, and some people with disabilities. Each state regulates who can receive Medicaid benefits and manages its own program.

TABLE 1.1 Snapshot of the 2018 HCCs for Medicare Advantage (MA) Reporting

Included is the community RAF for an enrollee who is aged but not disabled or eligible for Medicaid (non-low income, age >65).

HCC	HCC TITLE	RISK-ADJUSTMENT FACTOR
HCC 1	HIV/AIDS	0.312
HCC 2	Septicemia, Sepsis, Systemic Inflammatory Response Syndrome/Shock	0.455
HCC 6	Opportunistic Infections	0.435
HCC 8	Metastatic Cancer and Acute Leukemia	2.625
HCC 9	Lung and Other Severe Cancers	0.970
HCC 10	Lymphoma and Other Cancers	0.677
HCC 11	Colorectal, Bladder, and Other Cancers	0.301
HCC 12	Breast, Prostate, and Other Cancers and Tumors	0.146
HCC 17	Diabetes with Acute Complications	0.318
HCC 18	Diabetes with Chronic Complications	0.318
HCC 19	Diabetes without Complication	0.104
HCC 21	Protein-Calorie Malnutrition	0.545
HCC 22	Morbid Obesity	0.273
HCC 23	Other Significant Endocrine and Metabolic Disorders	0.228
HCC 27	End-Stage Liver Disease	0.962
HCC 28	Cirrhosis of Liver	0.390
HCC 29	Chronic Hepatitis	0.165
HCC 33	Intestinal Obstruction/Perforation	0.246
HCC 34	Chronic Pancreatitis	0.276
HCC 35	Inflammatory Bowel Disease	0.294

EXAMPLE

Martin McNally is an MA patient whose comorbidities are tallied into a RAF score for HCCs. He does not subscribe to Part D (prescription coverage).

RISK/PAYMENT FACTOR	HCC	RAF
66-year-old male	(community, nondual, aged)	0.300
Congestive heart failure (CHF)	85	0.323
Prostate cancer	12	0.146
Diabetes mellitus (DM), complicated	18	0.318
Peripheral vascular disease	108	0.298
Below-knee amputation	189	0.588
Morbid obesity	22	0.273
Interaction CHF & DM	NA	0.154
Total RAF		**2.400**

Nondual
A term used to describe Medicare beneficiaries who are not enrolled in Medicaid or Medicaid beneficiaries who are not enrolled in Medicare.

If we assume a CMS capitated rate for McNally's locality of $800 per month, the MAO would receive a payment of $9,600 per year for an enrollee without risk diagnoses. Multiply the capitated rate ($9,600) by 2.400 (McNally's RAF) to determine the CMS payment to the MAO to cover McNally's care. The total is $23,040 annually. RxHCCs would be calculated separately and added to payment, if the patient subscribed to Part D.

A patient with McNally's comorbidities would be at higher risk for resource-intensive care, including hospitalization. The MAO would pay for such care.

TABLE 1.2 Snapshot of the 2018 RxHCCs for Medicare Advantage (MA) Reporting

Included is the community RAF for an enrollee who is aged but not disabled or eligible for Medicaid (non-low income, age >65).

RxHCC	RxHCC TITLE	RISK-ADJUSTMENT FACTOR
RxHCC 1	HIV/AIDS	3.192
RxHCC 5	Opportunistic Infections	0.261
RxHCC 15	Chronic Myeloid Leukemia	67.383
RxHCC 16	Multiple Myeloma and Other Neoplastic Disorders	3.405
RxHCC 17	Secondary Cancers of Bone, Lung, Brain, and Other Specified Sites; Liver Cancer	1.435
RxHCC 18	Lung, Kidney, and Other Cancers	0.244
RxHCC 19	Breast and Other Cancers and Tumors	0.087
RxHCC 30	Diabetes with Complications	0.396
RxHCC 31	Diabetes without Complication	0.263
RxHCC 40	Specified Hereditary Metabolic/Immune Disorders	2.785
RxHCC 41	Pituitary, Adrenal Gland, and Other Endocrine and Metabolic Disorders	0.111
RxHCC 42	Thyroid Disorders	0.095
RxHCC 43	Morbid Obesity	0.067
RxHCC 45	Disorders of Lipoid Metabolism	0.054
RxHCC 54	Chronic Viral Hepatitis C	1.921
RxHCC 55	Chronic Viral Hepatitis, Except Hepatitis C	0.322
RxHCC 65	Chronic Pancreatitis	0.239
RxHCC 66	Pancreatic Disorders and Intestinal Malabsorption, Except Pancreatitis	0.094
RxHCC 67	Inflammatory Bowel Disease	0.470

HCCs and RxHCCs are not only used for determining risk and payment for MA enrollees; state-run Medicaid programs also use RA and rely on the HCC/RxHCC model.

Calculating Risk Scores

Multiple variables contribute to the risk score of a patient. Age and sex are assigned values, as is Social Security disability status and Medicaid status. The patient's housing status, whether in the community or in an institution, also contributes to the scoring. The RAFs from chronic or acute diagnoses also contribute. Long-term care and ESRD also affect payments. In addition, CMS has calculated that some diagnoses, when occurring together, have more resource intensity than the sum of the two diagnoses would suggest. For example, if a patient has heart failure in addition to diabetes, it is considered a synergistic risk, and this combination reimburses at a higher rate than the sum of the two HCCs separately. CMS provides a Disease Interactions Table that assigns additional RAFs for these combinations at the end of its HCC table, which is available in Appendix A.

Part C Risk Factors

Demographics contribute to RA calculations. In this example, we compare rates for a married couple with the same chronic illnesses: chronic obstructive pulmonary disease (COPD) and congestive heart failure (CHF). The husband, who is significantly older than his wife, is also disabled and living in an assisted-care center. Because his condition is more complex, it carries more risk and risk-adjusts at nearly twice the rate of his wife's condition.

PATIENT	AGE FACTOR	COPD HCC 111	CHF HCC 85	DISABLED, CHF, IN INSTITUTION	TOTAL RAF*
Martha Jones, 69, who lives at home	0.312	0.328	0.323	–	0.963
Matthew Jones, 92, disabled and lives in assisted living	0.964	0.305	0.191	0.321	1.781

TABLE 1.3. RxHCC List of Disease Hierarchies

Excerpts from Table V-5 List of Disease Hierarchies for RxHCC Model Calendar Year 2018

RxHCC	IF THE DISEASE GROUP IS LISTED IN THIS COLUMN . . .	. . . THEN DROP THE RXHCC(S) LISTED IN THIS COLUMN
17	Secondary Cancers of Bone, Lung, Brain, and Other Specified Sites; Liver Cancer	18 Lung, Kidney, and Other Cancers 19 Breast and Other Cancer and Tumors
18	Lung, Kidney, and Other Cancers	19 Breast and Other Cancer and Tumors
30	Diabetes with Complications	31 Diabetes without complication
54	Chronic Viral Hepatitis C	55 Chronic Viral Hepatitis, Except C
65	Chronic Pancreatitis	66 Pancreatic Disorders and Intestinal Malabsorption, Except Pancreatitis
82	Psoriatic Arthropathy and Systemic Sclerosis	83 Rheumatoid Arthritis and Other Inflammatory Polyarthropathy 84 Systemic Lupus Erythematosus, Other Connective Tissue Disorders, Inflammatory Spondylopathies 316 Psoriasis, Except with Arthropathy
83	Rheumatoid Arthritis and Other Inflammatory Polyarthropathy	84 Systemic Lupus Erythematosus, Other Connective Tissue Disorders, Inflammatory Spondylopathies
95	Sickle Cell Anemia	98 Aplastic Anemia and Other Significant Blood Disorders
96	Myelodysplastic Syndromes and Myelofibrosis	98 Aplastic Anemia and Other Significant Blood Disorders
111	Alzheimer's Disease	112 Dementia, Except Alzheimer's Disease

As previously mentioned, some HCCs/RxHCCs are grouped together when calculating risk scores, and only the most severe HCC is counted in the calculation. For example, a claim with both rheumatoid arthritis (RxHCC 83) and systemic sclerosis (RxHCC 82) would not consider the rheumatoid arthritis in the RA calculation. Only the systemic sclerosis would be counted, as it is higher in the disease hierarchy, as can be seen in the excerpt from the RxHCC List of Disease Hierarchies (Table 1.3).

In some circles, the elimination of the lower HCC value as shown in the Disease Hierarchies Table is referred to as "trumping." See Appendix A for the Disease Interactions Table and Disease Hierarchies Table for 2018.

Submissions to CMS

Because the MAO is accountable for the diagnostic codes submitted to CMS by the physician, CMS allows the MAOs to send updates to the government's RA processing system (RAPS) before completing annual risk calculations. RAPS is an electronic data warehouse for diagnostic information provided by the MAO. When the MAO submits data to RAPS, that data are included in the CMS risk calculations for affected enrollees, along with fee-for-service data from the enrollee's physicians, and demographic information captured in the Medicare database.

Similarly, because MAOs are held accountable for the accuracy of fee-for-service diagnostic coding (ie, for medical necessity), MAOs may review physician data to seek out troublesome patterns of coding (eg, acute stroke being treated in a physician's office, in which the MAO may suspect that the physician should have reported history of stroke, but did not). While an acute stroke diagnosis risk-adjusts, history of stroke does not. Such a discovery could lead to an MAO audit targeting certain physicians, dates of service, or patients. The MAO can submit new codes to RAPS to replace codes reported by the physician office in its fee-for-service claim.

MAOs may also perform data mining to sniff out missed diagnoses. For example, a chart for a patient who is prescribed brexpiprazole, a drug that

RA processing system (RAPS)
Electronic warehouse for diagnostic information provided by the MAO. When the MAO submits data to RAPS, that data is included in the CMS risk calculations for affected enrollees and demographic information captured in the Medicare database.

treats only schizophrenia, may be worth reviewing if the fee-for-service claim or encounter data for the patient does not include a diagnosis code for schizophrenia. An audit of that patient's medical record may uncover overlooked documentation that allows a diagnosis of schizophrenia to be added to the RAPS file.

CMS is slowly migrating from RAPS to encounter data submission (EDS). Before EDS was blended into RAPS in the current payment methodology, MAOs gathered and filtered their own diagnosis codes to create RAPS files. In EDS, the MAOs send unfiltered encounter data to CMS, meaning accurate documentation and coding of claims is more important than ever.

RAPS submissions are done in an organized manner, culminating in what the RA industry calls "sweeps." Sweeps are predetermined periods of intense scrutiny and revision of the data in claims before submission to RAPS. MAOs sometimes have internal auditors perform the reviews, or they sometimes hire outside auditing companies to review claims. Targeting claims for review may be done by the MAO or by the auditing company. Keeping in mind that the risk scores are prospective, so diagnoses from claims filed the previous year are used to calculate the risk score of an enrollee for the current year for MAOs, CMS accepts amended ICD-10-CM files from MAOs and makes payments to the MAOs based on the schedule for "sweeps" shown in Table 1.4.

Health Insurance Marketplace Risk Pools

The health exchanges created by the ACA have risk pools that also use an HCC model (see Figure 1.2). These risk pools were established to allow people who were not eligible for group plans through employers or Medicare to qualify for affordable insurance, despite pre-existing conditions. Not all enrollees in these risk pools are high risk; some enrollees simply were looking for the most cost-effective health insurance plan, and these risk pools offered low costs and tax credits from the federal government. Because these exchanges have a broader population base, the HCC code set has been augmented with diagnoses for neonatal, pediatric, and maternity disorders. This model is known as the HHS-HCC model.

TABLE 1.4 MAOs "Sweeps" Schedule

RISK SCORE RUN	DATES OF SERVICE	DEADLINE FOR SUBMISSION OF RA DATA	INITIAL OR FINAL REIMBURSEMENT DATE
2017 Initial	07/01/2015–06/30/2016	Friday, 09/09/2016	January 2017
2016 Final Run	01/01/2015–12/31/2015	Tuesday, 1/31/2017	July 2017
2017 Mid-Year	01/01/2016–12/31/2016	Friday, 03/03/2018	August 2017
2018 Initial	07/01/2016–06/30/2017	Friday, 09/08/2017	January 2018
2017 Final Run	01/01/2016–12/31/2016	Wednesday, 01/31/2018	July 2018
2018 Mid-Year	01/01/2017–12/31/2017	Friday, 03/01/2019	August 2018
2019 Initial	07/01/2017–06/30/2018	Friday, 09/07/2018	January 2019
2018 Final Run	01/01/2017–12/31/2017	Thursday, 01/31/2019	July 2019
2019 Mid-Year	01/01/2018–12/31/2018	Friday, 03/06/2020	August 2019

Sweeps
Predetermined periods of intense scrutiny and revision of the data in claims that culminate in a deadline submission to CMS for RA.

FIGURE 1.2 How ACA Risk Pools Work

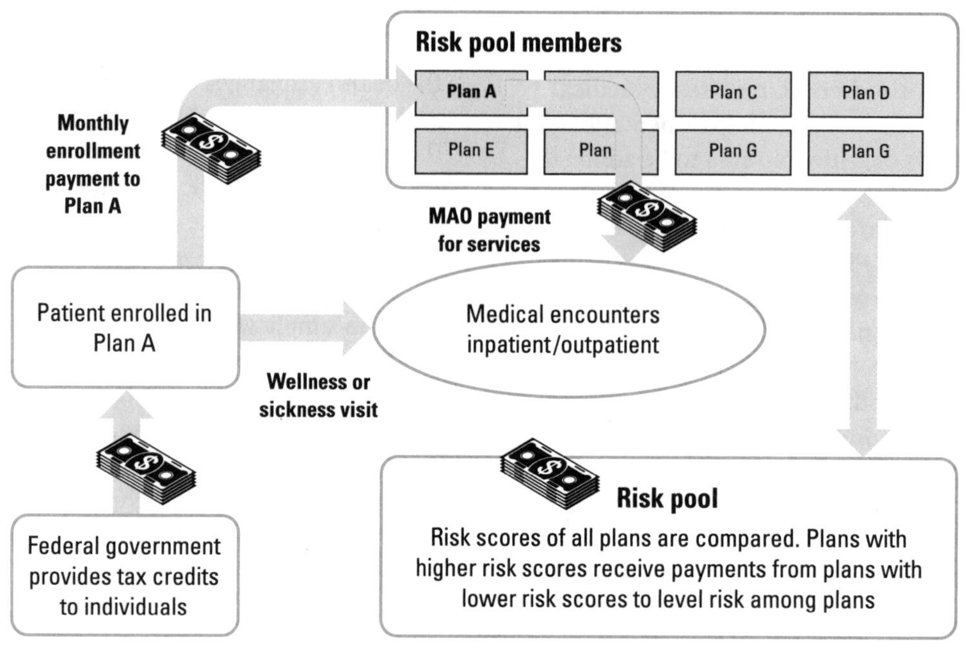

Value-Based Payment Modifier Program

The value modifier (VM) program assesses the quality and cost of care provided to Medicare beneficiaries by solo practitioners and medical groups. CMS uses RA in the evaluation of differences in Medicare spending per beneficiary (MSPB), to allow for more accurate evaluation of physicians based on the quality of their services and patient outcomes. Without RA, physicians who treat a sicker population of patients could perform worse on some quality and cost measures. The VM measures that risk-adjust include:

- **30-day all-cause hospital readmission.** This will risk-adjust for age and underlying risks associated with surgery/gynecology, general medicine, cardiorespiratory, cardiovascular, and neurology. For this given population, some readmissions are considered unavoidable. Planned readmissions are excluded from inclusion in this measure. More information on this methodology can be found at www.cms.gov/Medicare/Medicare-Fee-for-Service-Payment/PhysicianFeedbackProgram/Downloads/2015-ACR-MIF.pdf.
- **Hospital admissions for acute and chronic ambulatory care sensitive condition composite measures.** Age and sex both affect the likelihood of hospitalization for patients with acute and chronic conditions. Evaluation of these hospitalizations can identify physicians who are engaged in better primary care, care planning, and care coordination. Acute conditions measured are dehydration, bacterial pneumonia, and urinary tract infections. Chronic conditions include diabetes, chronic obstructive pulmonary disease or asthma, and heart failure. More information on this methodology can be found at www.cms.gov/Medicare/Medicare-Fee-for-Service-Payment/PhysicianFeedbackProgram/Downloads/2015-ACSC-MIF.pdf.
- **Per capita costs per member with specific diagnoses.** This measure compares projected costs for care against actual costs. More information can be found at www.cms.gov/Medicare/Medicare-Fee-for-Service-Payment/PhysicianFeedbackProgram/Downloads/2015-TPCC-MIF.pdf.

Value modifier (VM)
A calculation that considers the quality and cost of care provided to Medicare enrollees under the Medicare physician fee schedule (PFS) and compensates healthcare physicians for high-quality care and for care of patients with high risk due to comorbidities. It is also known as the *physician value-based modifier.*

- **Consumer assessment of health care physicians and systems for PQRS.** Case mix is a consideration in the scoring of the consumer surveys enrollees complete for their physicians. More information can be found on page 53 of the *CAHPS for PQRS Survey Quality Assurance Guidelines*, at www.pqrscahps.org/contentassets/6b04e492602b4bb58f80e3fb4e1e0676/cahps_for_pqrs_survey_qag_v1_july_2015.pdf.

Oversight of RA Programs

By law, if the Department of Health and Human Services (HHS) delegates administration of any of its programs, it is going to do so with significant oversight. For the MA program, oversight comes in two forms: ensure diagnoses reporting is performed correctly and without fraud or abuse, and ensure enrollees in the MA programs are receiving services and benefits that meet the standard set by HHS and CMS. Correct coding is evaluated through RA validation audits, and services and benefits are monitored through CMS' program integrity audits and measured through Five Star Quality Rating System. CMS also oversees the ACA risk pools for quality of coding, requiring initial and secondary validation audits for all plans.

MA RA Data Validation

MA RA data validation (RADV) is CMS' method to recoup improper payments, and the risk of a negative RADV audit works to ensure compliance among all participants in the MA program. Some MAOs are selected for audit because their enrollment had a higher-than-average risk score compared to other MAOs, because the MAO reported a high number of outlier HCCs, or a random selection.

An MAO selected for a RADV will be asked to provide a copy of a medical record from a patient encounter as evidence of a reported, patient-specific HCC-linked diagnosis during a proscribed reporting period. The medical record documentation must meet certain criteria and standards for CMS documentation and coding. If a diagnosis is not validated during an audit, CMS will use an extrapolation formula to determine the payment error rate for the MA contract. In many cases, the MAO is asked to refund millions of dollars when data validation is unsuccessful. Therefore, the MAO has a large stake in ensuring physicians enrolled in its programs are documenting and coding properly. An explanation of the payment formula is available at www.cms.gov/Medicare/Medicare-Advantage/Plan-Payment/Downloads/radvmethodology.pdf.

In addition to validation of HCCs in documentation, RADVs look at patient demographics to ensure data is correct for the enrollee. Review of administrative issues (eg, proper signature protocols) are also part of a RADV audit.

> **RA data validation (RADV)**
> Process of verifying by independent review the diagnosis codes submitted by an MAO for payment. Verification is performed by reviewing medical records. The purpose is to ensure risk-adjusted payment integrity and accuracy.[12]

MA Star Rating System

The MA Five Star Quality Rating System is designed to provide a twofold boost to MA enrollees. First, it measures the quality of care provided by MAOs to its members. In so doing, it tracks a variety of prevention metrics and rewards plans that encourage their physicians to be more proactive in preventive health. These preventive services include colonoscopies, mammograms, BMI calculations, cholesterol tests, influenza vaccines, and screenings for mental health. Also included are measures for elder care and diabetes. The second boost to MA enrollees comes in the ability of enrollees to evaluate their plan in surveys that look at issues like waiting-room time, customer service, responsiveness to complaints, and overall satisfaction.

The Five Star Quality Rating System is a five-star system that measures five areas: improvement, outcomes, intermediate outcomes, patient experience, and access to care and processes. Bonuses are awarded to MAOs that outperform their peers. The bonuses are computed on a per-enrollee basis. A plan must achieve at least four stars to qualify for a 5% bonus. In 2017, 4% of plans had five stars; 16% had 4.5 stars; and 21% had four stars, which means 41% of plans were eligible for bonuses. High performance has other rewards, namely being allowed to enroll beneficiaries throughout the year if a plan scores five stars. Other plans must wait until the open enrollment period, which runs from October 15 to December 7, to recruit new enrollees. For more information about the Stars Rating system, visit https://www.cms.gov/medicare/provider-enrollment-and-certification/certificationandcomplianc/fsqrs.html.

Initial Validation and Second Validation Audits

Initial validation audits (IVAs) are required by CMS for every plan participating in a health insurance marketplace risk pool. The payer organization selects the auditing company to perform the IVA. The audit reviews and validates the enrollee's demographic information and looks at coding and documentation for selected dates of service. Captured in the IVA are HCC errors of omission or commission and validation of the demographic information of enrollees. Administrative errors count against the codes captured in these audits as well.

Once the IVA has been completed, HHS may retain an independent second validation auditor (SVA) to review the IVA results and develop an error estimation based on the second validation. Payment to the insurance plan may be adjusted based on the audit results.

Quality and Cost

Appropriate RA, like all programs in healthcare, is dependent on the quality of the data. Clear and concise medical records are the cornerstone of quality. Without quality documentation, the abstraction of codes is flawed from the beginning. However, coders, too, play a pivotal role in quality. Proper use of the coding guidelines, conventions, and CMS policies promotes consistency in reporting across the country. Payers and the government use diagnostic codes to determine coverage decisions and to make funding determinations based on disease category or the locality of an outbreak. Most importantly, coding contributes data elements in evidence-based medicine (EBM). Consider the "evidence" in EBM: collective data on documented disorders, treatments, and outcomes are analyzed to determine patterns that can lead to a blueprint for better patient care in an effort to improve outcomes, reduce inappropriate care, and lower costs. What exactly is "evidence?" The foundation of EBM is the patient diagnosis and chosen treatment. In this way, medical documentation and coding comes full circle, as both the foundation of quality and outcome of quality.

The goal of RA programs like MA is to focus on resource-intensive chronic conditions and preventive measures. RA and quality reporting payments are carrots to ensure chronic conditions are addressed regularly. With quality care, precise documentation, and accurate coding, all facets of the healthcare system benefit: Physicians carry less risk and improve the outcomes of their patients. Costs are reduced. Data analytics provide accurate reports on population health for the appropriate distribution of health care dollars.

The complex guidelines for diagnostic coding and regulations surrounding use of the codes may seem overwhelming to clinicians or coders who are being asked to stretch their skillsets and learn RA documentation and coding, but it's a goal well worth pursuing. The guidance in this book should help readers start down that path.

References

1. Centers for Medicare & Medicaid Services. *2008 Risk Adjustment Data Technical Assistance For Medicare Advantage Organizations Participant Guide.* https://www.csscoperations.com/Internet/Cssc3.Nsf/files/participant-guide-publish_052909.pdf/$File/participant-guide-publish_052909.pdf. Accessed Sept 10, 2017.
2. Centers for Disease Control and Prevention. *ICD-10 Coordination and Maintenance Committee Meeting Summary of Diagnosis Presentations.* https://www.cdc.gov/nchs/data/icd/2015_09_23_2015_Summary_Final.pdf. Accessed September 10, 2017.
3. Mile High Healthcare Analytics. "Risk Adjustment in Medicaid." Posted on March 14, 2016. https://www.healthcareanalytics.expert/risk-adjustment-medicaid/. Accessed Oct 30, 2017.
4. Centers for Medicare & Medicaid Services. Value-Based Payment Modifier. https://www.cms.gov/medicare/medicare-fee-for-service-payment/physicianfeedbackprogram/valuebasedpaymentmodifier.html. Accessed Sept 10, 2017.
5. Centers for Medicare & Medicaid Services. Accountable Care Organizations (ACO). https://www.cms.gov/medicare/medicare-fee-for-service-payment/aco/. Accessed Sept 10, 2017.
6. US Congress. H.R.2015 - Balanced Budget Act of 1997. 105th Congress (1997-1998). https://www.congress.gov/bill/105th-congress/house-bill/2015. Accessed Sept 11, 2017.
7. Valderas JM, Starfield B, Sibbald B, Salisbury C, Roland M. Defining Comorbidity: Implications for Understanding Health and Health Services. *Ann Fam Med.* 2009;7(4):357-363. doi: 10.1370/afm.983. Accessed Sept 11, 2017.
8. Chronic Conditions Data Warehouse. Medicare Tables & Reports. https://www.ccwdata.org/web/guest/medicare-tables-reports. Accessed Sept 11, 2017.
9. Cubanski, J, Neuman T. "The Facts on Medicare Spending and Financing." July 18, 2017. http://kff.org/medicare/fact-sheet/medicare-spending-and-financing-fact-sheet/. Accessed Oct 27, 2017.
10. US Congress. H.R.1 - Medicare Prescription Drug, Improvement, and Modernization Act of 2003. 108th Congress (2003-2004). https://www.congress.gov/bill/108th-congress/house-bill/1. Accessed Oct 30, 2017.
11. Office of Inspector General. *Fiscal Year 2013 HHS OIG Work Plan.* https://oig.hhs.gov/reports-and-publications/archives/workplan/2013/. Accessed Oct 27, 2017.
12. Schamp R. "Risk Adjustment Data Validation (RADV) Guidelines for Medical Record Documentation." https://www.capstoneperformancesystems.com/articles/guidelines-for-medical-record-documentation-for-risk-adjustment-data-validation/. Accessed Oct 26 2017.

Evaluate Your Understanding

The following questions are critical checkpoints that are meant to let you apply your critical thinking and evaluate your understanding of the content covered in this chapter. The answers for the end-of-chapter exercises are available in Appendix C. In addition, the Internet-based Exercises are additional learning and research opportunities to learn more about the topics related to this chapter.

A Answer Questions

Provide the answer(s) to each of the following questions.

1. Who is responsible for the accuracy of the diagnostic codes submitted for payment for a patient who is participating in a Medicare Advantage plan?
   A. The patient
   B. The coder
   C. The physician
   D. The MAO
2. Medicare Advantage payments are prospective, which means:
   A. Future payments are based on previous diagnoses
   B. Current payments are based on current diagnoses
   C. MAOs must wait to be reimbursed for medical services rendered
   D. MAOs must preauthorize medical services with CMS in order to be paid
3. Which of the following payment systems does NOT reflect a risk-adjustment system?
   A. Part C
   B. Part D
   C. Pay for performance
   D. Health insurance marketplace
4. What contributes to the Medicare Advantage enrollee's risk score?
   A. The patient's age and sex
   B. The cumulative value of the HCCs associated with the patient
   C. The patient's disability status
   D. All of the above
5. HCC is an acronym for:
   A. HHS comorbidity categories
   B. Hierarchical condition category
   C. Health complication classifications
   D. Hierarchical complication category
6. In Medicare Advantage plans, who pays the physician for services performed?
   A. CMS
   B. HHS
   C. MAO
   D. Risk pool
7. What is the primary focus of a RADV audit?
   A. Medical documentation and coding
   B. Algorithms for RAF determination
   C. Proper assignment of HCCs by the physician office
   D. None of the above
8. MAOs are paid a capitated rate. What does this mean?
   A. Medicare discounts its payments to physicians
   B. Medicare pays the MAO based on the services provided to its enrollees
   C. Medicare pays the MAO a flat rate for each enrollee in the plan
   D. Medicare pays the MAO based on its Five Star Quality Rating System
9. Which of the following is NOT a CMS HCC?
   A. HCC 17 Diabetes with acute complications
   B. HCC 18 Diabetes with chronic complications
   C. HCC 19 Diabetes without complications
   D. HCC 20 Prediabetes
10. Which of the following Medicare programs is free to all citizens 65 years of age or older?
    A. Part A
    B. Part B
    C. Part C
    D. Part D

B True/False Questions

Answer true or false for the following statements.

1. Hospital coding of diagnoses is usually superior to physician office coding of diagnoses because diagnosis codes impact payment in hospitals.
2. Chronic diseases are usually predictive of more resource-intensive health care requirements.
3. Pull-down menus in EHRs are foolproof diagnostic coding tools.
4. NCHS is the federal agency chiefly responsible for managing HCC development.
5. Economic status, chronic disease, age, and disability are all elements that risk-adjust in Medicare Advantage.
6. When people enrolled in MA plans skip preventive care, lifelong chronic diseases may disappear from risk scores.
7. All risk factors are additive, meaning the risk scores for every chronic disease for an enrollee are tallied to determine the enrollee's final RAF score.
8. Coders should memorize all HCCs and their RAF values.
9. The health exchanges created by the ACA have risk pools that use the HHS-HCC model.
10. Value-based payment modifiers have a risk-adjusting element to identify health risks of the patient population.

C Internet-based Exercises 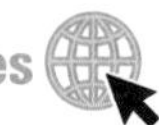

1. Interested in how popular Medicare Advantage plans are in your state and which types of programs are popular there? Go to http://kff.org/medicare/issue-brief/medicare-advantage-2016-spotlight-enrollment-market-update/.
2. Learn more about the history of Medicare and Medicaid at www.cms.gov/About-CMS/Agency-Information/History/index.html?redirect=/history/.
3. Read about RADV audits from the payer perspective in a paper issued by America's Health Insurance Plans (AHIP) at www.ahip.org/wp-content/uploads/2016/06/RADV_6.6.16.pdf.
4. Kaiser Family Foundation provides a snapshot of MAOs throughout the country in 2017 at http://kff.org/report-section/medicare-advantage-plans-in-2017-issue-brief/.
5. Understand more about the need to curb healthcare expenditures by reviewing www.cms.gov/research-statistics-data-and-systems/statistics-trends-and-reports/nationalhealthexpenddata/nhe-fact-sheet.html.

CHAPTER 2

Common Administrative Errors and Processes

Medical documentation and coding can be accurate and complete for a patient visit, but the Centers for Medicare & Medicaid Services (CMS) and other payers may reject the entire record and deny payment if the documentation contains administrative errors. For the purposes of this chapter, administrative errors are defined as nonclinical components of the patient chart that bring into question the authenticity of the encounter. Administrative questions might include: Was the encounter entered into the correct patient's chart? Has the record been properly authenticated by the physician?

Administrative issues do not stop with the identity of the patient and physician. Medical records are a hybrid collection of data as observed and recorded by physicians, nurses, medical assistants, and others. Coders are restricted to abstracting data only from acceptable sources, so separate identification of each author is necessary to avoid abstracting notes from unacceptable sources. Similarly, there are restrictions that apply specifically to electronic health record (EHR) documentation (eg, coders may not abstract diagnoses from cloned information in an EHR) and documents that are specifically excluded from abstraction for risk adjustment (RA) (eg, coders may not abstract diagnoses from laboratory or diagnostic radiology reports).

During a medical record review for Medicare Advantage organizations (MAOs), coders abstract codes from the chart only after they have reviewed the charts to verify the following information:

- The date of service (DOS) for a specific encounter is within the data collection period;
- The service was provided by an acceptable physician specialty or physician type;

Administrative errors
In medical documentation or coding and healthcare insurance adjudication, a mistake in documentation or reporting that usually does not directly affect patient care, but does call into question the authenticity of clinical documentation and coding and can result in claims denial. Common administrative errors involve signatures, dates of service, or reporting of an enrollee's identification or coverage.

- Each signature on the medical record is acceptable; and
- The documentation is legible and acceptable.

This chapter is a resource for clinicians seeking to identify and prevent administrative errors. Similarly, coders who review this chapter will better understand these administrative errors so they can take appropriate action when abstracting codes from a chart. Action by coders will vary according to whether they are working in the physician office, for a remote auditing firm, or directly for an MAO. Also included in this chapter is a brief review of some basic chart components for novice RA coders who may not be familiar with the diversity of medical record formats.

Most of the guidance provided in this chapter will apply to all medical coding, regardless of the insurance plan providing coverage. However, rules for data collection periods, acceptable physicians, and acceptable facilities presented in this chapter are specific to Medicare Advantage (MA), and may differ when dealing with other third-party payers.

CMS published an RA data-validation (RADV) checklist to assist auditors who are reviewing charts for MA validation audits. This checklist also offers guidance to MA coders, because the goal of any coder should be to abstract correctly and within the rules of the payer organization responsible for paying the claim. An MA record that passes the RADV checklist requirements will presumably succeed in a real RADV. Eight of the 11 items in the RADV checklist identify administrative errors that often cause failed RADVs. These questions should be answered for every coded chart.

YES	NO	
☐	☐	Is the record for the correct enrollee?
☐	☐	Is the record from the correct calendar year for the payment year being audited (i.e., for audits of 2011 payments, validating records should be from calendar year 2010)
☐	☐	Is the date of service present for the face to face visit?
☐	☐	Is the record legible?
☐	☐	Is the record from a valid provider type? (Hospital inpatient, hospital outpatient/ physician)
☐	☐	Are there valid credentials and/or is there a valid physician specialty documented on the record?
☐	☐	Does the record contain a signature from an acceptable type of physician specialist?
☐	☐	If the outpatient/physician record does not contain a valid credential and/or signature, is there a completed CMS-Generated Attestation for this date of service?

Within this chapter are explanations for what is considered "valid" or "acceptable," according to CMS standards.

Medical Record

The medical record contains an enormous amount of data in a variety of formats. Most of the data are maintained as clinical support for the physician responsible for care of the patient. History of past and current conditions; medication and allergy lists; preventive care and vaccination histories; electronic X ray, computerized tomography (CT), or magnetic resonance imaging (MRI) reports and images; pathology and laboratory test results; consult letters; and nursing notes are all components of the clinical record for the patient. Maintaining a complete and accurate health record for a patient is not only necessary for informed medical decision making (MDM), it is also a requirement under physicians' state licenses.

Each medical record also contains the administrative business record with the insurance member and group numbers, co-pay requirements, demographics, contact information, and name of the patient's primary care physician. These chart components are necessary for communicating with the patient, as well as for proper billing of insurance and collection of co-pays from patients.

All these elements are needed, but the volume of data requires a lot of parsing and sorting on the part of the coder. Even coders who work in a specific physician office and see the same chart format every day can find the volume of information daunting. For RA coders who abstract a variety of chart formats from a variety of physicians from all over the country, it is essential to quickly filter from the medical record the small percentage of codeable documents that can be abstracted. The RA–abstraction process begins with checking the administrative components of the medical chart. If a chart or record is too flawed to be acceptable to CMS, the RA coder will flag the record and move to the next one. In other cases, if administrative requirements are unmet, RA coders are instructed to complete the coding and flag the chart for errors. In any case, an administrative review of the chart is always the starting point because it is better to reject a chart before investing too much time coding it. A frequent reason for rejecting a chart in an MAO audit is if the chart contains records from more than one patient.

Patient Name and Demographics

Each encounter in the medical record must include the patient's full name and date of birth (DOB). For paper charts, the patient's full name should appear on every page of the record. For EHRs, best practices are that each printed or displayed page from the EHR contains the patient name. The goal is to ensure that the pages being reviewed are all part of the same encounter for the same patient. Presence of the patient name ensures that pages from other patient records are not interleaved with the other patient's notes. According to the American Health Information Management Association's (AHIMA's) *Integrity of the Healthcare Record: Best Practices for EHR Documentation*[1]:

> Documentation integrity is at risk when the wrong information is documented on the wrong patient health record. Errors in patient identification can affect clinical decision making and patient safety, impact a patient's privacy and security, and result in duplicate testing and increased costs to patients, providers, and payers. Patient identification errors can grow exponentially within the EHR, personal health record, and HIE [health information exchange] network(s) as the information proliferates.

For Medicare, the patient's name as it appears on the MA card is the name that must be included in the patient record. While it is acceptable to document the patient's name preference (eg, "Russell A. Corben, who prefers to be called Rusty"), the patient's full name must be entered in the record. Not all coders may understand that Rusty is a common nickname for Russell and could flag the encounter as for the wrong member. Far more important, the chart for Russell B. Corben is easily confused with Russell A. Corben if the full name is not used. Variations in spelling can also lead to mistakes in identification: Corben can also be spelled Corbin; Russell is sometimes spelled Russel. Physician practices and facilities should establish protocols in their policies and procedures for distinguishing between patients with identical or very similar names to prevent mistakes. The policies should also address corrective actions required by administrative staff, coders, or clinicians, when such errors are discovered.

Coders performing RA audits are abstracting targeted records from targeted enrollees, usually for an MAO. Coders must always validate the patient's full name and DOB against the audit demographics provided by the MAO before beginning an abstraction. If the name or DOB does not correspond to the MAO demographic information, the coder must flag the chart and discontinue the chart review for that enrollee. Continuing to review a chart with information from a wrong enrollee could be considered a privacy violation.

FYI

ECRI Institute is a not-for-profit US organization that performs evidence-based research to improve the safety of healthcare, completed an analysis of 7,613 patient identification errors at 181 organizations that occurred between January 2013 and August 2015 and determined that 33% of the errors involved diagnostic evaluations and 22% involved treatments and procedures. Another 13% of the errors occurred at registration.[2]

Date of Service

Date of service (DOS) is the date a patient receives care. In the outpatient environment, the DOS is a single date for most encounters; however, multiple dates may be reported for bedded overnight outpatient or observation care. For inpatient encounters, the DOS is a range of dates (eg, 12-11-2017 to 12-16-2017), representing the date of admission through the date of discharge from the facility. According to CMS' 2008 *Risk Adjustment Data Technical Assistance For Medicare Advantage Organizations Participant Guide (2008 RA Participant Guide)*, "a medical record that lacks a date or provider signature and credentials is invalid and will not be reviewed."[3]

ADVICE/ALERT NOTE

A medical record that lacks a date or provider signature and credentials is invalid and will not be reviewed.[3]

A qualifying encounter must include a face-to-face visit with a patient, or a telemedicine encounter that meets Medicare standards. A phone call to check a patient's response to a new medication does not qualify as a legitimate encounter for MA RA purposes. Medical documentation should contain evidence of the face-to-face visit (eg, a physical examination or observation regarding the patient's chief complaint). Evidence of an appointment time for the encounter is needed to meet the face-to-face requirement. Both of the encounters in the following Example are ineligible for RA because neither patient met face-to-face with an acceptable physician.

EXAMPLE

Encounter 1

Due to an earlier hypertensive event, John A. Clark, 72, returns to his physician's office every two days for a blood pressure (BP) check. Today, Joan Martien, LPN [licensed practical nurse], performed two BP readings on Clark. She informed Dr. Marx that Clark's readings were normal. Clark did not meet with Dr. Marx, although both Dr. Marx and Martien made notes in Clark's chart about the encounter.

Encounter 2

Mary Riggins, 67, has chronic obstructive pulmonary disease (COPD) and diabetes. Today, she is being seen for administration of an influenza vaccine, as she saw a news program promoting flu shots to seniors. Ron Bird, RN [registered nurse], asks Riggins to sign a release form, and documents that the shot was administered in the patient's upper left extremity. He also documents the vaccine and the dosage administered.

Date of service (DOS)
The calendar date a patient receives care. In the outpatient environment, the DOS is a single date (eg, 12-11-2017) for most encounters; however, multiple dates may be reported for bedded overnight outpatient or observation care. For inpatient encounters, the DOS is a range of dates (eg, 12-11-2017 through 12-16-2017), representing services from the date of admission through the date of discharge from the facility.

Telemedicine
Office visit or consultation in which an interactive, two-way telecommunication system with real-time audio and video is involved, allowing a physician or healthcare professional to treat or diagnose a patient who is at a remote healthcare facility. CMS' Medicare Learning Network (MLN) provides more information on telemedicine regulations and applicable sites of care.[4]

The DOS of the encounter is a crucial data element for various reasons:

- **All government and private payers require it.** An enrollee in an insurance plan has a coverage date range. Without the DOS, the payer cannot validate that the encounter occurred during a period in which the enrollee had coverage.
- **In an RA audit, DOS must be reconciled with the claims data filed by the physician.** CMS only risk-adjusts diagnoses that are the result of covered services, as represented by the Current Procedural Terminology (CPT®) or Healthcare Common Procedure Coding System (HCPCS) Level II codes submitted by the physician. If a physician's claim has been adjudicated by CMS and determined as payable, diagnoses from the encounter are eligible for RA. New diagnosis codes or code deletions submitted by the MAO must be aligned with an adjudicated claim in order to be eligible for RA. This is done by correlating data by physician, enrollee, and DOS. Without the DOS, correlation cannot occur, and MAO code changes will not be recognized and risk-adjusted.
- **In an RA audit, the audit period is for a specific date range, usually a calendar year.** The DOS for the encounter in the record must be within that date range. Any DOS outside the date range should not be abstracted.
- **Lack of a documented encounter in the medical record may flag a physician for audit.** Misrepresentation of DOS is a common fraud scheme, usually perpetrated by billing two encounters for a single office visit.
- **DOS is a component necessary to meet legal medical record standards.** Complete and accurate records are the best defense in a malpractice suit. Some state medical board rules provide for discipline against physicians with substandard documentation, including missing DOS.

Consultations

It is a common practice for consulting physicians to prepare a written report of findings for a referring physician. This consultation report is often written in the form of a letter to the referring physician, which describes reasons for the visit, the diagnostic tests or examinations performed on the referring physician's patient, as well as recommendations for future care of the patient. While these letters usually contain the date when written, many consultation letters fail to identify the DOS of the encounter during which the examination took place that led to the letter. If the DOS is not included in the consultation letter and there is no other documentation of date for that encounter, it fails to meet documentation requirements.

Many MAOs direct their auditors to abstract a consultation letter with a missing DOS, but also ask auditors to flag the record as having an error. Consultants are sought because they are experts, and so their records are valuable for RA. In some cases, the consultant's record may be the only note that documents a diagnosis sufficiently. If necessary, the MAO can seek out the consultant's medical record for the original encounter that led to the consultation letter, and use the documentation from the original encounter as evidence of the diagnosis.

Amending Medical Records

Because the medical record is a clinical and legal timeline of the diagnosis and treatment of a patient, any correction or addendum must be clearly and permanently identified by author and date. This is to protect the integrity of the medical record in the event of an audit or a lawsuit. CMS advised that an EHR system should have "the capability to identify changes to an original entry, such as 'addendums, corrections, deletions, and patient amendments.'"[5] Per the recordkeeping principles recommended by CMS, "[re]gardless of whether a documentation submission originates from a paper record or an electronic health record, documents submitted to MACs, CERT, Recovery Auditors, and ZPICs containing amendments, corrections or addenda must:

1. Clearly and permanently identify any amendment, correction or delayed entry as such, and
2. Clearly indicate the date and author of any amendment, correction or delayed entry, and
3. Not delete but instead clearly identify all original content."[6]

Consultation
A medical service provided by a physician whose advice regarding the care management of a specific patient has been sought by another physician. The consultant provides the referring physician with a written report of findings and recommendations for care.

In addition, CMS also advises that "[w]hen correcting a paper medical record, these principles are generally accomplished by using a single line strike through so that the original content is still readable. Further, the author of the alteration must sign and date the revision. Similarly, amendments or delayed entries to paper records must be clearly signed and dated upon entry into the record."[6]

Therefore, the date and author of any change must be easily differentiated from previous text. No content from the original record may be deleted. This includes not using correction fluid, ink, or other method to obliterate existing text in a handwritten chart, and no permanent deletion in an EHR. In paper records, the change may include a single line strikethrough of text, with author and date, so that the original entry is still legible.

 ADVICE/ALERT NOTE

Amending Entry Dates

- **EHRs**
  Be sure the EHR system has the capability to identify changes to an original entry, such as "addendums, corrections, deletions, and patient amendments." When making changes, the date, the time, the author making the change, and the reason for the change should be included.[6]
- **Paper records**
  When correcting a paper medical record, the record-keeping principles are generally accomplished by using a single line strikethrough so that the original content is still readable. In addition, the author of the alteration must sign and date the revision. Similarly, amendments or delayed entries to paper records must be clearly signed and dated upon entry into the record.[6]

Signatures

The Department of Health and Human Services (HHS) requires that physicians follow CMS regulations for signatures. These regulations aim to ensure that medical documentation is authenticated by its author, whether in an EHR or in a paper record. Without an authenticating signature from the author, the encounter may be rejected in an audit.

CMS does not provide specific guidance on the timeframe for the completion of the documentation and authentication for an encounter, except to require that it be "timely," and that "[p]roviders are encouraged to enter all relevant documents and entries into the medical record at the time they are rendering the service."[7] Any significant delay in timely completion and signature of a record must be explained in the record. Per CMS, "providers should not add late signatures to the medical record (beyond the short delay that occurs during the transcription process); but instead, should make use of the signature authentication process."[8] The only exception to this is for dictated reports, which should be signed within 180 days of the service, per CMS' *Contract-Level Risk Adjustment Data Validation Medical Record Reviewer Guidance (Contract-Level RADV Reviewer Guidance).*[9]

 ADVICE/ALERT NOTE

"Providers should not add late signatures to the medical record (beyond the short delay that occurs during the transcription process); instead, they should make use of the signature authentication process."[8]

While rules on acceptable signatures differ for paper records and EHRs, the person who performed the services during the encounter is responsible for documenting and authenticating the encounter. Even in cases in which the encounter is performed "incident to" by an advanced care practitioner (ACP) or by a resident in a teaching facility, the person performing the service and authoring the documentation should sign and date the record, attesting to its authenticity. A physician can then approve or release the record with a countersignature, in accordance with state regulations and facility policies.

"Incident to"
Physician services that are an integral part of the physician professional service, but performed by an ACP or other clinical staff member under the physician's direct supervision. These services may be performed in the course of diagnosis or treatment of the patient's condition, which was originally treated by the physician.

Advanced care practitioners (ACPs)
Clinicians including physician assistants (PAs), nurse practitioners (NPs), clinical nurse specialists (CNSs), certified nurse midwives (CNMs), and certified registered nurse anesthetists (CRNAs).

Teaching facility
A hospital or medical center providing education and training for clinical health careers. Federal and local regulations govern the oversight given by practicing physicians to physician residents being trained in clinical care and medical documentation.

Electronic Signatures

Physicians or practice managers should ensure that their EHRs contain compliant electronic signature elements to ensure records are properly authenticated. Otherwise, attestations, filled out and signed for each noncompliant encounter, would be necessary to authenticate the records in an audit. If the EHR is generating the faulty signature elements, virtually every encounter performed by a physician would need a separate attestation.

A completed signature in the EHR must include the author's:

- First name or initial;
- Last name;
- Credential(s) (initials associated with license, certification, or other education); and
- The date the record was validated (authenticated) by the physician.

A note indicating the record has been signed but not read is not evidence of authentication and is unacceptable to CMS. Language in the electronic signature must indicate that the author is taking responsibility for the contents of the record. (See the following Example on acceptable electronic signatures.) Authors using voice-recognition software may want to dictate a statement that a note was generated through voice-recognition, to account for any typographical errors or misspellings that may follow, but these authors, in signing the record, are attesting that they have read the record and it is correct.

EXAMPLE

Acceptable electronic signatures:

- *Electronically signed by* Mildred Monson, MD on 12/27/2017 2:45 PM
- *Authenticated by* Mildred Monson, MD on 12/27/2017 2:45 PM
- *Approved by* Mildred Monson, MD on 12/27/2017 2:45 PM
- *Completed by* Mildred Monson, MD on 12/27/2017 2:45 PM
- *Finalized by* Mildred Monson, MD on 12/27/2017 2:45 PM
- *Reviewed by* Mildred Monson, MD on 12/27/2017 2:45 PM
- *Validated by* Mildred Monson, MD on 12/27/2017 2:45 PM
- *Accepted by* Mildred Monson, MD on 12/27/2017 2:45 PM
- *Released by* Mildred Monson, MD on 12/27/2017 2:45 PM
- *Verified by* Mildred Monson, MD on 12/27/2017 2:45 PM
- *Authorized by* Mildred Monson, MD on 12/27/2017 2:45 PM
- *Confirmed by* Mildred Monson, MD on 12/27/2017 2:45 PM
- *Approved by* Mildred Monson, MD on 12/27/2017 2:45 PM
- *Electronically authored by* Mildred Monson, MD on 12/27/2017 2:45 PM
- *Entered data sealed by* Mildred Monson, MD on 12/27/2017 2:45 PM
- *Created by* Mildred Monson, MD on 12/27/2017 2:45 PM
- *Performed by* Mildred Monson, MD on 12/27/2017 2:45 PM

Unacceptable electronic signatures:

- Administratively signed by
- Dictated, but not signed
- Electronic signature on file [with no other indication of a date/time]
- Electronically signed to expedite delivery
- Proxy signature-signed via approval letter or statement, such as:
  - I authorize my name to be electronically affixed by using my unique dictation computer key
  - "Signature on file" or "Manually signed by" (The meaning of this is unknown. In some transcription/EMR systems, this might be acceptable, but it seems to mean the physician/practitioner will hand-sign the document after review.)

Electronic signature
Authentication of a record within an EHR system that identifies the author and provides verification that the record is accurate. The electronic signature contains the name and credential of the author, a statement of authentication, and a date/time stamp. Usually an electronic signature is tied directly to the login identity of the author.

Compliant EHRs are also expected to contain protections against modification, so that any alterations to a record are also date-stamped and identified by author and earlier versions of the record are maintained. In this way, an audit trail is evidence of the author of each version of the note.

Electronic signatures carry additional burdens of compliance associated with EHR systems because they need to safeguard the integrity of each record's entry time and authorship. When a medical assistant or nurse is entering information into the medical record, the EHR system should stamp that information as originating with that assistant or nurse. Similarly, the notes of the physician will be identified as the physician's work in a compliant EHR system. Authorship is not required to be visible in the EHR screen view, but the identity of the author must be recorded, retrievable, and available for submission if requested in an audit. Physicians should never share EHR login information with others in their practice, as this may lead to a misrepresentation of the medical record's or documentation's authorship.

FYI

Author identification

Different providers may add information to the same progress note, and when this occurs, each provider should be allowed to sign his or her entry, in order to enable verification of the amount of work performed and which provider performed the work.[5]

Several levels of author identification appear in the EHR. As noted, each entry is stamped with the time and author's login identification (ID). CMS also requires that the physician certify the completed record has been read and authenticated by the physician. Some EHRs perform an auto-authentication or auto-signature. Once a record has been closed, a "signature" of the author is appended to the end of the record. Auto-authentication is not acceptable, because CMS expects the physician to proactively approve and authenticate the documentation. Compliant authentication can be achieved with a single click of the mouse in some EHRs, ie, the login name, credentials, and date automatically populate. The physician, however, must attest to the veracity of the record. (See the following Example.)

EXAMPLE

Each EHR system has its own signature language and menu, and physicians must ensure they are using the signature menu compliantly.

Encounter Sign-Off

Encounter performed and documented by Jason Argo, PA

Encounter reviewed and signed by Mildred Monson, MD on 12/27/2017 2:50 PM

Encounter signed-off by Mildred Monson, MD on 12/27/2017 2:45 PM

This encounter was documented as "performed" by Jason Argo. The first line likely is auto-authenticated because there is no time and date stamp or attestation language. This first line is simply part of the audit trail the EHR system performs automatically. Such a note does not attest to the author checking documentation for completeness or accuracy. The record was "reviewed, signed, and signed-off" by Monson, who did not perform the work. This record is at risk in an audit because the author of the record, Jason Argo, did not authenticate it. Best practices would require Argo to "review and sign." Monson then could "sign-off" on the record, in accordance with local policy, facility rules, and licensing requirements.

Handwritten Signatures

The use of paper records has declined in recent years as government incentives have encouraged physicians to adopt EHR systems. Even so, there are occasions when a handwritten note is scanned into a chart, or paper charts are otherwise employed. In these instances, CMS has rules on acceptable authentication of the medical record. For a handwritten chart, the physician's name and credentials must be discernable in the record. The signature should appear at the end of the document. The signature does not need to be dated.

Often, signatures are illegible. This is acceptable if the printed page contains the physician name and credential, as in a header, or if the name and credentials are typed or handwritten under the illegible signature. To ensure proper authentication of an illegible signature, the physician office should create and maintain a signature log (see Figure 2.1). When audited, the signature log is provided to the auditor along with the charts under review. Signature logs are simple to create, and should be required within a practice's policies and procedures. In this way, the initials of the physician will always be sufficient to authenticate authorship of a paper chart. Signature logs often accompany charts that are under MAO or RADV review.

FIGURE 2.1 Examples of a Signature Log and Portion of a Paper Chart for Authentication

Valley Medical Signature Log

Name	Credentials	Signature	Initials
Martin A. Martin	PA	*Martin A. Martin*	*MAM*
Jeanne Jones	MD, FACS	*Jeanne Jones*	*JJ*
Albert Noisome	MD, FACS	*Albert Noisome*	*AN*

(bottom of paper chart)

A/P

1. GERD — stable on Ppi as asymptomatic

2. HTN — stable on metropropol and Lasix

3. Hyperlipidemia — order blood lipid panel, CMP, serum or plasma

RTC in three months

AN

With signature and initials on file in the signature log, this record is adequately authenticated as belonging to Albert Noisome, MD, FACS.

Signature log
List of physicians within an organization with their corresponding credentials, handwritten signature, and initials that can be used to establish signature identity of the author of medical documentation. Signature logs should be requested in chart audits.

In Chapter 3 (Verifying Potential Errors and Taking Corrective Actions) of the *Medicare Program Integrity Manual*, which is available at www.cms.gov/Regulations-andGuidance/Guidance/Manuals/Downloads/pim83c03.pdf, CMS provides clear advice on signature authentication. See Table 2.1

TABLE 2.1 Verifying Potential Errors and Taking Correction Actions: Signature Requirement Checklist

		SIGNATURE REQUIREMENT MET	CONTACT BILLING PROVIDER AND ASK A NON-STANDARDIZED FOLLOW-UP QUESTION
1	Legible full signature	X	
2	Legible first initial and last name	X	
3	Illegible signature over a typed or printed name **Example:** [signature] John Whigg, MD	X	
4	Illegible signature where the letterhead, addressograph, or other information on the page indicates the identity of the signatory **Example:** An illegible signature appears on a prescription. The letterhead of the prescription lists (3) physicians' names. One of the names is circled.	X	
5	Illegible signature **not** over a typed/printed name and **not** on letterhead, but the submitted documentation **is accompanied** by: a signature log, or an attestation statement	X	
6	Illegible signature **not** over a typed/printed name, **not** on letterhead, and the documentation is **unaccompanied** by: a signature log, or an attestation statement **Example:** [signature]		X
7	Initials over a typed or printed name	X	
8	Initials **not** over a typed/printed name but **accompanied** by: a signature log, or an attestation statement	X	
9	Initials **not** over a typed/printed name **unaccompanied** by: a signature log, or an attestation statement		X
10	Unsigned typed note with provider's typed name **Example:** John Whigg, MD		X
11	Unsigned typed note without providers typed/printed name		X
12	Unsigned handwritten note, the only entry on the page		X
13	Unsigned handwritten note where other entries on the same page in the same handwriting are signed	X	
14	"Signature on file"		X

Attestations

If a medical record is being audited and the record carries an unacceptable signature, RA coders are usually instructed to abstract the chart anyway and flag the record as having an unacceptable signature. CMS allows physicians to revisit outpatient records and complete attestation forms to authenticate these records. Should the flagged record ever be subjected to an audit from CMS, the flag would notify the MAO that an attestation from the author must be obtained before the medical record could be submitted.

The following language is typical of what would be seen in an attestation:

> "I, [*print full name of the provider*], hereby attest that the medical record entry for [*insert DOS*] accurately reflects signatures/notations that I made in my capacity as a(n) [*insert provider credentials, eg, MD*] when I treated/diagnosed the above-listed Medicare beneficiary [*patient's full name and Medicare number listed above*]. I do hereby attest that this information is true, accurate, and complete to the best of my knowledge, and I understand that any falsification, omission, or concealment of material fact may subject me to administrative, civil, or criminal liability."

This statement is to be followed by a signature with credential by the author of the record, and the date the attestation was signed.

No one (eg, another physician in the same group practice) except the author of the medical record may sign an attestation. In a RADV, instruction on attestations is available from the auditing entity.

ADVICE/ALERT NOTE

The CMS–generated attestation must be completed, signed, and dated by the physician/practitioner who provided those services. No other forms of an attestation will be accepted. The completed fields must include the printed physician's/practitioner's name, the date of service of the medical record to which they are attesting, the physician's/practitioner's specialty or credential, and must be signed and dated by the physician/practitioner who encountered the face-to-face visit.

Date ranges or multiple dates of service cannot be entered on a medical record coversheet from an outpatient record. A CMS-generated attestation may be completed by the attending physician/practitioner for a single date of service. If the date of service on the submitted CMS–generated attestation does not match the medical record submitted by the MAO with the medical record coversheet, it will be deemed invalid and will result in an error under the CMS RADV medical record–review process if the medical record lacks the necessary physician/practitioner signature and/or credentials.[9]

Inpatient Records

A recap of a patient's inpatient episode of care should be reflected in the hospital discharge summary. Ideally, the discharge summary identifies the reason for hospitalization, significant findings, treatments provided, the patient's condition at discharge, the patient's final diagnoses, and a record of instructions for care after discharge. The discharge summary is signed by the dictating physician. Of significance, unlike outpatient encounters and physician billing, the *ICD-10-CM Official Guidelines for Coding and Reporting* (*ICD-10-CM Guidelines*) allow for uncertain diagnoses, those qualified as possible, probable, likely, suspected, still to be ruled out, or other similar language, to be coded as if they were established if supported by reasonable clinical circumstances and documented in the discharge

Attestation
Formal statement asserting that a specific medical record, while not authenticated sufficiently by a physician at the time of care, is authentic. The attestation must be signed by the author of the medical record and include the name of the patient and the DOS. In Medicare RA, only outpatient-record signature errors may be corrected with an attestation.

Discharge summary
A written report identifying the reason for hospitalization, significant findings, treatments provided, the patient's condition at discharge, and a record of instructions for care after discharge. The physician who oversees the person's inpatient care must sign the report.

summary. These unconfirmed diagnoses are not acceptable when they are documented anywhere else in the inpatient record.

Although the components of an acceptable signature are the same for inpatient and outpatient encounters, CMS does not permit the use of an attestation for validation of inpatient charts with unacceptable signatures. However, CMS does not want to completely disallow the use of inpatient episodes of care for RA audits when the discharge summary does not have an acceptable signature. Therefore, CMS has developed a workaround. Inpatient records that are not authenticated with a compliantly signed discharge summary can be abstracted as individual physician encounters.

This means that instead of one date range and set of diagnoses for the encounter, each individual physician encounter, including progress notes, consultations, etc, for each day are abstracted. This exponentially increases the number of separate encounters to be coded, and those encounters must be abstracted using outpatient coding rules rather than inpatient coding rules. It can also mean that uncertain diagnoses documented at the time of discharge may not qualify for ICD-10-CM codes, thus affecting RA because the inpatient coding rules are not in effect. See the Example below for the differences between a compliant and noncompliant discharge summary.

According to CMS' *Risk Adjustment Data Validation (RADV) Medical Record Checklist and Guidance*, the minimum requirements for inpatient records must contain an admission and discharge date. In addition, inpatient records must include the signed discharge summary, stand-alone consultations must contain the consultation date, and stand-alone discharge summaries submitted as physician-provider type must contain the discharge date.[10]

ADVICE/ALERT NOTE

Minimum requirements for inpatient records state that these must contain an admission and discharge date. In addition,

- **inpatient records must include the signed discharge summary;**
- **stand-alone consultations must contain the consultation date; and**
- **stand-alone discharge summaries submitted as physician-provider type must contain the discharge date.[10]**

EXAMPLE

COMPLIANT DISCHARGE SUMMARY (SIGNED BY PHYSICIAN A)	NONCOMPLIANT DISCHARGE SUMMARY (CODED FOR ENCOUNTERS FOR HOSPITALIST, ENDOCRINOLOGIST, LICENSED CLINICAL SOCIAL WORKER, AND VASCULAR CONSULTANT)		
DOS Jan 1, 2018 through Jan 3, 2018	DOS Jan 1, 2018	DOS Jan 2, 2018	DOS Jan 3, 2018
Diagnoses: E11.59, I10, F32.9, I82.409	Physician A: E11.59, I10, F32.9, I82.409	Physician A: E11.59, I10, F32.9, I82.409	Physician A: E11.59, I10, F32.9, I82.409
	Physician B: E11.59, I10, I82.409	Physician B: E11.59, I10, I82.409	Physician B: E11.59, I10, I82.409
	Physician C: F32.9	Physician C: F32.9	Physician C: F32.9
	Physician D: E11.59, I10, F32.9, I82.409	Physician D: E11.59, I10, F32.9, I82.409	Physician D: E11.59, I10, F32.9, I82.409

Note that this example is much simpler than most inpatient encounters would be in the real world. The patient is diagnosed with diabetes with vascular complications; hypertension; depression; and an acute deep vein thrombosis. In this example, we see that the compliant discharge summary allowed the RA coder to abstract the entire hospitalization as one episode of care, ie, with four codes. With a noncompliant discharge summary, each individual note from each physician for each day must be abstracted separately, ie, with 36 codes.

Acceptable Providers for MA

CMS expects risk-adjusted diagnoses for MA to be documented by physicians who are directing the evaluation and/or treatment of those diagnoses. In Chapter 7 (Risk Adjustment) of CMS' *Medicare Managed Care Manual*, it states that "MA organizations should note that regardless of the type of diagnostic radiology bill (outpatient department or physician component), the diagnostic data associated with these services are not acceptable for RA. Diagnostic radiologists typically do not document confirmed diagnoses. Instead, the diagnosis confirmation comes from referring physicians or physician extenders and is, therefore, not assigned in the medical record documentation from diagnostic radiology services alone."[10] For that reason, radiologists and their records are excluded for consideration in an RA audit.

The logic lies in the fact that radiologists do not "treat" patients but merely provide a supporting service in the treatment and diagnosis of the patients' conditions. For example, a radiologist who reads and interprets an X ray is not going to treat a femoral fracture. Instead, an orthopedic surgeon will treat the femoral fracture. The radiologist provides diagnostic support to the orthopedic surgeon, who is in charge of the treatment. Radiologists are excluded from RA with the exception of interventional radiologists, who, as the name implies, are intervening and providing treatment to patients. In addition, other members of the care team may enter information into the chart but are also excluded (eg, medical assistants, licensed practice nurses, and registered nurses). This is because they are also not licensed to make diagnoses; instead, they provide clinical support to the physician or other qualified healthcare provider. CMS publishes a an annual list of physician specialties acceptable for RA. Be sure to obtain and review this list each year. New diagnoses must originate with the treating physician. A diagnosis from a pathologist, radiologist, or other diagnostic physician must be incorporated into the medical record of the treating physician in order for the diagnosis to be abstracted.

ADVICE/ALERT NOTE

"MA organizations should note that regardless of the type of diagnostic radiology bill (outpatient department or physician component), the diagnostic data associated with these services are not acceptable for RA. Diagnostic radiologists typically do not document confirmed diagnoses. Instead, the diagnosis confirmation comes from referring physicians or physician extenders and is, therefore, not assigned in the medical record documentation from diagnostic radiology services alone."[11]

Physicians whose documentation is acceptable for RA abstraction are identified in Table 2.2, along with their physician codes. Of note, pathologists are the only specialists who are not required to meet the face-to-face encounter rule in order for their records to be abstracted for RA.

Common Administrative Errors and Processes

Physician extenders
Healthcare providers who are not physicians but who perform medical activities that are typically performed by a physician. It is most commonly a nurse practitioner or physician assistant.

Face-to-face encounter
A visit between a physician and a patient during which both the physician and the patient are in the same room.

TABLE 2.2 Acceptable Physician Specialty Types for 2018 Payment Year (2017 Dates of Service) Risk Adjustment Data Submission[12]

CODE	SPECIALTY
1	General Practice
2	General Surgery
3	Allergy/Immunology
4	Otolaryngology
5	Anesthesiology
6	Cardiology
7	Dermatology
8	Family Practice
9	Interventional Pain Management (IPM)
10	Gastroenterology
11	Internal Medicine
12	Osteopathic Manipulative Medicine
13	Neurology
14	Neurosurgery
15	Speech Language Pathologist
16	Obstetrics/Gynecology
17	Hospice and Palliative Care
18	Ophthalmology
19	Oral Surgery (dentists only)
20	Orthopedic Surgery
21	Cardiac Electrophysiology
22	Pathology
23	Sports Medicine
24	Plastic and Reconstructive Surgery
25	Physical Medicine and Rehabilitation
26	Psychiatry
27	Geriatric Psychiatry
28	Colorectal Surgery (formerly Proctology)
29	Pulmonary Disease
33*	Thoracic Surgery
34	Urology
35	Chiropractic
36	Nuclear Medicine
37	Pediatric Medicine
38	Geriatric Medicine
39	Nephrology
40	Hand Surgery
41	Optometry
42	Certified Nurse Midwife
43	Certified Registered Nurse Anesthetist
44	Infectious Disease
46*	Endocrinology
48*	Podiatry
50*	Nurse Practitioner
62*	Psychologist
64*	Audiologist
65	Physical Therapist
66	Rheumatology
67	Occupational Therapist
68	Clinical Psychologist
72*	Pain Management
76*	Peripheral Vascular Disease
77	Vascular Surgery
78	Cardiac Surgery
79	Addiction Medicine
80	Licensed Clinical Social Worker
81	Critical care (intensivists)
82	Hematology
83	Hematology/Oncology
84	Preventive Medicine
85	Maxillofacial Surgery
86	Neuropsychiatry
89*	Certified Clinical Nurse Specialist
90	Medical Oncology
91	Surgical Oncology
92	Radiation Oncology
93	Emergency Medicine
94	Interventional Radiology
97*	Physician Assistant
98	Gynecologist/ Oncologist
99	Unknown Physician Specialty
C0	Sleep Medicine
C3	Interventional Cardiology
C5	Dentist
C6	Hospitalist
C7	Advanced Heart Failure and Transplant Cardiology
C8	Medical Toxicology
C9	Hematopoietic Cell Transplantation and Cellular Therapy

*Indicates that a number has been skipped.

Many other professions in the care-support team are excluded from RA audits, including ambulance-service providers, pharmacists, anesthesiology assistants, nutritionists, and registered dieticians. Some POS are excluded as well. (See Table 2.3 for an example of acceptable and unacceptable facilities.) All of these excluded groups can be linked to a treating physician, and it is the treating physician whose medical records would be useful to RA coders.

Physicians who are currently excluded from participating in Medicare, Medicaid, and other federal healthcare programs appear on the Office of Inspector General's (OIG's) list of excluded individuals/entities (LEIE). Physicians on the LEIE have been convicted of healthcare program–related crime, patient abuse or neglect, fraud in a healthcare program, or controlled substance charges. These physicians cannot be the authors of records for MAO audits. Similarly, medical coders who are on the LEIE are prohibited from participating in a federal RA audit.

List of excluded individuals/entities (LEIE)
A public, online listing of individuals and entities currently prohibited by the OIG from furnishing any services to federal healthcare programs, or to companies contracted to supply services to federal healthcare programs. The exclusion designation may be permanent or temporary.

TABLE 2.3 Examples of Acceptable and Unacceptable Facilities

RAPS PROVIDER TYPE	COVERED FACILITIES	NON-COVERED FACILITIES*
Hospital Inpatient	Short-term (general and specialty) Hospitals Religious Non-Medical Healthcare Institutions (formerly Christian Science Sanatoria) Long-term Hospitals Rehabilitation Hospitals Children's Hospitals Psychiatric Hospitals Medical Assistance Facilities/Critical Access Hospitals	Skilled Nursing Facilities (SNFs) Hospital Inpatient Swing Bed Components Intermediate Care Facilities Respite Care Hospice

*These are examples of non-covered facilities and not a comprehensive list.

Source: Pub. 100-16 Medicare Managed Care, Transmittal 116.

FYI Anyone who hires an individual on the LEIE to work on projects that are related in any way to CMS is subject to civil monetary penalties. To avoid liability, organizations should routinely check the LEIE to ensure compliance. The LEIE is updated monthly and can be downloaded from http://oig.hhs.gov/fraud/exclusions.asp.

Nurses Practitioners Certification Credentials

Nurse practitioners (NPs), code 50, and clinical nurse specialists (CNS), code 89, are ACPs with advanced-degree nursing certifications whose medical records are acceptable sources for MA abstraction. The clinical scope of these clinical nurse specialists is determined by state law. See Table 2.4 for credentials associated with these acceptable providers.

Nurse practitioners (NPs)
Advanced practice clinicians who are qualified to treat certain medical conditions without the direct supervision of a physician. NPs usually work in a private practice or office setting, but can also work on specialized inpatient units.

Clinical nurse specialists (CNS)
Advanced practice clinicians who are qualified to treat certain medical conditions without the direct supervision of a physician. CNS usually work in acute-care facilities (eg, hospitals).

Scribes

Scribe service is similar to real-time transcription during which a physician talks and an assistant transcribes the physician's words, usually typing directly into the EHR. There are currently no CMS regulations for scribes, however, according to CMS, "[s]cribes are not providers of items or services. When a scribe is used by a provider in documenting medical record entries (e.g., progress notes), CMS does not require the scribe to sign/date the documentation. The treating physician's/NPP's signature on a note indicates that the physician/NPP affirms the note adequately documents the care provided. Reviewers are only required to look for the signature (and date) of the treating physician/NPP on the note. Reviewers shall not deny claims for items or services because a scribe has not signed/dated a note."[12] Therefore, scribes are usually personnel who would be considered "unacceptable providers" if their notes were signed without authentication by a qualified physician. According to CMS, using a scribe is an acceptable practice if the physician signs the note, authenticating that is an accurate record of

Scribe
Any person who transcribes a physician's words during a patient encounter, doing so under the immediate supervision of the physician. There are no national standards for scribes, but some organizations have internal policies regarding their use.

TABLE 2.4 Certification Credentials[13]

CERTIFICATION	CREDENTIAL AWARDED
Nurse Practitioners	
Acute Care Nurse Practitioner	ACNP-BC
Adult Nurse Practitioner	ANP-BC
Adult-Gerontology Acute Care Nurse Practitioner	AGACNP-BC
Adult-Gerontology Primary Care Nurse Practitioner	AGPCNP-BC
Adult Psychiatric-Mental Health Nurse Practitioner	PMHNP-BC
Family Nurse Practitioner	FNP-BC
Gerontological Nurse Practitioner	GNP-BC
Psychiatric-Mental Health Nurse Practitioner (across the life span)	PMHNP-BC
Pediatric Primary Care Nurse Practitioner	PPCNP-BC
School Nurse Practitioner (retired exam)	SNP-BC
Advanced Diabetes Management (specialty certification, retired exam)	ADM-BC
Emergency Nurse Practitioner (specialty certification)	ENP-BC
Clinical Nurse Specialist	
Adult-Gerontology Clinical Nurse Specialist	AGCNS-BC
Adult Health Clinical Nurse Specialist	ACNS-BC
Adult Psychiatric-Mental Health Clinical Nurse Specialist	PMHCNS-BC
Child/Adolescent Psychiatric-Mental Health Clinical Nurse Specialist	PMHCNS-BC
Gerontological Clinical Nurse Specialist (retired exam)	GCNS-BC
Home Health Clinical Nurse Specialist (retired exam)	HHCNS-BC
Pediatric Clinical Nurse Specialist	PCNS-BC
Public/Community Health Clinical Nurse Specialist (retired exam)	PHCNS-BC

the encounter. This may be seen in paper or electronic records.

Many facilities have policies governing the use of scribes and require scribes to self-identify and sign the documents they transcribe for the physician. It becomes critical, then, for the coders to discern authorship when two signatures are listed with a note. In some cases, an acceptable provider (eg, NP or PA) may act as a scribe and sign the record stating he or she was acting as a scribe. Although the NP or PA is an acceptable provider, the self-described scribe's signature would not be acceptable as the signature of the author. Review the documentation to find the provider on record for the encounter and find the provider's signature, or flag the chart for attestation. A scribe cannot authenticate a record.

ADVICE/ALERT NOTE

Scribes are not providers of items or services. When a scribe is used by a provider in documenting medical record entries (eg, progress notes), CMS does not require the scribe to sign/date the documentation. The treating physician's or nonphysician practitioner's (NPP's) signature on a note indicates that the physician or NPP affirms the note adequately documents the care provided. Reviewers are only required to look for the signature (and date) of the treating physician or NPP on the note. Reviewers shall not deny claims for items or services because a scribe has not signed/dated a note.[14]

Acceptable Place of Service

MAOs are responsible to ensure that the facilities from which data are collected are acceptable to CMS for the RA process. Physician offices and inpatient or outpatient hospitals (including critical access) are acceptable places of service (POS) for MA, as are community mental health centers, rehabilitation hospitals, long-term hospitals, psychiatric hospitals, and freestanding, physician-based rural health clinics. When CMS addresses POS in RA, it is a different perspective than when CMS addresses POS in professional physician services. In professional physician billing, the POS may require the physician to share reimbursement for the service with the hosting facility if the service is not performed in the physician office. In RA, when CMS discusses POS, it is identifying the service provider. A physician is an acceptable provider in RA, and the physician can treat or diagnose patients in any POS. A billing document from an excluded POS would not be acceptable. Claims from skilled nursing facilities, hospital inpatient swing beds, intermediate care facilities, respite care, hospice, ambulatory surgery centers (ASCs), home healthcare, or freestanding renal dialysis facilities are not valid POS for RA. These facilities are excluded because CMS wants physician notes rather than the facility's record. Therefore, a physician's documentation and claim for service in any of these excluded facilities would be acceptable.

 **ADVICE/ALERT NOTE**

For long-term institutional (LTI) status, payment is recognized in the year in which LTI status occurs. Claims with LTI status are omitted as acceptable POS because in prospective audits, last year's claims are being evaluated. Instead, CMS collects and uses current year data for LTI status and factors them into current year payments.

Medical supply stores, durable medical equipment suppliers, and freestanding laboratories are also not acceptable as a POS or as an RA provider. The medical records originating with the prescribing physician should be sought, instead. See Table 2.5 for CMS' list of POS codes and descriptions that should be used on professional claims to specify the entity where service(s) were rendered. Always check with individual payers (eg, Medicare, Medicaid, other private insurance) for reimbursement policies regarding these codes from CMS.

Unacceptable Document Sources

Any documentation from an unacceptable provider is excluded from abstraction (eg, nursing notes or a radiologist's interpretation and report). However, coders will still want to review these documents, as they may provide clues for which diagnoses should be found in provider documentation. According to Chapter 7 (Risk Adjustment) of CMS' *Medicare Managed Care Manual*, practices should "implement procedures to ensure that diagnoses are from acceptable data sources. The only acceptable data sources are hospital inpatient facilities, hospital outpatient facilities, and physicians. Plan sponsors are responsible for determining provider type based on the source of the data."[11]

Diagnostic services support the work of the treating physician. Laboratories and radiologists perform diagnostic tests as ordered by the treating physician. The laboratory and radiology offices are not the treating physicians; therefore, their diagnoses are not accepted. Often, the primary care physician will include the diagnostic report in the paper or electronic record. The physician should make note of the results of the diagnostic test in the record as part of the documentation on MDM. If the results of a diagnostic report are not mentioned in the physician's record, it cannot contribute to the coding.

Like all rules, there are exceptions. There are specific circumstances under which the coder may abstract additional details from a radiology report. This occurs when the physician has documented a condition, and the radiology report in the patient record echoes the physician diagnosis,

Place of service (POS)
Location in which a medical encounter occurs. In RA, POS also refers to the entity reporting the service. CMS maintains POS codes so that the location is captured on each claim.

Swing beds
According to CMS, "[t]he Social Security Act (the Act) permits certain small, rural hospitals to enter into a swing bed agreement, under which the hospital can use its beds, as needed, to provide either acute or skilled nursing facility (SNF) care. As defined in the regulations, a swing bed hospital is a hospital or critical access hospital (CAH) participating in Medicare that has CMS approval to provide post-hospital SNF care and meets certain requirements. Medicare Part A (the hospital insurance program) covers post-hospital extended care services furnished in a swing bed hospital."[15]

TABLE 2.5 POS Codes and Descriptions[16]

CODE	DEFINITION
1	Pharmacy
2	Telehealth
3	School
4	Homeless Shelter
5	Indian Health Service Free-standing Facility
6	Indian Health Service Provider-based Facility
7	Tribal 638 Free-standing Facility
8	Tribal 638 Provider-based Facility
9	Prison/Correctional Facility
10	Unassigned
11	Office
12	Home
13	Assisted Living Facility
14	Group Home*
15	Mobile Unit
16	Temporary Lodging
17	Walk-in Retail Health Clinic
18	Place of Employment-Worksite
19	Off Campus-Outpatient Hospital
20	Urgent Care Facility
21	Inpatient Hospital
22	On Campus-Outpatient Hospital
23	Emergency Room – Hospital
24	Ambulatory Surgical Center
25	Birthing Center
26	Military Treatment Facility
27-30	Unassigned
31	Skilled Nursing Facility
32	Nursing Facility
33	Custodial Care Facility
34	Hospice
35-40	Unassigned
41	Ambulance – Land
42	Ambulance – Air or Water
43-48	Unassigned
49	Independent Clinic
50	Federally Qualified Health Center
51	Inpatient Psychiatric Facility
52	Psychiatric Facility-Partial Hospitalization
53	Community Mental Health Center
54	Intermediate Care Facility/ Individuals with Intellectual Disabilities
55	Residential Substance Abuse Treatment Facility
56	Psychiatric Residential Treatment Center
57	Non-residential Substance Abuse Treatment Facility
58-59	Unassigned
60	Mass Immunization Center
61	Comprehensive Inpatient Rehabilitation Facility
62	Comprehensive Outpatient Rehabilitation Facility
63-64	Unassigned
65	ESRD Treatment Facility
66-70	Unassigned
71	Public Health Clinic
72	Rural Health Clinic
73-80	Unassigned
81	Independent Laboratory
82-98	Unassigned
99	Other Place of Service

but offers more specificity. When the physician has not transferred the more specific information from the diagnostic report into the encounter note, the more specific details may be reported.[17] Consistency with the physician diagnosis is a requirement for using more specified details from a radiology report. If the diagnostic report from a pathologist or radiologist aligns with the physician diagnosis, but gives more specificity (eg, identifies the type of hip fracture more precisely), coders are permitted to use the more specific details of the physician-authored diagnostic reports. See the examples in Table 2.6.

ADVICE/ALERT NOTE

Implement procedures to ensure that diagnoses are from acceptable data sources. The only acceptable data sources are hospital inpatient facilities, hospital outpatient facilities, and physicians. Plan sponsors are responsible for determining provider type based on the source of the data.[11]

TABLE 2.6 Examples of Physician Diagnosis and Specified Diagnosis of Radiology Report

EXAMPLE	RATIONALE
Physician states "R scapula fracture" in a patient presenting for active treatment. Radiologist's report notes "displaced fracture of neck of right scapula."	Radiologist further specifies the physician's diagnosis of right scapular fracture. Report code S42.151A, *Displaced fracture of neck of scapula, right shoulder, initial encounter for closed fracture.*
Radiologist documents "nondisplaced fracture of neck of right scapula" while physician documents "scapular sprain" in a patient presenting for active treatment.	The diagnoses differ, and coders must report a diagnosis from the treating physician. Query the treating physician if possible. If not, report code S43.409A, *Unspecified sprain of unspecified shoulder joint, initial encounter.*
Physician documents pneumonia. Radiologist's report identifies abscess of lung without pneumonia.	The diagnoses differ. Abstract the physician's diagnosis and report code *J18.9, Pneumonia, unspecified organism.*

If the radiology report offers more details that do not align with the physician diagnosis, and the physician is not available for query, the physician diagnosis should be reported.

DOCUMENTATION TIP The physician who also assigns codes for an encounter must document the encounter in such a way that the diagnoses are recorded in the narrative of the medical record. Simply initialing the radiology or laboratory report and putting the report in the medical record is not enough. Simply writing a diagnosis code is not enough. The diagnosis must be written into the narrative unique to this encounter or the code cannot be reported.

Nurses and medical assistants often document in the physician's record, but their documentation may not be abstracted for the most part because they are not acceptable providers. However, there is an exception to this rule, too. ICD-10-CM Guideline Section 1(B.14) states that, "[f]or the Body Mass Index (BMI), depth of non-pressure chronic ulcers, pressure ulcer stage, coma scale, and NIH stroke scale (NIHSS) codes, code assignment may be based on medical record documentation from clinicians who are not the patient's provider (i.e., physician or other qualified healthcare practitioner legally accountable for establishing the patient's diagnosis), since this information is typically documented by other clinicians involved in the care of the patient (e.g., a dietitian often documents the BMI, a nurse often documents the pressure ulcer stages, and an emergency medical technician often documents the coma scale). However, the associated diagnosis (such as overweight, obesity, acute stroke, or pressure ulcer) must be documented by the patient's provider."[16]

Therefore, if a nurse documents that a pressure ulcer is at Stage 3, the presence of the ulcer cannot be coded in ICD-10-CM, unless a qualified provider corroborates it. Similarly, while a nurse may document an elevated BMI, it should only be coded using ICD-10-CM codes if an authorized provider documents a corresponding diagnosis, such as overweight, obesity, or morbid obesity. Without the accompanying weight-related diagnosis, the coder should not report the ICD-10-CM code for the elevated BMI, but instead ensure that the appropriate HCPCS Level II G code is captured for quality reporting.

Body mass index (BMI)
A computation based on a patient's weight and height that determines a patient's weight status as underweight, normal, overweight, obese, or morbidly obese. While ICD-10-CM codes for BMI may be based on documentation from a nonprovider, a corresponding diagnosis and its impact on patient care or treatment should be documented by a physician in order to substantiate the selected and reported ICD-10-CM code.

BMI

Use HCPCS Level II codes to report BMI status of patients to comply with quality reporting, which affects physician and payer payments. Some EHRs auto-generate quality reports, while other systems require the codes to be abstracted. There are physicians who do not participate in the BMI quality measure, in which case no BMI codes would be reported.

If the physician participates in a quality measure related to BMI and if a weight-related diagnosis is absent from the record, the HCPCS Level II codes for BMI status that should be used include:

G8417 BMI is documented above normal parameters and a follow-up plan is documented

G8418 BMI is documented below normal parameters and a follow-up plan is documented

G8419 BMI documented outside normal parameters, no follow-up plan documented, no reason given

G8420 BMI is documented within normal parameters and no follow-up plan is required

G8421 BMI not documented and no reason is given

G8422 BMI not documented, documentation the patient is not eligible for BMI calculation

G8938 BMI is documented as being outside of normal limits, follow-up plan is not documented, documentation the patient is not eligible

G9716 BMI is documented as being outside of normal limits, follow-up plan is not completed for documented reason

Problem List

According to CMS, "although the term, 'problem list' is commonly used with regard to ambulatory medical record documentation, a universal definition does not exist. The problem list is generally used by a coder to gain an overall clinical picture of a patient's condition(s). Problem lists are usually supported by other medical record documentation, such as SOAP [subjective, objective, assessment plan] notes, progress notes, consultation notes, and diagnostic reports."[3] A problem list is a menu item, which is segregated from the patient's progress or treatment notes that chronicles the injuries, illnesses, and other factors influencing a patient's health status. The problem list is valuable as a communication tool to ensure personnel active in the patient's care have access to the patient's health history. The list can be an aid to the busy physician regarding the patient's health history and chronic conditions, who can quickly review prior to the patient encounter. In facilities, the problem list is essential for the comprehensive treatment of the patient by multiple physicians.

Unlike diagnostic statements that are part of a physician's authenticated note, problem lists are segregated from the progress or treatment notes, which are usually carried forward from a previous encounter. They are unsigned, thus do not qualify for ICD-10-CM code assignment. In addition, diagnoses in a problem list incorporated into a properly authenticated treatment note do not qualify for ICD-10-CM codes unless the physician indicates how each affected the care or treatment the patient received for that visit. Per CMS' *2008 RA Participant Guide*, "[f]or CMS' risk-adjustment data-validation purposes, an acceptable problem list must be comprehensive and show evaluation and treatment for each condition that relates to a [ICD-10-CM] code on the date of service, and it must be signed and dated by the physician or physician extender."[3]

According to CMS, "[p]roblem lists are evaluated on a case-by-case basis when the problem list is not clearly dated as part of the face to face encounter . . . . EMR population of diagnoses in a list will be considered on a case-by-case basis for RADV once all other coding rules and checks for consistency have been applied."[9] Similarly, in a list of examples of unacceptable document sources, CMS instructs auditors to reject such a problem list as an "invalid source."

Problem lists have proliferated in recent years, having been a requirement in the federal Meaningful Use (MU) core measures for EHRs. While as an MU measure, the problem list was defined

Problem list

Chronicle of the injuries, illnesses, and other factors influencing health status that are specific to a patient, which is segregated from patient progress or treatment notes. The problem list is valuable as a communication tool to ensure individuals active in the patient's care have access to the patient's health history.

as an "up-to-date list of current and active diagnoses," maintenance of these lists has proven to be a challenge on different levels for various reasons. In many outpatient EHRs, the problem list self-populates from the previous medical encounter into the current one. If a new diagnosis develops, it is added to the existing list, but none of the old diagnoses is dropped or removed from the list. The CMS' *RADV Checklist and Guidance* cautioned/advised that, "[w]hen reviewing medical records, pay special attention to the problem list on electronic medical records. Often, in certain systems, a diagnosis never drops off the list, even if the patient is no longer suffering from the condition. Conversely, the problem list may not document the HCC [hierarchical condition categories] your MA contract submitted for payment."[10]

 **ADVICE/ALERT NOTE**

"When reviewing medical records, pay special attention to the problem list on electronic medical records. Often, in certain systems, a diagnosis never drops off the list, even if the patient is no longer suffering from the condition. Conversely, the problem list may not document the HCC your MA contract submitted for payment."[10]

Problem lists are as varied as the EHRs that support them. Some problem lists appear as diagnosis codes and code descriptions as a summary of all diagnoses that have appeared on encounters for the patient throughout the patient's care. Other problem lists include a date stamp identifying when the diagnosis was first made; still others identify when a diagnosis was most recently addressed.

CMS' *Contract-Level RADV Reviewer Guidance* directs auditors to "[e]valuate the problem list for evidence of whether the conditions are chronic or past and if they are consistent with the current encounter documentation (i.e., have they been changed or replaced by a related condition with different specificity). Evaluate conditions listed for chronicity and support in the full medical record, such as history, medications, and final assessment." It goes on to state that "[p]roblem lists are evaluated on a case-by-case basis when the problem list is not clearly dated as part of the face to face encounter indicated on the coversheet or there are multiple dates of conditions both before and after the DOS."[9]

CMS sees the problem with coding from problem lists as a practical one: If the problem list is not authored during the current encounter, how can it count toward the current encounter? For example, if the patient is noted in the problem list as having stage 4 chronic kidney disease (CKD), but no mention of CKD is made in the record of the current encounter, how could it be appropriate to report CKD for the current encounter? (See the following Clinical Examples for an example of a problem list in a patient's medical record that indicates many diagnoses, but that is ambiguous because it is unclear of the chronicity associated with those diagnoses.)

 **ADVICE/ALERT NOTE**

For CMS' RA data-validation purposes, an acceptable problem list must be comprehensive and show evaluation and treatment for each condition that relates to an ICD-10-CM code on the date of service, and it must be signed and dated by the physician or physician extender.[3]

CLINICAL EXAMPLES

WISE, CLARENCE DOB 7/27/1944 DOS 8/1/2017

HPI: Mr. Wise is a 74 YO WM with a PMH significant for CAD s/p CABG, HLD, HTN, arthritis, pulmonary HTN, DM, and chronic sinusitis who was referred to GI clinic by his primary care doctor. His PCP was concerned about a recent incidental finding on a CT chest from 7/16/2017, which showed a severely dilated esophagus with concern for dysmotility and aspiration risk.

PROBLEM LIST

1. Mild nonprolf db retnoph
2. Benign eyelid
3. Health maintenance
4. Diabetes mellitus without mention of complication, type II
5. CAD – native vessel
6. CABG
7. Sinusitis

continued

8. Pain, RT, surgery
9. Infection, high risk
10. Hyperlipidemia
11. Arthritis: mult sites
12. Hypertension, unspec
13. Allergic rhinitis
14. Impotence

COMMENTS: HPI is an acronym for "history of present illness." The HPI and problem list for Mr. Wise contain many diagnoses that may not be addressed elsewhere in the note. The use of the acronym "PMH" in the HPI references "past medical history." While the terms "past" and "history" do not indicate the presence or treatment of a current condition, many physicians were trained to use the phrase "history of" to indicate the presence of a condition (eg, "history of COPD and CHF"), creating a conflict with ICD-10-CM's definition of personal history codes. With problem list entries like "benign eyelid," "pain, RT, surgery," and "infection, high risk," it is impossible to prove the list represents current conditions that are being addressed or treated, unless each diagnosis is described in narrative elsewhere in the record. The only item in this note that is indisputably a current condition is the dilated esophagus (K22.6, *Other specified diseases of esophagus*). A few other diagnoses might be considered for abstraction depending on the individual organization's policies and procedures, which must comply with official ICD-10-CM conventions, guidelines, and advice. Policies and procedures will be addressed in Chapter 5.

Some problem lists allow the physician to enter "Resolved" with the diagnosis, or to click a field that moves the diagnosis from the patient's problem list to the patient's past medical history (PMH). A problem list that allows for transfer of a resolved diagnosis to PMH as well as allowing the addition of new problems is ideal, because it provides the most accurate clinical record. Even so, a diagnosis in a problem list, without more information, is not acceptable for RA, according to CMS.

Medication List

Medication lists can fall prey to the same process woes as problem lists. Often, it is impossible to determine if the list represents all historic prescriptions for a patient, or only those that are currently prescribed. Because only entries made during the current encounter can be considered for code abstraction, determining the origin of a list is critical.

Normally, the medication list would not be abstracted because it usually contains drugs, not diagnoses. Coders and physicians cannot abstract diagnoses based on the type of drug prescribed for the patient. For example, donepezil is commonly prescribed for patients with dementia, but donepezil in the patient's medication list does not translate into a diagnosis of dementia. The physician must document dementia in the record during an encounter in order for dementia to be abstracted by the physician or by the coder. However, some medication lists may include diagnoses within their format and may be appropriate for abstraction, if there is evidence the diagnoses on the list were addressed in the encounter, as in the case of documentation of reconciliation of the patient's current medications. (See the following medication reconciliation Clinical Examples.)

CLINICAL EXAMPLES

ACTIVE MEDICATIONS AND SUPPLIES

Speedy Cath, 14FR Male, 1 catheter 6x day, neurogenic bladder	ACTIVE
Diltiazem 120 mg one capsule every day for heart	ACTIVE
Hydrochlorothiazide 12.5 mg tab every day, diuretic, HTN	ACTIVE
Lisinopril 20 mg tab one every day for HTN	ACTIVE
Metoprolol tartrate 100 mg one tablet every 12 hours for HTN	ACTIVE
Sertraline HCL 50 mg tab one by mouth every day for mood	ACTIVE
Sildenafil citrate 50 mg tab 3x a day for pulmonary HTN	ACTIVE
Aspirin 81 mg tab by mouth per day	ACTIVE
Calcium 500 mg/ Vitamin D 200 unit tab every day	ACTIVE
Cholecalciferol (Vitamin D3) 1000 unit tab every day	ACTIVE
Miscellaneous magnesium tablet every day	ACTIVE
Ranitidine HCL 150 mg every day	ACTIVE

MEDICATION RECONCILIATION:

Completed general overview/reconciliation of medications and/or any OTC/herbals/supplements being taken: [ ] YES [ ] NO

COMMENTS: Note that most of the medications here are not linked to diagnoses, but neurogenic bladder, hypertension, and pulmonary hypertension are documented with their medication or supply. Although all prescriptions in this example are listed as "active," the physician failed to document that the medications had been reviewed and/or reconciled by checking the "Yes" box. There is no evidence of when "active" was noted in the chart. No diagnosis may be abstracted from this unreconciled list. Other EHRs may not document medication reconciliation, but may instead date-stamp the current encounter for each medication reviewed by the physician. With a current author and date stamp, the diagnoses can be abstracted from the medication list. Best practices would display an author and date stamp whenever the medication list is addressed in an encounter.

Due to routine auto-population of medication lists in EHRs, diagnoses listed on medication lists are usually rejected as unacceptable documentation. Diagnoses on the medication list may be abstracted, if the individual medication is noted to treat a specific disorder and the entry is dated and author-stamped for the current encounter by an acceptable physician. Diagnoses in a medication list may also be abstracted if they are linked to the treating medications, and the record specifically states that on this encounter, ie, the medication list was reviewed and/or reconciled.

Medication reconciliation

The process of reviewing all medications on file, including dosage and frequency, against the physician's orders, the patient's compliance, and the medication list in the record. Medication reconciliation is a quality measure for physicians and facilities.

ADVICE/ALERT NOTE

According to AHIMA, "[p]roviders must recognize each encounter as a stand-alone record, and ensure the documentation for that encounter reflects the level of service actually provided and meets payer requirements for billing and reimbursement."[1] However, it is important to note that according to *ICD-10-CM Guidelines*, documentation from previous encounters (eg, HIV disease [coded as ICD-10-CM code B20]) may not be used for ICD-10-CM coding of a current encounter, unless it is incorporated into the applicable documentation and affects care or treatment.

Diagnostic Reports

With few exceptions, only the comments made by the treating physician entered into the medical record are acceptable for code abstraction. Diagnostic reports and sometimes diagnostic images are commonly uploaded into EHRs. Copies of the printed reports are often interleaved into documentation in a paper record. It is the treating physician's responsibility to enter the pertinent aspects of the diagnostic report into the patient's diagnostic statement for that encounter.

The RA coder may abstract from the physician's note, but may not abstract directly from the test results. (See the following Clinical Examples.)

CLINICAL EXAMPLES

Radiology Report
AP Pelvis and Lateral Hip

FINDINGS: Inlet and outlet views as well as Judet views of the pelvis demonstrate multiple bilateral fractures. The most superior aspect of the right acetabulum is fractured and displaced. There is also a fracture extending across the left iliac bone. This latter fracture is displaced by approximately 6 mm. The femoral heads are well seated in the acetabulum.

IMPRESSION: Numerous insufficiency fractures of the pelvis bilaterally as described above. Bilateral fractures extend into the hip joints.

Treating Physician Note
(Excerpt from HPI)

X ray revealed numerous insufficiency fractures of the pelvis with fractures extending into the hip joints. Marked osteoporosis is noted on these films. Hip ROM decreased symmetrically with mild pain. Active ROM increases pain.

ASSESSMENT/PLAN:

Metabolic: Patient is obviously osteoporotic. Recommend DEXA bone scan to quantitate Z and T scores, followed by appropriate pharmacologic therapy.

Musculoskeletal: Both WB surfaces of patient's acetabuli appear to be intact.

There is a displaced pubic root fracture of L side. Recommend WBAT R and 50% WB L. Patient needs an assistive device at all times. After the patient has been mobilized, repeat Judet series.

COMMENTS: While the documentation from the radiologist may seem complete, it is unacceptable for RA abstraction. A radiology report does not contain evidence of medical decision-making and care treatment planning, and is from an excluded provider. In this example, the physician has sufficiently pulled the radiologist's assessment into the record, added his own assessment, and described the treatment plan. The patient's care is documented.

According to CMS' *Contract-Level RADV Reviewer Guidance*, another exception to the diagnostic testing rule is pathology reports, including surgical pathology, cytopathology, and other analyses with an interpretation by a pathologist:

> The interpretation of the findings by a pathologist as an acceptable physician specialty is acceptable. This is an exception to the face-to-face requirement.
>
> Examples of pathology reports include the following:
>
> - Pathology reports from a tissue biopsy (e.g., lung biopsy, bone biopsy, etc.)
> - Cell block report
> - Cytopathology report of fluids/brushings
> - PAP (Papanicolaou) smear report
> - Chromosome analysis[9]

Superbills

A superbill is a customized form that contains lists of diagnoses and procedures with their corresponding codes. Superbills are unacceptable document sources because they do not provide any documentation of how the diagnoses listed are being evaluated or treated. Similarly, CMS does not allow repetitive encounter flowsheets without physician notes for the day of treatment (eg, dialysis, infusion/ injections, chemotherapy, radiation, international normalized ratio prothrombin time (INR/Protime) test results).[9]

Hospital-specific Documents

The inpatient record under review is often hundreds of pages in length. Only documents authenticated by a physician with face-to-face contact with the patient may be coded. Inpatient radiology-interpretation reports may not be coded by the facility, unless validated in a treating physician's notes or a query document that is part of the permanent medical record. Many of these pages are ineligible for abstraction because they contain diagnostic test data, physician orders, medications, and nurses' notes.

> **MS-DRG coding summary**
> Inpatient tally sheet identifying the admission diagnosis and all other diagnoses or procedures abstracted from the inpatient encounter. This internal document is for resource utilization and financial planning, and is not an acceptable document source.

MS-DRG Coding Summary

One item that is usually included in an inpatient chart being audited for RA is the Medicare severity-diagnosis related group (MS-DRG) coding summary. An MS-DRG coding summary is a tool for resource management at the facility. The MS-DRG coding summary lists all ICD-10-CM/ PCS codes abstracted from the chart along with the various DRGs generated by these codes. It is the auditor's responsibility to review the MS-DRG coding summary, as it may provide a preview of what is revealed in the medical record. The RA auditor must, however, approach the chart independent of the codes abstracted by the hospital coder. RA auditors may find that the hospital coders may have made errors of omission or selected codes erroneously. RA auditors are engaged to improve upon physician or facility coding, not duplicate it.

Patient Transfers

Patient transfers are administrative papers that document a physician's or nurse's notes regarding the movement of a patient from one facility to another. Patient transfer documents are administrative documents that identify the patient who is being moved from one facility to another. Usually, diagnostic information is mentioned in a transfer, but because a transfer fulfills an administrative function, rather than detailing care for the patient, it is considered an unacceptable document source.

EHR-specific Issues

There are many things that physician offices and facilities can do to make their EHRs more audit-friendly and compliant. CMS regulations regarding EHRs continue to evolve and facilities and physician offices can expect an increased regulatory focus on EHRs in the future. In its January 2014 report, the OIG outlined the issues with program integrity and EHRs. The report began:

> Electronic health records (EHRs) replace traditional paper medical records with computerized recordkeeping to document and

store patient health information. Experts in health information technology caution that EHR technology can make it easier to commit fraud. For example, certain EHR technology features may be used to mask true authorship of the medical record and distort information to inflate healthcare claims. The transition from paper records to EHRs may present new vulnerabilities and require the Centers for Medicare & Medicaid Services (CMS) and its contractors to adjust their techniques for identifying improper payments and investigating fraud.[18]

Since that time, CMS did publish on its website a series of documents, which are known as the "EHR Toolkit." However, the Toolkit has since been removed from CMS' website. Some guidance can still be found in CMS' *Electronic Health Records Provider*, which is available at www.cms.gov/Medicare-Medicaid-Coordination/Fraud-Prevention/Medicaid-Integrity-Education/Downloads/docmatters-ehr-providerfactsheet.pdf.

FYI Documentation is often the communication tool used by and between providers. Documenting a patient's record with all relevant and important facts, and having that information readily available, allows providers to furnish correct and appropriate services that can improve quality, safety, and efficiency. EHRs can help improve communication between providers through real-time access to valuable information.[5]

Foremost, ensure the EHR's signature format complies with CMS requirements. EHRs have been known to have faulty signature formats or practices have faulty signature protocols that essentially negate the authenticity of every signature within the system. Ensure the signature language denotes approval of the record, contains a time and date stamp, and contains the physician's full name and credentials.

Login information (ie, username and password) ties directly to the audit-log data generated by EHRs, and the OIG has identified audit-log data as a valuable reference for medical records audits. Every line of data added to a record is time-stamped and identified by author in the audit log. This is essential for record integrity, and could be used to authenticate the medical record. No physician should share login information, as this information is uniquely linked to the physician's identity.

CMS, in its *Contract-Level RADV Reviewer Guidance*, specifically notes that the following are "unacceptable electronic signatures:

- Administratively signed by
- Dictated, but not signed
- Electronic signature on file (with no other indication of a date/time)
- Electronically signed to expedite delivery
- Proxy signature–signed via approval letter or statement, such as:
  - I authorize my name to be electronically affixed by using my unique dictation computer key
  - "Signature on file" or "Manually signed by" (The meaning of this is unknown. In some transcription/EMR systems, this might be acceptable, but it seems to mean the physician/practitioner will hand sign the document after review.)"[9]

Cloning

Once the hurdles of authorship and time stamp have been successfully completed, the one element that could solve a multitude of EHR issues is this: uniqueness. Each encounter should include unique information relevant to the encounter that is evidence the encounter occurred as documented. According to CMS in its publication, *Electronic Health Records Provider*, the "medical record must contain documentation showing the differences and the needs of the patient for each visit or encounter. Simply changing the date on the EHR without reflecting what occurred during the actual visit is not acceptable."[5] Physicians do this by updating information on duration, severity, location, quality, or other modifying factors of a diagnosis, by updating elements of the physical examination, and/or by updating elements in the patient's care plan.

Audit-log data
Record of all authors and dates for each entry into an EHR auto-generated and stored by the EHR to verify the validity of information entered.

Increasingly, CMS is focusing on the practice of cloned documentation. In cloned documentation, information from a past encounter is copied and pasted into the current encounter. Problem lists and medication lists, when "pulled forward" in the medical record from one encounter to the next, are examples of what could be considered cloning. In the 2013 OIG Work Plan, it was observed that "Medicare contractors have noted an increased frequency of medical records with identical documentation across services."[20] In this case, the OIG stated it would review Evaluation and Management (E/M) billing of physicians due to this issue. While this has had primarily a fee-for-service focus to date, and while MAOs are not currently the target of such EHR scrutiny, it is not hard to imagine that in the future this could become an issue.

ADVICE/ALERT NOTE

The medical record must contain documentation showing the differences and the needs of the patient for each visit or encounter. Simply changing the date on the EHR without reflecting what occurred during the actual visit is not acceptable. Using electronic signatures or a personal identification number may help deter some of the possible fraud, waste, and abuse that can occur with increased use of EHRs.[5]

Risk Adjustment Documentation & Coding offers two recommendations for safeguarding the documentation and coding associated with EHRs:

- **Be vigilant.** Watch for guidance from CMS, OIG, or other state and federal agencies regarding the features of EHRs that bring into question the authenticity of the encounter.
- **Be proactive.** Educate physicians and coders regarding ICD-10-CM guidelines and conventions, and reference the American Hospital Association's (AHA's) *Coding Clinic for ICD-10-CM and ICD-10-PCS* (*Coding Clinic*) frequently. Review Chapter 5 for tips on how to build a defensible EHR policies and procedures.

Cloned documentation
Selection of a segment of a medical record that is copied and pasted into another location in the record, either in the same patient's chart or in another patient's chart.

Chart Components

Because one of the goals of *Risk Adjustment Documentation & Coding* is to prepare new RA coders for the diversity of documentation seen during chart abstraction, a basic review of medical charts, their content, and organization is presented here. As noted in CMS' E/M Services 1995 and 1997 Documentation Guidelines, "[m]edical record documentation is required to record pertinent facts, findings, and observations about an individual's health history, including past and present illnesses, examinations, tests, treatments, and outcomes. The medical record chronologically documents the care of the patient, which is an important element that contributes to high quality care. The medical record facilitates:

- The ability of the physician and other healthcare professionals to evaluate and plan the patient's immediate treatment, and to monitor his or her healthcare over time;
- Communication and continuity of care among physicians and other healthcare professionals involved in the patient's care;
- Accurate and timely claims review and payment;
- Appropriate utilization review and quality of care evaluations; and
- Collection of data that may be useful for research and education.

An appropriately documented medical record can reduce many of the 'hassles' associated with claims processing and may serve as a legal document to verify the care provided, if necessary."[20]

Many medical chart templates are organized according to the elements in the E/M Services 1995 and 1997 Documentation Guidelines. These elements and their definitions include:

- **Chief complaint (CC):** Concise statement describing the symptom, problem, condition, diagnosis, physician recommended return, or other factor that is the reason for the encounter
- **History of present illness (HPI):** A chronological description of the development of the patient's present illness form the first sign and/or symptom or from the previous encounter to the present
- **Review of systems (ROS):** Inventory of body systems obtained through a series of questions seeking to identify signs and/or symptoms

that the patient may be experiencing or has experienced.

- **Past, family, and/or social history (PFSH):** Patient's past experiences with illnesses, operations, injuries, and treatments; review of medical events in the patient's family, including diseases that may be hereditary or place the patient at risk; and an age-appropriate review of past and current activities.
- **Physical exam (PE):** Visual and tactile examination of the body that may be focused on all systems or a subset of anatomical systems depending on the clinical judgment of the physician.

A well-documented patient encounter will include the reason for the encounter, relevant history, the findings of a physical exam, pertinent diagnostic test results, and the physician's assessment of the patient's condition and medical plan of care. This information will be collected and recorded in various ways. The note will have both subjective and objective findings, and coders must distinguish between the two.

A subjective finding is an observation from the patient. The CC is almost always a subjective finding, with the exception of an encounter for a proscribed purpose (eg, vaccination or medication refill or a follow-up in the continuum of care). Patients answer questions for an oral or paper review of symptoms. This is also a subjective finding. Usually, a patient will describe symptoms and let the physician know what is wrong (eg, how much pain the patient is experiencing). These subjective notes are valuable for the physician, who will use this information in MDM; however, most subjective observations are not abstracted by the coder. Exceptions include pertinent medical, social, allergy, surgical, and family histories. In these cases, the subjective history is all there is available. This HPI is the physician's documentation of the development of the patient's disorder.

Objective findings in the chart include vital statistics and the results of physical examination. These contribute to the MDM. MDM leads to the assessment and plan (A/P), usually found at or near the end of the notes for the encounter. The A/P identifies the diagnoses and the physician's care treatment plan. While the A/P contains key diagnostic information relative to the encounter, the coder cannot focus only on the A/P during abstraction, as other diagnoses may be found elsewhere (eg, in the HPI and PE). (See the following Clinical Examples.)

CLINICAL EXAMPLES

Report objective diagnoses from the medical record, but avoid coding most subjective diagnoses.

DOCUMENTATION	SUBJECTIVE/OBJECTIVE: TO CODE OR NOT TO CODE
Patient comes in today because "it feels like I have appendicitis."	Subjective observation of the patient. Do not code.
Patient complains today of a lump in her L breast. Patient is post-mastectomy, L side. On the L chest wall on the anterior axillary line, 1 inch above the mastectomy scar, is a palpable mass under the skin, approximately 1 cm × 1 cm.	Patient's "lump in breast," N63, *Unspecified lump in breast*, is subjective. Do not code. Objective documentation states chest mass, R22.2, *Localized swelling, mass and lump, trunk.*
Physician notes during the physical exam that the patient's ileostomy is without inflammation or excoriation.	Code this objective observation from direct visualization of the stoma site, Z93.2, *Ileostomy status.*
Chief complaint is pain in hands when performing work. Physician states in assessment, bilateral osteoarthritis in hand joints.	Do not code pain, M79.641, *Pain in right hand*, and M79.642 *Pain in left hand.* Instead, code objective diagnosis of osteoarthritis of hands, M19.041, *Primary osteoarthritis, right hand*, and M19.042, *Primary osteoarthritis, left hand.*

Subjective finding
In the medical record, a description of any observation or diagnosis that originates with the patient, as documented by the physician.

Objective finding
In the medical record, a description of any observation or diagnosis that originates with the physician, as documented by the physician.

Subjective and objective observations will take the physician to his assessment and plan. Together, these four components of a chart comprise the SOAP note. (See Table 2.7.)

TABLE 2.7 Sample SOAP Note

Michael Barbados, DOB 9/23/1951	Morris Kointy MD office visit 1/27/2018
SUBJECTIVE: A brief narrative of the patient's chief complaint, including the history and symptoms associated with the complaint	Sudden onset of R shoulder pain following slip and fall on ice last week. Patient has had mild, chronic R shoulder pain for 2 years with a diagnosis of chronic rotator cuff injury. Sleep following the fall has been difficult due to exacerbation of shoulder paint when lying down.
OBJECTIVE: Physician examination and testing to determine the patient's condition	Before this encounter, patient underwent shoulder MR without contrast. MRI revealed 1. 0.5 x 0.7 cm high-grade partial thickness bursal sided rotator-cuff tear of the distal supraspinatus tendon. PE reveals limited ROM and tenderness at the acromion, AC joint, clavicle, bicipital grove, scapular spine, humeral head, supraspinatus tendon, and over the coracoid process.
ASSESSMENT: The physician's determination of the diagnosis(es)	Acute on chronic rotator-cuff tear
PLAN: The treatment that will be undertaken to correct the patient's problem	Patient has agreed to begin ibuprophen therapy and today received a cortisone injection to the bursa in the R shoulder. This injection may reduce inflammation and discomfort. The possibility of the need for surgery in the future was discussed, but for the short-term, the patient wants to see how his shoulder responds to NSAIDs and cortisone injections.

ADVICE/ALERT NOTE

Medical record documentation is required to record pertinent facts, findings, and observations about an individual's health history, including past and present illnesses, examinations, tests, treatments, and outcomes. The medical record chronologically documents the care of the patient, which is an important element that contributes to high quality care. The medical record facilitates:

- The ability of the physician and other healthcare professionals to evaluate and plan the patient's immediate treatment, and to monitor his or her healthcare over time;
- Communication and continuity of care among physicians and other healthcare professionals involved in the patient's care;
- Accurate and timely claims review and payment;
- Appropriate utilization review and quality of care evaluations; and
- Collection of data that may be useful for research and education.

An appropriately documented medical record can reduce many of the "hassles" associated with claims processing and may serve as a legal document to verify the care provided, if necessary.[21]

Behavioral Disorder Charts

Charts for mental health usually follow a different format than a SOAP chart. The mental health chart will follow a multiaxial format in which each axis presents a health status component:

Axis 1 Acute clinical disorder
Other comorbidities than may require clinical attention

Axis 2 Personality disorder
Intellectual disability

Axis 3 General medical conditions that may influence behavioral issues

Axis 4 Psychosocial and environmental problems

Axis 5 World Health Organization (WHO) Disability Assessment Schedule (WHODAS 2.0)

See the following Example that shows a mental-health chart that uses the multiaxial format.

EXAMPLE

Axis 1	Major depressive episode, recurrent, severe without psychotic features Alcohol dependence, in remission
Axis 2	Avoidant personality disorder
Axis 3	Alcoholic cirrhosis Hypothyroidism Congestive heart failure
Axis 4	Smoker; lives alone
Axis 5	(not performed)

The axis information in a behavioral health chart is followed by a history, assessment, and plan, usually in narrative form. Anything from axis 1 to axis 4 or from the assessment and plan may be abstracted for RA. WHODAS 2.0 is a self-report by the patient, and results in a numeric value, so it cannot be abstracted.

Tips for RA Abstractors

When abstracting a chart for RA, utilize the following steps to ensure complete and efficient abstraction:

1. Verify the correct patient by checking the name and DOB of the patient against the file's demographics.
2. Go to the inpatient discharge summary or the outpatient "Assessment/Plan," because this is where the crux of the encounter will be found. The beginning of the note may include signs and symptoms that are intrinsic in the final diagnosis, so beginning with the final diagnoses is an important time-saver.
3. Skim the entire inpatient file, across all records, to ensure there are no unauthorized documents within the file (eg, another patient's record).
4. Go to the beginning and read the inpatient admission data or outpatient chief complaint.
5. Reconcile the admission/chief complaint with the discharge summary/assessment and plan, and abstract the pertinent and supported diagnoses.
6. Read through the rest of the record to determine if any other diagnoses are supported and should be coded.
7. Always code to the highest level of specificity, following the classification in the ICD-10-CM Alphabetic Index, the instructions in the ICD-10-CM Tabular List, the additional requirements in the ICD-10-CM guidelines, the official advice in the AHA's *Coding Clinic*, and appropriate local policies and procedures.

References

1. American Health Information Management Association. Integrity of the Healthcare Record: Best Practices for EHR Documentation. http://library.ahima.org/doc?oid=300257#.WSxnDdgzXIU. Accessed Sept 11, 2017.
2. ECRI Institute. Patient Identification Lessons Learned from ECRI Institute's 2016 Deep Dive. https://www.ecri.org/components/HRCAlerts/Pages/HRCAlerts092816_PatientID.aspx. Accessed Sept 11, 2017.
3. Centers for Medicare & Medicaid Services. *2008 Risk Adjustment Data Technical Assistance For Medicare Advantage Organizations Participant Guide.* https://www.csscoperations.com/Internet/Cssc3.Nsf/files/participant-guide-publish_052909.pdf/$File/participant-guide-publish_052909.pdf. Accessed Sept 10, 2017.
4. Medicare Learning Network. "New Place of Service (POS) Code for Telehealth and Distant Site Payment." *MLN Matters®*. 2016; (MM9726). https://www.cms.gov/Outreach-and-Education/Medicare-Learning-Network-MLN/MLNMattersArticles/Downloads/MM9726.pdf. Accessed Sept 11, 2017.
5. Centers for Medicare & Medicaid Services. Program Integrity: Documentation Matters Toolkit: Electronic Health Records Provider Fact Sheet. https://www.cms.gov/Medicare-Medicaid-Coordination/Fraud-Prevention/Medicaid-Integrity-Education/Downloads/docmatters-ehr-providerfactsheet.pdf. Accessed Sept 11, 2017.
6. Centers for Medicare & Medicaid Services. CMS Manual System: Pub. 100-08 Medicare Program Integrity. Pub. 100-08 Transmittal 442: December 12, 2012: Change Request 8105. https://www.cms.gov/Regulations-and-Guidance/Guidance/Transmittals/Downloads/R442PI.pdf. Accessed Oct 27, 2017.
7. Centers for Medicare & Medicaid Services. CMS Manual System: Pub. 100-08 Medicare Program Integrity. Pub. 100-08 Transmittal 442: December 7, 2012: Change Request 8105.
8. Centers for Medicare & Medicaid Services. CMS Manual System: Pub. 100-08 Medicare Program Integrity. Pub. 100-08 Transmittal 604: July 24, 2015: Change Request 9225. https://www.cms.gov/Regulations-and-Guidance/Guidance/Transmittals/downloads/R604PI.pdf. Accessed Oct 27, 2017.
9. Centers for Medicare & Medicaid Services. *Contract-Level Risk Adjustment Data Validation Medical Record Reviewer Guidance (As of 09/27/2017).* https://www.cms.gov/Research-Statistics-Data-and-Systems/Monitoring-Programs/Medicare-Risk-Adjustment-Data-Validation-Program/Other-Content-Types/RADV-Docs/Coders-Guidance.pdf. Accessed Oct 27, 2017.
10. Centers for Medicare & Medicaid Services. Risk Adjustment Data Validation (RADV) Medical Record Checklist and Guidance. https://www.cms.gov/Medicare/Medicare-Advantage/Plan-Payment/Downloads/radvchecklist.pdf. Accessed Oct 27, 2017.
11. Centers for Medicare & Medicaid Services. Chapter 7, Risk Adjustment. In: *Medicare Managed Care Manual.* https://www.cms.gov/Regulations-and-Guidance/Guidance/Manuals/Internet-Only-Manuals-IOMs-Items/CMS019326.html. Accessed Oct 26 2017.
12. Palmetto GBA. https://www.csscoperations.com/internet/cssc3.nsf/files/2018_Specialty_Code_List_5CR_100417.pdf/$FIle/2018_Specialty_Code_List_5CR_100417.pdf. Accessed Nov 20, 2017.
13. American Nurses Credentialing Center. Certification Credentials. http://www.nursecredentialing.org/CertificationCredentials. Accessed Oct 27, 2017.
14. Centers for Medicare & Medicaid Services. CMS Manual System: Pub. 100-08 Medicare Program Integrity. Pub. 100-08 Transmittal 713: May 25, 2017: Change Request 10076. https://www.cms.gov/Regulations-and-Guidance/Guidance/Transmittals/downloads/R604PI.pdf. Accessed Oct 27, 2017.
15. Centers for Medicare & Medicaid Services. Swing Bed Providers. https://www.cms.gov/Medicare/Medicare-Fee-for-Service-Payment/SNFPPS/SwingBed.html. Accessed Oct 27, 2017.
16. Centers for Medicare & Medicaid Services. Place of Service Code Set. https://www.cms.gov/Medicare/Coding/place-of-service-codes/Place_of_Service_Code_Set.html. Accessed Oct 27, 2017.
17. American Hospital Association. *Coding Clinic for ICD-10-CM and ICD-10-PCS.* 2016; 3(3):26.
18. Centers for Medicare & Medicaid Services. *ICD-10-CM Official Guidelines for Coding and Reporting* (FY 2018). https://www.cms.gov/Medicare/Coding/ICD10/Downloads/2018-ICD-10-CM-Coding-Guidelines.pdf. Accessed Oct 27, 2017.

19. Office of Inspector General. *CMS and Its Contractors Have Adopted Few Program Integrity Practices to Address Vulnerabilities in EHRs.* https://oig.hhs.gov/oei/reports/oei-01-11-00571.pdf. Accessed Oct 27, 2017.

20. Office of Inspector General. *Work Plan Fiscal Year 2013.* https://oig.hhs.gov/reports-and-publications/archives/workplan/2013/work-plan-2013.pdf. Accessed Oct 27, 2017.

21. Medicare Learning Network. *Evaluation and Management Services.* ICD006764; August 2017. https://www.cms.gov/Outreach-and-Education/Medicare-Learning-Network-MLN/MLNProducts/Downloads/eval-mgmt-serv-guide-ICN006764.pdf. Accessed Oct 27, 2017.

Evaluate Your Understanding

The following questions are critical checkpoints that are meant to let you apply your critical thinking and evaluate your understanding of the content covered in this chapter. The answers for the end-of-chapter exercises are available in Appendix C. In addition, the Internet-based Exercises are additional learning and research opportunities to learn more about the topics related to this chapter.

A Answer Questions

Provide the answer(s) to each of the following questions.

1. Which of the following represents an administrative error in risk adjustment?
   A. Missing radiology report
   B. Missing signature
   C. Missing subjective finding
   D. Missing ICD-10-CM code

2. What is the purpose of an attestation?
   A. To amend a medical record's diagnoses
   B. To identify the scribe of the record
   C. To authenticate the record by its author
   D. To mark a cloned document as reviewed in the current encounter

3. An audit log:
   A. Is a tool for RA coders working for an MAO
   B. Identifies all coding errors in a chart
   C. Is not acceptable evidence in any audit
   D. Is tied directly to login information

4. Documentation from a nurse is acceptable for diagnostic code abstraction for which of the following?
   A. BMI
   B. Staging of skin ulcer
   C. Chief complaint
   D. Both A and B

5. All of these are acceptable providers for RA review **except**:
   A. ACP
   B. GNP-BC
   C. RN, BSN
   D. CNS-BC

6. A diagnosis on a problem list:
   A. May represent a part of the patient's past medical history.
   B. May be an active, chronic condition.
   C. May be reported if supported elsewhere in the medical record.
   D. All of the above.

7. Which of the following is a subjective finding?
   A. BMI
   B. +3 edema
   C. Rhonchi
   D. Pain

8. Which of the following is considered an acceptable point of service (POS) for RA, under certain circumstances?
   A. Freestanding laboratory
   B. Telemedicine
   C. Hospice
   D. Durable medical equipment (DME) distribution center

9. Without a proper signature on a discharge summary,
   A. The chart should be flagged for attestation
   B. The chart should be flagged as invalid
   C. The chart should be coded as an inpatient chart
   D. The chart should be coded as an outpatient chart for each individual encounter

10. When abstracting codes in a letter from a consulting physician,
    A. Use the date the exam was performed as the DOS
    B. Use the date of the consult letter as the DOS
    C. Use the referring physician's follow-up encounter as the DOS
    D. Stop, because consultation letters are not acceptable document sources

B True/False Questions

Answer true or false for the following statements.

1. An interventional radiologist is an acceptable provider.
2. CMS requires a scribe to sign the document.
3. A consult letter to the referring physician should contain the date of the patient examination that was performed as part of the consultation.
4. A physician's documentation of "regular rate and rhythm, no rubs" is an objective observation.
5. A psychiatric inpatient hospital is not an acceptable POS.
6. A diagnosis on a problem list is evidence of a continuing, chronic condition.
7. In EHRs, physicians are permitted to share their login information with the scribe according to CMS standards.
8. If signed by an acceptable provider, a transfer is an acceptable source for abstraction in RA.
9. Without an acceptable signature on a discharge summary, an inpatient record must be coded as an outpatient encounter for MAO coding.
10. Diabetes mellitus would be appropriately reported in Axis 3 in the behavioral-health record of a patient with recurrent major depression.

C Internet-based Exercises 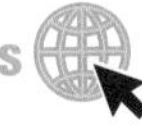

1. CMS published an Electronic Health Records Resource Guide containing dozens of links to information on the proper use of EHRs for physicians serving Medicaid patients. Peruse the list of Internet links at https://www.cms.gov/Medicare-Medicaid-Coordination/Fraud-Prevention/Medicaid-Integrity-Education/Downloads/docmatters-ehr-resourceguide.pdf.
2. Physicians interested in more information on documentation and signature requirements as they relate to "incident to" reporting can find an interesting perspective in this publication of the American Health Lawyers Association, https://www.sullivancotter.com/wp-content/uploads/2017/05/HTC_Resource_SullivanCotter.pdf.
3. Want more guidance from CMS on EHRs? Check out https://www.cms.gov/Medicare-Medicaid-Coordination/Fraud-Prevention/Medicaid-Integrity-Education/Downloads/ehr-providerfactsheet.pdf.
4. Access the most current and past ICD-10-CM Index, Table, Guidelines, and other supporting documents at https://www.cms.gov/Medicare/Coding/ICD10/Downloads/2018-ICD-10-CM-Coding-Guidelines.pdf.
5. Read the impact of EHRs on information integrity as analyzed by Sue Bowman of AHIMA here https://www.ncbi.nlm.nih.gov/pmc/articles/PMC3797550/.
6. Submit your own questions about ICD-10-CM coding to the American Hospital Association's Central Office. Access their site at https://www.codingclinicadvisor.com/. Whenever possible, send a redacted provider note to better clarify the question and to avoid a delay in receiving an answer.

CHAPTER 3

Clinical Documentation and Coding for RA

The Social Security Act and the Centers for Medicare & Medicaid Services (CMS) regulations require that services be medically necessary, have documentation to support the claims, and be ordered by physicians. Consistent, current, and complete documentation in the medical record is an essential component of quality patient care according to the National Committee for Quality Assurance. In addition to accreditation standards and federal regulations, medical record documentation must also comply with state licensure regulations and payer policies, as well as professional practice standards. Compliance and accurate reimbursement depend on the correct application of codes, which is based on physician documentation. In addition to the reimbursement implications, physician documentation is used in quality improvement initiatives and pay-for-performance programs. Therefore, the codes reported on health insurance claims must be supported by the documentation in the medical record. Most payers require reasonable documentation that services are consistent with the insurance coverage provided. Medicare specifically requires that all services billed must be supported by documentation that justifies payment. CMS has implemented numerous corrective actions to reduce improper payments along with efforts to educate physicians about the importance of thorough documentation to support the medical necessity of services and items. For Medicare Advantage programs, medical record documentation must comply with all legal and regulatory requirements applicable to Medicare claims. Documentation guidelines identify the minimal expectations of physician documentation for payment of services under the Medicare program. In addition, state or local laws, professional guidelines, and the policies of a practice or facility often require additional documentation.

Patient care, documentation, coding, and compliance go hand-in-hand. It is not possible to assign the most specific and most appropriate diagnosis code without complete, detailed documentation related to the patient's disease, injury, or other reason for the encounter/visit. Documentation must also support the medical necessity of any service provided or procedure performed. Detailed, consistent, complete documentation in the medical record is one of the cornerstones of compliance.

Medical Documentation

Lack of clarity is the enemy in medical documentation. In Chapter 2, one type of uncertainty was explored in a synopsis of administrative issues that can lead to failed audits: confusion regarding date of service (DOS), physician appropriateness, and document acceptability. Chapter 3 moves on to the medical record, and enumerates the unintended consequences of word choice in documentation. Many of these language choices are easily improved with a simple change to format or phrasing, leading to correct diagnostic code assignment. The goal is clarity in the medical record, as well as precision in ICD-10-CM coding. According to the Office of Inspector General's (OIG's) *Compliance Program for Individual and Small Group Physician Practices*, procedural and diagnostic codes "reported on the health insurance claims form should be supported by documentation in the medical record and the medical chart should contain all necessary information and coded in compliance with official conventions, guidelines, and advice."[1]

The Documentation Guidelines for Evaluation and Management Services developed by the American Medical Association (AMA) with CMS outline the fundamental elements of the patient record, and are the foundation for building solid documentation practices:

> **II. GENERAL PRINCIPLES OF MEDICAL RECORD DOCUMENTATION**
>
> The principles of documentation listed below are applicable to all types of medical and surgical services in all settings. For evaluation and management (E/M) services, the nature and amount of physician work and documentation varies by type of service, place of service and the patient's status. The general principles listed below may be modified to account for these variable circumstances in providing E/M services.
>
> 1. The medical record should be complete and legible.
> 2. The documentation of each patient encounter should include:
>   - reason for the encounter and relevant history, physical examination findings, and prior diagnostic test results;
>   - assessment, clinical impression, or diagnosis;
>   - plan for care; and
>   - date and legible identity of the observer.
> 3. If not documented, the rationale for ordering diagnostic and other ancillary services should be easily inferred.
> 4. Past and present diagnoses should be accessible to the treating and/or consulting physician.
> 5. Appropriate health risk factors should be identified.
> 6. The patient's progress, response to and changes in treatment, and revision of diagnosis should be documented.
> 7. The CPT and [ICD-10-CM] codes reported on the health insurance claim form or billing statement should be supported by the documentation in the medical record.[2]

The focus of this book is diagnosis-based risk adjustment (RA), therefore, this chapter will discuss documentation and coding for ICD-10-CM codes based on government-issued guidelines, such as the *ICD-10-CM Official Guidelines for Coding and Reporting* (*ICD-10-CM Guidelines*), E/M Documentation Guidelines, the American Hospital Association's (AHA's) *Coding Clinic for ICD-10-CM and ICD-10-PCS* (*Coding Clinic*), as well as widely accepted best practices in the healthcare industry. Whether the physician selects diagnosis codes, utilizes computer-assisted coding programs, or delegates code abstraction to coders, the physician needs to understand the criteria and process for ICD-10-CM code selection so that the documented record supports the diagnoses reported. In most cases, these are outlined in the *ICD-10-CM Guidelines* and/or the AHA's *Coding Clinic*. In other cases, they are derived from federal RA guidance. Some common practices reflect what is accepted as a risk standard by some, but may not be required by law. Although there are numerous official resources and guidelines for documentation, there are instances when there is no official guidance for those circumstances. In such instances, the recommendation in this chapter will be identified as "best practice."

> **Best practice**
> Technique, procedure, or methodology, which, through experience and research, is accepted or prescribed as being correct or most effective. In the case of medical record documentation, best practices have been proven to achieve regulatory compliance, disambiguation, and completeness. In the case of code abstraction, best practices consistently utilize the *ICD-10-CM Guidelines* and AHA's *Coding Clinic*.

Chapter 3 is not only directed to the physician who seeks to improve documentation, but to the person responsible for code abstraction (coder or physician). The general topics in this chapter are appropriate to all coders and physicians, as they are not diagnosis- or specialty-specific and outline guidance and best practices that can improve documentation and coding for all records, not only those that risk-adjust. In some instances, subtle shifts in word choice can ensure a record describes the patient's condition precisely, and a deeper understanding of the rules of ICD-10-CM can close loopholes in documentation that prevent accurate code abstraction. Coders and physicians who need to brush up on their coding skills will also be able to review ICD-10-CM coding conventions and code look-up protocols within this chapter. This foundation will prepare readers for Chapter 4, a review of clinical documentation improvement and coding compliance for specific risk-adjusted diagnoses.

The medical record serves a number of purposes. Foremost, it must chronicle the histories, diagnoses, and treatments of the patient to ensure the safety and efficacy of care, and to improve the patient's health. The record must reflect the decision making, consents, and professionalism that will protect the physician from medicolegal claims. The record must also be complete so that another physician could, if necessary, assume care of the patient based on the content of the medical chart.

Medical documentation that accurately and completely captures the services provided and the significant health conditions considered by the physician in medical decision making (MDM) serves the primary purpose of supporting ongoing care. Such documentation should also satisfy numerous other needs, such as reporting RA or billing data, quality metrics data, and medical/legal risk management. The Centers for Disease Control and Prevention (CDC) National Center for Health Statistics (NCHS) supervises the ICD-10-CM Index and Tabular Section. In cooperation with CMS, the AHA, and the American Health Information Management Association (AHIMA), the NCHS approves the *ICD-10-CM Official Guidelines for Coding and Reporting*. Official advice interpreting the ICD-10-CM conventions and guidelines is provided by the AHA's Central Office as a free service to individual requestors and, in cooperation with the NCHS, CMS, and AHIMA, in a paid publication, the AHA's *Coding Clinic*. As instructed in ICD-10-CM Guideline Section IV(C), "[f]or accurate reporting of ICD-10-CM diagnosis codes, the documentation should describe the patient's conditions, using terminology that includes specific diagnoses, as well as symptoms, problems, or reasons for the encounter. There are ICD-10-CM codes to describe all of these.[3]

ADVICE/ALERT NOTE

Per ICD-10-CM Guideline Section IV(C), "[f]or accurate reporting of ICD-10-CM diagnosis codes, the documentation should describe the patient's conditions, using terminology that includes specific diagnoses, as well as symptoms, problems, or reasons for the encounter. There are ICD-10-CM codes to describe all of these."[3]

The Concept of Support

Every physician must be familiar with the concept of medical necessity and the importance of ICD-10-CM codes to establish the reason a test or procedure is performed. The patient's nature of the presenting problem and comorbidities also contribute to the complexity of examinations and MDM when determining the level of E/M services of an encounter. These diagnoses establish the need for the care provided, and support the level of reported services.

In RA, CMS requires support for any reported diagnosis, but does not define what constitutes "support," as evidenced in the *2008 Risk Adjustment Data Technical Assistance for Medicare Advantage Organizations Participant Guide* (*2008 RA Participant Guide*), which states that "[a]s a basic risk adjustment rule, all risk adjustment diagnosis codes submitted by MA organizations must be supported by medical record documentation."[4] Similarly, in the Introduction to the *ICD-10-CM Guidelines*, the concept of documenting "support" for a diagnosis is stated thus: "The importance of consistent, complete documentation in the medical record cannot be overemphasized. Without such documentation,

Medical necessity
Established evidence of the appropriateness of resource use in the medical treatment of a patient, based on the patient's diagnosis and standards of care. Individual payers establish their own medical necessity requirements.

accurate coding cannot be achieved. The entire record should be reviewed to determine the specific reason for the encounter and the conditions treated."[3]

Still, the definition of "support" is elusive. Could CMS mean the diagnosis was simply listed somewhere in the medical record? In CMS' *Contract-Level Risk Adjustment Data Validation Medical Record Reviewer Guidance* (*Contract-Level RADV Reviewer Guidance*), a discussion of problem lists offers what might be interpreted as an answer. Problem lists are a list of conditions from the patient's history:

> Evaluate the problem list for evidence of whether the conditions are chronic or past and if they are consistent with the current encounter documentation (i.e., have they been changed or replaced by a related condition with different specificity). **Evaluate conditions listed for chronicity and support in the full medical record, such as history, medications, and final assessment** [emphasis added].[5]

In the ICD-10-CM code set, the guidelines presented in a specific chapter provide information on assigning codes, but it often includes information related to documentation. Most users think of the guidelines primarily as instructions on assigning and sequencing codes, but there are many references to information that must be included in the documentation to allow assignment of specific codes. In addition, the coding guidelines often indicate when the physician should be queried for additional information related to the diagnosis. Therefore, the chapter-specific guidelines are an important tool that must be used to ensure that the documentation supports assignment of a specific code. Although CMS has not specifically and clearly defined what constitutes supporting documentation for any reported diagnosis, based on the coding guidelines and requirements of the ICD-10-CM codes, the basic ICD-10-CM documentation requirements can be summarized as follows:

- Identify causal agents, as appropriate, with the documented diagnosis.
- Identify the documented condition as acute or chronic.
- Identify the location of the documented condition with as much specificity as possible.
- Document the clinical findings/indicators to support the diagnosis documented.
- Document manifestations whenever appropriate, and link them to the underlying documented diagnoses.

The volume of documentation for a diagnosis will vary depending on its complexity. At a minimum, the diagnosis should be documented somewhere in the medical record for the encounter. If documented only in the problem list for the encounter, the diagnosis must be supported elsewhere in the record (eg, for a problem-list entry stating "Type 2 diabetes mellitus," documentation that the patient's "blood sugars were high today at 305 mg/dL, so we will increase his insulin and monitor for ketones in his urine until he recovers from the flu."). Such documentation, though not specifically mentioning diabetes mellitus, supports the diagnosis in the patient's problem list and would be abstracted for RA, in keeping with the instructions from *Contract-Level RADV Reviewer Guidance* to "[e]valuate the problem list for evidence of whether the conditions are chronic or past and if they are consistent with the current encounter documentation (i.e., have they been changed or replaced by a related condition with different specificity). Evaluate conditions listed for chronicity and support in the full medical record, such as history, medications, and final assessment."[5] Some organizations have adopted constructs to aid coders in assessing sufficiency of documentation to support coding of diagnosis. One such construct is known as the MEAT criteria. This is a framework for coding outpatient encounters that requires documentation that a diagnosis has been evaluated, treated, or in some way measured during an encounter if that diagnosis is going to be abstracted by a coder. In some organizations, MEAT is applied only to chronic diseases seen in problem lists, while other organizations require MEAT for all diagnoses being abstracted. As a result, "support" is often taught using the concept of **m**onitor/measure, **e**valuate, **a**ssess/address, **t**reat, which makes up the acronym, MEAT.

MEAT
Evidence in medical documentation that resources have been expended in the care of a patient's diagnosis, either through monitoring, evaluating, assessing, treating, testing, or MDM. MEAT is required in order to abstract a chronic condition documented only in the problem list of the encounter.

It is defined as follows:

- Monitor—signs, symptoms, disease progression, disease regression
- Evaluate—test results, medication effectiveness, response to treatment
- Assess/Address—order tests, discussion of test results, review records, counseling
- Treat—prescribe medications, therapies, other modalities

Therefore, MEAT in a document means the physicians explicitly documents their critical thinking or treatment of the diagnosis in some way. According to the MEAT criteria, support must come from an acceptable physician and acceptable document source and be noted within the encounter being abstracted. The support may be found in the physical examination, an updated medication list that is part of the encounter, a note in the record interpreting diagnostic test results or ordering new tests, physician referral, or a discussion of a plan for that diagnosis. A diagnostic statement by the physician contained in the assessment of the progress note or other acceptable areas, such as the encounter diagnosis–field of the medical record, should suffice. If it is unclear that the documented condition meets ICD-10-CM's requirements for code assignment, the coder should query the physician for clarification, if possible. (See Table 3.1.)

Documenting MEAT for a patient's comorbidities sometimes slips through the cracks. Comorbidity refers to the existence of more than one disorder or disease process in the same patient. Documenting comorbidity(ies) beyond the problem list will capture a more appropriate patient acuity and assist in establishing medical necessity to the care provided. It is known that it is not necessary for a physician to be in charge of a patient's comorbidity in order for it to be abstracted; the comorbidity simply needs to affect decision-making or treatment in the current encounter. Therefore, noting that a patient has prostate cancer in the history of present illness (HPI) of an encounter for a patient with Crohn's disease may be all that is necessary or appropriate. However, if the physician is considering the prostate cancer while formulating a treatment plan for the Crohn's disease (eg, if the cancer treatment is exacerbating the Crohn's), the prostate cancer could be described in more detail, as clinically appropriate. This is a clinical best practice but it is not essential for RA data submission. For more information on comorbidity, see later discussion of comorbidity in this chapter. According to ICD-10-CM Guideline Section IV(G), physicians should "[l]ist first the ICD-10-CM code for the diagnosis, condition, problem, or other reason for encounter/visit shown in the medical record to be chiefly responsible for the services provided. List additional codes that describe any coexisting conditions."[3] In addition, Guideline Section IV(J) also clearly specify to "[c]ode all documented conditions that coexist at the time of the encounter/visit, and require or affect patient care treatment or management. Do not code conditions that were previously treated and no longer exist. However, history codes (categories Z80-Z87) may be used as secondary codes if the historical condition or family history has an impact on current care or influences treatment."[3] Furthermore, Guideline Section I(A.19) states that the "assignment of a diagnosis code is

TABLE 3.1 Examples of Support As Described by MEAT

MEAT ELEMENT	PROBLEM	SUPPORT
Measured, monitored	Morbid obesity	George is still unwilling to consider bariatric surgery, even though it would help his knees considerably.
	Diabetes mellitus.	A1C today is 6.7
Evaluated	CHF	+3 LE edema
	Pneumonia	Film shows R lung is clearing
Assessed, addressed	HTN	Blood pressure is controlled. Continue low sodium diet.
	Moderate reactive asthma	Breathing improved with weather change
Treated	Assessment: Hypothyroidism	New Rx for levothyroxine 125 mcg daily
	New diagnosis of Stage 3 CKD	Referred to nephrology clinic

Abbreviations: CHF indicates congestive heart failure; CKD = chronic kidney disease; HTN = hypertension; LE = lower extremity; and Rx = prescription.

based on the provider's diagnostic statement that the condition exists. The provider's statement that the patient has a particular condition is sufficient. Code assignment is not based on clinical criteria used by the provider to establish the diagnosis."[3]

It should also be noted that because there is a lack of federal direction, there is some variation in how organizations and coders are interpreting MEAT concepts and applying them, if at all. As noted, some organizations are using it as their standard for all coding. Others are using it more strategically to assist coders in decision-making related to diagnosis abstraction for those diagnoses that may be in the past medical history or problem lists, but were not already documented by the physician in the assessment portion of the progress note or other acceptable areas, such as the encounter diagnosis–field of the medical record. These organizations generally accept diagnoses documented in the assessment because the assessment portion of the encounter record is essentially the diagnostic statement by the physician of the diagnoses considered during the encounter, and were relevant to the care, treatment, or management provided at that encounter, as well as MDM. Because MEAT is not a federal requirement, any application of MEAT rules should be a subject of organizational policy-making, which is discussed further in Chapter 5. (See the following MEAT Clinical Coding Example.)

CLINICAL CODING EXAMPLE

A 75-year-old female has painful urination and lower abdomen discomfort. She reports a poor appetite. She has mild malnutrition, is frail, and has lost two pounds a month for the past nine months. Urinalysis performed today shows E. coli [Escherichia coli], white cells, leukocyte esterase, and microalbuminuria. Serum creatinine is 1.4. Patient complains of dry, itchy skin for the past three months.

Problem list: Stable DM [diabetes mellitus], recurrent major depression, CKD [chronic kidney disease] stage 3.

Plan:

- Glucophage 500 mg b.i.d. for DM.
- Cipro XR, 500 mg daily for UTI [urinary tract infection] due to E. coli.
- Ensure supplements for malnutrition.
- Referral to nephrologist for CKD.

Coding (per MEAT criteria)

B96.20 Unspecified Escherichia coli [E. coli] as the cause of diseases classified elsewhere

N39.0 Urinary tract infection, site not specified (urinalysis, Cipro XR)

E11.22 Type 2 diabetes mellitus with diabetic chronic kidney disease ("stable," glucophage)

N18.3 Chronic kidney disease stage 3 (laboratory tests, referral)

E44.1 Mild protein-calorie malnutrition (weight loss, Ensure)

COMMENTS: Itchy, dry skin is subjective and would not be reported. Recurrent major depression is a risk-adjusting disorder, but because there is no MEAT for depression and because it is only documented in the problem list of this note, it must be omitted.

 **ADVICE/ALERT NOTE**

Per ICD-10-CM Guideline Section IV(J), "[c]ode all documented conditions that coexist at the time of the encounter/visit that require or affect patient care treatment or management."[3]

All coding and clinical document improvement undertakings take time, effort, and resources. Organizations pondering adopting MEAT criteria need to recognize and be willing to accept the additional costs and work related to MEAT for both coders and physicians and should carefully assess the impact to clinical care and quality. They should work with physician leaders to guide documentation improvement efforts that enhance clinical care as well as accurate and complete code capture. There may be additional physician work related to the more stringent documentation requirements, and there should be the expectation of increased physician queries from coders, especially early on. RA coders require an extended knowledge of anatomy and pathophysiology in order to link diagnoses to MEAT. For example, signs and symptoms pertinent in a physical examination that relate to a patient with chronic obstructive pulmonary disease (COPD) in the problem list might include the use of neck muscles during breathing; barrel chest; bluish tinge to nail beds; and clubbing of fingers, or cachexia, in very severe cases. These are not obvious pulmonary symptoms, and require experience and study. Similarly, coders must have a deeper understanding of pharmacology, and access to a reliable reference resource for drugs or medications to be able to link diagnoses to prescription drugs when the physician does not provide that link. Support cannot be ambiguous. For example, if an assessment includes both rheumatoid arthritis and sarcoidosis, and prednisone is on the medication list, prednisone cannot be used as support for either condition because it could have been prescribed for either condition. A physician note occasionally documents support for two diagnoses using a single drug (eg, "The patient notes a reduction in her rheumatoid arthralgia since starting prednisone for her sarcoid"). This would be acceptable MEAT for both conditions. (See the following Clinical Examples.)

CLINICAL EXAMPLES

CC [chief complaint]: F/U hypertension

Vitals: Ht: 5"11 Wt: 200 BMI: 27.9 BP: 124/84 Pulse: 64 bpm

Medications, reconciled during today's encounter
Amlodipine 5 mg-benazepril 20 mg cap, once daily
Hydrochlorothiazide 12.5 cap, once daily
Metoprolol tartrate 25 mg tab, twice daily
Pantoprazole 40 mg tab, once daily
Potassium chloride ER 10 mEq tab, once daily
Sucralfate 1 gr tab, once daily
Rivaroxaban 20 mg tab, once daily

Problems

- Hyperlipidemia
- Rheumatoid arthritis
- Hypertension
- GERD
- Barrett's esophagus
- BPH
- Prostatitis
- Dyspnea
- Anterior chest wall pain
- Osteoporosis

ROS [review of systems]: None

PE [physical examination]: All findings normal

Assessment

1. Hypertension
2. Abnormal EKG
3. Barrett's esophagus
4. Rheumatoid arthritis
5. Osteoporosis

continued

Analysis of diagnoses and MEAT

1. Hypertension	blood pressure reading, amlodipine, hydrochlorothiazide
2. Abnormal EKG	none
3. Barrett's esophagus	pantoprazole
4. Rheumatoid arthritis	none
5. Osteoporosis	none
6. Hyperlipidemia	none

COMMENTS: Applying the strictest rules of MEAT, the rheumatoid arthritis, hyperlipidemia, osteoporosis, and abnormal EKG are unacceptable diagnoses for RA because they are not supported with MEAT in the record. However, depending on local policies regarding comorbidities, some or all of these diagnoses may be appropriate for submission to CMS because the physician has, by putting them in his assessment, indicated that they were considered and did affect the clinical encounter. No MEAT would be necessary. Of those, both rheumatoid arthritis and osteoporosis risk-adjust. Hyperlipidemia, a chronic condition that risk-adjusts, was not supported with MEAT in the record and appeared only in the problem list. As such, it would not be abstracted under some organizations' policies.

Most medical records follow a SOAP note format. SOAP notes are typically divided into four segments: subjective, objective, assessment, and plan. (See Chapter 2 for more about SOAP notes.)

 ADVICE/ALERT NOTE

SOAP NOTES

SOAP note format assists both the physician and record reviewer/coder in identifying documentation elements. SOAP stands for:

Subjective: How the patient describes the problem or illness.

Objective: Data obtained from examinations, laboratory results, vital signs, etc.

Assessment: Listing the patient's current condition and status of all chronic conditions. How the objective data relate to the patient's acute problem.

Plan: Next steps in diagnosing the problem further, prescriptions, consultation referrals, patient education, and recommended time to return for follow-up.[4]

FYI Coders must pay attention to who reports or provides the information in a medical record. Patients often self-diagnose, which the physician may note in the medical record. Such "self-diagnosis" by the patient is not acceptable for RA submission, unless the physician affirms the diagnosis.

One of the simplest ways to improve documentation is the adoption of a combined assessment/plan format for a SOAP note, combining the final two elements into one (see Table 3.2). The assessment/plan format is present in some electronic health record (EHR) systems, while those EHRs that do not have this function or format can be retooled. Depending on local policies and procedures, plan elements may also be linked to active diagnoses. Doing so brings clarity to the medical record and provides MEAT specific to each diagnosis in the assessment.

SOAP note

Method of medical record documentation communicating the patient's and physician's observations and the physician's diagnosis and treatment plan. SOAP notes are a widely used format for medical documentation because they are flexible and facilitate concise but comprehensive documentation.

TABLE 3.2. Sample Assessment/Plan

ASSESSMENT	PLAN
Hypertension	Propranolol ER 80 mg and continue home monitoring
Morbid obesity	Referral to bariatric clinic for initial interview for gastric bypass surgery
Hypercholesterolemia	Zetia, 10 mg daily, curb red meats and dairy
Major depressive disorder, recurrent, in partial remission	Continue fluoxetine and contact therapist

There are many different formats or approaches to link diagnoses and plan elements. One method is the grid method. By setting up an assessment/plan grid or similar approach, a physician can ensure that every diagnosis has a care treatment plan documented. A linkage between assessment and plan makes it clear which treatment is supporting which diagnosis. Consider how easily supported diagnoses could have been abstracted from the previous Clinical Examples' table of documentation had an assessment/plan format been utilized, and how the format would have given the physician the opportunity to address some of the diagnoses lacking MEAT in the note. Another method is the numbering method in which some physicians number the diagnoses in the assessment, followed by corresponding numbers in the plan. Note that this requires an additional level of attentiveness from the physician to ensure all numbers match up.

Communicating the Encounter

While a physician views the patient record as a continuum of care and often flips through the record to look at data from other office visits, the coder's perspective is limited to the specific encounter. All information used to abstract diagnoses from the encounter must be documented within the encounter. It is important to include all information pertinent to the encounter in the note to reduce the frequency of coder queries and to ensure all pertinent diagnoses can be abstracted. (See the following Clinical Coding Example.)

CLINICAL CODING EXAMPLE

DOS [date of service]: 1/4/2018

CC: Pneumonia follow-up

HPI [history of present illness]: Gilda Warren, 67, is seen today as a follow-up to her hospitalization for pneumonia. She is feeling very tired, but much better than when she was released from the hospital on 12/26/2017. A chest X ray today reveals only a small residual of the infection remaining in the lower right lobe. Her partial pressure of oxygen (pO_2) is at 91%. Her cough has greatly diminished and she reports no chest pain and a low fever only at night. I instructed her to continue with the antibiotic course.

A/P [assessment/plan]: Pneumonia. Continue oral ciprofloxacin and return to clinic in two weeks.

COMMENTS: Report the only diagnosis code for this encounter, which is code J18.9, *Pneumonia, unspecified organism*. While the discharge summary of the inpatient admission identified that the pneumonia was due to pseudomonas aeruginosa, and even though ciprofloxacin is an appropriate treatment for pseudomonas pneumonia, but because this is not documented on the 1/4/2018 visit, code J15.1, *Pneumonia due to Pseudomonas*, cannot be submitted for the 1/4/2018 visit. According to the AHA's *Coding Clinic for ICD-9-CM* (Third Quarter, 2013), code assignment is based only on what is documented on the current encounter because "conditions documented on previous encounters may not be clinically relevant on the current encounter."[6] In addition, it indicates that "[w]hen reporting recurring conditions and the recurring condition is still valid for the outpatient encounter or inpatient admission, the recurring condition should be documented in the medical record with each encounter/admission."[6] As such, the coder coding the encounter for 1/4/2018 cannot retrieve data from the hospital discharge summary, which identified *Pseudomonas aeruginosa* as the infectious agent causing the pneumonia. The *Pseudomonas* responded to intravenous ciprofloxacin and she was discharged with a

continued

prescription for oral ciprofloxacin to continue at home. The physician oversaw the care of this patient during hospitalization, but failed to note *Pseudomonas* as the infectious agent in the follow-up care at the 1/4/2018 office visit. If the physician is not available for query for the causal agent of the pneumonia for the 1/4/2018 encounter, report code J18.9, *Pneumonia, unspecified organism.* Had the physician documented the causal agent in the note on 1/4/2018, it would have been appropriate to report code J15.1, *Pneumonia due to Pseudomonas.* While unspecified pneumonia does not risk-adjust, many bacterial pneumonias do risk-adjust when the causal agent is identified. Code J15.1 risk-adjusts to HCC 114, *Aspiration and Specified Bacterial Pneumonias,* with a community nondual aged rate of 0.599. The hospitalization dates and the 1/4/2018 encounter occur in different RA cycles. Without the causal agent of pseudomonas documented in 2018 when the patient still is diagnosed with pneumonia, the 0.599 RA factor is lost for CY 2018 even though the patient had the condition and she was being treated for it.

FYI According to AHA's *Coding Clinic* (Third Quarter, 2013), the coder may not review previous encounters to code the encounter for the current DOS.[6] Each encounter must stand on its own documentation merits, and only the physician can determine if past diagnoses have any clinical relevance in the current DOS.

Lists

A problem list is a separate section of the medical record that chronicles a specific patient's chronic illness and may include transient or resolved illnesses and injuries. In some EHRs, this is a document that is generated by the physician; in others, it is a document that is an auto-generated compilation of all diagnoses that have ever been associated with a patient—a "cloned" element. Therefore, problem lists are not the best source for code abstraction (see the following Example for a typical problem list that itemizes every diagnosis ever assigned to a patient problem list). They do, however, inform a coder of what to look for in the medical record, and with MEAT, are acceptable for coding. CMS advises in its *Risk Adjustment Data Validation (RADV) Medical Record Checklist and Guidance,* "[w]hen reviewing medical records, pay special attention to the problem list on electronic medical records. Often, in certain systems, a diagnosis never drops off the list, even if the patient is no longer suffering from the condition. Conversely, the problem list may not document the condition supporting the HCC your organization submitted for payment."[7] It would be advisable for physicians to review a patient's problem list at the start of each encounter to ensure that information in the current DOS is complete and that all pertinent comorbidities are documented, if addressed. Again, as advised in the *2008 RA Participant Guide,* "[f]or CMS' RADV purposes, an acceptable problem list must be comprehensive and show evaluation and treatment for each condition that relates to an ICD-10-CM code on the date of service, and it must be signed and dated by the physician or physician extender."[4] If possible, physicians should monitor problem lists and delete or move diagnoses that no longer exist in the patient to past medical history, retaining only chronic or recurring diagnoses in the problem list.

Problem list
A separate section of the medical record that chronicles a specific patient's chronic diseases or may include transient or resolved illnesses and injuries.

EXAMPLE

This is a typical problem list itemizing every diagnosis ever assigned to a patient.

Problem List

- Hypothyroidism
- Hyperlipidemia, unspecified
- Mixed hyperlipidemia
- Hypoalbuminemia
- Glaucoma
- Cataract
- Tricuspid valve regurgitation
- Essential hypertension
- Benign essential hypertension
- Hypertensive emergency
- Coronary atherosclerosis
- Mitral valve disorder
- Valvular regurgitation

- Chronic atrial fibrillation
- Atrial fibrillation
- Deep venous thrombosis
- Pneumonia
- Frank hematuria
- Post-menopausal uterine bleeding
- Osteoarthritis
- Knee pain
- Fever
- Fatigue
- Unsteady gait
- Abnormal gait

It is impossible to tell which of these conditions have resolved, or which of similar descriptions is more accurate.

ADVICE/ALERT NOTE

Per CMS' *Risk Adjustment Data Validation (RADV) Medical Record Checklist and Guidance*, "[w]hen reviewing medical records, pay special attention to the problem list on electronic medical records. Often, in certain systems, a diagnosis never drops off the list, even if the patient is no longer suffering from the condition. Conversely, the problem list may not document the HCC your organization submitted for payment."[7]

ADVICE/ALERT NOTE

Per CMS' *2008 RA Participant Guide*, "[f]or CMS' RADV purposes, an acceptable problem list must be comprehensive and show evaluation and treatment for each condition that relates to an ICD-10-CM code on the date of service, and it must be signed and dated by the physician or physician extender."[4]

Medication lists are menus within the medical record that catalogs drugs, durable medical equipment, medical supplies, and over-the-counter vitamins and supplements that have been prescribed to the patient or that the patient reports using. These medication lists are a component of the EHR and the encounter that allows the physician to electronically prescribe or refill medications, or detect drug interactions or patient allergies.

Medication lists in the EHR populate each encounter with a list of drugs that have been historically prescribed to the patient. The same maintenance issues exist for medication lists as for problem lists. These lists are useful tools when regularly updated. Medication reconciliation has become a standard of care for physicians, and it is important for physicians to document this reconciliation when it occurs.

Coders are not clinicians and may not infer a diagnosis based on prescribed medication when it has not been documented for coding purposes. In its *Contract-Level RADV Reviewer Guidance*, CMS specifically states "[d]o not use prescription drug information on the order form to report conditions. The condition must be documented."[5]

A medication list can be a source of MEAT; however, for coders looking for support for a diagnosis, the medication list may also provide an inventory of diagnoses to anticipate in a chart. Some physicians identify in the medication list the indication for the drug:

- Amlodipine besylate 5 mg tab, twice daily for hypertension
- Triamterene/HCTZ 37.5/25 one tab daily for hypertension
- Ibuprofen 800 mg tab every six hours as needed for osteoarthritis
- Fenofibrate 160 mg, one tab daily for hypercholesterolemia

These documented diagnoses add clarity to the note, as many medications are used to treat a variety of diagnoses. Even so, without the physician adding a note directly to the medication list during the encounter, or referencing it as having been reviewed in the medical record for the encounter, a cloned medication list may not be accepted to support a diagnosis. The notation that a prescription is "current" in the EHR does not necessarily mean the physician has reviewed it; more likely, it means that the prescription is still valid according to its original prescribing date, and the note is autogenerated by the EHR. Coders should tread lightly regarding diagnoses listed on medication lists that are not addressed during the current encounter.

Medication lists
A separate menu within the medical record that catalogs drugs, durable medical equipment, medical supplies, and over-the-counter vitamins and supplements that have been prescribed to the patient or that the patient reports using. These medication lists are a component of the EHR and the encounter that allows the physician to electronically prescribe or refill medications, detect drug interactions or patient allergies.

These medication lists may be considered a type of problem list and dismissed in a validation audit. (See the following Clinical Examples.) In best practices, diagnoses are documented and supported during the current encounter.

CLINICAL EXAMPLES

This excerpt is from an urgent-care center visit for an 82-year-old.

Medications

1. Amitriptyline 25 to 50 mg p.o. q h.s.
2. Augmentin 500 mg 3 times a day.
3. Aspirin 81 mg once a day.

*4. Pulmicort 1 puff twice a day.

5. Calcium carbonate with vitamin D; 1 tablet twice a day.
6. Digoxin 0.25 mg once a day.
7. Diltiazem 120 mg once a day.
8. Folic acid 1 mg once a day.
9. Citrucel t.i.d. p.r.n.

*10. DuoNeb nebulizers q 4 hours p.r.n.

*11. Oxygen 4 liters.

12. Vitamin B12 1000 mg/mo.
13. Xalatan eye drops both eyes q h.s., 0.005%.

*14. Prednisone 25 mg, then taper to 20 mg p.o. daily.

*15. Salmeterol inhaler 1 puff twice a day.

16. Senokot 1 tablet twice a day.
17. Sulfasalazine 500 mg twice a day.

Abbreviations: *Per os* (p.o.) indicates by mouth; *quaque hora somni* (q.h.s) = every bedtime; *ter in die* (t.i.d) = three times a day; and *pro re nata* (p.r.n.) = as needed

Assessment

1. Syncope in shower causing fall with mild concussion and 3-cm laceration on patient's forehead, requiring sutures.
2. Patient lives alone; home health assists recommended for bathing. We are helping her set that up.

COMMENTS: All the medications with one asterisk (*) point to chronic obstructive pulmonary disease (COPD) or other serious pulmonary condition that may affect the patient's activities of daily living. This condition should have been documented and discussed, as the disease, its symptoms, or its medications would have been considered in the physician's MDM as they could have contributed to the patient's syncopal episode. With more thorough documentation, several additional risk-adjusting diagnoses linked to medications on this list may have been noted and abstracted. These include chronic hypoxemic respiratory failure justifying the use of chronic supplemental oxygen, digoxin for the treatment of heart failure or atrial fibrillation, amitriptyline for the treatment of major depression, and others. Without this documentation, ICD-10-CM codes affecting RA cannot be assigned. Coders may want to query physicians regarding prescriptions in circumstances such as these.

Test Values

Not only are coders forbidden to infer diagnoses from a medication list, they are forbidden to infer a diagnosis from any element in a medical record. Coders are not clinicians. Physicians must state the diagnosis, even when it seems obvious. A coder who believes a diagnosis was inadvertently omitted from the encounter documentation may query the physician, who can then amend the documentation, as appropriate.

FYI According to AHA's *Coding Clinic for ICD-10-CM and ICD-10-PCS* (First Quarter 2014), ICD-10-CM coding cannot be based on up and down arrows. For example, ⇩ hematocrit of 34 may signify anemia in a male but not in a female. Arrows have variable interpretations and the clinical judgment of the physician is necessary for a diagnosis that establishes the clinical significance of the arrows.[8]

A radiology or laboratory report uploaded into an EHR or copied into the paper record is included as a reference for the treating physician, but its contents are not acceptable document sources in most cases. The treating physician must note in the record the results of the test and document the diagnosis. If the treating physician documents laboratory values into the record but does not document a diagnosis, the coder may not code or assign a diagnosis code for this laboratory value. Arrows are also not acceptable documentation, as they require the coder to infer the meaning of the arrows. (See the following Clinical Examples.)

CLINICAL EXAMPLES

WHAT WAS DOCUMENTED	CLINICAL DIAGNOSIS INTENDED	CODER ABSTRACTION (ACCORDING TO GUIDELINES)
1. Diabetic, finger stick today BG 37	Diabetic hypoglycemia	E11.9, Type 2 diabetes mellitus without complications
2. Her mental frailty is stable, according to daughter	Alzheimer's disease	R41.81, Age-related cognitive decline
3. ⇧potassium	Hyperkalemia	No code

COMMENTS:

1. A blood glucose reading of 37 is clinically significant for hypoglycemia; but the coder cannot abstract hypoglycemia if it is not documented, even if the coder understands the significance of the value. Coders cannot abstract diagnoses based on laboratory values. They can, however, query the physician.
2. In the ICD-10-CM Alphabetic Index, frailty/mental is indexed to a symptom code for age-related cognitive decline. If the patient has a more specific diagnosis, it should be documented. A more specific diagnosis cannot be abstracted from the problem list from documentation in past encounters.
3. ⇧potassium may be indicative of elevated serum potassium (hyperkalemia); but it also may be indicative of improvement in a patient with depressed serum potassium (hypokalemia). Without more information, a diagnosis cannot be abstracted by the coder.

When documenting certain complex syndromes in the medical record, physicians may need to include all components of the syndrome and state which documented conditions are an integral part of the syndrome and which are not. ICD-10-CM Guideline Section 1(B.15) states, "Follow the Alphabetic Index guidance when coding syndromes. In the absence of Alphabetic Index guidance, assign codes for the documented manifestations of the syndrome. Additional codes for manifestations that are not an integral part of the disease process may also be assigned when the condition does not have a unique code."[3]

Lemierre syndrome, for example, is characterized in clinical literature by sepsis often evolving after a sore throat or tonsillitis and then complicated by various septic emboli and thrombosis of the internal jugular vein.[9-11] If a physician documents Lemierre syndrome, and then additionally documents a deep tissue abscess in the patient's right neck, a septic pulmonary embolism, and resultant sepsis, the coder would have to consider that the ICD-10-CM Alphabetic Index to Diseases classifies Lemierre syndrome only with code I80.9, *Phlebitis and thrombophlebitis of other specified sites,* and does not include codes for the manifestations that are an integral part of the disease process. Code I80.9 does not risk-adjust, whereas codes I26.90, *Septic pulmonary embolism without acute cor pulmonale,* and A41.9, *Sepsis, unspecified organism,* do risk-adjust. Because Lemierre syndrome does not have a unique code, it would be acceptable to code based on the documented individual elements, such as pharyngitis; cervical cellulitis and lymphadenitis; sepsis or severe sepsis (if acute organ dysfunction is present); and septic pulmonary embolism—all of which are easily coded and defended in the event of a retrospective audit.

ADVICE/ALERT NOTE

Per ICD-10-CM Guideline Section 1(B.15), "[f]ollow the Alphabetic Index guidance when coding syndromes. In the absence of Alphabetic Index guidance, assign codes for the documented manifestations of the syndrome. Additional codes for manifestations that are not an integral part of the disease process may also be assigned when the condition does not have a unique code.[3]

There is an exception to documentation rules regarding diagnostic radiology test results. Diagnostic radiology test results signed by a physician and interleaved into the medical record that provide further specificity to the diagnosis documented in the record by the treating physician are acceptable. The test result must corroborate the treating physician's diagnosis, which will provide greater specificity. If the test result conflicts with the treating physician's diagnosis (eg, the treating physician states "pneumonia" and the radiologist states "lung mass"), the coder must report the treating physician's diagnosis. When circumstances permit, coders may query physicians for more information. However, most RA coders do not have access to the authors of the charts they are abstracting. In any circumstance, no information can be appended to an encounter once it is under audit. Physicians should err on the side of inclusion.

According to CMS' *Risk Adjustment 101 Participant Guide,* "[m]edical history alone may not be used as a source of diagnoses for risk adjustment purposes. For a chronic condition to be accepted for risk adjustment, the patient must have a face-to-face visit each year with a provider/physician who assesses and documents that condition."[12] (See the following Clinical Coding Example.)

ADVICE/ALERT NOTE

Per CMS' *Risk Adjustment 101 Participant Guide,* "[m]edical history alone may not be used as a source of diagnoses for risk adjustment purposes. For a chronic condition to be accepted for risk adjustment, the patient must have a face-to-face visit with a physician who assesses and documents that condition on a yearly basis. In addition, the visit must be repeated and coded annually at a minimum in order to have a lasting effect on the patient's RAF score."[12]

CLINICAL CODING EXAMPLE

HPI: Mr Lucian went for a six-week vacation to Austria and Switzerland and did a lot of hiking. Reports no chest pain/ shortness of breath. Started canagliflozin before he left and he reports he had loose stools from the new medication, which have since resolved.

Problem List

- Hypothyroidism
- Type 2 diabetes uncontrolled
- Mixed hyperlipidemia
- Hypertension
- DVT [deep vein thrombosis]
- Pulmonary embolism
- Fever
- Cough

Medications

- Atorvastatin, 10 mg tab once daily — renewed 11/23/17
- Fenofibrate 145 mg tab once daily — renewed 11/23/17
- Canagliflozin 100 mg tab once daily — filled 3/15/18
- Levothyroxine 112 mcg tab once daily — prescribed 2/15/18
- Metformin 500 mg twice daily — renewed 11/23/17
- Warfarin 5 mg tab daily — renewed 11/23/17
- Valsartan 320 mg; HCl 25 mg daily — filled 3/15/18
- Nifedipine ER 90 mg tab daily — filled 3/15/18
- Metroprolol succinate ER 50 mg daily — renewed 11/23/17

Past Medical History

- DVT
- Hyperlipidemia
- Pulmonary embolism
- Hypertension
- Diverticulosis
- CKD4 [chronic kidney disease stage 4]
- MD2 [myotonic dystrophy type 2]
- Heart murmur
- MR [mitral regurgitation], LVEF [left ventricular ejection fraction] 45%

Laboratories Studies for Discussion

• Glycohemoglobin, total, blood 11/23/17	Result: A1C 7.4	NORMAL
• GFR, 11/23/17	Result: 28	LOW
• TSH, 11/23/17	Result: 4.930	HIGH

ROS: Mr Lucian reports a 6-lb weight loss since his last visit three months ago. He reports no chest pain or palpitations. He reports no cough, no abdominal pain, no loss of consciousness, and no numbness. He reports no depression, no fatigue, and no leg swelling.

Vitals: Ht. 5 ft 11 in; Wt. 230; BMI: 32.1; BP: 130/80; Pulse: 68

PE: Patient is a 66-year-old obese man with diabetes and hypertension. **Cardiovascular:** Normal S1 and S2 and RRR [respiratory rate and rhythm], no murmurs. No JVD [jugular venous distension]. No carotid bruits. Bilateral carotid pulses present. Normal DP pulses bilaterally. No edema. No shortness of breath.

Assessment/Plan

1. Acquired hypothyroidism	Perform TSH around 6/1/18
2. Hyperlipidemia	
3. Hypertension	Low salt diet
4. DM2	A1C slightly improved; continue canagliflozin

COMMENTS: The patient's past and current medical conditions are comingled in the Problem List and PMH of this note, requiring the coder to judge which diagnoses can correctly be abstracted from this encounter. In the assessment and plan, we have four diagnoses. Applying the strict rules of MEAT, there is no support for hyperlipidemia in this note. However, depending on local policies regarding comorbidities, this diagnosis may be appropriate for submission to CMS because the physician has, by putting them in his assessment, indicated that they were considered during and did impact the clinical

continued

encounter. The CKD listed in PMH is supported by a GFR result, but is not discussed anywhere in the "current" record. Therefore, CKD must be considered as "past history," unless local policies and procedures say otherwise. ICD-10-CM coding guidelines instruct us to link CKD to diabetes because CKD is subclassified in the Alphabetic Index under the term, "Diabetes," using the word "with." However, in this scenario, the CKD is listed in the PMH and by some local coding policies, would not be reported.

Risk-adjusting diagnoses validated in this record:

E78.5 Hyperlipidemia, unspecified [RxHCC:0.038] (assuming codes in assessment require no MEAT)

E03.9 Hypothyroidism, unspecified [RxHCC: 0.101]

I10 Hypertension [RxHCC: 0.123]

E11.9 Type 2 diabetes mellitus without complications [HCC: 0.104, RxHCC: 0.280]

Potential risk-adjusting and under-documented diagnoses:

N18.4 Chronic kidney disease, stage 4 (severe) [HCC 137 0.237, RxHCC 0.093]

E11.29 Type 2 diabetes mellitus with other diabetic kidney complication (HCC: 0.318, RxHCC: 0.425

Code E11.22 would replace code E11.9. With documentation improvements, the RAF for these diagnoses goes from 0.504 to 0.780 for RxHCCs, and from 0.104 to 0.555 for HCCs. HCCs and RxHCCs are based on 2018 community, non-low income rates.

Comorbidities

Many patients in Medicare have multiple comorbidities, and these comorbidities contribute to the MDM for all but the most minor of encounters. Diabetes, eg, is a risk factor in any illness, infection, or injury: It affects treatment choices, anticipated duration of an acute illness, resource consumption, and potential complications. Patients with multiple comorbidities will require a greater degree of MDM, and this service should be represented in the medical record. The existence of a diagnosis in a problem list is not sufficient to capture this service, as problem lists are not acceptable documents for RA without support.

Using best practices, physicians should review the patient's problem list and document all conditions that co-exist at the time of an encounter that affect MDM or the care-treatment plan. As indicated in the ICD-10-CM Guideline Section IV(J), "[c]ode all documented conditions that coexist at the time of the encounter/visit, and require or affect patient care treatment or management. Do not code conditions that were previously treated and no longer exist. However, history codes (categories Z80-Z87) may be used as secondary codes if the historical condition or family history has an impact on current care or influences treatment."[3] Sometimes, the patient's complication/comorbidity is minor, but comorbidities add complexity to the case. Something as simple as candidal intertrigo (yeast infection in the fold of redundant skin) can be associated with comobidities. Treatment for intertrigo includes consistent application of topical medication and preventive measures, such as glucose control, good hygiene, daily monitoring of site, and weight loss. On the other hand, a patient with rheumatoid arthritis, diabetes, and dementia has additional risks that affect the treatment plan for intertrigo: Is the patient's diabetic control sufficient? Can the patient apply the cream herself? Are her rheumatoid arthritis medications exacerbating the infection? Can the patient remember the instructions and perform adequate self-care? Ideally, these risks and their effect on care should be documented.

In its 2008 *RA Participant Guide*, CMS lists eight diagnoses that are chronic, ongoing conditions generally managed with long-term medication and have the potential for exacerbation, particularly if the patient has an acute condition:

- Diabetes
- Atrial fibrillation
- Congestive heart failure

- Chronic obstructive pulmonary disease
- Multiple sclerosis
- Hemiplegia
- Rheumatoid arthritis
- Parkinson's disease

CMS' *2008 RA Participant Guide* states that these "diseases are generally managed by ongoing medication and have the potential for acute exacerbations if not treated properly, particularly if the patient is experiencing other acute conditions. Although they may not impact every minor healthcare episode, it is likely that patients having these conditions would have their general health status evaluated within a data-reporting period."[13] These eight diagnoses have been the basis of many RA coding policies, with some consulting organizations determining that these eight conditions can be coded without MEAT, or even abstracted from past medical history. However, this list is flawed. For example, atrial fibrillation can, in fact, be cured with ablation; thus, if it is not treated with any medications, a code for a personal history of atrial fibrillation, Z86.79, *Personal history of other diseases of the circulatory system*, would be assigned. Post-ablation, atrial fibrillation may still appear in a patient's past medical history, but coding the condition as an active condition would be a mistake. In addition, one could ask, if the list of the "chronic eight" is substantive, why Parkinson's disease is included while Huntington's disease and amyotrophic lateral sclerosis, also significant neurological disorders, are not included. Clearly, the list of "chronic eight" is incomplete. This book will explore how CMS' guidance on comorbidities can be used to develop sensible and defensible policies and procedures for documenting and coding chronic, incurable conditions in Chapter 5.

Keep in mind that the Medicare Advantage organization (MAO) is going to receive additional monies from CMS for the management of a patient with reported comorbidities. In exchange, CMS expects the MAO to ensure the patient's comorbidities are being appropriately monitored, treated, and/or considered in MDM during the year. MAOs monitor what have come to be called "disappearing diagnoses," ie, incurable conditions that disappear, year over year, from a patient's claims data. Often, this is not because the diagnoses have not been treated or addressed, but because the patient has missed appointments, because documentation was insufficient for coders to abstract the diagnoses, or the physicians failed to enter the diagnosis into the billing software. In some cases, MAOs contact physicians who have patients whose historic comorbidities have not been reported in recent months. These physicians may be asked by the MAOs to contact the patients to schedule encounters to address these comorbidities. In some cases, these encounters are conducted in the patient's home. These health-risk assessments (HRAs) are usually wellness examinations performed by a nurse practitioner or other qualified healthcare provider, who are licensed within their scope of practice to make diagnoses allowable for billing purposes. This practice is good for all involved:

- **The patient,** whose chronic conditions will receive more frequent attention;
- **The physician,** who will be perceived as proactive and attentive, will be reimbursed for the encounter, and will be deemed more cost efficient in the Medicare Access and CHIP Reauthorization Act (MACRA) of 2015 related methodologies;
- **The MAO,** which receives higher payments from CMS to offset a higher level of care for high-risk patients; and
- **CMS,** whose goal is the improved health of Medicare enrollees to improve their lives and reduce future costs.

"History of"

Physicians are taught a very different use of the words "history of" than the ICD-10-CM code set uses, and this discrepancy is a great source of confusion for coders. While most medical dictionaries describe "history" as an "account of a patient's family and personal background and past and present health," ICD-10-CM defines "history of" as "explain a patient's past medical condition that no longer exists and is not receiving any treatment."[3] Therefore, when the physician documents a "history" of a condition, the coder's default is not to abstract the condition. On the other hand, if from the documentation, the coder can infer the "history of" a condition is still active, if the condition is one that is chronic and incurable, or if it is still being treated (eg, toremifene as an adjuvant treatment for breast cancer), the coder might abstract the code for that diagnosis, but is taking a risk in doing so. If possible, coders should query the physician when these questions arise.

Physicians should not rely on the coder's initiative or knowledge of pathophysiology to determine what is meant; instead, physicians should recognize the ICD-10-CM coding convention for personal history and document accordingly. According to the *2008 RA Participant Guide*, "history of" means the patient no longer has the condition and the diagnosis often indexes to a history code not in the HCC models. A physician can make errors in one of two ways with respect to these codes. One error is to document or code a past condition as active. The opposite error is document or code as "history of" a condition when that condition is still active or being treated. Both of these errors can impact RA values.[13] (See the following Coding Example.)

CODING EXAMPLE

DOCUMENTATION	COMPLIANT CODING AND HCC
History of opioid dependence	F11.21, Opioid dependence, in remission (HCC 55, 0.383)
History of opioid abuse	F11.11, Opioid abuse, in remission Does not map for RA
Current methadone maintenance for opioid dependence	F11.20, Opioid dependence, uncomplicated (HCC 55; 0.383)
History of diabetic foot ulcer	Z86.31, Personal history of diabetic foot ulcer (no HCC)
Diabetic foot ulcer, exposed fat layer, R midfoot	E11.621, Type 2 diabetes mellitus with foot ulcer (HCC 18; 0.318) L97.412, Non-pressure chronic ulcer of right heel and midfoot with fat layer exposed (HCC 161; 0.535)
History of prostate cancer	Z85.46, Personal history of malignant neoplasm of prostate (no HCC)
Prostate cancer stable on leuprolide	C61, Malignant neoplasm of prostate (HCC 12; 0.146)
History of pulmonary embolism	Z86.711, Personal history of pulmonary embolism (no HCC)
Pulmonary embolism responding favorably to anticoagulation therapy	I26.99, Other pulmonary embolism without acute cor pulmonale (HCC 107; 0.400)

Education of physicians in documentation best practices could help limit physician documentation of "history of" to resolved conditions that no longer require treatment. Instead of documenting "history of" in describing an active condition, quantify the continuum of care: for example, "Mr Ashoff is being seen today for his Parkinson's disease, first diagnosed seven years ago." (See the following Documentation Tip using the ICD-10-CM nomenclature for "history of" and "remission.") Alternatively, the EHR documentation infrastructure may be structured under the "past medical history" section to explicitly outline those that have resolved (eg, mumps when 5 years old; myocardial infarction one year ago) and those that are currently present (eg, chronic kidney disease, stage 4; a hypercoagulable state requiring chronic anticoagulation).

DOCUMENTATION TIP To follow ICD-10-CM nomenclature for "history of" and "remission":

- Become familiar with the personal history classification of the ICD-10-CM Alphabetic Index to Diseases and the instructions for personal history in the *ICD-10-CM Official Guidelines for Coding and Reporting*.
- Do not use the term "history of" if a condition is still present or not manifested because it is still being treated (eg, atrial fibrillation, currently maintained in normal sinus rhythm with amiodarone; diabetes mellitus with a hemoglobin A1C of less than 6.0 that is still being treated with metformin and glyburide; metastatic breast cancer that is receiving adjuvant chemotherapy). State that the patient has the condition and/or that it is controlled with the treatment.
- Do not use "history of" to describe a liquid malignancy (eg, leukemia or multiple myeloma) in remission unless one believes that the patient has been completely cured of the illness, such as a child who had acute lymphoblastic leukemia and who has been disease-free for over 10 years. Instead, document "in remission."
- Do not use "remission" to describe a malignancy that has been excised and for which all treatment has been completed and the patient has no evidence of disease (eg, breast cancer in remission). Instead, document "history of."

According to the *ICD-10-CM guidelines*, physicians and coders are instructed not to "code conditions that were previously treated and no longer exist. However, history codes (categories Z80-Z87) may be used as secondary codes if the historical condition or family history has an impact on current care or influences treatment."[3] In addition, Guideline Section I(C.21.c.4) states that "[p]ersonal history codes may be used in conjunction with follow-up codes and family history codes may be used in conjunction with screening codes to explain the need for a test or procedure. History codes are also acceptable on any medical record regardless of the reason for visit. A history of an illness, even if no longer present, is important information that may alter the type of treatment ordered."[3] (See the following Clinical Coding Example.)

CLINICAL CODING EXAMPLE

HPI: The patient is a 64-year-old female with a past medical history significant for diabetes, DVTs, and thyroid cancer, referred to the urology clinic due to a history of recurrent UTIs.

Current medications: Levothyroxine, warfarin, nortriptyline.

A/P: The patient is a 64-year-old female with a past medical history significant for diabetes, DVTs, and thyroid cancer, referred to the clinic because of her history of recurrent UTIs. Patient is sexually active and denies any incontinence symptoms. Educated patient regarding post-menopausal changes to genitourinary flora, and prescribed nitrofuantoin macro 50 mg, one capsule daily after intercourse. If the UTIs continue, we will add a topical estrogen. RTC [return to clinic] in six months.

COMMENTS: In this example, all diagnoses are documented as "past medical histories." The record does not support current diabetes as an active condition, thus, a code cannot be abstracted. The record neither documents DVTs as a current condition, thus, it should not be abstracted. In addition, it is not documented whether the warfarin is prophylaxis against a new clot or is treatment for a current clot. The patient has a history of thyroid cancer, and is on thyroid replacement therapy (levothyroxine); however, its relevance to this encounter is not clear. Without a documented diagnosis of hypothyroidism, an ICD-10-CM code for this condition cannot be reported. Given that the physician has documented in his assessment the history of thyroid cancer, history of diabetes, and history of DVTs, these histories could be appropriate for reporting to CMS depending on organizational policies. There is no evidence of a current urinary tract infection (UTI) documented. The ICD-10-CM coding for this outpatient encounter is: Z87.440, *Personal history of urinary (tract) infections.* Other history codes can be abstracted according to local policies. In this example, a physician query could be helpful to clarify which diagnoses are active diagnoses.

 **ADVICE/ALERT NOTE**

History (of)

Per ICD-10-CM Guideline Section 1(C.21.c.4), there are "two types of history Z codes, personal and family. Personal history codes explain a patient's past medical condition that no longer exists and is not receiving any treatment, but that has the potential for recurrence, and therefore may require continued monitoring.

Family history codes are for use when a patient has a family member(s) who has had a particular disease that causes the patient to be at higher risk of also contracting the disease.

Personal history codes may be used in conjunction with follow-up codes and family history codes may be used in conjunction with screening codes to explain the need for a test or procedure. History codes are also acceptable on any medical record regardless of the reason for visit. A history of an illness, even if no longer present, is important information that may alter the type of treatment ordered."[3]

Causal Relationship

Causal relationships occur when an underlying condition or etiology is documented to symptoms or manifestations, or when assumed to be related to each other by the ICD-10-CM Alphabetic Index to Diseases with the word "with," or when another guideline for coding and reporting so instructs. For example, the ICD-10-CM Alphabetic Index to Diseases classifies diabetes mellitus with chronic kidney disease as E11.22; however, vaginal candidiasis is not assumed to be caused by or a complication of diabetes, unless it is explicitly documented as such, due to the lack of a listing for diabetes "with" vaginal candidiasis in the ICD-10-CM Alphabetic Index.

Physicians with the best documentation regularly use phrases like "due to," "caused by," "resulting in," and other similar language to link conditions. When documenting a condition, these physicians consider whether there should be an attribution that further refines the diagnosis:

Aphasia	due to	cerebral infarction
Hip fracture	due to	car accident
Cirrhosis	due to	alcohol dependence
Anemia	due to	antineoplastic medication (not "status post" antineoplastic Rx)
Cellulitis	due to	methicillin resistant Staphylococcus aureus

In some cases, physicians **include two levels of attribution:**

Aphasia	due to	cerebral infarction due to atherosclerotic cerebral vessels
Anemia	due to	antineoplastic medication due to malignant neoplasm, R breast
Gastroparesis	due to	diabetes due to pancreatectomy

These details contribute scope to the documented diagnoses, allow for clarity in code abstraction, and correctly capture the risks associated with the patients' conditions. Not only does "due to" link two diagnoses to show the causal relationship between them, the term also prevents causal links from being reported where they do not exist.

As discussed earlier, ICD-10-CM convention requires physicians and coders to link two conditions together if certain circumstances occur. The convention is based on a coding guideline in Guideline Section 1(A.15), which reads:

> The word "with" or "in" should be interpreted to mean "associated with" or "due to" when it appears in a code title, the Alphabetic Index, or an instructional note in the Tabular List. The classification presumes a causal relationship between the two conditions linked by these terms in the Alphabetic Index or Tabular List. These conditions should be coded as related even in the absence of provider documentation explicitly linking them, unless the documentation clearly states the conditions are unrelated or when another guideline exists that specifically requires a documented linkage between two conditions (e.g., sepsis guideline for "acute organ dysfunction that is not clearly associated with the sepsis").[3]

The dozens of diagnoses following "Diabetes/with" in the ICD-10-CM Alphabetic Index are automatically linked to diabetes if they coexist in the physician's documentation, regardless of whether the physician documents a causal relationship. It is the physician's responsibility to specifically document relationships that are ***not*** due to diabetes (eg, a pressure ulcer in the heel of a diabetic patient), so that they are appropriately linked to another condition for ICD-10-CM coding purposes. Physicians who get in the habit of including "due to" in their notes, even for complications of diabetes, will find fewer queries in their in boxes and their practices will generate fewer claims containing diagnosis-coding errors. (See the following Clinical Examples.)

Causal relationships
Medical scenarios in which an underlying condition is directly responsible for a second condition (eg, pneumonia due to pseudomonas or heart failure due to hypertension).

Etiology
For ICD-10-CM, a disease or condition that originates or causes a problem; an underlying condition (eg, follicular carcinoma of the thyroid [etiology] causing thyrotoxicosis).

Manifestations
For ICD-10-CM, signs, symptoms, or complications from an underlying disease (eg, thyrotoxicosis [manifestation] caused by follicular carcinoma of the thyroid).

CLINICAL EXAMPLES

An established patient has a current medical history of tubulo-interstitial nephritis and CKD stage 4 on the problem list. The CKD is due to the tubulo-interstitial nephritis due to a sulfa allergy, but this is not in the record. During today's encounter, the patient is diagnosed with type 2 diabetes.

COMMENTS: It becomes critical that the tubulo-interstitial nephritis and CKD are linked in the language of the medical record; otherwise, the coder will follow guidelines and link the diabetes to the CKD.

Physicians who want to control the diagnoses assigned to their patients must consider these causal relationships, because without proper causal attributions in the record, the ICD-10-CM conventions will become applicable and diagnoses will be assigned accordingly. For physicians who are selecting the codes themselves, proper documentation of causal relationships will substantiate coding in an audit. Just because the physician selects a diagnosis code in the billing software does not mean the code is substantiated in the medical record or with a proper application of ICD-10-CM coding conventions, guidelines, or official advice. The diagnosis selected by the physician must be supported in the medical record.

FYI Diabetes is the most commonly documented diagnosis with causal relationships assumed by the ICD-10-CM Alphabetic Index. The use of "with" in the index entry establishes the causal relationship without it being documented. If there is a different causal relationship, it must be documented by the physician so the disorder is not linked to the diabetes.

Diabetes, diabetic (mellitus) (sugar) E11.9
- with
  - amyotrophy E11.44
  - arthropathy NEC E11.618
  - autonomic (poly) neuropathy E11.43
  - cataract E11.36
  - Charcot's joints E11.610
  - chronic kidney disease E11.22
  - circulatory complication NEC E11.59
  - complication E11.8
    - specified NEC E11.69
  - dermatitis E11.620
  - foot ulcer E11.621
  - gangrene E11.52
  - gastroparalysis E11.43
  - gastroparesis E11.43
  - glomerulonephrosis, intracapillary E11.21
  - glomerulosclerosis, intercapillary E11.21
  - hyperglycemia E11.65
  - hyperosmolarity E11.00
    - with coma E11.01
  - hypoglycemia E11.649
    - with coma E11.641
  - kidney complications NEC E11.29
  - Kimmelsteil-Wilson disease E11.21
  - loss of protective sensation (LOPS)—see Diabetes, by type, with neuropathy
  - mononeuropathy E11.41
  - myasthenia E11.44
  - necrobiosis lipoidica E11.620
  - nephropathy E11.21
  - neuralgia E11.42
  - neurologic complication NEC E11.49
  - neuropathic arthropathy E11.610
  - neuropathy E11.40
  - ophthalmic complication NEC E11.39
  - oral complication NEC E11.638
  - osteomyelitis E11.69
  - periodontal disease E11.630
  - peripheral angiopathy E11.51
    - with gangrene E11.52
  - polyneuropathy E11.42
  - renal complication NEC E11.29
  - renal tubular degeneration E11.29
  - retinopathy E11.319
    - with macular edema E11.311
      - resolved following treatment E11.37
    - nonproliferative E11.329
      - with macular edema E11.321
      - mild E11.329
        - with macular edema E11.321
      - moderate E11.339
        - with macular edema E11.331
      - severe E11.349
        - with macular edema E11.341
    - proliferative E11.359
      - with
        - combined traction retinal detachment and rhegmatogenous retinal detachment E11.354
        - macular edema E11.351
        - stable proliferative diabetic retinopathy E11.355
        - traction retinal detachment involving the macula E11.352
        - traction retinal detachment not involving the macula E11.353
  - skin complication NEC E11.628
  - skin ulcer NEC E11.622

If a physician does not want a causal relationship coded between diabetes and the disorders on this list, the documentation must either state that the two are unrelated or state another causal agent for the disorder.

Clinical Documentation and Coding for RA

Consulting the Alphabetic Index is crucial for correct coding of causal relationships with the "with" rule. Dementia, for example, is due to Parkinson's disease when both occur, according to the Alphabetic Index, and alcohol abuse is the default cause of sexual dysfunction when both conditions are documented in the same encounter.

The strict application of the MEAT criteria creates an interesting dilemma in causal relationship coding: What sort of MEAT is required for causal relationships? In a causal relationship, does each diagnosis require MEAT in order to be abstracted as etiology and manifestation? As there is no official guidance from *ICD-10-CM Guidelines*, AHA's *Coding Clinic*, or specific RA guidance from CMS, some organizations choose to accept both diagnoses if support is documented for one; while others require both diagnoses to be supported in the record, and if one of the two diagnoses does not have support, the causal relationship dissolves. This is another area for organizational policymaking, which is discussed in Chapter 5.

ADVICE/ALERT NOTE

Per ICD-10-CM Guideline Section I(B.9), "[m]ultiple coding should not be used when the classification provides a combination code that clearly identifies all the elements documented in the diagnosis. When the combination code lacks necessary specificity in describing the manifestation or complication, an additional code should be used as a secondary code."[3]

Physicians who make it a habit to "think in ink" may find that their documentation is more robust and offers a better record of the clinical picture. CMS' *2008 RA Participant Guide* states that "[c]linical specificity involves having a diagnosis fully documented in the source medical record instead of routinely defaulting to a general term for the diagnosis."[13] Use free-text boxes when they are available to augment the note so that a note of "positive for cough" becomes "positive for chronic, dry cough that is worse at night," and "type 2 diabetes" becomes "type 2 diabetes with blood sugars responding well to daily exercise." When physicians "think in ink," there will always be clear support for RA, and plenty of evidence showing the work involved in patient care.

ADVICE/ALERT NOTE

Per CMS' *2008 RA Participant Guide*, "[c]linical specificity involves having a diagnosis fully documented in the source medical record instead of routinely defaulting to a general term for the diagnosis."[13]

Complete Documentation

Physicians should take advantage of narrative opportunities in the HPI to expand upon the patient's chief complaint and chronic conditions. By following the 1995 or 1997 Documentation Guidelines for Evaluation and Management Services and the ICD-10-CM code assignment ("decoded" as documentation requirements), these conditions will be adequately documented and will include the information needed for code abstraction or direct submission for RA purposes.

The HPI is a chronological description of the development of the patient's present illness from the first sign and/or symptom or from the previous encounter to the present. It includes the following elements:

- location;
- quality;
- severity;
- duration;
- timing;
- context;
- modifying factors; and
- associated signs and symptoms.[14]

Not all elements are required in every illness or encounter, but when appropriate, these elements should be included. These elements are not limited to HPI; they can also be included in the assessment as appropriate.

Location. Laterality and site of a disease or injury. Laterality is expressed as right or left, but location can be more detailed (eg, S72.461S, *Displaced supracondylar fracture with intracondylar extension of lower end of right femur, sequela,* and C25.2, *Malignant neoplasm of tail of pancreas*). A common problem with location documentation is that it is very specific in the initial encounter, but that specificity is lost in subsequent encounters, and so must be coded as "unspecified."

Quality. Characteristics of the symptom, injury, or disease. Quality is expressed with adjectives. In the case of pain, it might be described as sharp, dull, throbbing, severe, stinging, aching, or stabbing.

Severity. Intensity of the symptom. This commonly is established by asking the patient to assign a severity level based on a scale of 1 to 10. The severity of behavioral disorders is often identified as mild, moderate, severe, or in partial or complete relapse. Drug and alcohol use disorders are qualified as use (without evidence of a use disorder), abuse (mild use disorder), or dependence (moderate or severe use disorder), as currently active or in remission, and according to its coexisting consequences (eg, insomnia; sexual dysfunction) as listed in the ICD-10-CM Alphabetic Index to Diseases. Drug or alcohol use disorders not specified as being mild, moderate, or severe may not be coded in ICD-10-CM, unless documented as being "in remission," and require clarification.

Duration. Length of time the problem persisted, whether describing how many years the patient has had multiple sclerosis, or how long the patient has had gross hematuria. If the physician has established that the condition is acute or chronic, this element should be documented, as the distinction contributes to many code decisions.

Timing. Different from duration, timing addresses when the symptom occurs (eg, leg pain that starts when walking starts and stops when walking stops).

Context. Circumstances that caused the problem to worsen or recede (eg, shortness of breath only when lying flat or back pain following moving sacks of compost from the truck to the back yard).

Modifying factors. Circumstances that can improve or worsen a symptom (eg, the patient's diabetes is responding well to the new prescription of Lantus or the physical therapy was helping at first, but now her symptoms are returning).

Associated signs and symptoms. For example, cough, fever, and chest pain with pneumonia. Associated signs and symptoms are not reported when there is a definitive diagnosis, unless they are not routinely associated with that diagnosis (eg, hypoxia with COPD). Under no circumstances can a probable or uncertain differential diagnosis be abstracted from the record in any physician (including inpatient physician) or outpatient billing. However, for inpatient facility billing, an uncertain diagnosis (eg, one qualified as possible, probable, likely, suspected, still to be ruled out) may be coded, if documented (not established, but documented) at the time of discharge (eg, discharge note, discharge order, discharge summary), except for limited exceptions (eg, HIV infections, certain influenza infections). Otherwise, physicians should document to the level of their certainty the definitive diagnosis or the signs and symptoms for which there is no final diagnosis.

ADVICE/ALERT NOTE

Per ICD-10-CM Guideline Section IV(H), "[d]o not code diagnoses documented as 'probable,' 'suspected,' 'questionable,' 'rule out,' or 'working diagnosis' or other similar terms indicating uncertainty. Rather, code the condition(s) to the highest degree of certainty for that encounter/visit, such as symptoms, signs, abnormal test results, or other reason for the visit for physician or outpatient billing."[3]

Definitive diagnosis
Final diagnosis that is the result of MDM and the review of signs, symptoms, and test results.

Differential diagnosis
Working diagnosis early in the MDM process as the physician considers signs, symptoms, and test results to determine the patient's final diagnosis. Usually, there are more than one differential diagnoses being considered.

Quick List of Dos and Don'ts

Some documentation and coding best practices for RA seem obvious, and some do not. Highlighted here are some quick changes to documentation habits that can translate into big improvements in the communication of diagnoses.

Acronyms or Abbreviations

Acronyms, regardless how commonly used, are ambiguous. A hospitalist documenting a diagnosis of "ARF" for a patient being treated for severe sepsis would not be identifying whether the patient's kidneys (acute renal failure) or pulmonary system (acute respiratory failure) had been damaged by the sepsis. A review of tests and context may not be enough for clarity in the medical record. Best practices would have physicians spelling out the first use of an acronym in every DOS. Alternately, a practice can create a policy on commonly accepted acronyms and follow that list, so long as the list is shared in any audit. According to CMS' *Contract-Level RADV Reviewer Guidance,* auditors are given the discretion in accepting or rejecting coding based on ambiguous acronyms or abbreviations: "If more than one meaning applies or documentation is too limited to differentiate, and this is the only diagnosis listed within the record, evaluate on a case-by-case basis. Otherwise, use discretion to report or not based on other circumstances in the record."[5] (See the following Example in which an acronym used has multiple meanings.)

EXAMPLE

The patient's AD is stable, on meds.

AD	Alzheimer's disease
AD	Androgen deprivation
AD	Atopic dermatitis
AD	Autistic disorder

Status Conditions

Status condition is defined as the element within a patient's medical profile that is significant for current or future medical risk, as identified by a status code in ICD-10-CM. A significant number of medical-status codes risk-adjust, and these Z codes are among the most often overlooked codes in RA abstraction. The fault may lie with the physician in which the conditions may simply be omitted from documentation (eg, the patient's status as having a lower-extremity amputation may not seem significant during an encounter to treat pneumonia). When the patient has significant underlying health issues, these should be addressed at least annually; ideally, twice yearly. Lower extremity amputation status is usually the result of vascular disease, but even if it is the result of a traumatic event, the amputation status will affect the patient's ambulation and, therefore, circulation. Hence, it should be reported at least annually.

The fault may lie with the coder, who sometimes overlooks these conditions during abstraction. Coders must always review the entire note. The PE often harbors status information as the physician reviews the patient's stoma site (pink, warm, skin intact) or lower extremity amputation.

Always abstract these status conditions when they are documented in the record:

- HIV-positive status (HCC 1, 0.312): Z21, *Asymptomatic human immunodeficiency virus [HIV] infection status,* may not be reported in the state of California. To obtain the risk-adjustment for HCC 1 in California, the physician must document that the patient qualifies for B20, *Human immunodeficiency virus [HIV] disease.*
- Stoma status or attention to stoma (HCC 188, 0.571): This is appropriate for urinary or intestinal stomas. Tracheostomy also should be documented and coded (HCC 82, 1.055).
- Lower extremity amputation status, even of a single toe; or fitting/adjustment of an artificial limb (HCC 189, 0.588)
- Major organ or stem cell transplant status (HCC 186, 1.00)
- BMI 40 or greater (HCC 22, 0.273): While a code for BMI of 40 or more may be obtained from nursing documentation, an associated diagnosis (eg, morbid obesity) should also be documented by the physician and abstracted from the chart.
- Presence of heart assist device (HCC 186. 1.00)
- Dependence on respirator status (HCC 82, 1.055)
- Dialysis status (HCC 134, 0.422)
- Long-term use of insulin (HCC 19, 0.104)

Problem Lists

Problem lists present an opportunity for physicians to incorporate into their HPI the status of the patient's chronic conditions, ensuring these chronic conditions are evaluated regularly. According to ICD-10-CM Guideline Section IV(I), "[c]hronic diseases treated on an ongoing basis may be coded and reported as many times as the patient receives treatment and care for the condition(s)."[3] See the following Example of how to use the problem list to capture the status of the patient's chronic conditions and incorporated into the HPI.

EXAMPLE

PROBLEM LIST	PROBLEMS INCORPORATED INTO HPI
1. Diabetes mellitus, type 2 2. Hypertension 3. GERD [gastroesophageal reflux disease] 4. Rheumatoid arthritis	Katherine Hawze, a 67-year-old woman with stable DM, well-controlled hypertension, and asymptomatic GERD was seen today due to a rheumatoid nodule on her R elbow that is large and being subjected to repeated trauma. She requests surgical removal, having undergone a similar procedure on her L elbow last year.

 ADVICE/ALERT NOTE

Per ICD-10-CM Guideline Section IV(I), "[c]hronic diseases treated on an ongoing basis may be coded and reported as many times as the patient receives treatment and care for the condition(s)."[3]

Training

With the advent of EHRs, physicians and administrative staff have come to believe that code selection is a simple process, and that pick-lists are sufficient for accurate and compliant coding. However, anyone engaging in ICD-10-CM code abstraction must understand and implement the conventions of the ICD-10-CM code set, their official guidelines and advice, and CMS regulations for diagnostic coding. Codes and guidelines are updated annually, whereas official advice is published quarterly in AHA's *Coding Clinic*. While some may find it more efficient to employ or outsource the coding portion of their practice to professional coders, who must earn continuing education units every year and stay updated on constantly evolving regulations and code sets, physicians should definitely understand the coding and documentation needs of ICD-10-CM, especially in the ambulatory environment in which the physician may be simultaneously documenting and coding the diagnosis in the process of care. In addition, physicians and practices may wish to consider licensing ICD-10-CM coding software that includes the ICD-10-CM Alphabetic Index, Tabular section, Guidelines, and the AHA's *Coding Clinic*, which is regularly updated, to facilitate time-efficiency for themselves and their coding professionals. According to the Office of Inspector General's (OIG's) publication, *Compliance Program for Individual and Small Group Physician Practices*, "it is in the practice's best interest to ensure that individuals who are directly involved with billing, coding, or other aspects of the federal healthcare programs receive extensive education specific to that individual's responsibilities. Some examples of items that could be covered in coding and billing training include:

- Coding requirements;
- Claim development and submission processes;
- Signing a form for a physician without the physician's authorization;
- Proper documentation of services rendered;
- Proper billing standards and procedures and submission of accurate bills for services or items rendered to federal healthcare program beneficiaries; and
- The legal sanctions for submitting deliberately false or reckless billings."[1]

ADVICE/ALERT NOTE

Coding and billing training on the federal healthcare program requirements may be necessary for certain members of the physician practice staff depending on their respective responsibilities. The OIG understands that most physician practices do not employ a professional coder and that the physician is often primarily responsible for all coding and billing. However, it is in the practice's best interest to ensure that individuals who are directly involved with billing, coding, or other aspects of the federal healthcare programs receive extensive education specific to that individual's responsibilities. Some examples of items that could be covered in coding and billing training include:

- Coding requirements;
- Claim development and submission processes;
- Signing a form for a physician without the physician's authorization;
- Proper documentation of services rendered;
- Proper billing standards and procedures and submission of accurate bills for services or items rendered to federal healthcare program beneficiaries; and
- The legal sanctions for submitting deliberately false or reckless billings.[1]

Codes in Documentation

Coders should check the coding performed by physicians, and correct it as necessary. Codes are not *documentation*, so coders do not need to be concerned they are changing documentation. Correct coding and billing is a joint effort between physicians and coders, wherein the physician's primary focus is on the patient and the documentation that follows from an encounter, while the coder's focus is on the abstraction after the encounter. One supports and reinforces the other, which is supported by the *Contract-Level RADV Reviewer Guidance*, which states that ICD-10-CM codes "without narrative are not acceptable to report in place of a diagnosis to support a CMS-HCC. It is the codes that are being validated by medical record written documentation."[5] (See the following Coding Example to see what can and cannot be abstracted from the physician documentation.)

CODING EXAMPLE

The physician treated the patient for an acute exacerbation of COPD. The coder must abstract the text. Codes cannot be abstracted from the simple documentation of a code number in the medical record.

DOCUMENTATION	WHAT CAN BE ABSTRACTED (ASSUMING THERE IS MEAT)	RATIONALE
J44.1	No code	No text to abstract
J44.1 COPD	J44.9 Chronic obstructive pulmonary disease, unspecified	COPD is documented. J44.1, which reports COPD with exacerbation, is rightly ignored.
J44.1 COPD w/exacerbation	J44.1 Chronic obstructive pulmonary disease with (acute) exacerbation	The text contains enough information to abstract with specificity.

A stand-alone code without written documentation will be rejected by CMS. Physicians who use pick-lists in their EHRs to document an ICD-10-CM code instead of a narrative description of the diagnosis are doing so in error. Codes cannot be substituted for documentation of a diagnosis, and codes do not have the same descriptive quality of documented narrative. Failure to support diagnoses with narrative will result in negative audit results. According to the Introduction to the *ICD-10-CM Guidelines*, a "joint effort between the healthcare provider and the coder is essential to achieve complete and accurate documentation, code assignment, and reporting of diagnoses and procedures. These guidelines have been developed to assist both the healthcare provider and the coder in identifying those diagnoses that are to be reported. The importance of consistent, complete documentation in the medical record cannot be overemphasized. Without such documentation, accurate coding cannot be achieved. The entire record should be reviewed to determine the specific reason for the encounter and the conditions treated."[3]

ICD-10-CM Coding Conventions

ICD-10-CM is a code set managed by the CDC's National Center for Health Statistics (NCHS) within the framework of the scientific classification system developed and maintained by the World Health Organization (WHO). WHO's goal is to provide codes for reporting of disease for analysis of world population health. In the United States, the clinical modification of the WHO's international ICD-10 code set (ICD-10-CM) is expanded to more closely align with healthcare reporting here, and in addition to disease tracking, is used in claims reporting and adjudication.

CMS and the NCHS, in cooperation with the AHA and AHIMA, provide guidelines for coding and reporting using ICD-10-CM. The *ICD-10-CM Guidelines*, in addition to containing diagnosis-specific coding advice, describe conventions for understanding the information within ICD-10-CM, and rules for using the Alphabetic Index and Tabular sections within the coding system.

An understanding of the conventions of ICD-10-CM, which are found in Section I of the guidelines, is essential for proper use of its codes:

> **Section I. Conventions, general coding guidelines and chapter specific guidelines**
> The conventions, general guidelines and chapter-specific guidelines are applicable to all health care settings unless otherwise indicated. The conventions and instructions of the classification take precedence over guidelines.
>
> **A. Conventions for the ICD-10-CM**
> The conventions for the ICD-10-CM are the general rules for use of the classification independent of the guidelines. These conventions are incorporated within the Alphabetic Index and Tabular List of the ICD-10-CM as instructional notes.
>
> **1. The Alphabetic Index and Tabular List**
> The ICD-10-CM is divided into the Alphabetic Index, an alphabetical list of terms and their corresponding code, and the Tabular List, a structured list of codes divided into chapters based on body system or condition. The Alphabetic Index consists of the following parts: the Index of Diseases and Injury, the Index of External Causes of Injury, the Table of Neoplasms and the Table of Drugs and Chemicals.

Scientific classification
In the case of ICD-10-CM, a system for categorizing the etiology of illness and injury by their shared characteristics. In the alphanumeric system of ICD-10-CM, all types of glaucoma are grouped together in the Diseases of the Eye and Adnexa chapter, with category H40 containing all glaucoma codes. The codes are further divided into subcategories to describe etiology, severity, stage, and laterality.

World Health Organization (WHO)
Organization established by the United Nations to lead efforts in improving international public health. WHO developed and maintains the International Classification of Disease (ICD)'s current Tenth Edition (ICD-10), which is clinically modified in the United States (US) to become ICD-10-CM. While the WHO's ICD-11 is slated for release in 2018 (not in the US), its modification by the National Center for Health Statistics (NCHS), ICD-11-CM, will not be used by physicians in the US until it is developed and approved by the Secretary of the Health and Human Services.

2. Format and Structure:
The ICD-10-CM Tabular List contains categories, subcategories and codes. Characters for categories, subcategories and codes may be either a letter or a number. All categories are 3 characters. A three-character category that has no further subdivision is equivalent to a code. Subcategories are either 4 or 5 characters. Codes may be 3, 4, 5, 6 or 7 characters. That is, each level of subdivision after a category is a subcategory. The final level of subdivision is a code. Codes that have applicable 7th characters are still referred to as codes, not subcategories. A code that has an applicable 7th character is considered invalid without the 7th character.

The ICD-10-CM uses an indented format for ease in reference.

3. Use of codes for reporting purposes
For reporting purposes only codes are permissible, not categories or subcategories, and any applicable 7th character is required.

4. Placeholder character
The ICD-10-CM utilizes a placeholder character "X." The "X" is used as a placeholder at certain codes to allow for future expansion. An example of this is at the poisoning, adverse effect and underdosing codes, categories T36-T50.

Where a placeholder exists, the "X" must be used in order for the code to be considered a valid code.

5. 7th Characters
Certain ICD-10-CM categories have applicable 7th characters. The applicable 7th character is required for all codes within the category, or as the notes in the Tabular List instruct. The 7th character must always be the 7th character in the data field. If a code that requires a 7th character is not 6 characters, a placeholder "X" must be used to fill in the empty characters.

FYI A placeholder "X" is an alpha character added to an ICD-10-CM code to ensure it retains the structural integrity of the classification. The "X" may be preassigned, or it may be assigned by the coder.

If preassigned, the placeholder "X" allows for future expansion of the code set.

T38.3X1 Poisoning by insulin and oral hypoglycemic [antidiabetic] drugs, accidental (unintentional)

In this case, the classification assigned the "X" allow for future identification of specific types of insulins and oral hypoglycemic causing adverse effects. The placeholder "X" would allow this breakout without affecting the sixth-digit convention of assigning a cause to the event, in this case, accidental. A seventh character is added to these codes to describe the circumstances of the encounter (initial treatment, subsequent encounter, or sequela).

The coder assigns the second type of placeholder "X." The "X" assigned by a coder will always be assigned to accommodate a seventh character. For example:

Z72.21 Displaced subtrochanteric fracture of right femur

A seventh character is required to identify the circumstance of the encounter, in this case, "A," *initial encounter for closed fracture.*

If the "A" is applied to Z72.21, then "A" would be the sixth character. If submitted on a claim, Z72.21A would be rejected as an invalid code. Placeholder "X" is used to fill in the empty character space. The correct code is:

Z72.21XA Displaced subtrochanteric fracture of right femur, initial encounter for closed fracture

In some cases, the coder may need to assign more than one "X" in order for the seventh character to be accommodated:

S33.4 Traumatic rupture of symphysis pubis

Correctly coded:

S33.4XXA Traumatic rupture of symphysis pubis, initial encounter

6. Abbreviations

a. Alphabetic Index abbreviations
NEC "Not elsewhere classifiable"

This abbreviation in the Alphabetic Index represents "other specified." When a specific code is not available for a condition, the Alphabetic Index directs the coder to the "other specified" code in the Tabular List.

NOS "Not otherwise specified"

This abbreviation is the equivalent of unspecified.

FYI NEC, not elsewhere classified, indicates that the classification does not have a code specific to the condition being reported, so a general code must be used. NOS, not otherwise specified, indicates there is not enough information available to choose a more specific code, usually because the diagnostic process is still under way, or because the documentation is insufficient.

b. Tabular List abbreviations
NEC "Not elsewhere classifiable"

This abbreviation in the Tabular List represents "other specified". When a specific code is not available for a condition, the Tabular List includes an NEC entry under a code to identify the code as the "other specified" code.

NOS "Not otherwise specified"

This abbreviation is the equivalent of unspecified.

7. Punctuation

[ ] Brackets are used in the Tabular List to enclose synonyms, alternative wording or explanatory phrases. Brackets are used in the Alphabetic Index to identify manifestation codes.

( ) Parentheses are used in both the Alphabetic Index and Tabular List to enclose supplementary words that may be present or absent in the statement of a disease or procedure without affecting the code number to which it is assigned. The terms within the parentheses are referred to as nonessential modifiers. The nonessential modifiers in the Alphabetic Index to Diseases apply to subterms following a main term, except when a nonessential modifier and a subentry are mutually exclusive, the subentry takes precedence. For example, in the ICD-10-CM Alphabetic Index under the main term Enteritis, "acute" is a nonessential modifier and "chronic" is a subentry. In this case, the nonessential modifier "acute" does not apply to the subentry "chronic."

: Colons are used in the Tabular List after an incomplete term, which needs one or more of the modifiers following the colon to make it assignable to a given category.

8. Use of "and"
See Section I.A.14. Use of the term "And"

9. Other and Unspecified codes

a. "Other" codes
Codes titled "other" or "other specified" are for use when the information in the medical record provides detail for which a specific code does not exist. Alphabetic Index entries with NEC in the line designate "other" codes in the Tabular List. These Alphabetic Index entries represent specific disease entities for which no specific code exists so the term is included within an "other" code.

b. "Unspecified" codes
Codes titled "unspecified" are for use when the information in the medical record is insufficient to assign a more specific code. For those categories for which an unspecified code is not provided, the "other specified" code may represent both other and unspecified.

10. Includes Notes
This note appears immediately under a three character code title to further define, or give examples of, the content of the category.

11. Inclusion terms
List of terms is included under some codes. These terms are the conditions for which that code is to be used. The terms may be synonyms of the code title, or, in the case of "other specified" codes, the terms are a list of the various conditions assigned to that

code. The inclusion terms are not necessarily exhaustive. Additional terms found only in the Alphabetic Index may also be assigned to a code.

FYI Do not be confused by inclusion terms or includes notes. These diagnostic phrases are affirmations if the diagnosis the coder seeks is listed, but the absence of the sought diagnosis from an inclusion term or note does not indicate the diagnosis is excluded.

12. Excludes Notes
The ICD-10-CM has two types of excludes notes. Each type of note has a different definition for use but they are all similar in that they indicate that codes excluded from each other are independent of each other.

a. Excludes 1
An Excludes 1 note is a pure excludes note. It means "NOT CODED HERE!" An Excludes 1 note indicates that the code excluded should never be used at the same time as the code above the Excludes 1 note. An Excludes 1 is used when two conditions cannot occur together, such as a congenital form versus an acquired form of the same condition.

An exception to the Excludes 1 definition is the circumstance when the two conditions are unrelated to each other. If it is not clear whether the two conditions involving an Excludes 1 note are related, query the physician. For example, code F45.8, *Other somatoform disorders*, has an Excludes 1 note for "sleep related teeth grinding (G47.63)," because "teeth grinding" is an inclusion term under code F45.8. Only one of these two codes should be assigned for teeth grinding. However, psychogenic dysmenorrhea is also an inclusion term under code F45.8, and a patient could have both this condition and sleep-related teeth grinding. In this case, the two conditions are clearly unrelated to each other, and so it would be appropriate to report codes F45.8 and G47.63 together.

b. Excludes 2
An Excludes 2 note represents "Not included here." An Excludes 2 note indicates that the condition excluded is not part of the condition represented by the code, but a patient may have both conditions at the same time. When an Excludes 2 note appears under a code, it is acceptable to use both the code and the excluded code together, when appropriate.

13. Etiology/Manifestation Convention ("Code First," "Use Additional Code," and "In Diseases Classified Elsewhere" Notes)
Certain conditions have both an underlying etiology and multiple body system manifestations due to the underlying etiology. For such conditions, the ICD-10-CM has a coding convention that requires the underlying condition be sequenced first, if applicable, followed by the manifestation. Wherever such a combination exists, there is a "use additional code" note at the etiology code, and a "code first" note at the manifestation code. These instructional notes indicate the proper sequencing order of the codes, etiology followed by manifestation.

In most cases, the manifestation codes will have in the code title, "in diseases classified elsewhere." Codes with this title are a component of the etiology/manifestation convention. The code title indicates that it is a manifestation code. "In diseases classified elsewhere" codes are never permitted to be used as first-listed or principal diagnosis codes. They must be used in conjunction with an underlying condition code and they must be listed following the underlying condition. See category F02, *Dementia in other diseases classified elsewhere*, for an example of this convention.

There are manifestation codes that do not have "in diseases classified elsewhere" in the title. For such codes, there is a "use additional code" note at the etiology code and a "code first" note at the manifestation code, and the rules for sequencing apply.

In addition to the notes in the Tabular List, these conditions also have a specific Alphabetic Index entry structure. In the Alphabetic Index both conditions are listed together with the etiology code first followed by the manifestation codes in brackets. The code in brackets is always to be sequenced second.

An example of the etiology/manifestation convention is dementia in Parkinson's disease. In the Alphabetic Index, code G20 is listed first, followed by code F02.80 or F02.81 in brackets. Code G20 represents the underlying etiology, Parkinson's disease, and must be sequenced first, whereas codes F02.80 and F02.81 represent the manifestation of dementia in diseases classified elsewhere, with or without behavioral disturbance.

"Code first" and "Use additional code" notes are also used as sequencing rules in the classification for certain codes that are not part of an etiology/manifestation combination.

ADVICE/ALERT NOTE

When a code in the Alphabetic Index is followed by a second code in brackets, ICD-10-CM convention is indicating that two codes are required to correctly report the etiology and manifestation (eg, Pick's disease G31.01 [F02.80], requiring a second code to report dementia in Pick's disease [F02.80]). The second code, F02.80 cannot be omitted, according to ICD-10-CM convention.

14. "And"

The word "and" should be interpreted to mean either "and" or "or" when it appears in a title.

For example, cases of "tuberculosis of bones," "tuberculosis of joints," and "tuberculosis of bones and joints" are classified to subcategory A18.0, *Tuberculosis of bones and joints.*

15. "With"

The word "with" or "in" should be interpreted to mean "associated with" or "due to" when it appears in a code title, the Alphabetic Index, or an instructional note in the Tabular List. The classification presumes a causal relationship between the two conditions linked by these terms in the Alphabetic Index or Tabular List. These conditions should be coded as related even in the absence of physician documentation explicitly linking them, unless the documentation clearly states the conditions are unrelated or when another guideline exists that specifically requires a documented linkage between two conditions (eg, sepsis guideline for "acute organ dysfunction that is not clearly associated with the sepsis").

For conditions not specifically linked by these relational terms in the classification or when a guideline requires that a linkage between two conditions be explicitly documented, physician documentation must link the conditions in order for them to be coded as related.

The word "with" in the Alphabetic Index is sequenced immediately following the main term, not in alphabetical order.

16. "See" and "See Also"

The "see" instruction following a main term in the Alphabetic Index indicates that another term should be referenced. It is necessary to go to the main term referenced with the "see" note to locate the correct code.

A "see also" instruction following a main term in the Alphabetic Index instructs that there is another main term that may also be referenced, which may provide additional Alphabetic Index entries that may be useful. It is not necessary to follow the "see also" note when the original main term provides the necessary code.

17. "Code Also" note

A "code also" note instructs that two codes may be required to fully describe a condition, but this note does not provide sequencing direction. The sequencing depends on the circumstances of the encounter.

ADVICE/ALERT NOTE

If the Tabular instructions state, "Code First," a second code is mandatory. If Tabular instructions state, "Code Also," a second code is optional.

18. Default codes
A code listed next to a main term in the ICD-10-CM Alphabetic Index is referred to as a default code. The default code represents the condition that is most commonly associated with the main term, or is the unspecified code for the condition. If a condition is documented in a medical record (eg, appendicitis) without any additional information, such as acute or chronic, the default code should be assigned.

19. Code Assignment and Clinical Criteria
The assignment of a diagnosis code is based on the physician's diagnostic statement that the condition exists. The physician's statement that the patient has a particular condition is sufficient. Code assignment is not based on clinical criteria used by the physician to establish the diagnosis.

Start with the Alphabetic Index

The ICD-10-CM code set provides tidbits of information during the code-lookup process, and to skip any of these steps is to invite the possibility of error into coding. The ICD-10-CM code set is divided into two main sections: an Alphabetic Index of terms and the codes associated with them, and the Tabular List of codes, organized by body system in a scientific classification and including coding advice. ICD-10-CM Guideline Section I(B.1) states:

> To select a code in the classification that corresponds to a diagnosis or reason for visit documented in a medical record, first locate the term in the Alphabetic Index, and then verify the code in the Tabular List. Read and be guided by instructional notations that appear in both the Alphabetic Index and the Tabular List.
>
> It is essential to use both the Alphabetic Index and Tabular List when locating and assigning a code. The Alphabetic Index does not always provide the full code. Selection of the full code, including laterality and any applicable 7th character can only be done in the Tabular List. A dash (-) at the end of an Alphabetic Index entry indicates that additional characters are required. Even if a dash is not included at the Alphabetic Index entry, it is necessary to refer to the Tabular List to verify that no 7th character is required.[3]

ADVICE/ALERT NOTE

Per ICD-10-CM Guideline Section IV(A), the "most critical rule involves beginning the search for the correct code assignment through the Alphabetic Index. Never begin searching initially in the Tabular List as this will lead to coding errors."[3]

Default code
The ICD-10-CM code listed directly after a main term in the index, representing the most common form of the disorder, and used when further specificity is not documented. Examples of defaults are chronic rotator-cuff tear for "tear, rotator cuff" and chronic sinusitis for "sinusitis."

Code Assignment and Clinical Criteria

ICD-10-CM Guideline Section I (A.19) entitled, **Code Assignment and Clinical Criteria**, requires the attention of all invested in ICD-10-CM coding compliance, and its interpretation is underscored by coding advice from the AHA's *Coding Clinic* (Fourth Quarter, 2016).[16] The ICD-10-CM Guideline Section I (A.19) states that the "assignment of a diagnosis code is based on the provider's diagnostic statement that the condition exists. The provider's statement that the patient has a particular condition is sufficient. Code assignment is not based on clinical criteria used by the provider to establish the diagnosis."[3] This guideline has prompted some to interpret this guideline "to mean that clinical documentation improvement (CDI) specialists should no longer question diagnostic statements that don't meet clinical criteria."[15] According to the AHA's *Coding Clinic* (Fourth Quarter, 2016):

> Coding must be based on provider documentation. This guideline is not a new concept, although it had not been explicitly included in the official coding guidelines until now. *Coding Clinic* and the official coding guidelines have always stated that code assignment should be based on provider documentation. As has been repeatedly stated in *Coding Clinic* over the years, diagnosing a patient's condition is solely the responsibility of the provider. Only the physician, or other qualified healthcare practitioner legally accountable for establishing the patient's diagnosis, can "diagnose" the patient.
>
> As also stated in *Coding Clinic* in the past, clinical information published in *Coding Clinic* does not constitute clinical criteria for establishing a diagnosis, substitute for the provider's clinical judgment, or eliminate the need for provider documentation regarding the clinical significance of a patient's medical condition.
>
> The guideline noted addresses coding, not clinical validation. It is appropriate for facilities to ensure that documentation is complete, accurate, and appropriately reflects the patient's clinical conditions. Although ultimately related to the accuracy of the coding, clinical validation is a separate function from the coding process and clinical skill. The distinction is described in the Centers for Medicare & Medicaid (CMS) definition of clinical validation from the Recovery Audit Contractors Scope of Work document and cited in the AHIMA Practice Brief ("Clinical Validation: Next Level of CDI") published in the August issue of *JAHIMA*: "Clinical validation is an additional process that may be performed along with DRG validation." Clinical validation involves a clinical review of the case to see whether or not the patient truly possesses the conditions that were documented in the medical record. Clinical validation is performed by a clinician (RN, CMD, or therapist). Clinical validation is beyond the scope of DRG (coding) validation, and the skills of a certified coder. This type of review can only be performed by a clinician or may be performed by a clinician with approved coding credentials.
>
> While physicians may use a particular clinical definition or set of clinical criteria to establish a diagnosis, the code is based on his/her documentation, not on a particular clinical definition or criteria. In other words, regardless of whether a physician uses the new clinical criteria for sepsis, the old criteria [for sepsis], his [or her] personal clinical judgment, or something else to decide [if] a patient has sepsis (and documents it as such), the code for sepsis is the same—as long as sepsis is documented, regardless of how the diagnosis was arrived at, the code for sepsis can be assigned. Coders should not be disregarding physician documentation and deciding on their own, based on clinical criteria, abnormal test results, etc., whether or not a condition should be coded. For example, if the physician documents sepsis and the coder assigns the code for sepsis, and a clinical validation reviewer later disagrees with the physician's diagnosis, that is a clinical issue, but it is not a coding error. By the same token, coders shouldn't be coding sepsis in the absence of physician documentation because they believe the patient meets sepsis clinical criteria. A facility or a payer may require that a physician use a particular clinical definition or set of criteria when establishing a diagnosis, but that is a clinical issue outside the coding system."[16]

In essence, while coding is based only on what the physician documents in the medical record and not an interpretation of the clinical circumstances by the coder (eg, hematocrit of 25 being coded as anemia; potassium level of 2.6 being coded as hypokalemia), this presumes that the physician documentation is clinically valid based on the patient's clinical indicators, which are based on criteria established by a facility or a payer. In supporting ICD-10-CM coding essential to RA, physicians and their facilities must work closely with each other to establish criteria that would defend clinical validity of documented diagnoses reported with ICD-10-CM codes and be prepared to address differences of opinion between the physician and any auditing entity (eg, the Office of Inspector General, the Department of Justice, or an RA Data Validator).

CLINICAL CODING EXAMPLE

A common mistake for physicians coding from an EHR pick-list or drop-down menu is to choose the top diagnosis in the pick-list of diagnoses (eg, as a diagnosis of alcoholic esophageal varices with bleeding):

Esophageal varices, I85.00

However, I85.00, *Esophageal varices without bleeding,* does not describe the patient with bleeding varices secondary to alcoholic liver disease in the setting of alcohol dependence. The pick-list does not include crucial instructions. In referencing the full code set, the entries in the Alphabetic Index for esophageal varices read:

Index

Varix (lower limb) (ruptured) I83.90
  esophagus (idiopathic) (primary) (ulcerated) I85.00
    bleeding I84.01
    congenital Q27.8
    in (due to)
      alcoholic liver disease I85.10
        bleeding I85.11

By using the Alphabetic index, the reader discovers that there are codes specific to bleeding varices of the esophagus, in addition to codes specifying varices due to alcohol dependence. Following the instructions from the guideline, the reader next reviews the Tabular List entry:

Tabular List

I85 Esophageal varices
  Use additional code to identify:
    alcohol abuse and dependence (F10.-)

  I85.0 Esophageal varices
    Idiopathic esophageal varices
    Primary esophageal varices

    I85.00 Esophageal varices without bleeding
      Esophageal varices NOS

    I85.01 Esophageal varices with bleeding

  I85.1 Secondary esophageal varices
    Esophageal varices secondary to alcoholic liver disease
    Esophageal varices secondary to cirrhosis of liver
    Esophageal varices secondary to schistosomiasis
    Esophageal varices secondary to toxic liver disease
    Code first underlying disease

    I85.10 Secondary esophageal varices without bleeding

    I85.11 Secondary esophageal varices with bleeding

Following the Tabular entry to I85.11, the coder finds an instruction to "Code first underlying disease." In this case, it would be the underlying documented liver disease, given its listing in the ICD-10-CM Alphabetic Index. In addition, use an additional code to capture any documented alcohol abuse or dependence. As such, alcohol dependence (F10.288, *Alcohol dependence with other alcohol-induced disorders*) would be coded and sequenced after the esophageal varices code. A diagnosis of esophageal varices risk-adjusts to HCC 27, with a weight of 0.962, and the alcohol dependence risk-adjusts to HCC 55, with a value of 0.383. A query would be needed to determine what the nature of the underlying alcoholic liver disease is so that it may be coded based on physician documentation.

Documented Nomenclature

Coders should never make assumptions regarding the language of the record. Accuracy demands that the documented language record be abstracted exactly. If the physician describes a "mass," use the term "mass" in the Alphabetic Index look-up. The term "mass" may produce different results than "lump," "tumor," or "lesion," depending on the site.

EXAMPLE

Coders must use the language in the record. Physicians choose their nomenclature carefully. Different terms yield different results from the ICD-10-CM Alphabetic Index. It would be a mistake, eg, to assume that "mass" is a synonym for "tumor" in code lookup:

Mass, liver
R16.0 Hepatomegaly, not elsewhere classified

Lesion, liver
K76.9 Liver disease, unspecified

Lump, see Mass
R16.0 Hepatomegaly, not elsewhere classified

Tumor, liver (see also Neoplasm, unspecified behavior, by site)
D49.0 Neoplasm of unspecified behavior of digestive system

 ADVICE/ALERT NOTE

"It is reasonable for physicians (and other providers) to ask: what duty do they owe the federal healthcare programs? The answer is that all healthcare providers have a duty to reasonably ensure that the claims submitted to Medicare and other federal healthcare programs are true and accurate."[1]

The Right Resources

ICD-10-CM Guidelines are essential to proper code abstraction, but they are not embedded in the code set or most EHRs. It is the responsibility of anyone assigning diagnostic codes to ensure the Guidelines are being followed, and that code selection aligns with the advice of AHA's *Coding Clinic*. AHA's *Coding Clinic* is a quarterly publication that provides advice in addition to those found in the Guidelines.

In addition, AHA's *Coding Clinic* offers a free service of providing official ICD-10-CM coding advice through their website at https://www.codingclinicadvisor.com/, which may be used in defining and defending coding policies and procedures. CMS expects AHA's *Coding Clinic* advice to be followed in light of the current or recently amended conventions outlined in the ICD-10-CM Alphabetic Index, Tabular List, and the ICD-10-CM Guidelines. Failure to do so can affect the accuracy of RA.

EXAMPLE

AHA *Coding Clinic*® *for ICD-10-CM and ICD-10-PCS* (First Quarter, 2017)[17]

Upper or Lower Extremity Weakness Following Acute Cerebrovascular Accident

Question: A patient presented with weakness of the right arm due to an old cerebrovascular accident (CVA). The provider documented, "h/o CVA with mild residual right arm weakness." How would weakness of one extremity (upper or lower) be coded in a patient who is post CVA?

Answer: Assign the appropriate code from subcategory I69.33-, *Monoplegia of upper limb following cerebral infarction*, or I69.34-, *Monoplegia of lower limb following cerebral infarction*, for upper or lower limb weakness that is clearly associated with a CVA.

Note how this advice is crucial to RA in that there is no listing in the ICD-10-CM Alphabetic Index to Diseases for the term "monoparesis"; however, this advice allows a coder to equate the clinical indicators of monoparesis (weakness instead of paralysis of one extremity) with "monoplegia," when one upper or lower extremity's weakness is clearly associated with a CVA.

In addition, it is important to note that the previous advice in AHA's *Coding Clinic* (First Quarter, 2015) states that "[w]hen unilateral weakness is clearly documented as being associated with a stroke, it is considered synonymous with hemiparesis or hemiplegia. Unilateral weakness outside of this clear association cannot be assumed as hemiparesis/hemiplegia, unless it is associated with some other brain disorder or injury."[18] This same logic would apply to upper or lower limb weakness that is clearly associated with a stroke.

References

1. Office of Inspector General. OIG Compliance Program for Individual and Small Group Physician Practices. *Fed Regist.* 2000;65(194). https://oig.hhs.gov/authorities/docs/physician.pdf. Accessed Oct 20, 2017.
2. Centers for Medicare & Medicaid Services. 1995 Documentation Guidelines for Evaluation and Management Services. In: *Medicare Physician Guide.* https://www.cms.gov/outreach-and-education/medicare-learning-network-mln/mlnedwebguide/downloads/95docguidelines.pdf. Accessed Oct 20, 2017.
3. Centers for Disease Control and Prevention. *ICD-10-CM Official Guidelines for Coding and Reporting* (FY 2018). https://www.cdc.gov/nchs/data/icd/10cmguidelines_fy2018_final.pdf. Accessed Oct 30, 2017.
4. Centers for Medicare & Medicaid Services. Module 7.1.1 RADV–Purpose, Method, and Objectives. In: *2008 Risk Adjustment Data Technical Assistance for Medicare Advantage Organizations Participant Guide.* https://www.csscoperations.com/internet/Cssc.nsf/files/2008-resource-guide_060109.pdf/$FIle/2008-resource-guide_060109.pdf. Accessed Nov 1, 2017.
5. Centers for Medicare & Medicaid Services. *Contract-Level Risk Adjustment Data Validation Medical Record Reviewer Guidance (As of 09/27/2017*).* https://www.cms.gov/Research-Statistics-Data-and-Systems/Monitoring-Programs/Medicare-Risk-Adjustment-Data-Validation-Program/Other-Content-Types/RADV-Docs/Coders-Guidance.pdf. Accessed Nov 1, 2017.
6. American Hospital Association. *Coding Clinic® for ICD-9-CM Q3.* 2013;30(3): 27-28.
7. Centers for Medicare & Medicaid Services. *Risk Adjustment Data Validation (RADV) Medical Record Checklist and Guidance.* https://www.cms.gov/Medicare/Medicare-Advantage/Plan-Payment/Downloads/radvchecklist.pdf. Accessed Nov 1, 2017.
8. American Hospital Association. *Coding Clinic® for ICD-10-CM and ICD-10-PCS Q1.* 2014;1(1):13.
9. Johannesen KM, Bodtger U. Lemierre's Syndrome: Current Perspectives on Diagnosis and Management. *Infect Drug Resist.* 2016;9:221-227. https://doi.org/10.2147/IDR.S95050. Accessed Nov 1, 2017.
10. Lemierre A. On Certain Septicaemia Due to Anaerobic Organisms. *Lancet.* 1936;227:701-703.
11. Alfreijat M. A Case of Lemierre's Syndrome with a Brief Literature Review. *J Infect Public Health.* 2016;9(5):681-3. http://dx.doi.org/10.1016/j.jiph.2016.01.006. Accessed Nov 1, 2017.
12. Centers for Medicare & Medicaid Services. *Risk Adjustment 101 Participant Guide (2013 National Technical Assistance).* https://www.csscoperations.com/Internet/Cssc3.Nsf/files/2013_RA101ParticipantGuide_5CR_081513.pdf/$File/2013_RA101ParticipantGuide_5CR_081513.pdf. Accessed Nov 1, 2017.
13. Centers for Medicare & Medicaid Services. *2008 Risk Adjustment Data Technical Assistance for Medicare Advantage Organizations Participant Guide.* https://www.csscoperations.com/mwg-internal/de5fs23hu73ds/progress?id=04WTUGzH8NVu7krDOTYPeYjddO9VvdH6yE8I9-B9MLA. Accessed Nov 1, 2017.
14. Medicare Learning Network. 1997 Documentation Guidelines for Evaluation and Management Services. In: *Evaluation and Management Services.* https://www.cms.gov/Outreach-and-Education/Medicare-Learning-Network-MLN/MLNProducts/Downloads/eval-mgmt-serv-guide-ICN006764.pdf. Accessed Oct 20, 2017.
15. American Hospital Association. *Coding Clinic® for ICD-10-CM and ICD-10-PCS Q4.* 2016;3(4): 27-28.
16. American Hospital Association. *Coding Clinic® for ICD-10-CM and ICD-10-PCS Q4.* 2016;3(4):147-149.
17. American Hospital Association. *Coding Clinic® for ICD-10-CM and ICD-10-PCS Q1.* 2017;4(1):47-48.
18. American Hospital Association. *Coding Clinic® for ICD-10-CM and ICD-10-PCS Q1.* 2015;2(1):25.

Evaluate Your Understanding

The following questions are critical checkpoints that are meant to let you apply your critical thinking and evaluate your understanding of the content covered in this chapter. The answers for the end-of-chapter exercises are available in Appendix C. In addition, the Internet-based Exercises are additional learning and research opportunities to learn more about the topics related to this chapter.

A Answer Questions

Provide the answer(s) to each of the following questions.

1. Etiology and manifestation have a relationship that is:
   A. Irrelevant
   B. Assumed
   C. Causal
   D. History
2. Which of the following is an acceptable source for coding?
   A. PMH
   B. Cloned problem list
   C. HPI
   D. Medication list
3. In a SOAP note, "Refer to neurology clinic" would fall into which category?
   A. S
   B. O
   C. A
   D. P
4. Which of the following is a risk-adjusting condition?
   A. Personal history of immunosuppression therapy
   B. Personal history of excision of right forefoot
   C. Personal history of removal of kidney
   D. Personal history of colon cancer
5. This term(s), when it appears in the ICD-10-CM Alphabetic Index, links two conditions together as etiology and manifestation even without explicit documentation by the physician.
   A. Due to
   B. And
   C. And/or
   D. With
6. When the following phrase appears with a code, a second code is required for complete code assignment:
   A. Code first
   B. Code also
   C. Use additional code
   D. And
7. The patient is documented as having history of breast cancer on 1/1/2018; breast cancer on 2/1/2018; and history of breast cancer on 3/1/2018. Without the ability to query the physician, the coder should:
   A. Report history of breast cancer for January, breast cancer for February, and history of breast cancer for March.
   B. Report breast cancer for January and February, and history of breast cancer for March.
   C. Report history of breast cancer for all three months.
   D. Report breast cancer for all three months.
8. The physician documents "F01.51 dementia, stable." In an audit, the correct coding would be:
   A. No code
   B. F03.90, *Unspecified dementia without behavioral disturbance*
   C. F01.50, *Vascular dementia without behavioral disturbance*
   D. F01.51, *Vascular dementia with behavioral disturbance*
9. When abstracting a code using ICD-10-CM, start in the:
   A. Guidelines
   B. Tabular section
   C. Index
   D. Pick list
10. Under which of the following circumstances may acronyms safely be used in the medical record?
   A. When they are commonly accepted in that specialty
   B. When the practice develops a list of acceptable acronyms or the acronym is in the ICD-10-CM Alphabetic Index to Diseases
   C. When the first reference is spelled out
   D. B and C

B Internet-based Exercises

1. Medication lookup sources are available at www.rxlist.com and www.drugs.com. Note that the Indications section identifies diagnoses for a specific prescribed drug.
2. To find out more about the origins of and information about WHO's ICD-10 code set, visit www.who.int/classifications/icd/en/.
3. Learn about Great Britain's approach to risk adjustment at www.apixio.com/what-america-can-learn-from-the-u-k-s-experience-with-risk-adjustment-and-population-health/.
4. *For the Record* magazine discusses support for secondary diagnoses in RA coding at www.fortherecordmag.com/archives/0916p10.shtml.
5. Download a PDF of the *ICD-10-CM Official Guidelines* at https://www.cdc.gov/nchs/icd/icd10cm.htm.

C Audit Exercises

Review the following clinical scenario and answer the questions that follow.

Megan Boyd (76 YO [year old]) DOS [date of service] 3/1/2018 DOB [date of birth] 2/15/1942

Past Medical History
- Mixed hyperlipidemia
- Cerebrovascular accident
- Congestive heart failure (CHF)
- Atrial fibrillation
- Aortic valve regurgitation
- Cardiomyopathy
- Osteoporosis

Medication List: Reconciled 3/1/2018
- Atorvastatin 10 mg tab once weekly
- Lisinopril 2.5 mg tab twice daily
- Digoxin 125 mcg tab every other day
- Metoprolol succinate ER 50 mg tab twice daily
- Rivaroxaban 20 mg tab daily
- Vitamin D 1000 unit cap daily
- Ensure shakes

Laboratory Studies
CMP, Serum or Plasma

Results:
- Sodium: 138 (Normal)
- Potassium: 4.4 (Normal)
- Chloride: 102 (Normal)
- Carbon Dioxide: 24 (Normal)
- Creatinine: 0.9 (Normal)
- Glomerular Filtration Rate: 60 (Normal)
- Glucose: 189 (High)
- Calcium: 9.3 (Normal)
- Total Bilirubin: 0.6 (Normal)
- Aspartate Amino Transferase: 15 (Normal)
- Alanine Aminotransferase: 42 (Normal)
- Total Protein: 7.6 (Normal)
- Albumin: 3.9 (Normal)
- Alkaline Phosphatase: 95 (Normal)

S: Patient is being seen today for a check-up for her CHF, mixed hyperlipidemia, and atrial fibrillation. Ms Boyd reports she has been feeling well, a little dizzy at times, but less now that she has stopped taking furosemide. She states her left-sided weakness is improving with physical therapy. She reports no chest pain or palpitations. She reports no abdominal pain or swelling. She reports no depression. She does report problems sleeping more than three hours a night, and she has no appetite.

Clinical Documentation and Coding for RA

O: Patient is a 76-year-old underweight female.

VITALS: Ht: 5 ft 4 in Wt 109 lb BMI 18.7

Psychiatric: Good judgment and affect [display of emotions in facial expressions]. Normal mood.

Neck: No carotid bruit.

Lungs: Auscultation: breath sounds normal. Good air movement. No wheeze, rhonchi, or rales.

Cardiovascular: Auscultation: normal S1, S2. Murmur and irregular beat. No JVD [jugular vein distention].

Abdomen: Bowel sounds normal.

Musculoskeletal: 3/5 strength L upper and lower extremities. No cyanosis or edema.

Neurological: Irregular gait. Cranial nerves intact.

A/P:

1. Cerebrovascular accident. Continue PT for left-sided weakness.
2. Atrial fibrillation. Continue rivaroxaban, metopropol, digoxin.
3. Congestive heart failure. Continue without furosemide provided she has no edema.
4. Hyperlipidemia. Continue weekly statin.

This chart was electronically signed by Orville Hawkins at 12:49 p.m. on 3/1/2018

Codes submitted:

I50.9 Heart failure unspecified

I48.91 Unspecified atrial fibrillation

I63.9 Cerebral infarction, unspecified

R00.9 Unspecified abnormalities of heart beat

E78.5 Hyperlipidemia, unspecified

1. Which codes, as reported, are supported and correctly abstracted?
   A. I50.9, I48.91, I63.9, R00.9, E78.5
   B. I50.9, I48.91, I63.9, R00.9
   C. I50.9, I48.91, I63.9
   D. I50.9, I48.91
2. Should the patient's left-sided weakness be reported, and if so, with which code?
   A. No, left-sided weakness is not in the assessment. Omit this diagnosis.
   B. Yes, I69.954, *Hemiplegia and hemiparesis following unspecified cerebrovascular disease affecting left non-dominant side*
   C. Yes, R26.89, *Other abnormalities of gait and mobility*
   D. Yes, R53.1, *Weakness*
3. From a clinical documentation improvement perspective, are there any measurements or test values in this note that could be further addressed?
   A. BMI
   B. JVD
   C. Glucose
   D. A and C

4. Osteoporosis, a chronic condition, is noted in the PMH but nowhere else in the note, and so it is not reported. Supposing local coding policy allows diagnoses in PMH to be reported when supported in the medical record, which documentation element in this note might support a PMH of osteoporosis?
   A. Vitamin D 1000 unit cap daily
   B. Calcium: 9.3 Normal
   C. 3/5 strength L upper and lower extremities
   D. None of the above

5. Are there any administrative errors in this record?
   A. Yes, the patient is not authenticated.
   B. Yes, the DOS is not authenticated.
   C. Yes, the provider is not authenticated.
   D. No, this record is administratively correct.

CHAPTER 4

Clinical Documentation Integrity and Coding

PART 1: TOPICS A–C

The illusion of expertise is something to watch out for in the ever-evolving world of medical coding and documentation. Rules change, and inattentive coders break them. Codes change, and documentation crucial to code selection is not entered into the medical record. Adaptability is essential, but everyone must also develop proper habits—not only physicians but also coding and documentation experts. Take the time to be logical, methodical, and resourceful, and resolution to a risk-adjustment (RA) puzzle can usually be found. Make assumptions, and errors will follow.

The goal of this chapter is to reduce documentation and coding errors of commission and omission by centralizing guidance for ICD-10-CM–pertinent documentation and coding of conditions that risk-adjust for Medicare Advantage (MA). Organized alphabetically by diagnostic topic, it is a quick look-up tool for guidance and tips pertaining to the documentation and coding for ICD-10-CM. While HHS-HCCs for Affordable Care Act risk pools are not addressed individually in this publication, many of the same diagnoses are included in both payment systems, and coding and documentation guidance applies to either one. For simplicity, CMS-HCCs and RxHCCs for MA plans will be identified simply as HCCs and RxHCCs.

Sometimes a topic in this chapter covers a single HCC or RxHCC, and sometimes multiple HCCs and RxHCCs are grouped together under one topic. In some instances, HCCs and RxHCCs share the same title and codes (eg, HCC 1, *HIV/AIDS*, and RxHCC 1, *HIV/AIDS*). For other diagnoses, HCCs and RxHCCs are not defined identically (eg, HCC 58, *Major depressive, bipolar, and paranoid disorders*, but RxHCC 132, *Major depression*, and RxHCC 134, *Depression*). When the HCC and RxHCC titles differ, the RxHCC is listed on a separate line from the associated HCC. Some topics are grouped together for discussion, for example, HIV/AIDS and opportunistic infections.

For quick reference, a single RA value representing only the 2018 community aged rate, non-low income group, is provided for each HCC and RxHCC discussed in this chapter. See Appendix A for the complete contents of the 2017 Attachment IV and 2018 Table VII-5 from the Medicare Advantage and

Part D payment policies, both of which are current for reporting in calendar year 2018. The Appendix A tables contain the unabridged table of factors for calculating RA. (Appendix B contains a table with all ICD-10-CM codes that risk-adjust for Medicare Advantage in alphanumeric order, with their associated HCCs and RxHCCs.)

In this chapter, when the HCC or RxHCC value is listed as N/A, it indicates there is no HCC for the community, non-low-income, aged category; however, the low income or disabled category for that HCC or RxHCC has a value (see Table 4-1.1).

TABLE 4-1.1 2017 CMS-HCC Model Relative Factors for Community and Institutional Beneficiaries

VARIABLE	DISEASE GROUP	COMMUNITY, NON-LOW INCOME, AGE ≥ 65	COMMUNITY, NON-LOW INCOME, AGE <65	COMMUNITY, LOW INCOME, AGE ≥ 65	COMMUNITY, LOW INCOME, AGE < 65	INSTITUTIONAL
RxHCC 146	Profound or Severe Intellectual Disability/ Developmental disorder	–	0.172	0.368	0.334	N/A
RxHCC 147	Moderate Intellectual Disability/ Developmental disorder	–	–	0.240	0.158	N/A
RxHCC 148	Mild or Unspecified Intellectual Disability/ Developmental disorder	–	–	0.098	0.033	

In some cases, two HCCs or RxHCCs may have the same RA factor (RAF) listed. These HCCs or RxHCCs are not combined because their RAFs differ in value in other categories (see Table 4-1.2).

TABLE 4-1.2 2017 CMS-HCC Model Relative Factors for Community and Institutional Beneficiaries

VARIABLE	DISEASE GROUP	COMMUNITY, NON-LOW INCOME, AGE≥65	COMMUNITY, NON-LOW INCOME, AGE<65	COMMUNITY, LOW INCOME, AGE ≥65	COMMUNITY, LOW INCOME, AGE<65	INSTITUTIONAL
RxHCC 133	Specified Anxiety, Personality, and Behavioral Disorders	0.127	0.172	0.143	0.311	0.108
RxHCC 134	Depression	0.127	0.172	0.137	0.206	0.108

Most diagnoses and HCCs are illustrated with examples of good and bad documentation and contain coding exercises that are either abbreviated scenarios or complete encounter notes. Answers to all exercises are in Appendix C. Rare disorders or those uncommon in the Medicare population (eg, hereditary metabolic disorders and cystic fibrosis) will be brief and not include any documentation or coding examples. Resources instead will focus on common HCC and RxHCC diagnoses (eg, hypertension, chronic obstructive pulmonary disease [COPD], neoplasms, ischemic heart disease, and congestive heart failure) and on diagnoses that are prone to documentation or coding errors or omissions (eg, diabetes mellitus, depression, renal failure, drug/alcohol use disorders, cerebrovascular disease, and peripheral vascular disease).

There will be some guidance included in this chapter for codes that may not risk-adjust. In some cases, these codes illustrate how word choice in documentation can change the coding from a RA diagnosis to a diagnosis that does not risk-adjust. In some cases, the codes will reflect ICD-10-CM conventions (eg, a "Use additional code" note/guidance in the circulatory and respiratory system chapters indicates that tobacco disorders must be reported in addition to the circulatory or respiratory condition). Organizations that choose to abstract only those codes that risk-adjust may want to consider the implications of this decision, since this can negatively affect compliant coding. For example, a patient with cardiomyopathy caused by gout would normally be reported with codes I43, *Cardiomyopathy in diseases classified elsewhere,* and M10.00, *Idiopathic gout, unspecified site*. While code I43 maps for RA, code M10.00 does not. A note under code I43 instructs coders to "Code first underlying condition." Without the gout code, the cardiomyopathy code would be rejected as an unsupported manifestation code. ICD-10-CM Guideline Section I(A.13) states, "'In diseases classified elsewhere' codes are never permitted to be used as first-listed or principal diagnosis codes. They must be used in conjunction with an underlying condition code."[1]

The information in this chapter is current as of January 1, 2018. Any subsequent advice from the National Centers for Health Statistics, the American Hospital Association's (AHA's) *Coding Clinic for ICD-10-CM and ICD-10-PCS* (*Coding Clinic*), or the Centers for Medicare & Medicaid Services (CMS) advice supersedes what is written here. As with all coding resources, confirm codes in the current year's ICD-10-CM, and read all pertinent instructions within the codebook and official guidelines and advice before making a final code selection. The guidance within this chapter does not negate the responsibility of the physician or coder to document and abstract compliantly.

AIDS *see* HIV and Opportunistic Infections

Alcohol Use Disorders *see* Drug/ Alcohol Use Disorders

Alzheimer's Disease *see* Dementia

Amputation

Traumatic amputations and complications
HCC 173 0.266

Amputation status, lower limb/amputation complications
HCC 189 0.588

Lower-limb amputation status is a commonly missed HCC in RA documentation and coding. According to the Centers for Disease Control and Prevention (CDC), 60% of non-traumatic lower-limb amputations of adults occur in patients with diabetes. The National Limb Loss Information Center reports that dysvascular amputations have historically accounted for 82% of hospital discharges related to limb loss.[2] Dysvascular amputations almost always affect lower limbs. Peripheral arterial disease (PAD) is a common complication of diabetes, and a common form of dysvascular disease. In PAD, the arterial blood supply to the extremities is compromised, and as the PAD progresses, it may cause ischemic injury to lower extremity (LE) tissue. Lower-limb loss increases a patient's risk for obesity, cardiovascular disease, and depression. The five-year mortality rate following lower-limb amputation due to disease is more than 50%, and the one-year mortality rate for patients over 65 is 36%. Patients with lower-limb amputation are at a much higher risk of subsequent amputation of their remaining intact limbs, according to the Amputee Coalition.[3]

Dysvascular
Poor or impaired vascular systems, usually relating to ischemic lower extremities as seen in patients with diabetes and peripheral arterial disease.

Physician Documentation

Because a lower-limb amputation puts the patient at risk for further lower-limb loss, physicians should perform regular examinations of the patient's lower extremities and document the existence of any lower-limb amputation including its level, laterality, and its impact on the patient's current health. Even stating that the patient is coping well with the amputation demonstrates the physician's assessment of the patient's current status.

DOCUMENTATION TIP Amputation status for LE body parts (except the knee joint and/or hip joint alone) is a significant CMS-HCC and must be addressed and reported annually to capture the condition. While not affecting CMS-HCCs for physicians and MA plans, upper-extremity amputation status affects the RA for companies offering insurance on the HHS healthcare exchange (HHS-HCCs). CMS' methodology for RA is to start each enrollee's year with zero HCCs assigned to a patient, and comorbidities are tallied only when the physician addresses them and the care is documented and abstracted from the chart and submitted to CMS each new year. Physicians who are not "treating" the patient's existing and healed amputation are nevertheless considering the amputation when weighing the patient's health status as the amputation relates to overall health and wellness, vascular disease, neuropathy, ambulation, and behavioral health. The amputation should be noted and coded.

Address and document the root cause of the amputation, as the underlying condition(s) (PAD, diabetes, etc) may require ongoing treatment to preserve the contralateral leg. If the patient has diabetes and PAD, document both conditions. Also note any current foot ulcer and specify whether it is due to diabetes or a pressure sore, as 85% of diabetes-related amputations are preceded by a foot ulcer. The Amputee Coalition recommends routine foot inspection, proper shoes and orthotics, and patient education to reduce the incidence of wounds and secondary infections, which may lead to subsequent amputations among the diabetic population. Document any current nicotine or tobacco dependence (note that ICD-10-CM classifies the documentation of "smoker" as nicotine dependence) or previous history of tobacco use or nicotine dependence that is currently in remission and any hyperlipidemia, autonomic or peripheral neuropathy, or hypertension (see Table 4-1.3). Along with diabetes, all of these conditions can contribute to the patient's health status and impact circulatory health.

TABLE 4-1.3 Common Tobacco Use and History Codes

CODE	DESCRIPTION
F17.210	Nicotine dependence, cigarettes, uncomplicated
F17.211	Nicotine dependence, cigarettes, in remission
F17.218	Nicotine dependence, cigarettes with other nicotine-induced disorders
Z72.0	Tobacco use
Z77.22	Contact with and (suspected) exposure to environmental tobacco smoke (acute) (chronic)
Z87.891	Personal history of nicotine dependence

Late effects of amputation (eg, phantom limb syndrome or neuroma of amputation stump) are risk-adjusting diagnoses, regardless of site. These, too, should be documented at least annually. Describe the late effect and document that it is linked to the amputation. Document a care treatment plan.

CLINICAL EXAMPLES

NONSPECIFIC DOCUMENTATION	SPECIFIC DOCUMENTATION
Example 1 67-year-old needs prosthesis evaluation.[a]	**Example 1** 67-year-old with right below-knee amputation (BKA) is here today to evaluate advancing from a wheelchair to a prosthesis now that his wound site has healed.[b]
Example 2 Physical Examination Lower extremities: No change[c]	**Example 2** Physical Examination Lower extremities: Left ankle discoloration and diminished pedal pulses associated with atherosclerosis of native arteries of the lower extremities. Right extremity: BKA status without evidence of pressure ulcers or skin irritation at the stump. Gait seems stable.[d]

[a] It is unknown whether the patient has an amputation, because a prosthesis can also be implanted. The site of the amputation must be noted in the record, and some description of the amputation and its appearance should also be noted.

[b] BKA is a widely accepted acronym for below-knee amputation, and the reason for the visit is clear in this note. Laterality is addressed, and the physician has also documented the condition of the patient's surgical site.

[c] "No change" is not acceptable documentation. Every date of service must stand on its own; so "No change" raises the question, "No change from what?"

[d] Symptoms of the atherosclerosis are clearly described, and the physician states the patient has atherosclerosis of left lower extremity, rather than a generic diagnosis of peripheral vascular disease. The amputation site is noted and its cause is described, and a reference to the effect of the amputation on the patient's gait is further evidence that the physician evaluated this amputation.

Coding

The most commonly overlooked sites for documentation of a lower-limb amputation in the medical record is the physical examination (PE) notes. Always read the entire note, and capture the LE amputation any time it is documented anywhere in the record by an acceptable physician. It may be appropriate to report LE amputation status based on past medical history (PMH) or a problem list in the physician's documentation, depending on internal policies at the workplace. Coding for an acquired absence of part or the entire lower limb is based on the site, or extent, of the amputation and laterality (see Table 4-1.4).

TABLE 4-1.4 LE Amputation Codes

SITE	RIGHT	LEFT	UNSPECIFIED
Great toe	Z89.411	Z89.412	Z89.419
Other toe(s)	Z89.421	Z89.422	Z89.429
Foot	Z89.431	Z89.432	Z89.439
Ankle	Z89.441	Z89.442	Z89.449
Below knee	Z89.511	Z89.512	Z89.519
Above knee	Z89.611	Z89.612	Z89.619

CODING TIP Most patients with amputations have related comorbidities. It is not always possible to link the amputation to the comorbidity(ies) in the coding, but the comorbidities are generally significant disorders that should be documented and coded. Examples of comorbidities often seen with amputations include diabetes, atherosclerosis, hyperlipidemia, PAD, hypertension, and nicotine dependence.

Report the acquired absence of an LE even when it was caused by trauma or a malignant neoplasm. Because the muscles used in ambulation assist in the return of venous blood to the heart, any disruption in the ability to walk can affect circulation. Amputees tend to exercise less. Amputation status always affects the health of a lower-leg amputee, even when the loss is not due to a comorbid condition, as the patient's ambulation and exercise level are usually affected.

Acquired absence of limb codes are not to be reported for congenital absence of limbs. Acquired absence of limb codes cannot be reported for the encounter during which amputation occurs; amputation status codes are reported only for subsequent encounters. Traumatic amputations also risk-adjust, but at a significantly lower rate than amputation status, capturing risks associated with the acute condition rather than the long-term effects of amputation status. Once the acute episode of care is completed for the patient with a traumatic amputation, that patient's amputation status would be reported instead, thus capturing the higher risk.

ABSTRACT & CODE IT!

Abstract and code the clinical coding example below. Check your answers against the answers in Appendix C.

Patient 1

67-year-old with right BKA is here today for fitting of his first prosthesis, now that his wound-site has healed.

Patient 2

Physical Examination

Lower extremities: bilateral ankle discoloration and diminished pedal pulses associated with peripheral vascular disease.

Left extremity: great toe absent due to surgical amputation. Gait seems stable.

Patient 3

The patient is a 69-year-old diabetic male with peripheral vascular disease, who has developed gangrene of his right fifth toe requiring a right fifth ray amputation. His blood glucose at the time of surgery is in fair control, at 163 mg/dl.

Anemia *see* Blood Disorders

Angina Pectoris *see* Ischemic Heart Disease

Anxiety Disorders *see* Behavioral Disorders

Arrest, Shock, Ventilator Status

Respiratory arrest
HCC 83 0.658

Cardio-respiratory failure and shock
HCC 84 0.302

Respirator/tracheostomy status
HCC 82 1.055

Most of the codes in this HCC grouping represent acute and life-threatening conditions for the patient, due to acute respiratory or cardiac conditions. The exceptions are chronic respiratory failure and dependence on respirator or presence of tracheostomy.

Among the conditions that map to HCC 84 are ventricular fibrillation and flutter, acute or chronic hypoxemic or hypercapnic respiratory failure (not just "oxygen dependent"), acute pulmonary (note: the documentation must be "pulmonary," not "respiratory") insufficiency that occurs after surgery, acute respiratory distress *syndrome* (not just "acute respiratory distress"), and cardiac or respiratory arrest. Cardiogenic and unspecified shock also maps to HCC 84 whereas other septic or many other specified shock maps to other HCCs (eg, HCC 2). Cardiac arrest occurs when the electrical system in the heart stops firing and contractions stop, known as asystole. The heart stops beating. There are many causes of cardiac arrest, but the most common one is ventricular fibrillation.

Physician Documentation

Respiratory failure, shock, and cardiac arrest do not occur without cause, and the cause of these conditions should be well cited in the medical record if known. Because many of these patients are hospitalized, this discussion should be explicitly documented in the inpatient record, especially the discharge summary. Unlike physician or outpatient coding, inpatient facilities may submit ICD-10-CM

Ventricular fibrillation and flutter
Life-threatening rapid and ineffectual arrhythmia in the ventricular heart and a common cause of cardiac arrest. In fibrillation, the contractions are chaotic and fast; in flutter, they are less irregular. Ventricular flutter can progress to ventricular fibrillation.

Respiratory failure
Insufficiency in the gas exchange occurring in the lungs, resulting in a low level of oxygen and/or high level of carbon dioxide in the blood. Failure may be an acute or chronic diagnosis. Respiratory failure may be due to a number of causes, including acute conditions, such as pulmonary embolism, pulmonary hypertension, pulmonary edema, acute lung injury, or shock, and/or chronic conditions, such as airway obstruction, muscular dystrophy, atelectasis, fibrosis, COPD, neurological damage, pneumothorax, or defects in the alveoli.

Pulmonary edema
Fluid collection in the alveoli of the lungs. Pulmonary edema may be cardiogenic (eg, due to congestive heart failure) or noncardiogenic (eg, due to fluid overload, aspiration, lung injury, allergic reaction, or adult respiratory distress syndrome [ARDS]).

Respiratory arrest
The cessation of independent breathing, leading to no uptake of oxygen and no elimination of carbon dioxide. This may require interventions including supply of oxygen, clearing the airway, and artificial ventilation. Respiratory arrest differs from respiratory failure in that failure has gradations; the lungs still operate, but their function is impaired, affecting oxygen and/or carbon dioxide exchange.

Shock
Shock is best defined as a life-threatening, generalized form of acute circulatory failure associated with inadequate oxygen utilization by the cells. It is a state in which the circulation is unable to deliver sufficient oxygen to meet the demands of the tissues, resulting in cellular dysfunction and dysoxia. Some clinical symptoms and signs suggest an impaired microcirculation, including mottled skin, acrocyanosis, slow capillary refill time, an increased central-to-toe temperature gradient, and elevated lactate levels.[4] While hypotension is commonly present, in the proper clinical setting, it is not required to make the diagnosis, especially if the serum lactate level is elevated.

codes based on uncertain diagnoses (eg, those qualified as possible, probable, likely, suspected) if they are documented and not just established at the time of discharge and if it is clinically congruent with the patient's treatment. It is the physician's responsibility to document the clinical evidence supporting the diagnosis and the etiology of respiratory failure, shock, or cardiac arrest or failure. For shock, proper documentation requires that the physician document its underlying cause, such as sepsis, hypovolemia, distributive mechanisms (eg, as in a systemic inflammatory response syndrome due to pancreatitis), reduced cardiac output (cardiogenic), or obstruction of the pulmonary artery as in a massive saddle pulmonary embolus.

DOCUMENTATION TIP "Acute respiratory distress" has a new code in the ICD-10-CM 2018 code set, R06.03, *Acute respiratory distress.* If more information is known about the patient's condition (eg, the patient is diagnosed with acute respiratory distress syndrome [J80], acute or chronic respiratory failure, respiratory arrest, or dependence on a respirator, document the more specific condition). Document the conditions contributing to the medical decision making (MDM) and diagnosis. "Acute respiratory distress" and "respiratory insufficiency" are symptom diagnoses that do not risk-adjust.

ICD-10-CM classifies "pulmonary insufficiency" to code J98.4, *Other disorders of lung*, unless documented as acute or chronic following surgery or involving leakage of pulmonary valve. There is no one clinical definition of "pulmonary insufficiency" especially after surgery that differentiates it from respiratory insufficiency or failure. AHA's *Coding Clinic for ICD-9-CM* (Fourth Quarter, 2011) describes pulmonary insufficiency as "conditions that only require supplemental oxygen or intensified observation."[5] "Pulmonary insufficiency" does not risk-adjust.

A coder cannot determine from diagnostic test results that a patient has respiratory failure; it must be documented by the physician. When describing respiratory failure, document as many of these elements as appropriate:

- Acute, chronic, or acute on chronic
- Presence of hypoxia or hypercapnia
- Specific respiratory status as failure, insufficiency, ARDS, or arrest
- Etiology, eg, COPD, emphysema, pneumonia (cite the organism, if known or suspected based on the antibiotics selected), or pneumoconiosis (identify external agent)
- If due to sequela of a smoke inhalation or drug overdose (identify drug)
- Chemical pneumonitis due to anesthesia
- Intubation or dependence on ventilator
- Presence of tracheostoma

In critical care records, the language of documentation is especially important because there is often an abundance of nuanced language. For example, for a patient with respiratory complications related to thoracic surgery who will require ventilation, multiple codes exist, and the language of record will aid in determining which code is appropriate, based on *insufficiency* vs *failure* or *distress*, and *acute* vs *chronic*:

J95.1	Acute pulmonary insufficiency following thoracic surgery
J95.3	Chronic pulmonary insufficiency following surgery
J95.821	Acute postprocedural respiratory failure
J95.822	Acute and chronic postprocedural respiratory failure
R06.03	Acute respiratory distress
R09.2	Respiratory arrest

It is not enough to document a code as a way of documenting the diagnosis. Codes cannot be abstracted from codes. It is the physician's responsibility to describe the diagnosis and its etiology, acuity, and manifestations. The physician's language, in combination with the ICD-10-CM Alphabetical Index, should take the abstractor to the correct code. Because many of these codes affect the hospital's Medicare severity diagnosis-related group (MS-DRG) payment and quality scores, physician practices should collaborate with their hospital's coding and clinical documentation integrity teams to assure that the physician's documentation adheres to the facility's coding compliance initiatives. Always document any existing tobacco status for a patient with any cardio-respiratory diagnosis.

DOCUMENTATION TIP Do not document acute respiratory failure (ARF) when a patient is maintained on a ventilator following surgery when the ventilator is a routine aspect of the surgery (eg, less than 48 hours or another time period negotiated with the surgical facility). Instead, report acute respiratory failure when weaning the patient from the respirator does not occur in the anticipated timeframe, when complications prevent weaning, or if the patient requires reintubation. Identify the respiratory failure as acute or chronic, whether it is a complication of the surgery, of a medication or anesthesia, or of another disease (eg, decompensated systolic or diastolic heart failure), and identify the nature of the surgery during which the patient was placed on a ventilator (eg, thoracic or neurosurgery).

Sometimes, patients are documented as being intubated "for airway protection," especially in cases of acute lung trauma. If the patient is unable to maintain the airway for ventilation, this is likely respiratory failure. If the ventilation is for prophylaxis (eg, to ensure continued breathing in the case of tracheal edema), the patient does not have respiratory failure. Be sure to the patient's condition is well documented regarding failure status so there is no error in code abstraction.

Tracheostomy status should be noted. Document if the tracheostoma is being cleansed, reformed, or closed. If there are complications, identify:

- Hemorrhage from tracheostoma
- Tracheostoma infection, and any presence of cellulitis; document infectious agent, if known
- Malfunction of tracheostoma
- Presence of tracheostoma fistula

For cardiac arrest, document the etiology (eg, ventricular fibrillation or flutter, ischemic heart disease [especially if a myocardial infarction occurred], pulmonary embolism, or long QT syndrome). ICD-10-CM instructs coders to first code the underlying condition for category I46, *Cardiac arrest*, if it is known. If cardiac arrest is the result of a procedure, document whether the arrest occurred intra-operatively or postoperatively. Document the nature of the procedure, too.

In critical care, document the diagnosis in addition to the signs and symptoms that lead to it. For example, in this documentation excerpt, "72 year old woman with CAD, hypotension, and dyspnea requires hemodynamic monitoring. A PA catheter reveals significantly low CO_2 [carbon dioxide]," the documentation is detailed, but it provides no diagnosis. If the patient has a diagnosis of cardiogenic shock, note it and any coexisting systolic or diastolic heart failure, as well as its underlying cause specifically. To avoid confusion, spell out the first reference of a diagnosis (eg, cardiac arrest [CA]).

CLINICAL EXAMPLES

NONSPECIFIC DOCUMENTATION	SPECIFIC DOCUMENTATION
Example 1 Severe sepsis with ARF[a]	**Example 1** Severe sepsis due to methicillin resistant *Staphylococcus aureus* (MRSA) intertrigo of groin with acute on chronic respiratory failure with hypoxia[b]
Example 2 Procedure: Tracheostomy creation Preoperative diagnosis: Respiratory failure[c]	**Example 2** Procedure: Tracheostomy creation Preoperative diagnosis: Acute on chronic respiratory failure with hypoxemia secondary to amyotrophic lateral sclerosis (ALS)[d]

[a] ARF is ambiguous and may be interpreted as acute respiratory failure, acute renal failure, or acute rheumatic fever.

[b] With a few words, much information is conveyed here. The infective agent for the sepsis, the infection site, and the type of organ failure, as well as the presence of hypoxia.

[c] More information on the etiology of the respiratory failure and its severity is needed.

[d] Noted here is the acuity of the respiratory failure, the presence of hypoxemia, and the etiology of the failure (ALS).

Coding

Signs and symptoms of respiratory failure include hypercapnia, hypoxemia, tachypnea, accessory muscle use, and asynchronous respirations. Intubation or tracheostoma is not required for a respiratory failure diagnosis. Codes for respiratory distress and failure that are included in the CMS RA model are in Table 4-1.5.

TABLE 4-1.5 Respiratory Distress and Failure Codes Included in CMS RA Model

DESCRIPTION	CODE
Acute respiratory distress syndrome	J80
Acute pulmonary insufficiency following thoracic surgery	J95.1
Acute pulmonary insufficiency following nonthoracic surgery	J95.2
Chronic pulmonary insufficiency following surgery	J95.3
Acute postprocedural respiratory failure	J95.821
Acute and chronic postprocedural respiratory failure	J95.822
Acute respiratory failure, unspecified whether with hypoxia or hypercapnia	J96.00
Acute respiratory failure with hypoxia	J96.01
Acute respiratory failure with hypercapnia	J96.02
Chronic respiratory failure, unspecified whether with hypoxia or hypercapnia	J96.10
Chronic respiratory failure with hypoxia	J96.11
Chronic respiratory failure with hypercapnia	J96.12
Acute and chronic respiratory failure, unspecified whether with hypoxia or hypercapnia	J96.20
Acute and chronic respiratory failure with hypoxia	J96.21
Acute and chronic respiratory failure with hypercapnia	J96.22
Respiratory failure unspecified, unspecified whether with hypoxia or hypercapnia	J96.90
Respiratory failure, unspecified with hypoxia	J96.91
Respiratory failure, unspecified with hypercapnia	J96.92
Respiratory arrest	R09.2

According to ICD-10-CM Guideline Section I(C.10.d.1), "[c]ode J95.851, *Ventilator associated pneumonia*, should be assigned only when the physician has documented ventilator associated pneumonia (VAP). An additional code to identify the organism (e.g., *Pseudomonas aeruginosa*, code B96.5) should also be assigned. Do not assign an additional code from categories J12-J18 to identify the type of pneumonia.

Code J95.851 should not be assigned for cases where the patient has pneumonia and is on a mechanical ventilator and the physician has not specifically stated that the pneumonia is ventilator-associated pneumonia."[1]

CODING TIP Oxygen delivered via a tracheal mask, nasal cannula, CPAP, or BiPAP does not constitute ventilator status.

CODING TIP Code R06.03, *Acute respiratory distress,* is new for 2018 and represents labored breathing without evidence of respiratory failure. This code may be reported for a child or an adult. Note that while code J80, *Acute respiratory distress syndrome*, risk-adjusts, code R06.03 describes a symptom and does not risk-adjust.

ADVICE/ALERT NOTE

Per ICD-10-CM Guideline Section I(C.10.d.1), "[c]ode J95.851, *Ventilator associated pneumonia*, should be assigned only when the physician has documented ventilator associated pneumonia (VAP). An additional code to identify the organism (e.g., *Pseudomonas aeruginosa*, code B96.5) should also be assigned. Do not assign an additional code from categories J12-J18 to identify the type of pneumonia.

Code J95.851 should not be assigned for cases where the patient has pneumonia and is on a mechanical ventilator and the physician has not specifically stated that the pneumonia is ventilator-associated pneumonia."[1]

Do not report code J80, *Acute respiratory distress syndrome* (ARDS), when "respiratory distress" is documented. Instead, report code R06.03, *Acute respiratory distress.* ARDS describes a life-threatening inflammatory lung condition with hypoxemia in a critically ill patient, usually occurring in conjunction with another acute condition (eg, sepsis, near-drowning, pneumonia, drug overdose, or inhalation of toxins or irritants). Do not report ARDS in conjunction with a code from category J96, *Respiratory failure, not elsewhere classified,* as instructed by Excludes1 note conventions.

A patient who has acute respiratory failure due to smoke inhalation requires at least three codes:

- One for the respiratory condition (eg, J96.00, *Acute respiratory failure, unspecified whether with hypoxemia or hypercapnia);*
- One to attribute the condition to smoke inhalation (eg, J70.5, *Respiratory conditions due to smoke inhalation);* and

Ventilator status
In patients with reduced or absent respiratory effort, mechanical inflation and deflation of the lungs for delivery of oxygen and removal of carbon dioxide is likely reduced or absent. The patient is either intubated or has a tracheostomy and placed on ventilator support. If a patient is ventilated during surgery, this does not qualify as ventilator status.

- one to identify the episode of care and external cause (eg, T59.811A, *Toxic effect of smoke, accidental [unintentional], initial encounter*).

Thoracic and other major surgery patients may be managed on a ventilator during and immediately after surgery. This does not constitute postprocedural respiratory failure. Usually, a patient will be weaned off a ventilator within 48 hours or so of surgery. Look for documentation that the patient's ventilator use is prolonged or that weaning was not successful, that it is a complication of surgery, or that the patient was re-ventilated following surgery before assigning a code for dependence on ventilation. Consult with the facility's clinical documentation integrity and coding teams as well, given that acute postprocedural respiratory failure impacts certain quality measures, such as the Agency for Healthcare Research and Quality's (AHRQ's) patient safety indicators, affecting facility quality measurements and performance.

CODING TIP AHA's *Coding Clinic* (Third Quarter, 2013) advises that catecholaminergic polymorphic tachycardia (CPVT) is reported with code I47.2, *Ventricular tachycardia*.[6] CPVT is a form of ventricular tachycardia induced by natural adrenalines during times of emotional or physical stress. CPVT occurs in a heart that is structurally normal.

ABSTRACT & CODE IT!

Abstract and code the clinical coding example below. Check your answers against the answers in Appendix C.

Patient 1

Patient with acute on chronic respiratory failure due to end-stage panlobular emphysema is admitted to the ICU with hypoxia and hypercapnia and required mechanical ventilation. The patient has a history of tobacco dependence.

Patient 2

Patient with ARDS and septic shock due to *Klebsiella pneumoniae*.

Patient 3

Patient develops acute respiratory failure two days following a left lower lobectomy for lung cancer and requires mechanical ventilation.

Arthritis and Inflammatory Disorders

Rheumatoid arthritis and inflammatory connective tissue disease
HCC 40 0.423

Psoriatic arthropathy and systemic sclerosis
RxHCC 82 0.769

Rheumatoid arthritis and other inflammatory polyarthropathy
RxHCC 83 0.377

Systemic lupus erythematosus, other connective tissue disorders, and inflammatory spondylopathies
RxHCC 84 0.212

Psoriasis, except with arthropathy
RxHCC 316 0.205

Both psoriatic and rheumatoid arthritis are chronic, systemic autoimmune disorders, presenting with painful swelling and inflammation of joints that often lead to permanent joint damage. They respond well to disease-modifying anti-rheumatic drugs (DMARDs) and pain and swelling may also be treated with anti-inflammatory medications or low-dose corticosteroids. Biologic agents are used to treat more serious cases.

While these disorders are characterized as joint disorders, they have systemic implications. The autoimmune disease that attacks the patient's joints can also damage the eyes, lungs, or heart of a patient with rheumatoid arthritis. A diagnosis of rheumatoid arthritis is based on a combination of symptoms rather than a single, definitive test. The erythrocyte sedimentation rate (ESR) and/or the C-reactive protein will likely be elevated, and the physician may also look for elevation in the rheumatoid factor, antibodies to cyclic citrullinated peptides, or other serological assays. The arthritis is bilateral. Adult rheumatoid arthritis has periods of low and high activity but is a chronic disease that will be with the patient for the patient's lifespan. Juvenile rheumatoid arthritis (JRA), also known as juvenile idiopathic arthritis, is the most common form of arthritis in children and often has a complete recovery. Recovery depends on a number of factors, including the severity of the disease at onset, damage done to joints, and the type and timing of treatment. Children who continue to have rheumatoid arthritis as they become adults still carry a diagnosis of JRA, as it is a distinct variation from other rheumatoid arthritis.

In psoriatic arthritis, the patient experiences joint pain, erythematous plaques, and changes in the nails. The arthritis is asymmetrical. Most patients will have a negative rheumatoid factor.

Psoriasis occurring without arthropathy is also an immune-mediated disorder. The most common form is plaque psoriasis, in which raised patches of dead skin develop. These can crack and bleed, causing pain and itching. Psoriasis risk-adjusts for RxHCCs. Psoriasis responds well to immunosuppressants.

Systemic lupus erythematosus (SLE) describes a systemic autoimmune disease that affects joints and organs, which usually presents as a series of flare-ups and remission, like rheumatoid and psoriatic arthritis. In SLE, inflammation and damage may be limited to the joints or may involve one or more organs. The Lupus Foundation of America estimates that about 1.5 million Americans have SLE.[7] While SLE is incurable, its symptoms are usually manageable and people usually live a normal lifespan.

Systemic sclerosis is another autoimmune rheumatic disease. Approximately 100,000 people have systemic sclerosis in the United States (US). In systemic sclerosis, collagen invades the connective tissue in an autoimmune response and causes a thickening and stiffening of the skin, esophagus, and some organs. It is incurable and life shortening. Symptoms of systemic sclerosis are treated individually and the systemic condition may be treated with immunosuppressants. Systemic sclerosis is sometimes called scleroderma.

Physician Documentation

The ICD-10-CM Alphabetic Index default for a simple note of "arthritis" is a code for unspecified osteoarthritis, unspecified site, which does not capture the severity of rheumatoid arthritis or psoriatic arthritis, or the resources required for treatment. The effects of osteoarthritis on a patient's cardiovascular system or vision are insignificant. Rheumatoid arthritis and psoriatic arthritis, conversely, can cause serious complications to many organ systems (eg, cranial nerve palsies, keratitis, retinopathy, or scleritis [seen by an ophthalmologist]). Also, treatment of rheumatoid arthritis with long-term steroids can cause cataracts. The physician, regardless of specialty, should assess how the autoimmune arthritis is affecting the rheumatoid arthritis patient. This is best for outcomes, and for medicolegal protection of the practice. It is also best for generating accurate RA scores, as only rheumatoid and psoriatic varieties of arthritis risk-adjust.

Etiology of arthritis is a critical element to documentation, but it is only the beginning. For arthritis, physicians should document the acuity as acute, chronic, or intermittent. The severity should be noted as mild, moderate, or severe. Identify the location as well as laterality, and include any associated symptoms described by the patient and current medication treating the arthritis. Do not scrimp on details in documentation. All of these elements support the medical necessity of the proscribed care treatment plan. Focus on clear documentation of arthritis regardless of whether the condition maps for RA. See Table 4-1.6 for crucial documentation elements for arthritis.

TABLE 4-1.6 Crucial Documentation Elements for Arthritis

TYPE OF ARTHRITIS	CODE CATEGORY(IES)
Pyogenic • Site(s) and laterality • Infective agent • Direct or indirect infection • Postinfective with cause, or reactive	**M00-M02**
Rheumatoid arthritis • Site(s) and laterality • Positive or negative for rheumatoid factor • Type, as juvenile type, Felty's syndrome • Manifestations, ie, organ or system involvement, bursitis, nodules, myopathy, polyneuropathy	**M05, M06, M08**
Psoriatic arthritis • Juvenile or adult • Site and laterality • Identify psoriatic arthritis mutilans, if present	**L40.5-**
Gout • Site(s) and laterality • Etiology (renal, drug, lead, idiopathic, other secondary) • Chronic or acute • With tophus	**M1A, M10**
Other crystal arthropathies • Site(s) and laterality • Type (hydroxyapatite deposition disease, familial chondrocalcinosis, or other crystal arthropathy)	**M11**
Arthritis in disease classified elsewhere • Site(s) and laterality • Etiology, eg, in infectious arthritis	**M14**
Osteoarthritis • Site(s) and laterality • Bilateral of single joint • Primary, secondary, post-traumatic (identify trauma)	**M15-M19**
Other • Site(s) and laterality • Document etiology as postrheumatic and chronic, Kaschin-Beck, villonodular synovitis, palindromic rheumatism, intermittent hydrarthrosis, transient, allergic, monoarthritis NOS	**M12, M13**

DOCUMENTATION TIP JRA is not simply a childhood version of rheumatoid arthritis. The juvenile variant of rheumatoid arthritis can completely resolve or continue into adulthood. Rheumatoid arthritis, conversely, is a lifelong disease. For patients with rheumatoid arthritis, identify the type as adult-onset or juvenile onset. If an adult patient has a form of rheumatoid arthritis that originated in childhood, document JRA. The age of onset determines whether the patient has rheumatoid arthritis or JRA.

Do not rely on the medication list to document the patient's current long-term medications. Address in the note for the current encounter the drugs being used to treat the patient's condition by documenting any current use of aspirin, NSAIDs, opioids, steroids, biologics, or immunosuppressive drugs. If a patient has joint pain, stiffness, or effusion, document the specific joint and laterality.

There are four different forms of lupus: systemic lupus erythematosus (SLE), cutaneous lupus, drug-induced lupus, and neonatal lupus. In drug-induced lupus, identify the drug causing the adverse effect. Identify the type of lupus, and for SLE, identify any organ involvement. For cutaneous lupus, specify discoid lupus erythematous, subacute cutaneous erythematosus, lupus panniculitis, or lupus erythematosus profundus. Systemic scleroderma is the default for "scleroderma." Specify cutaneous scleroderma in patients with localized disease.

DOCUMENTATION TIP When the patient tests positive or negative for rheumatoid factor, document this in the note. A coder cannot infer rheumatoid arthritis with rheumatoid factor from a test value. Any interpretation of an abnormal laboratory value must be documented by the physician, in order for it to be coded compliantly.

Simply documenting "lupus" does not provide enough information for ICD-10-CM code abstraction. Define the lupus as systemic, systemic erythematous, or discoid, and by the site or organ involvement (eg, endocarditis, pericarditis, renal, or pulmonary).

CLINICAL EXAMPLES

NONSPECIFIC DOCUMENTATION	SPECIFIC DOCUMENTATION
Example 1 John Doe, 24, has had rheumatoid arthritis[a] for 12 years.	**Example 1** John Doe, 24, has had systemic juvenile arthritis for 12 years and is being seen today for bilateral arthropathies in his wrists and hands.[b]
Example 2 Rheumatoid factor results are 31 U/ml with bilateral rheumatoid arthritis of the hands and shoulders.[c]	**Example 2** Rheumatoid factor results are 31 U/ml with bilateral rheumatoid arthritis with rheumatoid factor of the hands and shoulders.[d]

[a] Document the juvenile version of rheumatoid arthritis when an adult patient has had the disease since childhood. Document joints affected and the reason for the encounter. Document the type of juvenile rheumatoid arthritis.

[b] In this case, the type (systemic), location (hands and wrists), and juvenile status of the arthritis have been captured.

[c] Rheumatoid factor cannot be interpreted by the coder, and must be documented for specificity. Document specifically rheumatoid arthritis with rheumatoid factor.

[d] Location of the arthritis is identified as well as the rheumatoid factor.

Coding

In ICD-10-CM, "arthritis" defaults to unspecified osteoarthritis of an unspecified site. Read all ICD-10-CM notes carefully and capture codes that fully report the etiology of conditions. Start with the Alphabetic Index. Although most types of arthritis are reported with codes from the ICD-10-CM musculoskeletal chapter, some forms of arthritis are reported with codes from other chapters. Notably, psoriatic arthritis is reported with codes from the Skin and Subcutaneous Tissue chapter because this type of arthritis occurs with psoriasis. Forms of infective arthritis are reported with codes from the Infectious Disease chapter (eg, A02.23, *Salmonella arthritis*).

CODING TIP The ICD-10-CM code set differentiates between patients who are immunocompromised as a result of immunosuppressants and those who are naturally immunocompromised. AHA's *Coding Clinic* (Third Quarter, 2015) advises that patients who are immunocompromised therapeutically to treat autoimmune disease do not have a diagnosis related to the immunosuppression. Instead, code the long-term use of immunosupressants with Z79.899, *Other long term (current) drug therapy.* For patients who are otherwise immunocompromised, report with code D89.9, *Disorder involving the immune mechanism, unspecified.*[8]

CODING TIP There is no available code to report bilateral rheumatoid arthritis of any joint. If the condition is bilateral, report two codes.

JRA describes a form of rheumatoid arthritis with onset in childhood. If rheumatoid arthritis is documented in a patient under 16 years old, query the physician regarding the type of rheumatoid arthritis if it is not documented as JRA. A patient diagnosed with JRA in childhood may continue to have JRA in adulthood. JRA is synonymous with juvenile idiopathic arthritis (JIA), according to the Arthritis Foundation.[9]

CODING TIP For systemic autoimmune diseases, support may be found in disease-modifying anti-rheumatic drugs (DMARDs) including methotrexate, hydroxychloroquine, azathioprine, sulfasalazine, leflunomide, cyclosporine, gold salts, D-penicillamine, and minocycline. Biologic tumor necrosis factor (TNF)-inhibiting DMARDs include etanercept, infliximab, adalimumab, certolizumab, and golimumab. Biologic no-TNF DMARDs include Rituximab, anakinra, abatacept, tocilzumab, sarlilumab, and tofacitnib.

Charcot's arthropathy in diabetes is reported with code E--.610, *Diabetes with diabetic neuropathic arthropathy*, rather than a code from category M14.6, *Charcot's joint.* A patient with rheumatoid factor in juvenile rheumatoid arthritis is reported with a code from category M08, *Juvenile arthritis*, and not category M05, *Rheumatoid arthritis with rheumatoid factor.*

CODING TIP The default for documented "scleroderma" is systemic sclerosis. There is no default for documented "lupus," but "lupus erythematosus" defaults to the local condition, code L93.0, *Discoid lupus erythematosus*. To report systemic or disseminated lupus erythematosus, the physician must document it as such. According to the ICD-10-CM Alphabetic Index, joint involvement in rheumatoid arthritis can only be reported if the physician documents that it is seropositive or seronegative for rheumatoid factor. The ICD-10-CM Tabular List does not consider antibodies to cyclic citrullinated peptides (CCPs) to be positive serologies; "seropositive" and "seronegative" referred only to the reporting of positive or negative rheumatoid factor serologies. Antibodies to anti-CCPs may be classified in subcategory M06.8, *Other specified rheumatoid arthritis*. If the physician's diagnostic statement does not discuss the presence or absence of rheumatoid factor or other antibodies or use the terms "seropositive" or "seronegative," only code M06.9, *Rheumatoid arthritis, unspecified*, may be reported.

The ICD-10-CM Alphabetic Index classifies rheumatoid arthritis as juvenile, seronegative, or seropositive, or with organ involvement. The lack of documentation of rheumatoid factor does not constitute "seronegative" rheumatoid arthritis. When rheumatoid-factor status is not documented, report code M06.9 *Rheumatoid arthritis, unspecified*, unless rheumatoid nodules or bursitis are documented. Even when affected joints are specified, documented rheumatoid arthritis without noting the rheumatoid factor is reported with code M06.9. Specific rheumatoid arthritis codes are also classified in the ICD-10-CM Alphabetic Index under "nodule" and "bursitis."

ABSTRACT & CODE IT!

Abstract and code the clinical coding example below. Check your answers against the answers in Appendix C.

CC [chief complaint]: A 46-year-old male presents for treatment of suspected rheumatoid arthritis. He describes bilateral aching joint pain and swelling that began four months ago and has been steadily worsening. He has also been experiencing fatigue and low-grade fevers.

Family History: Rheumatoid arthritis, maternal grandmother

ROS [review of systems]: All normal, with the exception of pain and swelling in upper extremities.

PE: BP Standing: 120/84 HR: 79 Temp: 99.9 Ht: 5 ft, 8 in Wt: 168 lb BMI: 25.5

Patient is a pleasant and well-nourished male with good attention to hygiene and body habitus. Skin: No skin rash, subcutaneous nodules, lesions, or ulcers observed. Palpation of skin shows no abnormalities.

HEENT [head, ears, eyes, nose, throat]: No abnormalities. Hair growth and distribution is normal. Examination of scalp shows no abnormalities. Conjunctiva and lids reveal no signs or symptoms of infection. PERRLA [pupils equal, round, reactive to light and accommodation]. Ocular motility examination reveals gross orthotropia with full ductions and versions bilateral. Bilateral retinas reveal normal color, contour, and cupping. Inspection of ears reveals no abnormalities. Otoscopic examination reveals no abnormalities. Normal oropharynx and ears.

Neck: Neck supple and trachea that is midline, without adenopathy or crepitance. Thyroid smooth and symmetric gland with no enlargement, tenderness, or masses noted. Neck lymph nodes are normal.

Respiratory: Auscultation of lungs reveals clear lung fields and no rubs noted.

Cardiovascular: Normal S1 and S2 and no murmurs, gallop, rubs, or clicks.

Abdomen: Abdominal contour is slightly rounded. Abdomen soft, nontender, bowel sounds present x4 without palpable masses. Palpation of liver reveals no abnormalities. Palpation of spleen reveals no abnormalities.

continued

Musculoskeletal: Gait and station normal. Muscle tone is normal. Some swelling and tenderness noted in each hand.

Psychiatric: Oriented to person, place, and time. Mood and affect normal.

Test Results: Rheumatoid factor: 54 U/ml. Sed rate: 34 mm/hr. C4 complement: 19 mg/dl.

Assessment: Rheumatoid arthritis, seronegative

Plan: ESR ordered; automated. Ordered RBC. Ordered quantitative rheumatoid factor. Return to clinic in 2 week(s).

Prescriptions: Rofecoxib 12.5 mg tab b.i.d.; dispense: 30, refills: 2. Referral to rheumatology clinic.

Atrial Fibrillation *see* Heart Arrhythmias

Autism

Autism
RxHCC 145 0.127

Autism spectrum disorder (ASD) begins to be noticeable once an infant is old enough to begin interacting and communicating, usually by 18 months, but the condition is usually not diagnosed until age 2 or 3 years, when the symptoms are more evident. A developmental disorder, autism affects social interaction and communication with others, greatly impairing a person's ability to develop or sustain relationships. ASD also contains an element of restrictive, repetitive patterns of behavior that affect the patient's quality of life. ASD persists throughout life, although some therapies during childhood are believed to mitigate the severity of some autism symptoms. The autism "spectrum" refers to the wide range of symptoms and severity in the disorder. Supplement the ASD diagnosis with other codes to identify its manifestations, as appropriate.

Physician Documentation

Because ASD affects many facets of a patient's physical and behavioral health, ASD should be reported as often as the diagnosis contributes to the MDM during the encounter. For example, if the patient's ASD impedes the physical examination of a child, or limits the ability to collect the medical history of an adult, the ASD should be documented as affecting the encounter. Similarly, if any disorder commonly linked to autism is addressed in the visit (eg, attention deficit disorder), the autism should be documented as the underlying cause.

Always spell out the first reference (eg, autism spectrum disorder [ASD]), as ASD can also refer to atrial septal defect, which may also be diagnosed as a congenital disorder in early childhood.

The spectrum of symptoms in autism is vast. Physicians should clearly document any behavioral or emotional comorbidities associated with ASD. Among the disorders often occurring with autism are insomnia, intellectual disabilities, epilepsy and seizure, wandering, speech or language delays, or attention deficit or hyperactivity disorders. Documenting these disorders in addition to the autism provides a complete clinical picture of the severity of the patient's condition.

CLINICAL EXAMPLES

NONSPECIFIC DOCUMENTATION	SPECIFIC DOCUMENTATION
Example 1 The patient was not forthcoming about his medical history due to his being on the spectrum.[a]	**Example 1** The patient was not forthcoming due to his being on the spectrum. His autism is relatively mild, but even so, he was not able to describe the onset of his fever.[b]
Example 2 The patient also has ASD, diagnosed when he was 3 years old.[c]	**Example 2** The patient also has autistic spectrum disorder (ASD), diagnosed when he was 3 years old.[d]

[a] The coder cannot infer words in the record. Without the word "autism," the coder cannot abstract this order.

[b] Noting autism was an impediment to obtaining the history of present illness clarifies the circumstances and protects the physician.

[c] Atrial septal defect or autism spectrum disorder? Both uses of ASD are common for pediatric patients.

[d] Acronym spelled out at first reference clarifies the diagnosis.

Coding

A diagnosis of ASD usually comes from a clinician qualified under the health plan for behavioral healthcare (eg, a licensed clinical social worker, neurologist, psychiatrist, psychologist, or physician specializing in ASD). The clinician performs an applied behavioral analysis (ABA) and develops a treatment plan.

Autism may be mild or severe; the patient with autism may be able to perform activities of daily living or may require round-the-clock supervision and support. Codes specifically for autism offer little detail about the disorder and are selected based on physician documentation:

- F84.0 Autism, NOS (**Note:** Autism spectrum disorder also uses this code)
- F84.5 Asperger's syndrome
- F84.8 Other pervasive developmental disorders
- F84.9 Pervasive developmental disorder, unspecified

Because the spectrum of comorbidities in autism varies widely, coders also should report any behavioral or emotional disorders documented in the medical record in addition to the autism. Among the pertinent disorders often occurring with ASD are insomnia, intellectual disabilities, epilepsy and/or seizure disorders, speech or language delays, and attention deficit or hyperactivity disorders.

ABSTRACT & CODE IT!

Abstract and code the clinical coding example below. Check your answers against the answers in Appendix C.

Patient 1
The psychologist has diagnosed the patient with atypical autism and mild intellectual disabilities.

Patient 2
Seven-year-old Mary, who has been diagnosed with Fragile X syndrome and autism spectrum disorder, is here today for evaluation of new onset seizures. She has had three, each lasting about 60 seconds, according to her mother.

Patient 3
Tom is 2 years old and his mother is concerned because he has no interest in communicating with his parents. I suspect autism, and have referred her to Ted Rice, pediatric psychologist, for evaluation.

Behavioral Disorders

Schizophrenia
HCC 57 0.608
RxHCC 130 0.261

Major depressive, bipolar, and paranoid disorders
HCC 58 0.395

Bipolar disorders
RxHCC 131 0.255

Major depression
RxHCC 132 0.127

Depression
RxHCC 134 0.127

Specified anxiety, personality and behavior disorders
RxHCC 133 0.127

Anxiety disorders
RxHCC 135 0.051

Many behavioral disorders risk-adjust only for RxHCCs because the conditions are managed well with prescription drugs and the conditions do not have a significant impact on the physical health of the patient or costs of care beyond medication. Schizophrenia, major depressive episodes, mania, and bipolar disorders also map to HCCs. The most severe of these conditions is schizophrenia.

Schizophrenia is a disorder in which the patient has a faulty perception of reality. Onset usually follows puberty. Approximately 3.5 million people in the US have schizophrenia, according to the Schizophrenia and Related Disorders Alliance of America.[10] Schizophrenia can be managed with antipsychotic medication, such as clozapine (Clozaril), which must be administered for one's lifetime, even if its manifestations are well controlled. One of the highest risks of schizophrenia is the risk of suicide. Between one-third and one-half of homeless adults in the US have schizophrenia.

Major depression affects 6.7% of US adults, with a significantly higher rate of depression among women than men. Bipolar disorder prevalence is 4%.[11] While substance abuse disorders are classified as behavioral disorders, they are addressed separately here under the heading, Drug/Alcohol Use Disorders, as the documentation and coding issues associated with substance abuse differ from those of other behavioral disorders.

Physician Documentation

Psychiatric conditions often affect the health and wellness of the patient and influence how well the patient will comply with any treatment plan. The trend today is to a more holistic approach toward the patient, thus psychiatric conditions are being diagnosed or treated by primary caregivers in increasing numbers. Prevention, screening, and coordination of care with behavioral health specialists help provide opportunities for earlier intervention and improved outcomes.

When a behavioral disorder is suspected but not yet confirmed, document it as "rule out" or "probable" so that the coder does not abstract the diagnosis as being established from the record. Also identify any differential diagnoses (eg, paranoid schizophrenia/paranoid personality disorder) as "probable" or "rule out" to prevent the coder from abstracting both disorders. Once a behavioral disease is confirmed, preferably using *Diagnostic and Statistical Manual of Mental Disorders , Fifth Edition* (DSM-5) criteria, document its presence even if its manifestations are well controlled with medication or active psychotherapy. Document the medications and types of therapy in use. Documentation and coding of behavioral syndromes that resolve is tricky. For example, ICD-10-CM classifies single episodes and recurrent major depressive disorders, bipolar disorders, manic episodes, alcohol and drug abuse, and alcohol and drug dependence as being "in remission" as opposed to being described as a "personal history." For behavioral disorders that resolve and do not require treatment, such as anxiety disorders, agoraphobia, personality disorders, dysthymia, and conversion disorders, it is appropriate to report code Z86.59, *Personal history of other mental and behavioral disorders*. This code does not risk-adjust.

The medical record for each date of service must stand on its own. A diagnosis in the problem list or PMH cannot be abstracted, unless it is addressed in the record for the current encounter. Use the following descriptors when documenting mood disorders:

- **Type**: Depressive, manic, or bipolar disorder
- **Episode**: Single episode or recurrent
- **Status**: Partial remission or full remission; identify most recent episode as manic, depressed, or mixed
- **Severity**: Mild, moderate, severe, or with psychotic elements

Self-harm risk-adjusts and should be documented when it occurs or when sequela is being treated. Make a note regarding the administration and results of a depression screening, and if suicide risk was assessed. Document any suicidal ideation. Document the specific treatment plan and time invested in counseling and coordination of care.

Psychosocial Circumstances and Encounters

ICD-10-CM provides codes for behaviors that have not yet been classified to behavioral disorders, but that may contribute to the need for further treatment or study. See the following table for examples of those codes, which do not risk-adjust.

Code	Description
R41.0	Disorientation, unspecified
R41.82	Altered mental status, unspecified
R41.840	Attention and concentration deficit
R44.3	Hallucinations, unspecified
R45.83	Excessive crying of child, adolescent or adult
R45.84	Anhedonia
R45.86	Emotional lability
R45.87	Impulsiveness
R46.0	Very low level of personal hygiene
R46.2	Strange and inexplicable behavior
R46.81	Obsessive-compulsive behavior

Identify post-traumatic stress disorder (PTSD) as acute or chronic. In obsessive-compulsive disorder, note any hoarding, skin-picking, obsessive acts, or neuroses. The acronym MDD may be interpreted as manic depressive disorder or major depressive disorder. Always identify an acronym by spelling it out the first time it is used (eg, major depressive disorder [MDD]).

CLINICAL EXAMPLES

NONSPECIFIC DOCUMENTATION	SPECIFIC DOCUMENTATION
Example 1 Patient is psychotic.[a]	**Example 1** Patient has paranoid psychosis.[b]
Example 2 Anorexia[c]	**Example 2** Anorexia nervosa, with purging[d]

[a] Psychotic is a vague adjective that classifies to F29, *Unspecified psychosis not due to a substance or known physiological condition.* It does not risk-adjust.

[b] This diagnoisis is indexed to F22, *Delusional disorders,* a specific diagnosis that risk-adjusts.

[c] Anorexia is a symptom, not a behavioral diagnosis. There are several codes associated with anorexia nervosa.

[d] The physician has differentiated the patient's anorexia nervosa as purging rather than the type in which the patient restricts her diet.

Coding

Behavioral health diagnoses may come from a clinician qualified under the health plan to evaluate and counsel the patient; eg, a licensed clinical social worker, neurologist, psychologist, or psychiatrist. A licensed professional counselor (LPC) is not a valid provider, however. The clinician performs an applied behavioral analysis and develops a treatment plan. Behavioral disorders are increasingly diagnosed and treated by the patient's general practitioner, and should be reported as often as they are documented and assessed or treated. Behavioral health issues are often documented secondary to the patient's chief complaint or final assessment. A patient's mental status contributes to MDM and should be considered when coding the record. Evaluation of the patient's confusion, depression, anxiety, fatigue, or hysteria by the physician should be abstracted when documented, unless there is a diagnosis for which these conditions would be considered symptoms.

According to the *2008 Risk Adjustment Data Technical Assistance for Medicare Advantage Organizations Participant Guide* (*2008 RA Participant Guide*), "[m]ental disorders in the HCC models require particular attention to specific wording in documentation and coding. Episodic mood disorders are mental diseases that include mood disturbances such as major depression. Physicians are encouraged to carefully document the characteristics of the mood disturbance (e.g., mania, depression, single episode, recurrent episode, circular) and use specific mental disorder terminology in the final diagnosis. The coder is cautioned to exactly code only the narrative provided by the physician in the final diagnosis and not make any further assumptions based on the patient work-up."[12]

When behavioral health services are rendered at behavioral health clinics, the care providers differ from what RA coders consider the norm. CMS allows clinical social workers and clinical psychologists to provide behavioral health services in addition to the acceptable providers discussed in Chapter 2. Individual and group services are covered.

ADVICE/ALERT NOTE

Per the *2008 RA Participant Guide,* "[m]ental disorders in the HCC models require particular attention to specific wording in documentation and coding. Episodic mood disorders are mental diseases that include mood disturbances such as major depression. Physicians are encouraged to carefully document the characteristics of the mood disturbance (e.g., mania, depression, single episode, recurrent episode, circular) and use specific mental disorder terminology in the final diagnosis. The coder is cautioned to exactly code only the narrative provided by the physician in the final diagnosis and not make any further assumptions based on the patient work-up."[12]

Documentation of "traits" is not documentation of a disorder. For example, if a patient is said to have "borderline personality traits," the physician has not documented borderline personality disorder. Do not make assumptions regarding the language physicians use in describing patient conditions. Use the ICD-10-CM Alphabetic Index and look up the exact terminology from the medical record to properly abstract the diagnosis code. A note that the patient "seems depressed" is not a diagnosis of depression. The only "Depressed" entry in the ICD-10-CM Alphabetic Index is for HDL cholesterol.

Per the *2008 RA Participant Guide* (6.4.3), "[c]linical specificity involves having a diagnosis fully documented in the source medical record instead of routinely defaulting to a general term for the diagnosis. It is important to understand medical terminology in order to identify terms in the medical record that may be a more specific description of a general term. Communication with the physician is perhaps one of the key elements in improving documentation skills that allow for more specific coding."[12]

ADVICE/ALERT NOTE

Per the *2008 RA Participant Guide* (6.4.3), "[c]linical specificity involves having a diagnosis fully documented in the source medical record instead of routinely defaulting to a general term for the diagnosis. It is important to understand medical terminology in order to identify terms in the medical record that may be a more specific description of a general term. Communication with the physician is perhaps one of the key elements in improving documentation skills that allow for more specific coding."[12]

Diagnoses for children are, at times, found in what seems to be an "adult" area of diagnoses in ICD-10-CM, and diagnoses for adults, in the "children's" section. For example, the diagnosis for an adult with new onset attention deficit disorder is reported with a code from category F90, in a section entitled "Behavioral and emotional disorders with onset usually occurring in childhood and adolescence."

ABSTRACT & CODE IT!

Abstract and code the clinical coding example below. Check your answers against the answers in Appendix C.

Patient 1
The patient had a positive score on the PHQ-9 depression questionnaire.

Patient 2
The patient discontinued his aripiprazole and bupropion six weeks ago. His sister brought him in today due to anorexia and outbreaks of violence at home. He is being admitted with severe depression with reactive depressive psychosis.

Patient 3
The patient's depression is responding well to citalopram.

Bipolar Disorders *see* Behavioral Disorders

Blood Disorders

Severe hematological disorders
HCC 46 1.388

Disorders of immunity
HCC 47 0.625
RxHCC 97 0.428

Coagulation defects and other specified hematological disorders
HCC 48 0.625

Sickle cell anemia
RxHCC 95 0.086

Myelodysplastic syndromes and myelofibrosis
RxHCC 96 0.959

Aplastic anemia and other significant blood disorders
RxHCC 98 0.086

Blood disorders include a diverse grouping of diseases characterized by blood defects. Errors in the bone marrow's production of blood products may occur due to genetics, to autoimmune disorders, disease, or adverse effects of medication. Bone marrow produces red blood cells, white blood cells, and platelets. Errors in production may relate to clotting abilities, anemias, immunity issues, or other related problems. Types of errors that may occur are varied, and include:

- New cells malformed, as in sickle cell disease (SCD)
- Bone marrow unable to produce a certain type of cell, as in pure red cell aplasia
- New cells defective and malfunctioning, as in myelodysplastic syndrome
- Too many new cells produced, as in polycythemia vera or essential thrombocythemia
- Too few new cells produced, as in iron or vitamin B_{12} deficiency anemia

Anemia
Reduction of hemoglobin concentration or red cell mass in the blood, leading to pallor, weakness, and breathlessness. Anemia has three potential causes: blood loss, red blood cell production errors, or destruction of red blood cells.

Sickle cell disease
An inherited autosomal recessive disease in which a proliferation of abnormal red blood cells affects oxygen delivery and blood flow. Sickle cell disease causes anemia, because the defective red blood cells have a shorter life span than normal cells. Carriers of the sickle cell gene without sickle cell anemia have the sickle cell trait.

Physician Documentation

Under-documentation of anemia specificity is a chronic problem in RA documentation and coding. The most common diagnosis in this grouping of HCCs is a diagnosis of anemia. There are dozens of causes for anemia, and scores of codes. Some codes risk-adjust, while others (eg, all nutritional anemias, blood-loss anemias and anemias in chronic diseases classified elsewhere) do not.

The physician must assign diagnoses to the laboratory values in order for them to be abstracted. Coders cannot abstract anemia based on laboratory values reported in the record. When documenting other types of anemia, capture the following elements:

- Is the condition primary or secondary? In either case, specify the exact cause.
- In nutritional anemia, what is the deficiency?
- Is the condition acute or chronic?
- In thalassemia, what type (alpha, beta, delta-beta, E-beta, minor)?
- In sickle cell, what type? (Hb-SS, Hb-C, Hb-SD, Hb-Se, thalassemia, trait), and if in crisis, specify acute chest, splenic sequestration, etc.

The codes for SCD show the level of detail needed in documentation (see Table 4-1.7).

Thalassemia
Genetic disorder resulting in the manufacture of red blood cells with abnormal hemoglobin.

TABLE 4-1.7 Sickle Cell Disease (SCD)

CODE	DESCRIPTION
D57.00	Hb-SS disease with crisis, unspecified
D57.01	Hb-SS disease with acute chest syndrome
D57.02	Hb-SS disease with splenic sequestration
D57.1	Sickle-cell disease without crisis
D57.20	Sickle-cell/Hb-C disease without crisis
D57.211	Sickle-cell/Hb-C disease with acute chest syndrome
D57.212	Sickle-cell/Hb-C disease with splenic sequestration
D57.219	Sickle-cell/Hb-C disease with crisis, unspecified
D57.3	Sickle-cell trait
D57.40	Sickle-cell thalassemia without crisis
D57.411	Sickle-cell thalassemia with acute chest syndrome
D57.412	Sickle-cell thalassemia with splenic sequestration
D57.419	Sickle-cell thalassemia with crisis, unspecified
D57.80	Other sickle-cell disorders without crisis
D57.811	Other sickle-cell disorders with acute chest syndrome
D57.812	Other sickle-cell disorders with splenic sequestration
D57.819	Other sickle-cell disorders with crisis, unspecified

The CDC estimates there are about 100,000 people diagnosed with SCD living in the US.[13] SCD is a common acronym for sickle cell disease, but SCD is also used to describe spinal cord disease, sudden cardiac death, and other medical conditions. To avoid confusion, always spell out the first reference to an acronym; eg, sickle cell disease (SCD).

The CDC estimates there are about 20,000 people who have been diagnosed with hemophilia in the US.[14] The default for documented "hemophilia" is code D66, *Hereditary factor VIII deficiency*, or classical hemophilia A, because the majority of hemophilia patients have this type of hemophilia. Document the type of hemophilia or the coder must assign hemophilia A by default, according to the ICD-10-CM Alphabetic Index (see Table 4-1.8). Link any chronic joint disease or pain to the underlying hemophilia, as appropriate.

TABLE 4-1.8 Coagulation Defects Including Hemophilia

CODE	DESCRIPTION
D65	Disseminated intravascular coagulation [defibrination syndrome]
D68.0	Von Willebrand's disease
D68.1	Hereditary factor XI deficiency
D68.2	Hereditary deficiency of other clotting factors
D68.311	Acquired hemophilia
D68.312	Antiphospholipid antibody with hemorrhagic disorder
D68.318	Other hemorrhagic disorder due to intrinsic circulating anticoagulants, antibodies, or inhibitors
D68.32	Hemorrhagic disorder due to extrinsic circulating anticoagulants
D68.4	Acquired coagulation factor deficiency
D68.8	Other specified coagulation defects
D68.9	Coagulation defect, unspecified

The clinical circumstances supporting the assignment of code D68.32, *Hemorrhagic disorder due to extrinsic circulating anticoagulants,* are often under-documented and/or not recognized by the coder. ICD-10-CM classifies any hemorrhagic disorder or bleeding (eg, hematuria, epistaxis, gastrointestinal bleeding) due to a medication affecting the coagulation system, such as an antiplatelet agent (eg, aspirin, dipyridamole), an anticoagulant (eg, warfarin), or other similar drugs (eg, a direct thrombin inhibitor), with ICD-10-CM code D68.32, *Hemorrhagic disorder due to extrinsic circulating anticoagulants*, which risk-adjusts to HCC 48, *Coagulation Defects and Other Specified Hematological Disorders.* Physician documentation must be clear that the medication contributed to or caused the patient's bleeding, not just that the patient was taking the medication.

Acute chest syndrome
Emergent fever, respiratory symptoms, abnormal chest radiographs, and chest pain in a patient with sickle cell disease, caused by intrapulmonary vaso-occlusion, usually leading to respiratory failure.

Hemophilia
Coagulation disorder due to the impaired production of coagulation factors (eg, Factor VIII), leading to prolonged or continuous bleeding. Hemophilia is usually genetic, but there is an acquired autoimmune form that occurs in adulthood.

CLINICAL EXAMPLES

NONSPECIFIC DOCUMENTATION	SPECIFIC DOCUMENTATION
Example 1 Acute chest syndrome[a]	**Example 1** Sickle cell Hb-SS disease with acute chest syndrome[b]
Example 2 Aplastic anemia[c]	**Example 2** Aplastic anemia due to antineoplastic radiotherapy for primary hepatocellular carcinoma.[d]

[a] While acute chest syndrome is defined as a lung-related complication of sickle cell disease, without sickle cell disease also noted in the documentation, acute chest syndrome cannot be coded. In ICD-10-CM, there is no entry under "syndrome," "chest," or "acute" classifying acute chest syndrome; it is only classified in subterms under sickle cell disease.

[b] Identify the type of sickle cell disease to capture the acute chest syndrome completely. Other comorbidities during the crisis would be reported secondarily (eg, any lung infection, embolus, pulmonary hypertension, respiratory failure, or atelectasis).

[c] There are more than 10 codes for aplastic anemia in ICD-10-CM. If there is enough data to document aplastic, is there enough data to provide a cause?

[d] In this case, the physician has documented the cause of aplastic anemia as well as the type of cancer that was being treated with radiotherapy.

Coding

Patients with hemophilia will usually perform home infusion of clotting factor to replace the clotting factor that is absent in their blood. This therapy may be performed as prophylaxis, or may occur only to stop bleeding when it occurs (demand therapy). Antifibrinolytics, tranexamic acid, or epsilon aminocaproic acid may be taken orally during home infusions to help keep blood clots from dissolving. Desmopressin may be prescribed as a nasal spray or injection, for self-treatment in emergent situations. Medications to treat hemophilia and Von Willebrand's disease may be used as support in RA. Often, support for hemophilia can also be found in the physical examination, as in notation of bruising or joint swelling or pain.

Pallor, icterus, erythema, edema, or splenomegaly all support SCD. The physician may note functional abnormalities in bones and joints. Oral hydroxyurea may be prescribed to prevent complications of SCD and reduce transfusion requirements. Sickle cell trait may cause some symptoms if the patient becomes hot and dehydrated. Documentation of physician queries into these symptoms can be used as support when abstracting sickle cell trait.

CODING TIP ICD-10-CM differentiates between patients who are immunocompromised as a result of immunosuppressants and those who are naturally immunocompromised. AHA's *Coding Clinic* (Third Quarter, 2015) advises that patients who are immunocompromised therapeutically to treat autoimmune disease do not have a diagnosis related with the immunosuppression.[8] Instead, code the long-term use of immunosupressants with Z79.899, *Other long term (current) drug therapy*. For patients who are otherwise immunocompromised, report with code D89.9, *Disorder involving the immune mechanism, unspecified*.[8]

ABSTRACT & CODE IT!

Abstract and code the clinical coding example below. Check your answers against the answers in Appendix C.

Patient 1
Bleeding of esophageal varices secondary to alcoholic liver disease and portal hypertension with acute blood-loss anemia, requiring the transfusion of two liters of blood. Patient's alcoholism is in remission and the liver disease is otherwise stable.

Patient 2
Aplastic anemia due to antineoplastic radiotherapy for primary hepatocellular carcinoma. After conferring with his oncologist, we have decided to perform blood and platelet transfusions to relieve his symptoms. He has one more radiotherapy session to complete.

Patient 3
Acute duodenal ulcer with bleeding due to warfarin therapy taken as directed resulting in acute blood-loss anemia.

Cachexia *see* Malnutrition

Cerebral Palsy

Cerebral palsy
HCC 74 0.280

Cerebral palsy (CP) describes a group of neurological disorders that affect movement, posture, and balance. CP may be a congenital condition in which the brain has not developed normally during fetal growth, a condition arising from a birth injury, or from damage occurring in infancy or early childhood. In CP, the cerebral cortex, that layer of the brain controlling muscle movement, is damaged. There is no cure for CP, which affects 3.3 children per 1,000 live births, according to the National Institutes of Health (NIH).[15] Even though CP is a disease of infancy or childhood, some patients are not diagnosed with milder forms of CP until later in life.

There are several forms of CP, and each has a unique code (see Table 4-1.9):

- Spastic CP with quadriplegia (full-body weakness, most severe form)
- Spastic CP with hemiplegia (right- or left-sided weakness)
- Spastic CP with diplegia (bilateral leg weakness)
- Athetoid CP (uncontrollable writhing movement of hands, feet, arms, or legs with hyperactivity of facial muscles and tongue)
- Ataxic CP (balance and depth perception issues causing wide gait and unsteady walking)

TABLE 4-1.9 Cerebral Palsy Codes

CODE	DESCRIPTION
G80.0	Spastic quadriplegic cerebral palsy
G80.1	Spastic diplegic cerebral palsy
G80.2	Spastic hemiplegic cerebral palsy
G80.3	Athetoid cerebral palsy
G80.4	Ataxic cerebral palsy
G80.8	Other cerebral palsy
G80.9	Cerebral palsy, unspecified

Physician Documentation

Document all comorbidities of CP (eg, seizure disorder, developmental delays, hearing loss, impaired vision, intellectual disability, incontinence, learning disability, osteopenia, and spinal deformities) as none of these conditions is inherent in CP and would be separate diagnoses.

Adults with CP sometimes experience post-impairment syndrome, a CP-specific disorder that captures the repetitive motion injuries, pain, bone deformities, osteoarthritis, fatigue, and weakness brought on by years of CP. There is no specific code in ICD-10-CM for post-impairment syndrome, but Guideline Section I(B.15) states that, "[i]n the absence of Alphabetic Index guidance, assign codes for the documented manifestations of the syndrome."[1] Therefore, when a patient is diagnosed with post-impairment syndrome, it is important to document the manifestations of the syndrome so these can be coded. CP is a common acronym for cerebral palsy, cleft palate, cor pulmonale, chronic pancreatitis, and chest pain. Always spell out the first instance (eg, cerebral palsy [CP]).

CLINICAL EXAMPLES

NONSPECIFIC DOCUMENTATION	SPECIFIC DOCUMENTATION
Example 1 Patient's gait is asymmetrical due to scoliosis and mild CP.[a]	**Example 1** Patient's gait is asymmetrical due to the patient's mild spastic diplegic cerebral palsy and its sequela, lumbosacral scoliosis.[b]
Example 2 Assessment: 1. Calcaneal fracture 2. Osteoporosis 3. Seizure disorder 4. Cerebral palsy[c]	**Example 2** 1. Pathological left calcaneal fracture due to osteoporosis; nondisplaced so treated with boot. 2. Osteoporosis due to long-term use of Dilantin; last DEXA 2 years ago. 3. Focal idiopathic epilepsy, stable on Dilantin. 4. Spastic quadriplegic cerebral palsy; requires wheelchair. 5. Mild intellectual disability.[d] Caregiver accompanied her to office visit (OV).

[a] The cause of the scoliosis and the type of CP should be documented. Spell out cerebral palsy in first reference.

[b] The type of CP has been identified and linked to the scoliosis.

[c] While these conditions are likely linked, there is no linkage in documentation. The seizure disorder and CP are not further specified. The laterality of the fracture is missing, and the circumstances would determine whether the fracture and the osteoporosis are linked. Any other manifestations of the CP should be documented in addition to the CP.

[d] Here, the fracture is noted as caused by osteoporosis, and the osteoporosis due to the long-term epilepsy medication. The type of epilepsy and CP are identified, and the patient's intellectual disability is documented.

Coding

"Toe walking," commonly seen in children with CP, would be separately reported if it is being treated (eg, with Botox injections). There is no entry in the Alphabetic Index specific to toe walking, but there are codes for difficulty in walking (R26.2) and abnormalities of gait (R26.89). Symptom codes for pain or instability could also be considered. Refer to documentation. Report G80.8, *Other cerebral palsy,* for monoplegic, triplegic, or mixed cerebral palsy, and for non-spastic cerebral palsy.

ABSTRACT & CODE IT!

Abstract and code the clinical coding example below. Check your answers against the answers in Appendix C.

Patient 1
Patient's gait is asymmetrical due to the patient's mild spastic diplegic cerebral palsy and its sequela, lumbosacral scoliosis.

Patient 2
Assessment:
1. Pathological left calcaneal fracture due to osteoporosis; nondisplaced so treated with boot.
2. Osteoporosis due to long-term use of Dilantin; last DEXA 2 years ago.
3. Focal idiopathic epilepsy, stable on Dilantin.
4. Spastic quadriplegic cerebral palsy; requires wheelchair.
5. Mild intellectual disability. Caregiver accompanied her to OV.

Patient 3
The 2-year-old child was diagnosed last week with congenital triplegia and is here today for a consultation regarding physical and occupational therapy. She is not yet walking.

Cerebrovascular Disease

Cerebral hemorrhage
HCC 99 0.263

Ischemic or unspecified stroke
HCC 100 0263

Cerebrovascular disease, except hemorrhage or aneurysm
RxHCC 206 0.044

A stroke occurs when tissue in the brain dies due to a lack of oxygen or if there is bleeding within the brain. The flow of oxygen-rich blood to brain tissue may be disrupted when an arterial vessel suffers occlusion by an embolus or thrombus or when blood flow is severely restricted by stenosis, or when a cerebral blood vessel bursts and blood flows out of circulation and into brain tissue. Strokes are defined as ischemic, caused by a clot; or hemorrhagic, caused by a rupture of a cerebral vessel. Hemorrhagic strokes may be caused by hypertension or by the rupture of an aneurysm.

About 90% of strokes are ischemic. A stroke is an urgent condition requiring emergency care. Strokes can cause transient disabilities (eg, cerebral edema), permanent late-effects (eg, hemiparesis), or death. By comparison, a transient ischemic attack (TIA) does not lead to brain tissue death; thus, by definition, has no sequela that lasts more than 24 hours. In a TIA, a small clot temporarily blocks a vessel, but quickly resolves. TIAs increase the stroke risk in a patient, but TIAs are not strokes.

Excluded from this topic are HCCs for monoplegia and hemiplegia due to stroke. These conditions are briefly mentioned here, but are discussed more fully in the topic, *Paralysis, Malformation of Brain/ Spinal Cord.*

Occlusion
Complete blockage of a lumen.

Embolus
A blockage or plug (eg, blood clot, air bubble, or other clot or matter) that obstructs a blood vessel.

Thrombus
Stationary blood clot lodged in the vessel where it developed, obstructing blood flow.

Stenosis
Abnormal narrowing of a lumen.

Physician Documentation

Classification of stroke in ICD-10-CM requires more information than many physicians have traditionally documented, and coding of sequelae of stroke and infarction also demands a level of detail often missing in medical records. Do not just document "CVA" (I63.9, *Cerebral infarction, unspecified*). Its etiology and site of stroke or infarction affect outcomes, so document as thoroughly as possible during emergent and ongoing care. Identify the etiology of a stroke, infarction, or TIA by category (see Table 4-1.10). In addition to the stroke or infarction type, document the vessel and its laterality, if known.

TABLE 4-1.10 Etiology of Stroke, Infarction, or TIA by Category

CODES OR SUBCATEGORIES	STROKE TYPE
I60.-	Nontraumatic (spontaneous) subarachnoid hemorrhage
I61.-	Nontraumatic (spontaneous) intracerebral hemorrhage
I62.-	Nontraumatic (spontaneous) subdural hemorrhage
I63.0- to I63.2-	Thrombosis/embolus precerebral arteries
I63.3- to I63.5-	Thrombosis/embolus cerebral arteries
I63.6	Cerebral infarction due to cerebral venous thrombosis, nonpyogenic
I63.8	Other cerebral infarction
I63.9	Cerebral infarction, unspecified
G45.9	Transient cerebral ischemic attack, unspecified (TIA)

Once a patient has been released from the acute care facility following the initial stroke or infarction, the stroke or infarction is classified by its type and by late effects. A common documentation error is to refer to the stroke as an acute condition after the patient is discharged from the inpatient facility. In nearly all cases in which a stroke patient is seen in the physician office, the patient is seen for follow-up care or sequelae, as defined by ICD-10-CM, not for acute stroke. Specify each encounter as an acute event or as treatment of sequelae. The site and type of stroke should be documented at every encounter in which sequelae are addressed. Identify whether the initial event was hemorrhagic or ischemic. The coder cannot refer to past encounters to find the details relating to a current diagnosis. This information must be re-entered with every encounter.

Document specific symptoms of cognitive deficit following stroke (eg, attention, memory, executive function, psychomotor, visuospatial, social, emotional) and specifically link them to the cerebrovascular event. Emphasize all extremities that are weak from the stroke, such as monoparesis, hemiparesis, or even quadriparesis for patients who have had multiple strokes. (Refer to topic, *Paralysis, Malformation of Brain/Spinal Cord.*) For patients experiencing hemiplegia or hemiparesis from stroke or infarction, document which side is dominant, and which is affected. If documentation does not inform the coder, the *ICD-10-CM Guidelines* will provide specificity to the coding.

According to ICD-10-CM Guideline Section I(C.9.d):

> Category I69 is used to indicate conditions classifiable to categories I60-I67 as the causes of sequela (neurologic deficits), themselves classified elsewhere. These "late effects" include neurologic deficits that persist after initial onset of conditions classifiable to categories I60-I67. The neurologic deficits caused by cerebrovascular disease may be present from the onset or may arise at any time after the onset of the condition classifiable to categories I60-I67.
>
> Codes from category I69, *Sequelae of cerebrovascular disease*, that specify hemiplegia, hemiparesis, and monoplegia identify whether the dominant or nondominant side is affected. Should the affected side be documented, but not specified as dominant or nondominant, and the classification system does not indicate a default, code selection is as follows:
>
> - For ambidextrous patients, the default should be dominant.
> - If the left side is affected, the default is non-dominant.
> - If the right side is affected, the default is dominant.[1]

ADVICE/ALERT NOTE

Per ICD-10-CM Guideline Section I(C.9.d), "[c]ategory I69, *Sequelae of cerebrovascular disease*, is used to indicate conditions that are a direct consequence of cerebrovascular diseases classified to categories I60-I67. These "late effects" include neurologic deficits that persist after initial onset of conditions classifiable to categories I60-I67. The neurologic deficits caused by cerebrovascular disease may be present from the onset or may arise at any time after the onset of the condition classifiable to categories I60-I67.

In addition, codes from category I69, *Sequelae of cerebrovascular disease*, that specify hemiplegia, hemiparesis, and monoplegia identify whether the dominant or nondominant side is affected. Should the affected side be documented, but not specified as dominant or nondominant, and the classification system does not indicate a default, code selection is as follows:

- For ambidextrous patients, the default should be dominant.
- If the left side is affected, the default is non-dominant.
- If the right side is affected, the default is dominant."[1]

Unfortunately, there is no code to classify the sequelae of spinal cord strokes, thus AHA's *Coding Clinic* (Third Quarter, 2017) recommended the use of various codes from Chapter 6, Diseases of the Nervous System, G00-G99, such as code G82.20, *Paraplegia, unspecified,* to describe the sequelae of spinal cord strokes.[16]

ICD-10-CM classifies weakness of an extremity (eg, paraparesis, hemiparesis, quadriparesis) as a complete paralysis of that extremity (eg, paraplegia, hemiplegia, and quadriplegia, respectively).[1] While the ICD-10-CM Alphabetic Index and Tabular List have no listing for the term "monoparesis," AHA's *Coding Clinic* (First Quarter, 2017) advised assigning the appropriate code from subcategory I69.33-, *Monoplegia of upper limb following cerebral infarction,* or I69.34-, *Monoplegia of lower limb following cerebral infarction,* for upper- or lower-limb weakness that is clearly associated with a CVA.[17] Given that many physicians select codes from billing software or computer programs that may only represent paralysis of one or more extremities (eg, quadriplegia), they must be informed that ICD-10-CM allows them to use "plegia" codes implying paralysis to report the weakness or paresis of one or more extremities. Clearly identify the cause and effect relationship of any cerebrovascular disease that occurs due to a surgical intervention. Specify whether the event occurred intraoperatively or post-procedurally, whether it involved an infarction or hemorrhage, the vessel involved, and the brain tissue affected, if known. For cerebral hemorrhage, the type of surgery that was being performed must also be documented. Document any tissue plasminogen activator (tPa) administered at the local or the referring facility and the time started. If the stroke was aborted, meaning that there were no neurological sequelae after 24 hours from the time of onset, document that fact. ICD-10-CM allows for the term "aborted stroke" to be coded as a stroke (which does affect HCC), whereas transient ischemic attacks are not coded as strokes. Consultation with a neurologist may be needed to ensure the clinical validity of the stroke or transient ischemic attack code being submitted.

Identify tobacco use history, as appropriate. Documentation of the term "smoker" is considered to be nicotine dependence (see Table 4-1.11). Document any coexisting hypertension, atrial fibrillation, CAD, or hypertension, as these conditions are vascular health risks.

TABLE 4-1.11 Common Tobacco Use and History Codes

CODE	DESCRIPTION
F17.210	Nicotine dependence, cigarettes, uncomplicated
F17.211	Nicotine dependence, cigarettes, in remission
F17.218	Nicotine dependence, cigarettes, with nicotine-induced disorders
Z72.0	Tobacco use
Z77.22	Exposure to environmental tobacco smoke (acute) (chronic)
Z87.891	Personal history of nicotine dependence

National Institutes of Health Stroke Scale (NIHSS) Score

The National Institutes of Health Stroke Scale (NIHSS) score was developed to help physicians objectively determine the severity of an ischemic stroke in an acute setting. This score is often taken by first responders, and repeated at intervals during the patient's hospitalization and recovery. Unlike most diagnosis codes, NIHSS scores may be compliantly reported based on nonphysician documentation, such as emergency medical technicians or nurses.

Higher scores in NIHSS indicate more severe symptoms associated with the stroke. Scoring is based on level of consciousness; if the patient knows the month and own age; whether patient can respond to commands to open and close eyes; best gaze with horizontal eye movement; visual field testing; face symmetry; motor function of each extremity; limb ataxia; sensory to pinprick; language; dysarthria; and extinction/inattention.

While NIHSS scores are useful to report, physicians must still document as a diagnosis the consequences of cerebrovascular diseases (eg, hemianopsia, aphasia, stupor, coma) as to promote complete and compliant ICD-10-CM coding. Details of the NIHSS scoring process can be accessed at https://stroke.nih.gov/resources/scale.htm.

Glasgow coma scales are another useful tool in measuring severity of strokes or any disease resulting in an altered mental status or level of consciousness and, unlike the NIHSS stroke scale, risk-adjust. Glasgow coma scales are divided into three sections, eye (1 to 4), verbal (1 to 5), and motor (1 to 6), each of which has its own ICD-10-CM code and crosswalks for adults and pediatric patients. It is best to report each individual element, given that ICD-10-CM codes for total scores do not affect HCC RA. Like the NIHSS score, ICD-10-CM coding for the Glasgow coma scale can be based on nonphysician (eg, nurse or EMT) documentation. A reference from the CDC describing the Glasgow coma scale is available at https://www.cdc.gov/masstrauma/resources/gcs.pdf.

CLINICAL EXAMPLES

NONSPECIFIC DOCUMENTATION	SPECIFIC DOCUMENTATION
Example 1 Assessment: 1. Stroke. Continue her PT for weakness. 2. Atrial fibrillation. We discussed the Watchman device and she would like to pursue this approach to treatment of her LAA. I referred her to Dr. Kent.[a]	**Example 1** Assessment: 1. Residual right-sided weakness as sequela of cerebral infarction. Continue physical therapy for gait and dexterity. She is left-handed. 2. Chronic atrial fibrillation. We discussed occlusion of the left atrial appendage with the Watchman device and she would like to pursue this approach. I referred her to Dr. Kent.[b]
Example 2 CVA with an NIHSS score of 12[c] with resultant right-handed clumsiness, impaired gait, and dizziness.	**Example 2** Cerebellar infarction, right cerebellar artery, in a right-handed individual with an NIHSS score of 12 as performed by me at admission[d] resulting in persistent ataxia, vertigo, and right-handed monoparesis.

[a] This entry omits many elements crucial to coding. "Stroke" is vague and not identified as a past event. "Weakness" is not linked directly to the stroke and is vague and without laterality. The atrial fibrillation is unspecified.

[b] In this example, we know that this encounter is for sequela of stroke. Laterality of the hemiplegia is noted and linked to the stroke. Dominant left side is noted. The type of atrial fibrillation is noted. The left atrial appendage is spelled out, rather than an acronym.

[c] CVA is a generic term that will classify to 163.9, *Cerebral infarction unspecified.* The NIHSS score needs to include some time context, and identify who performed the test.

[d] Be as specific as possible about the site of the infarction. Identify the timing of the NIHSS scoring and who performed the test.

Coding

According to ICD-10-CM Guideline Section I(C. 9.d.3), codes from "category I69 should not be assigned if the patient does not have neurologic deficits."[1] Seek answers to three questions when coding a stroke. First, determine if the cerebral event is acute. Acute cerebrovascular events are rarely managed in a physician office. Second, find in the medical record details for the site and laterality of the cerebrovascular event. Third, determine if the stroke is ischemic or hemorrhagic.

CODING TIP Hemiplegia is not inherent to a stroke and should be reported separately, according to AHA's *Coding Clinic* (First Quarter, 2014).[18] "Right-sided weakness" or "left-sided weakness" should be reported as hemiplegia when a causal relationship is documented between the weakness and a cerebral infarct or hemorrhage, according to AHA's *Coding Clinic* (First Quarter, 2015).[19] The linkage between weakness and cerebrovascular disease cannot be assumed.

ADVICE/ALERT NOTE

Per ICD-10-CM Guideline Section I(C.19.i), the "NIH stroke scale (NIHSS) codes (R29.7-) can be used in conjunction with acute cerebral infarct codes (I63) to identify the patient's neurological status and the severity of the stroke. The stroke scale codes should be sequenced after the acute stroke diagnosis code(s)."[1]

If the physician is not specific in recording the site of a stroke or infarction, it is permissible for coders to use CT scans or other radiological reports in the patient's record to report the specific anatomic site. These radiological reports must be part of the official medical record and signed by the authoring physician. Codes in category I69 identify the specific paralysis or other sequelae of the cerebrovascular event, including dysarthria, dysphagia, aphasia, dysphasia, spatial neglect, and apraxia.

If during hospitalization manifestations of a stroke resolve (eg, right-sided weakness or aphasia that was present on admission but the patient completely recovered her strength and ability to talk before discharge), code these conditions as active conditions since they were present during hospitalization. The conditions need not be treated in order for them to be reported, as their presence would have affected the patient's need for a diagnostic assessment, nursing time, and/or a longer length of stay. Do not report new neurological deficits of a newly diagnosed cerebrovascular disease during an initial hospitalization with codes from category I69, *Sequelae of cerebrovascular disease.* Instead, report each stroke manifestation or symptom separately (eg, G81.91, *Hemiplegia, unspecified affecting right dominant side,* and R13.11, *Dysphagia, oral phase*). Once the patient has completed the initial treatment for stroke and is released from acute care, report deficits with codes from category I69 (eg, I69.151, *Hemiplegia and hemiparesis following nontraumatic intracerebral hemorrhage affecting right dominant side,* and I69.191, *Dysphagia following nontraumatic intracerebral hemorrhage*). Report a second code from subcategory R13.1-, *Dysphagia,* to identify the dysphagia with more specificity, if known. Neurologic deficits may be present at the time of the acute event, or may arise at any time after the condition was initially reported with a code from categories I60-I67.

 **ADVICE/ALERT NOTE**

Per ICD-10-CM Guideline Section I(C.9.3), "[c]odes from category I69 should not be assigned if the patient does not have neurologic deficits."[1]

CODING TIP Remember the difference between dysphagia and dysphasia with this simple mnemonic device: dysphagia is difficulty swallowing and G identifies gastrointestinal system. Dysphasia is difficulty in speech and S identifies speech.

According to ICD-10-CM Guideline Section I(C.9.c), "[m]edical record documentation should clearly specify the cause-and-effect relationship between the medical intervention and the cerebrovascular accident in order to assign a code for an intraoperative or postprocedural cerebrovascular accident."[1] If the patient's dominant side is not documented, the default is for the right side to be dominant, except for ambidextrous patients. In ambidextrous patients, identify the affected side as dominant, whether it is right or left. The patient's health status may be documented with codes from category R29.7, *National Institutes of Health Stroke Scale (NIHSS) score,* or from the coma scale (R40.2-). It is appropriate to abstract either score when it is documented. The coma scale risk-adjusts; the stroke scores do not. Codes from categories I60-I69 should never be used to report traumatic intracranial events.

Dysarthria
Slurred or slow speech caused by a neurological disorder (eg, stroke or brain tumor).

Dysphagia
Difficulty or inability to swallow; may be due to neurological disorder or stenosis of esophagus.

Aphasia
Inability or deficiency in understanding or expressing speech due to a neurological disorder (eg, stroke or brain tumor).

Dysphasia
Inability or deficiency in generating speech due to neurological disorder (eg, stroke or brain tumor).

Spatial neglect
A phenomenon following brain injury in which the patient fails to see objects or people on one side of the body and is unaware of the defect. Also called hemispatial neglect or hemiagnosia.

Apraxia
Inability to perform actions with purpose or under direction due to a neurological disorder (eg, stroke or brain tumor).

ADVICE/ALERT NOTE

Per ICD-10-CM Guideline Section I(C.9.c), "[m]edical record documentation should clearly specify the cause-and-effect relationship between the medical intervention and the cerebrovascular accident in order to assign a code for an intraoperative or postprocedural cerebrovascular accident."[1]

Normally, codes from categories I60-I67 are not reported with codes from category I69. However, if the patient has deficits from an old cerebrovascular event and is currently having a new cerebrovascular event, both may be reported. If a patient has a history of a past cerebrovascular event and has no residual sequelae, report code Z86.73, *Personal history of transient ischemic attack (TIA), and cerebral infarction without residual deficits.*

If a patient is diagnosed with bilateral nontraumatic intracerebral hemorrhages, report code I61.6, *Nontraumatic intracerebral hemorrhage, multiple localized.* For bilateral subarachnoid hemorrhage, assign a code for each site. Categories I65 and I66 have unique codes for bilateral conditions. Also code any documented atrial fibrillation, coronary artery disease, diabetes, or hypertension, as these comorbidities are stroke risk factors. "Residual weakness" of one right or left extremity due to an old cerebrovascular accident is reported with a code from subcategory I69.33, *Monoplegia of upper limb following cerebral infarction,* or I69.34, *Monoplegia of lower limb following cerebral infarction,* according to AHA's *Coding Clinic* (First Quarter, 2017).[17]

CODING TIP "Residual weakness" of one right or left extremity due to an old cerebrovascular accident is reported with a code from subcategory I69.33, *Monoplegia of upper limb following cerebral infarction*, or I69.34, *Monoplegia of lower limb following cerebral infarction*, according to AHA's *Coding Clinic* (First Quarter, 2017).[17]

ABSTRACT & CODE IT!

Abstract and code the clinical coding example below. Check your answers against the answers in Appendix C.

DOS: 9/27/2017 **Patient:** Terry Bird
DOB: 7/17/47

Terry was referred to the Medical Center's Outpatient Rehabilitation Department for speech therapy, status post-cerebral infarction. She is here today for an assessment. Her husband, Ted, accompanied her.

Medical Diagnosis: Global aphasia, sequela of CVA on 8/22/17. The family removed her from Morton Long Term Care Facility because they were not satisfied with the treatment the patient was receiving, and the facility was 30 miles from her home.

Assessment: Based on the result of the Weston aphasia battery, global aphasia best describes Terry's deficits. Her most appropriate response was a thumb's up; otherwise she was able only to say "no," whether appropriate or not. She scored 4 out of 60 on the auditor word recognition subtest, and 8 out of 80 on the sequential commands. She stated repeatedly during the testing, "No." When the patient attempted speech, it was often unintelligible. Sometimes, however, she was understood by her husband. She was able to count to five. She has significant issues with both speech and receptive communications and appears very frustrated and unhappy with her speech status. She suffers from attention and concentration deficits, aphasia, dysphasia, and dysarthria, all linked to the cerebral infarction on 8/22/17. She has some left-sided weakness as well, and is seeing a physical therapist here at the clinic.

Plan: I will meet with Terry twice weekly for the next 12 weeks. She will receive treatment here, and also perform home activities with guidance from her husband.

Our goal for the next eight weeks, agreed upon by Ted and Terry, is for Terry to perform the following tasks with at least 80% accuracy:

- Correctly answer simple yes/no questions
- Complete simple sentences
- Follow one-step commands
- Name at least 10 everyday objects

She will return to clinic on Tuesday at 10 a.m.

Electronically signed by Herman Horton, DPT at 8:20 a.m. 9/28/2017

Chromosomal Abnormalities, Intellectual Disabilities, and Other Developmental Disorders

Profound or severe intellectual disability/ developmental disorder
RxHCC 146 N/A

Moderate intellectual disability/developmental disorder
RxHCC 147 N/A

Mild or unspecified intellectual disability/ developmental disorder
RxHCC 148 N/A

Adults with developmental and intellectual disabilities are more likely to have poorer health outcomes than people without disabilities because they are often unable to manage the chronic, complex health conditions they have, they usually have fewer financial resources, and their physical limitations (eg, obesity and poor eyesight or hearing) interfere with communication and understanding. According to the Chronic Conditions Data Warehouse evaluation of Medicare data from 2014, 1% of the Medicare population has an intellectual disability.[20]

Physician Documentation

Intellectual disabilities affect the ability of the patient to describe PMH and chief complaint, or to follow a care plan as directed by the physician. Document the intellectual disabilities of a patient in every encounter, as each encounter is a stand-alone document and the intellectual disability of the patient is going to be pertinent to care planning and MDM.

If the etiology and severity of the intellectual disability are known, document them. In some cases, each diagnosis carries its own RA; in other cases, only the intellectual disability will risk-adjust. Down syndrome, for example, does not risk-adjust, but the intellectual disabilities and other manifestations of Down syndrome (eg, heart defects, gastroesophageal reflux disease, hypothyroidism, and dementia) do risk-adjust. Dementia is common in adults with Down syndrome. Any dementia in a patient with an intellectual disability is reported in addition to the disability.

WHO ICD-10 Guide for Mental Retardation

The following is excerpted from the World Health Organization's (WHO's) *ICD-10 Guide for Mental Retardation* as instruction for documentation and coding for people with intellectual disabilities. (**Note:** Per WHO, the terms "retardation" and "retarded" are under consideration for a change in ICD-11.)

> People with mental retardation usually have multiple problems. To describe these problems adequately, it is usually necessary to use several diagnoses taken from different parts of the classification. It is necessary to record the degree of mental retardation and the presence of associated physical and mental disorders; to record the degree of psychosocial disability; and to note relevant abnormal psychosocial situations. These factors can be recorded in a systematic and orderly way by using a multiaxial system. The axes in a multiaxial system are not axes in the sense of statistically divided axes; they are means of recording different kinds of features of the case. The following axes form the structure of the ICD-10-CM scheme of classification for the mentally retarded.
>
> Axis I Severity of retardation and problem behaviors
>
> Axis II Associated medical conditions
>
> Axis III Associated psychiatric disorders
>
> Axis IV Global assessment of psychosocial disability
>
> Axis V Associated abnormal psychosocial situations
>
> The diagnostic codes to be recorded on each of these axes are part contained in the International Classification of Diseases. However most are scattered through the main volume and some are difficult to treat.[21]

DOCUMENTATION TIP ICD-10 classifies intellectual disabilities as follows:

F70 Mild intellectual disabilities
IQ level of 50-55 to approximately 70

F71 Moderate intellectual disabilities
IQ level of 35-40 to 50-55

F72 Severe intellectual disabilities
IQ level of 20-25 to 35-40

F73 Profound intellectual disabilities
IQ level of less than 20-25

CLINICAL EXAMPLES

NONSPECIFIC DOCUMENTATION	SPECIFIC DOCUMENTATION
Example 1 John's X ray shows pneumonia. We are culturing his sputum. His mother says that although he has been living independently for two years, she will bring him home until he recovers, since he has Down syndrome.[a]	**Example 1** John's X ray shows lobar pneumonia. We are culturing his sputum. His mother says that although he has been living independently for two years, she will bring him home until he recovers, since he has Down syndrome. She reports he has mild intellectual disabilities,[b] but will need help managing his fluid intake and medication schedule.
2. The patient has some intellectual disability as sequela to childhood meningitis, but functions very well in a group home environment.[c]	2. The patient has mild intellectual disability as sequela to childhood meningitis, but functions very well in a group home environment.[d]

[a] Provide status on the intellectual disability associated with Down syndrome during each encounter. Lobar pneumonia adds specificity to the diagnosis, even though the etiology of the infection is not yet determined.

[b] The Down syndrome and intellectual disability are both captured. There is no specificity available at this encounter for the pneumonia, so the unspecified diagnosis is OK.

[c] Qualitative information about the disability is missing.

[d] The disability is adequately described here.

Coding

In addition to capturing a patient's intellectual disability, report all comorbidities that manifest as physical conditions and the etiology of the intellectual disability, if known. Many intellectual disabilities are components of congenital syndromes. In many cases, multiple codes are required to capture the nature of the syndrome (eg, for Nager syndrome, report separate codes for the congenital anomalies of the face, microtia, cleft palate, reduced stature, mild intellectual disability, and hip dislocation).

ABSTRACT & CODE IT!

Abstract and code the clinical coding example below. Check your answers against the answers in Appendix C.

Patient 1

The social worker reports the patient's IQ is mildly subnormal, at 59.

Patient 2

John's X ray shows lobar pneumonia. We are culturing his sputum. His mother says that although he has been living independently for two years, she will bring him home until he recovers because he has Down syndrome. He has mild intellectual disabilities, but will need help managing his fluid intake and medication schedule.

Patient 3

The patient is being seen today for acute bronchitis due to *Mycoplasma pneumoniae.* She has moderate intellectual disability as sequela to childhood meningitis, but functions very well in a group-home environment.

Chronic Obstructive Pulmonary Disease *see* Pulmonary Disorders: Chronic

Cirrhosis of Liver *see* Liver Disease

Coma, Brain Damage

Coma, brain compression, anoxic damage
HCC 80 0.584

Injury to the brain can disrupt normal brain function and lead to coma, a prolonged and deep state of unconsciousness. The coma may be the result of traumatic injury or a brain injury secondary to swelling, ischemia, or other internal forces. A patient who is completely unresponsive to stimuli and has no evidence of higher brain function is said to be in a persistent vegetative state.

Codes reporting the coma scale or Glasgow coma scale are primarily used for trauma registries, but they do provide insight into to the severity of a patient's condition and should be reported when they are documented in the patient record. Coma-scale scores may risk-adjust. See Table 4-1.12 for other risk-adjusting coma diagnoses.

TABLE 4-1.12 Other Risk-Adjusting Coma Diagnoses

CODE	DESCRIPTION
G93.1	Anoxic brain damage, not elsewhere classified
G93.5	Compression of brain
G93.6	Cerebral edema
R40.3	Persistent vegetative state

Physician Documentation

To complete a Glasgow coma scale, a code is needed from each of three categories: eyes open, best verbal response, best motor response, and document the circumstance in which the evaluation was performed. This circumstance becomes the 7th character in the coma code:

0 Unspecified time
1 In the field [EMT or ambulance]
2 At arrival to emergency department
3 At hospital admission
4 24 hours or more after hospital admission

The Glasgow coma scale structured assessment can be downloaded at http://www.glasgowcomascale.org/. The eye, verbal, and motor scores individually provide more information than a total gross score. Include the three individual scores in documentation when possible. Physicians should be aware that "unconsciousness" is indexed to unspecified coma in ICD-10-CM.

Glasgow Coma Scale

CRITERION	RATING	SCORE	CODE
Eye Opening			
Open before stimulus	Spontaneous	4	R40.214-
After spoken or shouted request	To sound	3	R40.213-
After finger-tip stimulus	To pressure	2	R40.212-
No opening at any time, no interfering factors	None	1	R40.211-
Closed by local factor	Non-testable	NT	—
Verbal Response			
Correctly gives name, place, and date	Oriented	5	R40.225-
Not oriented but communication coherently	Confused	4	R40.224-
Intelligible single words	Words	3	R44.223-
Only moans, groans	Sounds	2	R44.222-
No audible response, no interfering factor	None	1	R44.221-
Factor interfering with communication	Non-testable	NT	—
Best Motor Response			
Obey 2-part request	Obeys commands	6	R40.236-
Brings hand above clavicle to stimulus on head neck	Localizing	5	R40.235-
Bends arm at elbow rapidly but features not predominantly abnormal	Normal flexion	4	R40.234-
Bends arm at elbow, features clearly predominantly abnormal	Abnormal flexion	3	R40.233-
Extends arm at elbow	Extension	2	R40.232-
No movement in arms/legs, no interfering factor	None	1	R40.231-
Paralyzed or other limiting factor	Non-testable	NT	—

Coding

The coma scale may be abstracted from the chart when it is not documented by physicians or other qualified health care personnel. An EMT often documents the coma or stroke scales. These scales should only be reported as secondary diagnoses. According to ICD-10-CM Guideline Section I(C.18.e):

> The coma scale codes (R40.2-) may be used in conjunction with traumatic brain injury codes, acute cerebrovascular disease or sequelae of cerebrovascular disease codes. These codes are primarily for use by trauma registries, but they may be used in any setting where this information is collected. The coma scale may also be used to assess the status of the central nervous system for other non-trauma conditions, such as monitoring patients in the intensive care unit regardless of medical condition. The coma scale codes should be sequenced after the diagnosis code(s).
>
> These codes, one from each subcategory, are needed to complete the scale. The 7th character indicates when the scale was recorded. The 7th character should match for all three codes.
>
> At a minimum, report the initial score documented on presentation at your facility. This may be a score from the emergency medicine technician (EMT) or in the emergency department. If desired, a facility may choose to capture multiple coma scale scores.
>
> Assign code R40.24, Glasgow coma scale, total score, when only the total score is documented in the medical record and not the individual score(s).[1]

Codes from subcategory R40.2, *Coma*, are typically used by trauma registries. Report code R40.24, *Glasgow coma scale, total score*, only when a total score is documented in the medical record, ie, coders are not to tally individual scores to determine a total score, but code the three scores from R40.21, R40.22, and R40.23, if available.

ADVICE/ALERT NOTE

Per ICD-10-CM Guideline Section I(C.18.e) "[t]he coma scale codes (R40.2-) may be used in conjunction with traumatic brain injury codes, acute cerebrovascular disease or sequelae of cerebrovascular disease codes. These codes are primarily for use by trauma registries, but they may be used in any setting where this information is collected. The coma scale may also be used to assess the status of the central nervous system for other non-trauma conditions, such as monitoring patients in the intensive care unit regardless of medical condition. The coma scale codes should be sequenced after the diagnosis code(s).

These codes, one from each subcategory, are needed to complete the scale. The 7th character indicates when the scale was recorded. The 7th character should match for all three codes.

At a minimum, report the initial score documented on presentation at your facility. This may be a score from the emergency medicine technician (EMT) or in the emergency department. If desired, a facility may choose to capture multiple coma scale scores.

Assign code R40.24, *Glasgow coma scale, total score,* when only the total score is documented in the medical record and not the individual score(s)."[1]

According to AHA's *Coding Clinic* (Fourth Quarter, 2017), a Glasgow coma score should never be reported for patients in medically induced comas.[22] A coma may be induced to protect the brain from swelling by reducing blood flow and the metabolic rate following injury. Because induced comas are intentional and therapeutic, they are not reported with coma scale codes.

CODING TIP According to AHA's *Coding Clinic* (Fourth Quarter, 2017), a Glasgow coma score should never be reported for patients in medically induced comas.[22]

Complications

Complications of specified implanted device or graft
HCC 176 0.597

Complications of care can be divided into two categories: intraoperative and postprocedural. Codes mapping to HCC 176 report postprocedural complications of implants or stomas. Included are codes related to mechanical complications, displacements, and infections and inflammatory reactions of urinary stomas, fixation devices, electronic devices, prosthetic joints, implants, and grafts that were previously placed.

Physician Documentation

Clearly document the relationship between the implant and the complication. ICD-10-CM Guideline Section I(B.16) states:

> **Documentation of Complications of Care**
>
> Code assignment is based on the provider's documentation of the relationship between the condition and the care or procedure, unless otherwise instructed by the classification. The guideline extends to any complications of care, regardless of the chapter the code is located in. It is important to note that not all conditions that occur during or following medical care or surgery are classified as complications. There must be a cause-and-effect relationship between the care provided and the condition, and an indication in the documentation that it is a complication. Query the provider for clarification, if the complication is not clearly documented.[1]

For complications of devices, identify the body system and the type of device. For clarity, identify the condition or diagnosis associated with the device. Specify the type of complication as breakdown, infection, displacement, leakage, hemorrhage, pain, embolism, fibrosis, etc. Note whether the patient is receiving care for the initial problem, or follow-up care in a subsequent encounter. Identify the complication as sequela, as appropriate.

CLINICAL EXAMPLES

NONSPECIFIC DOCUMENTATION	SPECIFIC DOCUMENTATION
Example 1 HPI: Patient has developed a PermaCath infection.[a]	**Example 1** HPI: Patient has developed a methicillin-resistant *Staphylococcus aureus* infection of her PermaCath, with sepsis. The patient is on hemodialysis for end-stage renal disease secondary to diabetic nephropathy.[b]
Example 2 Past history of cystocele repair with vaginal mesh implant 10 years ago. Being seen today for vaginal pain.[c]	**Example 2** Past history of cystocele repair with vaginal mesh implant 10 years ago. As a result, she has developed vaginal pain, as a complication of the extrusion of mesh into the vagina.[d]

[a] The etiology of the infection is missing, as well as the purpose of the PermaCath.

[b] In this instance, the infection is identified as MRSA and the catheter is documented as the cause of the infection. Furthermore, the reason for the catheter is documented, as is the cause of the patient's ESRD, all pertinent to this encounter and including multiple risk-adjusting codes.

[c] While the relationship between the mesh and the patient's ailment may seem obvious, a link has not been documented.

[d] Here, the patient's cellulitis and pain is clearly linked to the pelvic mesh.

Coding

Not all medical events during or following surgery are complications of surgical care. Hemorrhage, for example, may not be associated with surgical or procedural care, but with the underlying medical condition or as an adverse effect of a medication. In addition, an expected end-of-life of an implanted device also is not a complication of care. This distinction is drilled into coders and makes coders wary when assigning codes for complications of care. The codes in this HCC address complications of stomas or implanted devices. Malfunctions with stomas and implanted devices are considered implicit complications, ie, the implant or stoma would not be present without medical intervention; so, if the implant or stoma is malfunctioning, it is by definition a complication of medical care. This is supported by the classifications found under "Malfunction" in the Alphabetic Index and the placement of malfunction codes under categories for "Complication" in the ICD-10-CM Tabular List.

There is no time limit defining a complication of care. A graft or implant may fail or cause an infection immediately or years after surgery. Complications due to the presence of an implant are divided into two main categories: mechanical and non-mechanical. Mechanical failure indicates that the device malfunctioned in some way (eg, became broken, occluded, or displaced). Non-mechanical malfunctions include infection, fibrosis, or pain.

CODING TIP Finding the proper Alphabetic Index entry for device complication can be time consuming. In some cases, performing an electronic search of a PDF file of the *ICD-10-CM Official Guidelines for Coding and Reporting* may yield quicker and more accurate results (eg, for PICC line, nephroureteral stent, or penile prosthesis). This PDF can be downloaded from https://www.cms.gov/Medicare/Coding/ICD10/2018-ICD-10-CM-and-GEMs.html. First open the list entitled 2018 Code Tables and Index. Within that zipped file, save the file entitled icd10cm_index_2018.pdf.

ABSTRACT & CODE IT!

Abstract and code the clinical coding example below. Check your answers against the answers in Appendix C.

Patient 1

HPI: Patient has developed a methicillin-resistant *Staphylococcus aureus* infection of her PermaCath, with sepsis. The patient is on hemodialysis for end-stage renal disease secondary to diabetic nephropathy.

Patient 2

Past history of cystocele repair with vaginal mesh implant 10 years ago. As a result, she has developed vaginal pain related to extrusion of mesh into the vagina.

Patient 3

A patient undergoes a resection of the small intestine for Crohn's disease due to an obstruction. After surgery, the patient is noted to have acute blood-loss anemia.

Congestive Heart Failure

Congestive heart failure
HCC 85 **0.323**
RxHCC 186 **0.166**

Primary pulmonary hypertension
RxHCC 185 **0.740**

Heart failure is the condition in which the heart cannot pump sufficiently to keep up with the demands of the body, leading to tissue hypoperfusion, edema, and metabolic deficiencies. Normally, oxygen-rich blood is pumped out of the left side of the heart into the body, and carbon dioxide-rich blood returns to the right side of the heart to be pumped into the lungs for gas exchange. Oxygen-rich blood from the lungs enters the left side of the heart to be pumped into the body again. The right and left sides of the heart have separate functions, and when either side is dysfunctional, heart failure can result.

In the earliest stages of heart failure, the heart may try to compensate by beating faster and working harder, or it may develop more muscle mass in the ventricle. At this point, the physician may document systolic or diastolic dysfunction; however, if there is no documentation of heart failure, then a heart failure code from I50.- cannot be assigned.

When heart failure has advanced to a symptomatic state, it can be described as right-sided alone, left-sided alone, or biventricular. In addition, left-sided failure may be described as heart failure with reduced ejection fraction (HFrEF, usually less than 40% to 50%), otherwise known as systolic heart failure, or heart failure with preserved ejection fraction (HFpEF, usually greater than 40% to 50%), otherwise known as diastolic heart failure. The terms "systolic" and "diastolic" only apply to left-side heart failure.

Heart failure can even occur in what may appear to be a normal heart. Labeled as "high output heart failure," this occurs when the cardiac output is higher than normal due to increased peripheral demand. Circulatory overload ensues, which may lead to pulmonary edema secondary to an elevated diastolic pressure in the left ventricle. Common causes of high output heart failure include arteriovenous shunts in patients with end-stage renal disease, severe anemia, or Paget's disease of the bone.

"Congestive" heart failure describes the congestion of blood in the lungs and extremities when the heart cannot pump sufficiently. Congestive heart failure (CHF) is an unspecified description of heart failure. Common symptoms of heart failure are edema of the lower extremities or abdomen, shortness of breath (especially with exertion or when lying down flat), cough, loss of stamina, and difficulty sleeping. When symptoms are controlled, heart failure is considered to be compensated or chronic. If symptoms are uncontrolled, heart failure is considered to be decompensated or acute. Risk factors for congestive heart failure include obesity, tobacco use, coronary artery disease, hypertension, diabetes, and lung disease.

Pulmonary hypertension is classified in the congestive heart failure HCC and should be documented and coded when present. Pulmonary hypertension is defined as a mean pulmonary artery pressure ≥25 mm Hg at rest, measured during right heart catheterization.[23] Its presence, however, can be inferred if its consequences, right ventricular hypertrophy, and/or isolated right heart failure in the absence of left ventricular disease, are present in appropriate circumstances.

Cor pulmonale is right ventricular hypertrophy or dilation due to isolated pulmonary hypertension, implying that the left ventricular physiology does not contribute. It can be acute due to the rapid onset of pulmonary hypertension in the setting of a pulmonary embolus, manifested as right ventricular dilation and possibly a rise in the serum troponin levels, or chronic due to chronic pulmonary hypertension, manifested by right ventricular hypertrophy. Chronic (compensated) or acute (decompensated) right heart failure is not integral to the definition of acute or chronic cor pulmonale; however, it commonly occurs, which should be documented and coded with it occurs. ICD-10-CM has multiple codes for primary or secondary pulmonary hypertension based on its underlying cause. When present, use an additional code for cor pulmonale.

Physician Documentation

Heart health is critical to overall health, and treatments may include pharmacologic, nonpharmacologic, and surgical approaches. Details are important when documenting cardiac conditions, as treatment approaches vary depending on etiology, and because ICD-10-CM subdivides many heart ailments that were once bundled into a single code. Avoid using the phrase "history of CHF," as it may be interpreted as a current condition when it has resolved, or as a resolved condition when it is current. Instead, be specific in describing the duration of the CHF (eg, "The patient was first diagnosed with CHF in 2001 and currently requires furosemide for afterload reduction").

DOCUMENTATION TIP The physician must link a diastolic dysfunction or systolic dysfunction with heart failure in order for it to be reported as diastolic or systolic heart failure. Alternatively, HFpEF may be coded as diastolic heart failure and HFrEF may be coded as systolic heart failure. Other acronyms, such as HFrecEF (heart failure with recovered ejection fraction), require alternative documentation by the physician.

Heart failure is documented as left ventricular, right-sided, systolic, diastolic, or combined. Note whether acute (decompensated), chronic, or acute (decompensated) on chronic. New classifications for heart failure were added to the ICD-10-CM code set in 2018 and documentation should specifically describe these conditions when they occur (see Table 4-1.13).

TABLE 4-1.13 New Heart Failure Codes for 2018

CODE	DESCRIPTION
I50.810	Right heart failure, unspecified
I50.811	Acute right heart failure
I50.812	Chronic right heart failure
I50.813	Acute on chronic right heart failure
I50.814	Right heart failure due to left heart failure
I50.82	Biventricular heart failure
I50.83	High output heart failure
I50.84	End stage heart failure
I50.89	Other heart failure

For a diagnosis of biventricular and end-stage heart failure, two codes are required: one to report the biventricular or end-stage heart failure, and one to identify the type of heart failure. The National Center for Health Statistics (NCHS) described end-stage heart failure in its proposal for the new code:

> Patients with end stage heart failure fall into stage D of the ABCD classification of the American College of Cardiology (ACC)/American Heart Association (AHA), and are characterized by advanced structural heart disease and pronounced symptoms of heart failure at rest or upon minimal physical exertion, despite maximal medical treatment. They frequently develop intolerance to medical therapy and are developing worsening renal function and diuretic resistance according to current guidelines. This patient population has a 1-year mortality rate of approximately 50%, is at highest risk for re-hospitalization and requires special therapeutic interventions such as ventricular assist devices, artificial hearts and heart transplantation or hospice care.[24]

The ICD assumes a causal link between heart failure and hypertension unless the physician explicitly documents that heart failure is due to another cause (eg, an ischemic or alcoholic cardiomyopathy). This means that if hypertension and heart failure coexist, a code from I11, *Hypertensive heart disease,* or I13, *Hypertensive heart and chronic kidney disease* (if chronic kidney disease is also present that is not ascribed to another cause), must be used. If the heart failure is not due to hypertension, the physician must document the cause to prevent it from being abstracted as hypertensive heart disease.

Document pertinent symptoms related to the patient's CHF (eg, non-exertional dyspnea, fatigue, edema, or weight gain). (See Table 4-1.14.) The codes themselves would only be reported absent a heart diagnosis, as they are symptom codes, which do not risk-adjust.

TABLE 4-1.14 Common Heart-associated Symptom Codes

CODE	SYMPTOM
R00.0	Tachycardia, NOS
R00.1	Bradycardia, NOS
R00.2	Palpitations
R01.0	Benign murmur
R01.1	Murmur, NOS
R06.01	Orthopnea
R06.02	Shortness of breath
R18.8	Other ascites
R42	Dizziness
R53.83	Fatigue NOS
R60.0	Localized edema
R94.31	Abnormal ECG

In addition, document any tobacco exposure, dependence, or history for patients with heart disease (see Table 4-1.15).

TABLE 4-1.15 Common Tobacco Use and History Codes

CODE	DESCRIPTION
F17.210	Nicotine dependence, cigarettes, uncomplicated
F17.211	Nicotine dependence, cigarettes, in remission
F17.218	Nicotine dependence, cigarettes, with other nicotine-induced disorders
Z72.0	Tobacco use
Z77.22	Exposure to environmental tobacco smoke (acute) (chronic)
Z87.891	Personal history of nicotine dependence

Do not document "CHF" alone. CHF is a non-specific diagnosis, and there is a risk for an acronym to be misinterpreted. Spell out the first reference (eg, congestive heart failure [CHF]). Provide more specificity in the diagnosis, if possible.

CLINICAL EXAMPLES

NONSPECIFIC DOCUMENTATION	SPECIFIC DOCUMENTATION
Example 1 Echocardiography in combination with the patient's symptoms lead to a diagnosis of biventricular heart failure.[a]	**Example 1** Echocardiography in combination with the patient's symptoms lead to a diagnosis of acute on chronic systolic biventricular heart failure.[b]
Example 2 Hypertensive heart disease with heart failure.[c] We have increased his diuretics and he is now on full-time supplemental oxygen.	**Example 2** Hypertensive heart disease with end-stage heart failure with chronic diastolic and systolic heart failure that is now somewhat decompensated. We have increased his diuretics and he is now on full-time supplemental oxygen for chronic hyoxemic respiratory failure due to his pulmonary edema. He has requested and signed a DNR [do not resuscitate].[d]

[a] In addition to reporting the biventricular heart failure, the type of heart failure and its acuity must be documented. There isn't enough information for complete reporting here.

[b] With this information, the coder can now abstract the biventricular heart failure as well as the acute on chronic systolic heart failure.

[c] The physician echoed the language of the code description for the hypertension code, but it doesn't provide any details about the heart failure.

[d] The acuity of the patient's specific clinical condition is captured well here, with the documentation of chronic diastolic and systolic heart failure along with the end-stage heart failure.

Coding

Heart failure and heart dysfunction are not synonymous. Documentation of systolic or diastolic heart dysfunction is not documentation of systolic or diastolic heart failure. On the other hand, "heart failure with systolic dysfunction" or "heart failure and diastolic dysfunction" are sufficient linkage between heart failure and systolic or diastolic nature of the heart failure. AHA's *Coding Clinic* (First Quarter, 2017) advises that the documentation of "acutely decompensated congestive heart failure with diastolic dysfunction" may be coded as "I50.31, *Acute diastolic (congestive) heart failure.*" On the other hand, if the physician writes "CHF" on one line and "diastolic dysfunction" on another line and does not link the two together with the word "with," only I50.9, *Heart failure, unspecified*, may be reported.[17]

Support for CHF is often found in the physical exam, with noted third or fourth heart sounds, jugular vein distension, or extremity edema. Diagnostic tests (eg, electrocardiography, chest radiography, echocardiography, and angiography) also support heart failure. Medications to treat CHF include beta blockers, channel blockers, angiotension-converting enzyme (ACE) inhibitors, diuretics, digoxin, or spironolactone. It is important to find support that is specific to CHF in patients who have other heart conditions, as some medications may be used to treat both (eg, CHF and coronary artery disease).

Pleural effusion is a sign and symptom of congestive heart failure, which is not coded unless it is the subject of therapeutic intervention or diagnostic testing, according to AHA's *Coding Clinic* (Second Quarter, 2015).[25] When pleural effusion is part of an intervention or test, report code J91.8, *Pleural effusion in other conditions classified elsewhere,* in addition to the heart failure. Absent a heart-failure diagnosis, pulmonary edema is reported with a code from category J81, *Pulmonary edema.* This category of codes is not to be reported with heart-failure codes, unless the physician has explicitly documented that the pulmonary edema is noncardiogenic in nature, such as in an end-stage renal disease patient with fluid overload from noncompliance with hemodialysis.

Advanced structural heart disease and symptoms with little or no physical exertion are the hallmark of end-stage heart failure. According to AHA's *Coding Clinic* (Fourth Quarter, 2017), the ACC and AHA classify heart failure in stages, with end-stage heart failure falling into stage D. End-stage heart failure also falls into class III or IV of the New York Heart Association (NYHA) functional classification, as determined by the limitations the heart failure puts on physical activity. Patients with end-stage heart failure often develop intolerance to medical therapy, worsening renal function, and resistance to diuretics.[26] Stage A heart failure is a risk of heart failure, but it is not heart failure. Report Stage A heart failure with code Z91.89, *Other specified personal risk factors, not elsewhere classified*, according to AHA's *Coding Clinic* (First Quarter, 2017).[17] Never report Stage A heart failure with I50.9, *Heart failure, unspecified.*

For 2018, there is a new ICD-10-CM code for end-stage heart failure. I50.84, *End stage heart failure,* should be reported only when end-stage or Stage D heart failure is so stated in documentation. Report a second code to identify the patient's specific form of heart failure with I50.84, *End stage heart failure.* In addition, there are multiple new ICD-10-CM codes for secondary pulmonary hypertension categorized by its underlying cause, which must be explicitly documented (see Table 4-1.16).

TABLE 4-1.16 Secondary Pulmonary Hypertension Codes

CODE	DESCRIPTION
I27.20	Pulmonary hypertension, unspecified
I27.21	Secondary pulmonary arterial hypertension
I27.22	Pulmonary hypertension due to left heart disease
I27.23	Pulmonary hypertension due to lung diseases and hypoxia
I27.24	Chronic thromboembolic pulmonary hypertension
I27.29	Other secondary pulmonary hypertension

CODING TIP Advanced structural heart disease and symptoms with little or no physical exertion are the hallmark of end-stage heart failure. According to AHA's *Coding Clinic* (Fourth Quarter, 2017), the American College of Cardiology (ACC) and American Heart Association (AHA) classify heart failure in stages, with end-stage heart failure falling into stage D. End-stage heart failure also falls into class III or IV of the New York Heart Association (NYHA) functional classification, as determined by the limitations the heart failure puts on physical activity. Patients with end-stage heart failure often develop intolerance to medical therapy, worsening renal function, and resistance to diuretics.[25]

There are numerous instructions with each of the new secondary pulmonary hypertension codes, identifying other codes that should be reported in addition to the code for the pulmonary hypertension as well as inclusion terms with each entry.

CODING TIP AHA's *Coding Clinic* (Fourth Quarter, 2017) advises coders to also report any adverse effects of drugs or toxics, or associated conditions, such as HIV disease, thromboemboli, etc, when reporting codes from subcategory I27.2, *Secondary pulmonary hypertension*, if applicable.[26]

Chronic and acute cor pulmonale have separate codes that risk-adjust as congestive heart failure when present and coded. While it has multiple causes, ICD-10-CM only recognizes acute cor pulmonale when it is due to a pulmonary embolus. When a patient is diagnosed with acute cor pulmonale without pulmonary embolism, AHA's *Coding Clinic* (Fourth Quarter, 2014) advised that this condition should be reported with code I27.81, *Cor pulmonale (chronic)*, because "chronic" is a nonessential modifier, and code I26.09, *Other pulmonary embolism with acute cor pulmonale,* which is ICD-10-CM's only acute cor pulmonale code, includes pulmonary embolism.[27] According to AHA's *Coding Clinic* (Second Quarter, 2013), report decompensated heart failure as an acute on chronic heart failure.[28]

CODING TIP Never report code I10, *Essential (primary) hypertension,* with a code for CHF. There is a causal relationship between CHF and hypertension, ie, a code from either category I11, *Hypertensive heart disease,* or I13, *Hypertensive heart and chronic kidney disease,* should be reported instead, when hypertension and heart failure coexist with each other. The only exception is if the physician states in the record that the two conditions are not linked, in which case the physician would document another cause for the CHF.

Before the release of the 2018 changes to the Alphabetic Index, RA coders wondered if the *ICD-10-CM Guidelines* included heart failure in the rule regarding the assumed causal relationship to hypertension. That question is now resolved, and all of category I50, *Heart failure,* plus codes I51.4 through I51.9 have a causal relationship to hypertension:

I51.4	Myocarditis, unspecified
I51.5	Myocardial degeneration
I51.81	Takotsubo syndrome
I51.89	Other ill-defined heart diseases
I51.9	Heart disease, unspecified

New inclusion notes at the beginning of codes I50.2, *Systolic (congestive) heart failure,* and I50.3, *Diastolic (congestive) heart failure,* in the 2018 ICD-10-CM code set allow coders to report systolic or diastolic heart failure without these words being present in documentation. These inclusion terms reflect AHA's *Coding Clinic* (First Quarter, 2017) advice.[17]

Report systolic heart failure for documented:

- Heart failure with reduced ejection fraction
- HFrEF
- Systolic left ventricular heart failure

Report diastolic heart failure for documented:

- Diastolic left ventricular heart failure
- Heart failure with normal ejection fraction
- Heart failure with preserved ejection fraction (HFpEF)

Remember that these terms only apply to left heart failure, not isolated right heart failure.

ABSTRACT & CODE IT!

Abstract and code the clinical coding example below. Check your answers against the answers in Appendix C.

Patient 1
Assessment:

1. Hypertension. Bring record of home BP checks to next appointment.
2. Ventricular dilatation; unchanged in today's chest X ray.
3. Congestive heart failure. Continue diuretics and use of wedge pillow while sleeping.

Patient 2
Electrocardiography in combination with the patient's symptoms lead to a diagnosis of acute on chronic systolic biventricular heart failure.

Patient 3
Hypertensive heart disease with end-stage heart failure in chronic diastolic and systolic heart failure with mild decompensation. We have increased his diuretics and he is now on full-time supplemental oxygen for chronic hypoxemic respiratory failure. He has requested and signed a DNR.

Coronary Artery Disease *see* Ischemic Heart Disease

Crohn's Disease *see* Intestinal Disorders

Cystic Fibrosis

Cystic fibrosis
HCC 110 0.620
RxHCC 225 0.745

Cystic fibrosis (CF) is a genetic disorder of the exocrine glands that leads to malabsorption as a result of pancreatic deficiencies and to respiratory disorders as a result of deficiencies in secretions in the respiratory system. It is a life-shortening, incurable disorder affecting approximately 30,000 people in the US, with 2,500 new diagnoses each year.[29] In some cases, the diagnosis is made soon after birth in association with an intestinal blockage, when thick mucus prevents the passage of feces in the patient's ileum. This is called meconium ileus. In other cases, the diagnosis comes years later.

Patients with CF undergo daily percussive therapy to loosen thick mucus in the lungs. Pancreatic enzyme replacements improve nutritional uptake and are taken with every meal. Thick mucus not only affects the respiratory system, but the digestive system and its organs. Some patients with CF develop diabetes secondary to pancreatic damage.

Physician Documentation

In the neonate, note any meconium ileus. For CF patients with pneumonia, document the causal agent. If the patient is prescribed pancreatic enzymes for nutrient uptake, document the exocrine pancreatic insufficiency. It is reported in addition to the CF, and represents a different and additive RxHCC.

It is not uncommon for CF patients to develop pneumonia that is more commonly due to pseudomonas or methicillin-resistant *Staphylococcus aureus* (MRSA) that requires broader-spectrum or more specific antibiotics (eg, tobramycin) than patients without CF. The physician must explicitly state that the pneumonia or bronchitis is due to a specific organism if the pneumonia is to be captured for RA (see Table 4-1.17).

TABLE 4-1.17 Cystic Fibrosis Codes

CODE	DESCRIPTION
E84.0	Cystic fibrosis with pulmonary manifestations
E84.11	Meconium ileus in cystic fibrosis
E84.19	Cystic fibrosis with other intestinal manifestations
E84.8	Cystic fibrosis with other manifestations
E84.9	Cystic fibrosis, unspecified

Coding

Support for CF can be found in prescribed medications including bronchodilators, mucus-thinners, and digestive enzymes, as well as percussive therapies to loosen mucus. Close attention is paid in any encounter with a CF patient to the patient's pulmonary health, since pneumonia is a common problem for patients with CF. Percussive therapy is performed daily. For some patients, this therapy takes the form of a vest that contains a high-frequency chest-wall oscillation device. Code all comorbidities with CF.

CODING TIP Code K86.81, *Exocrine pancreatic insufficiency,* describes the inability to digest food properly due to an insufficiency in exocrine pancreatic digestive enzymes as seen in many patients with CF, according to AHA's *Coding Clinic* (Fourth Quarter, 2016).[30] The condition causes abdominal pain, diarrhea, gas, and weight loss. Treatment of this disorder with oral enzymes is called pancreatic enzyme replacement therapy (PERT).

References

1. Centers for Medicare & Medicaid Services. *ICD-10-CM Official Guidelines for Coding and Reporting* (FY 2018): Guideline I.A.13. https://www.cms.gov/Medicare/Coding/ICD10/2018-ICD-10-PCS-and-GEMs.html. Accessed Oct 27, 2017.
2. National Limb Loss Information Center. Amputation Statistics by Cause: Limb Loss in the Unites States. http://www.figeducation.com/nlcp/resources/section-4/ACA%20Statistics.pdf. Accessed Oct 27, 2017.
3. Amputee Coalition™. Roadmap for Preventing Limb Loss in America: *Recommendations From the 2012 Limb Loss Task Force.* http://www.amputee-coalition.org/wp-content/uploads/2014/09/lsp_Roadmap-for-Limb-Loss-Prevention-and-Amputee-Care-Improvement_241014-092312.pdf. Accessed Nov 20, 2017.
4. Cecconi M, De Backer D, Antonelli M. et al. Consensus on circulatory shock and hemodynamic monitoring. Task force of the European Society of Intensive Care Medicine. *Intensive Care Med* 2014;40(12):1795-1815. https://doi.org/10.1007/s00134-014-3525-z. Accessed Nov 20, 2017.
5. American Hospital Association. *Coding Clinic® for ICD-9-CM Q4.* 2011;28(4):123-125.
6. American Hospital Association. *Coding Clinic® for ICD-9-CM Q3.* 2013;30(3):23.
7. Lupus Foundation of America (National Resource Center on Lupus). Lupus Facts and Statistics. https://resources.lupus.org/entry/facts-and-statistics. Accessed Nov 21, 2017.
8. American Hospital Association. *Coding Clinic® for ICD-10-CM and ICD-10-PCS Q3.* 2015;2(3):21-22.
9. Arthritis Foundation®. What is Juvenile Idiopathic Arthritis? http://www.arthritis.org/about-arthritis/types/juvenile-idiopathic-arthritis-jia/what-is-juvenile-idiopathic-arthritis.php. Accessed Oct 27, 2017.
10. Schizophrenia and Related Disorders Alliance of America. About Schizophrenia. https://sardaa.org/resources/about-schizophrenia/. Accessed Nov 21, 2017.
11. Centers for Disease Control and Prevention. Burden of Mental Illness. https://www.cdc.gov/mentalhealth/basics/burden.htm. Accessed Nov 21, 2017.
12. Centers for Medicare & Medicaid Services. *2008 Risk Adjustment Data Technical Assistance for Medicare Advantage Organizations Participant Guide.* https://www.csscoperations.com/Internet/Cssc3.Nsf/files/participant-guide-publish_052909.pdf/$File/participant-guide-publish_052909.pdf. Accessed Nov 1, 2017.
13. Centers for Disease Control and Prevention. Sickle Cell Disease (SCD). https://www.cdc.gov/ncbddd/sicklecell/data.html. Accessed Nov 21, 2017.
14. Centers for Disease Control and Prevention. Hemophilia. https://www.cdc.gov/ncbddd/hemophilia/facts.html. Accessed Nov 21, 2017.
15. National Institute of Neurological Disorders and Stroke. What is Cerebral Palsy? https://www.ninds.nih.gov/Disorders/Patient-Caregiver-Education/Hope-Through-Research/Cerebral-Palsy-Hope-Through-Research. Accessed Nov 21, 2017.
16. American Hospital Association. *Coding Clinic® for ICD-10-CM and ICD-10 PSC Q3.* 2017;4(3):3.
17. American Hospital Association. *Coding Clinic® for ICD-10-CM and ICD-10 PCS Q1.* 2017;4(1):45-48.
18. American Hospital Association. *Coding Clinic® for ICD-10-CM and ICD-10-PCS Q1.* 2014;1(1):23.
19. American Hospital Association. *Coding Clinic® for ICD-10-CM and ICD-10-PCS Q1.* 2015;2(1):25.
20. Chronic Conditions Data Warehouse. Medicare Tables & Reports. https://www.ccwdata.org/web/guest/medicare-charts/medicare-other-chronic-and-disabling-conditions. Accessed Nov 1, 2017.
21. World Health Organization. *ICD-10 Guide for Mental Retardation.* Geneva, Switzerland: Division of Mental Health and Prevention of Substance Abuse; 1996. http://www.who.int/mental_health/media/en/69.pdf. Accessed Nov 21, 2017.
22. American Hospital Association. *Coding Clinic® for ICD-10-CM and ICD-10-PCS Q4.* 2017;4(4):95.
23. Hoeper MM, Bogaard J, Condliffe R, et al. Definitions and Diagnosis of Pulmonary Hypertension. *J Am Coll Cardiol.* 2013 Dec 24;62(25 Suppl):D42-50. doi: 10.1016/j.jacc.2013.10.032. Accessed Nov 20, 2017.

24. Centers for Disease Control and Prevention. End Stage Heart Failure, Right Heart Failure and Biventricular Heart Failure. In: ICD-10 Coordination and Maintenance Committee Meeting. September 22-23, 2015. Diagnosis Agenda. https://www.cdc.gov/nchs/data/icd/Topic_Packet_09_22_23_15.pdf. Accessed Nov 20, 2017.

25. American Hospital Association. *Coding Clinic® for ICD-10-CM and ICD-10-PCS Q2*. 2015;1(2):15-16.

26. American Hospital Association. *Coding Clinic for ICD-10-CM and ICD-10-PCS Q4*. 2017;4(4):15-16.

27. American Hospital Association. *Coding Clinic® for ICD-10-CM and ICD-10-PCS Q4*. 2014;1(4):21-22.

28. American Hospital Association. *Coding Clinic® for ICD-9-CM Q2*. 2013;30(2):33.

29. Centers for Disease Control and Prevention. Cystic Fibrosis. https://www.cdc.gov/scienceambassador/documents/cystic-fibrosis-fact-sheet.pdf. Accessed Nov 21, 2017.

30. American Hospital Association. *Coding Clinic® for ICD-10-CM and ICD-10-PCS Q4*. 2016;3(4):34-35.

CHAPTER 4

Clinical Documentation Integrity and Coding

PART 2: TOPICS D–M

Dementia

Alzheimer's disease
RxHCC 111 0.476

Dementia, except Alzheimer's disease
RxHCC 112 0.196

Dementia occurs in conjunction with degenerative conditions or damage to the brain. Changes to the blood supply to cerebral issue can cause ischemic disease and vascular dementia. HIV and some other infectious disorders, and noninfectious brain disorders like Parkinson's and Huntington's diseases can also result in dementia, as can direct trauma to the brain. Plaque deposits that occur in aging also can be a source of dementia, as in Alzheimer's disease. The neurodegeneration that causes dementia can come in many forms, affect different cerebral functions, and result in different symptoms. Diagnosis of dementia is often made based on the symptoms the patient exhibits or on the patient's underlying diagnosed diseases.

According to the National Institutes of Health (NIH), Alzheimer's disease is the most common cause of dementia in adults, and the third leading cause of death in older adults.[1] Most people with Alzheimer's disease develop the late form, which can occur after 65 years of age. Early onset disease can begin in a person's 30s to mid-60s, and represents less than 10% of all Alzheimer's disease. Most people with Down syndrome will develop Alzheimer's disease as adults.[1]

A patient with dementia has memory deficits and confusion or lapses in judgment. The degree of dementia can vary from hour to hour, or day to day. Over time, however, the patient becomes progressively confused. A caregiver or family member will usually accompany dementia patients to medical encounters, and provide the patient's history and chief complaint.

Physician Documentation

Documentation of mental health and decline is an important concept in senior care. Note all counseling services provided for driving alternatives, safety issues, neuropsychiatric referrals, interventions, or end-of-life decisions, and any medication changes. Note and document if any part of the patient's history is provided by someone other than the patient, as well as when the patient is accompanied to the encounter by another person. Be as specific as possible in describing the patient's mental capabilities, symptoms, or diagnosis.

Dementia is a progressive decline in cognition along with a short- and long-term memory loss due to brain damage or disease. It is always going to affect the health of the patient and should be documented for all encounters, as it affects care planning. See Table 4-2.1 for the ICD-10-CM common nomenclature for symptoms seen in patients at risk for dementia and the associated codes (of these, only the sequelae of stroke codes risk-adjust).

TABLE 4-2.1 ICD-10-CM Nomenclature for Dementia Symptoms and Codes

SYMPTOMS THAT MAY EVOLVE TOWARD DEMENTIA	CODE(S)
Altered mental status, unspecified	R41.82
Mild cognitive impairment, so stated	G31.84
Age-associated cognitive decline	R41.81
Cognitive communication deficit	R41.841
White matter disease, diagnostic imaging, NOS	R90.82
Cognitive deficit following stroke, specify deficit; specify origin as intracerebral/subarachnoid bleed vs infarction	I69.-
Personal history of traumatic brain injury	Z87.820
Frontal lobe and executive function deficit	R41.844

Often, there is a discrepancy between the nomenclature used by physicians in documentation and the nomenclature required for abstracting a specific dementia diagnosis. See Table 4-2.2 for the ICD-10-CM common nomenclature for the etiology of dementia and its associated codes.

TABLE 4-2.2 ICD-10-CM Nomenclature for Dementia Etiology and Codes

DEMENTIA ETIOLOGY	CODE(S)
Alcoholic dementia, state dependence, abuse	F10.27, F10.97,
Alzheimer's disease, state early or late onset	G30.-
Cerebral lipidoses	E75.-
Epilepsy	G40.-
Frontotemporal dementia	G31.09
Huntington's disease	G10
Lewy body disease	G31.83
Multiple sclerosis	G35
Parkinson's disease	G20
Pick's disease	G31.01
Senile dementia, not otherwise specified	F03.9-
Unspecified dementia	F03.9-
Vascular dementia	F01.5-

For most forms of dementia, one code identifies the etiology, and a second code describes dementia with or without behavioral disturbance. Document violent, combative, or aggressive behavior to capture the extra work required in serving a patient with behavioral disorders in dementia. This will be reported as dementia with behavioral disturbance. Also document any wandering (Z91.83) or sundowning (F05), so that the full scope of the patient's symptoms are captured.

DOCUMENTATION TIP The age of onset of Alzheimer's disease is pertinent to outcomes. Younger patients have a greater impairment in neocortical temporal function, affecting practical application of knowledge. Later onset results in greater impairment in limbic disorders affecting visual memory and orientation. Document the patient's Alzheimer's disease as early onset (before age 65) or late onset (after age 65).

Some conditions may be perceived as inherent in dementia or advanced dementia, but the classification does not capture these conditions in the dementia codes. These conditions (eg, depression, sleep disorders, cachexia, or frailty) may risk-adjust and should be documented when they occur. It's important to capture and treat these diagnoses for the patient's comfort, and the coding of these documented diagnoses provides reimbursement to the payer that is covering a member who has complications from his or her dementia.

Always spell out first references when using acronyms (eg, Alzheimer's disease [AD] and age-associated cognitive decline [AACD]), to prevent confusion and elevate the accuracy of documentation.

Dementia is always going to affect the care of a patient. The subjective record may not be accurate, or may be provided by someone other than the patient. Adherence to a treatment plan may be more difficult. Dementia and its underlying cause should be reported for every face-to-face encounter, as well as any reliance on a third party's provision of the patient's history, and any behavioral disturbance witnessed or reported.

Functional quadriplegia may be the reason that a patient with dementia is admitted to costly intermediate care facilities or have a longer length of stay in an inpatient facility. Physician recognition of this ICD-10-CM term and its documentation in the record is essential to proper HCC risk adjustment (RA).

CLINICAL EXAMPLES

NONSPECIFIC DOCUMENTATION	SPECIFIC DOCUMENTATION
Example 1 I have determined that the best course of care is to place a PEG tube for enteral feeding. Mrs. Doe has lost 32 lbs. in the past 12 months due to Alzheimer's disease.[a]	**Example 1** I have determined that the best course of care is to place a PEG tube for enteral feeding to see if the additional nourishment will improve Mrs. Doe's moderate malnutrition. Mrs. Doe has lost 32 lbs. in the past 12 months due to a lack of interest in food caused by her early Alzheimer's disease. Her current BMI is 16.8.[b]
Example 2 The patient is a long-term resident of the Acme Alzheimer's Center on Harmon Avenue and was transported to the Emergency Department for evaluation of urosepsis.[c]	**Example 2** The patient is a long-term resident of the Acme Alzheimer's Center on Harmon Avenue and was transported to the Emergency Department for evaluation of a suspected urinary tract infection (UTI). The nurse who accompanied the patient reported that the patient has Alzheimer's disease and has been in the facility for two years, as he was too combative to remain at home with his wife. Today, the patient is obtunded, with a low-grade fever. The facility suspects the patient has "another" UTI. These recur about three times a year.[d] The lab confirms UTI and sepsis, both due to *E. coli.*

[a] The type of Alzheimer's disease is not identified here. More importantly, there is no diagnosis associated with the patient's weight loss. A coder cannot infer a diagnosis of cachexia or malnutrition from statistics or the presence of Alzheimer's or any other disorder. The patient's BMI is missing, too.

[b] All critical elements of this patient's risks are addressed: early Alzheimer's; abnormal BMI; moderate malnutrition; and long-term weight loss.

[c] While it is stated that the patient is a resident of an Alzheimer's facility, this documentation neglects to connect the dots and state that the patient has Alzheimer's disease. Further, the term "urosepsis" is outdated. The ICD-10-CM Alphabetic Index directs coders under "Urosepsis" to "code to condition." If no condition other than urosepsis is listed, none can be captured.

[d] Key elements capture the patient's Alzheimer's disease, and that the patient has behavioral disturbances associated with his Alzheimer's condition. Also documented is that the person giving the patient's history is not the patient. The UTI and sepsis are both linked to an infective agent, and the history states the patient has recurring UTIs.

Coding

Dementia is inherent in Alzheimer's disease. If the physician does not document dementia, but documents Alzheimer's disease, report codes G30.9, *Alzheimer's disease, unspecified,* and F02.80, *Dementia in other diseases classified elsewhere without behavioral disturbance.* This is based on the Alphabetic Index entry requiring two codes, one bracketed. This convention also affects Lewy body and Pick's disease when dementia is not noted. Report behavioral status for any patient with dementia. The patient who is violent, aggressive, or uncooperative should be coded with behavioral disturbance. In some cases, the behavioral disturbance, dementia, and etiology are captured with one code. In other instances, two codes are required.

CODING TIP The Alphabetic Index entry, "Parkinson's disease, syndrome or tremor – *see* Parkinsonism," can be misleading. Parkinsonism is defined as tremor and abnormalities in movement. Patients with Parkinson's disease, a specific neurological disorder, have parkinsonism, but not all patients with parkinsonism have Parkinson's disease. It is best to ignore the Parkinson's disease entry in the Alphabetic Index, and code Parkinson's disease or parkinsonism with dementia without behavioral disturbance as follows:

Dementia due to Parkinson's disease:

G20	Parkinson's disease
F02.80	Dementia in diseases classified elsewhere without behavioral disturbance

Dementia due to parkinsonism:

G31.83	Dementia with Lewy bodies
F20.80	Dementia in diseases classified elsewhere without behavioral disturbance

Wandering is common in dementia, especially in Alzheimer's disease. Wandering is reported in addition to dementia with Z91.83, *Wandering in diseases classified elsewhere.* Sundowning, in which the patient becomes increasingly confused during the day so that the patient ends the day in delirium, is reported in addition to dementia with F05, *Delirium due to known physiological condition.* While there is no official ICD-10-CM guidance regarding whether sundowning and wandering constitute "behavioral disturbance," *Diagnostic and Statistical Manual of Mental Disorders, Fifth Edition* (DSM-5) states that clinically significant psychotic symptoms, mood disturbance, agitation, apathy, or other behavioral symptoms do. As inclusion terms for dementia with behavioral disturbance include only "aggressive," "violent," or "combative" behaviors, query the physician or report "without behavioral disturbance" if wandering or sundowning is documented in dementia.

> **CODING TIP** The ICD-10-CM assumes a link between persistent dementia and alcohol use, dependence, or unspecified use. For example, report code F10.27, *Alcohol dependence with alcohol-induced persisting dementia,* whenever documentation states persistent dementia in a patient who is also noted to be alcohol dependent, unless the physician documents another etiology for the persistent dementia.

Dementia is inherent in some neurological conditions (eg, Alzheimer's, Lewy body disease, and Pick's disease). If Alzheimer's disease is documented, report the Alzheimer's and code F02.80, *Dementia in diseases classified elsewhere,* even when documentation does not mention dementia. This is based on ICD-10-CM guidelines and the Alphabetic Index entry for Alzheimer's disease.

To understand why the index entries are important for capturing both codes for these conditions, see the etiology/manifestation convention in ICD-10-CM Guideline Section I(A.13), which states:

> Certain conditions have both an underlying etiology and multiple body system manifestations due to the underlying etiology. For such conditions, the ICD-10-CM has a coding convention that requires the underlying condition be sequenced first, if applicable, followed by the manifestation. Wherever such a combination exists, there is a "use additional code" note at the etiology code, and a "code first" note at the manifestation code. These instructional notes indicate the proper sequencing order of the codes, etiology followed by manifestation.[2]

The *ICD-10-CM Guidelines'* etiology/manifestation convention dictates that two codes are required to report Alzheimer's disease (Disease/Alzheimer's G30.9 *[F02.80]*). The Alphabetic Index also provides two codes for Disease/Lewy body (G31.83 *[F02.80]*), and Disease/Pick's (G31.01 *[F02.80]*). See Huntington's disease, Parkinson's disease, and Cruetzfeldt-Jakob disease for examples of neurological orders that may cause dementia, but for which dementia is not always a manifestation. The American Hospital Association's (AHA's) *Coding Clinic for ICD-10-CM and ICD-10-PCS (Coding Clinic)* (First Quarter, 2017) also addresses Alzheimer's disease and dementia, advising that dementia must be coded even when it is not documented with the Alzheimer's disease.[3]

> **CODING TIP** If vascular dementia is documented as a sequela of cerebral infarction or hemorrhage, report the vascular dementia with F01.5-, *Vascular dementia,* and the sequela with I69.398, *Other sequelae of cerebral infarction.* There is no time limit on when a late effect code can be used to report a cognitive deficit from a stroke. Once the patient has been released from the hospital following an acute infarct or hemorrhage, the codes from category I69 may be used to report any deficits.

Delirium and other symptoms similar to dementia may be present in an elderly patient who has a urinary tract infection or other malady. Do not make assumptions regarding the diagnosis; query the physician to answer any questions. Also code any noted dementia comorbidities (eg, E44.1, *Mild protein-calorie malnutrition,* F32.9, *Major depressive disorder, single episode, unspecified,* F51.05, *Insomnia due to other mental disorder,* or R54, *Age related physical debility*).

One of the most devastating consequences of a neurodegenerative illness is the loss of one's mobility, resulting in frequent falls and trauma and requiring total care that is quite expensive. Some patients with dementia become so incapacitated that they become bedridden, chair-ridden, or wheelchair confined. They cannot move from one place to another without total assistance.

ABSTRACT & CODE IT!

Abstract and code the clinical coding example below. Check your answers against the answers in Appendix C.

Patient 1

Pre-senile Alzheimer's disease, early onset. We will start the patient on donepezil.

Patient 2

Generalized atherosclerosis with vascular dementia. Patient also has a history of multiple transient ischemic attacks. She is being transferred to a long-term care facility.

Patient 3

Patient brought in by daughter who reports her mother has been disoriented and very confused for two days. The patient is determined to have a urinary tract infection due to *K. pneumoniae,* and is prescribed antibiotics.

Depression *see* Behavioral Disorders

Diabetes Mellitus

Diabetes with acute complications

HCC 17 **0.318**
RxHCC 30 **0.425**

Diabetes with chronic complications

HCC 18 **0.318**
RxHCC 30 **0.425**

Diabetes without complications

HCC 19 **0.104**
RxHCC 31 **0.280**

Proliferative diabetic retinopathy and vitreous hemorrhage

HCC 122 **0.217**

Diabetic retinopathy

RxHCC 241 **0.307**

Diabetes mellitus (DM) is a chronic, lifelong metabolic disorder affecting uptake and storage of carbohydrate, protein, and fat. Twenty-three million people have a diagnosis of diabetes in the United States (US), and 7.2 million have undiagnosed diabetes, according to the NIH *National Diabetes Statistics Report, 2017.*[4] Sustained high blood glucose levels lead to the diagnosis. One in four patients 65 years or older have diabetes. DM should be addressed in every encounter with the diabetic patient, as it will always affect outcomes and care.

Diabetes occurs when the supply of insulin cannot keep up with the body's demand or when the body becomes resistant to the insulin being produced. Insulin is a hormone produced by islet cells in the pancreas and is necessary for the conversion of sugars in the bloodstream into energy or fat. Without insulin, the sugars circulate in the blood until they are filtered by the kidneys and eliminated in urine. Because the sugar is eliminated through urination, polyuria and excessive thirst are often the first symptoms of diabetes. Because the body cannot take up the sugars that are digested, but instead eliminates them through urine, excessive hunger is another common symptom. Many patients have unexplained weight loss before the diagnosis of diabetes.

DM is actually a grouping of a couple of disorders with dissimilar etiologies, but because the resultant metabolic changes are similar, they are all called "diabetes mellitus." Chiefly, diabetes can be divided into two subgroups: diabetes with insulin production and diabetes absent insulin production. Type 2 DM is the most common form of DM, accounting for more than 90% of DM. In type 2 DM, insulin is manufactured by the pancreas. However, the patient has hyperglycemia because there exist problems in insulin production, transport, or uptake. Type 2 DM is usually seen in elderly or overweight adults; however, it may occur in juveniles. Type 1 DM, accounting for 5% of diabetic patients, is caused by an autoimmune response that results in the ultimate destruction of all insulin-producing cells in the pancreas. Type 1 DM usually begins in childhood but may first be diagnosed in young adults.[4]

There is a newer diagnosis of diabetes, type 1.5, thought to be the more correct diagnosis in as many as 10% of type 2 DM patients. Type 1.5 is a combination of types 1 and 2: the patient may not be overweight or elderly, and initially requires only oral medications for management of the diabetes. However, eventually the patient requires insulin, as an autoimmune process destroys the insulin-producing cells.

CODING TIP Diabetes insipidus (DI) is a completely different disease from diabetes mellitus, with its own codes. DI is a disorder affecting fluid balance in the body, and risk-adjusts to HCC 23 and RxHCC 41.

 **ADVICE/ALERT NOTE**

If the type of diabetes mellitus is not documented in the medical record, the default is E11.-, *Type 2 diabetes mellitus.*

Secondary forms of diabetes may occur because the pancreas has become diseased, as in cystic fibrosis (CF) or long-term use of corticosteroids; or due to pancreatectomy. In secondary diabetes, the patient may or may not produce insulin. Gestational diabetes is a temporary form of diabetes brought on by the burden of pregnancy on insulin production and transport. Delivery usually resolves the diabetes. Patients with diabetes may be treated with oral antihyperglycemics or insulin.

Type 1 patients will always be prescribed insulin; without it, they would likely develop ketoacidosis and die without treatment. Type 2 patients can be treated with oral medications to improve their sensitivity to insulin and/or with insulin as needed to achieve and maintain adequate control. While it is uncommon, a Type 2 diabetic may develop ketoacidosis. Type 1 and type 2 diabetic patients usually perform daily blood glucose tests at home to ensure their blood glucose is in good control. Studies have shown that controlled blood sugars can reduce the incidence of long-term complications of diabetes, which occur due to inflammation and damage, over time, to the small blood vessels in the body.

Physician Documentation

According to ICD-10-CM Guideline Section I(C.4.a.2), "[i]f the type of diabetes mellitus is not documented in the medical record the default is E11.-, Type 2 diabetes mellitus."[2]

Document the type of diabetes as:

- Type 1 (autoimmune; no insulin production)
- Type 2 (insulin resistance or low production; most common form)
- Secondary
  - Document underlying condition (eg, CF, cancer, pancreatitis, Cushing's syndrome, or disease not caused by pharmaceutical)
  - Document drug or chemical causing the adverse effect (eg, corticosteroids, streptozotocin, alloxan, Vacor rodenticide)
  - Document postpancreatectomy

Type 1.5 does not have its own code. Physicians should identify how the coder should abstract DM type 1.5 (eg, as type 1 or type 2). Only one type of diabetes should be documented in each encounter for one patient. A coder cannot look at other encounter notes to determine which type of diabetes a patient has, so it should be documented at every encounter. Prediabetes and borderline diabetes are classified to R73.03, *Prediabetes.*

Document whether the diabetes is controlled by diet and exercise, anti-diabetic medications, insulin, or a combination of these modalities. These outdated terms should be avoided in documentation:

- Insulin-dependent diabetes mellitus (IDDM)
- Noninsulin–dependent diabetes mellitus (NIDDM)
- Juvenile onset diabetes
- Adult onset diabetes
- Brittle diabetes

The ICD-10-CM instructs coders to assume a causal link between most systemic disorders and diabetes, meaning that if they coexist, ICD-10-CM considers these a complication of diabetes unless explicitly documented otherwise. While neuropathies, nephropathies, retinopathies, and the like are commonly encountered, ICD-10-CM also considers cataracts, osteomyelitis, periodontal diseases, and skin ulcers to be diabetic complications when they coexist. Physicians should document when a comorbidity is not due to diabetes, or it will be reported as a complication of diabetes. If the patient's chronic kidney disease (CKD) has another cause, be sure to document it, using clear language; eg, CKD stage 5 due to polycystic congenital kidney disease. Regardless of ICD-10-CM rules, best practices would have physicians always linking each complication to the diabetes in their documentation. This can be accomplished by adding the adjective "diabetic" before the complication (eg, diabetic nephropathy).

Provide qualitative information regarding diabetic control (eg, "Diabetes is in good control despite pneumonia. Blood glucose today is 105. Patient's A1C is 7.6, and his goal is 6.5.").

Address all complications of diabetes with qualitative language that documents the extent or severity of the complication; eg, "diabetic neuropathy has progressed to loss of protective sensation (LOPS)." Document any status resulting from diabetes. Ensure that the patient's vision loss, amputation, or dialysis status is documented during the encounter at least once a year.

Hyperglycemia is no longer considered a symptom of diabetes and should be noted in the medical record when it exists, as it is a complication of diabetes that changes the HCC. Similarly, document any hypoglycemia. State the obvious. Do not document "BG of 495." Instead, document, "patient's blood glucose indicates hyperglycemia at 495." Coders cannot code from laboratory values. Documented "poorly controlled" or "out-of-control" DM is reported as hyperglycemia, according to the ICD-10-CM Alphabetic Index. Documented "uncontrolled" diabetes is insufficient information for coding, as it could indicate hyper- or hypoglycemia and defaults to diabetes without complication.

DOCUMENTATION TIP When documenting diabetic retinopathy and macular edema, the following elements are necessary for complete reporting:

- Laterality
- Proliferative/nonproliferative
- With/without macular edema
- In proliferative: presence of traction retinal detachment; rhegmatogenous retinal attachment

Document resolved macular edema, including laterality, when present. The presence of *resolved* macular edema of diabetes is reported as an ongoing complication of diabetes.

Document all referrals for dietetic counseling, foot care, or other therapies. Avoid the acronym DM, as it may be misinterpreted. If using the acronym, spell it out in first reference (eg, diabetes mellitus [DM]).

CLINICAL EXAMPLES

NONSPECIFIC DOCUMENTATION	SPECIFIC DOCUMENTATION
Example 1 Assessment/Plan: 1. Hypertensive heart and renal disease with (congestive) heart failure.[a] I13.0, *Hypertensive heart and chronic kidney disease with heart failure and stage 1 through stage 4 chronic kidney disease, or unspecified chronic kidney disease* 2. Renal disorder due to type 2 diabetes mellitus. E11.29, *Type 2 diabetes mellitus with other diabetic kidney complication* Basic metabolic panel and HGB A1C ordered.	**Example 1** Assessment/Plan: 1. Controlled hypertension. Blood pressure today 125/81. Keep on current medications since they seem to be doing the job. 2. Improved chronic systolic heart failure. Edema is down, and patient is no longer SOB at rest. Significant improvement. 3. Stable CKD, stage 4. Most recent GFR 22; will retest next visit. 4. Controlled diabetes mellitus, type 2 Today's A1C was 7.1. Her BG was 105. Continue metformin. Basic metabolic panel and HGB A1C ordered.[b]
Example 2 Patient has had diabetes since he was 10.[c]	**Example 2** Patient has had type 1 diabetes since he was 10.[d]

[a] This assessment says a lot without providing much information. It is noted that the patient has hypertensive heart disease, but no heart disease is documented and no heart failure is noted. The renal disorder due to diabetes is not identified. The stage of CKD is not specified. It is usually a mistake to use diagnostic codes in the assessment. This practice tends to lead to under-documentation.

[b] The physician has given some context for each diagnosis, as improved, controlled, stable, etc, and identified in narrative the plan for each diagnosis. By listing each diagnosis separately, a more detailed picture of the individual diagnosis is provided (eg, the heart failure and CKD). The type of medication used by the patient is also documented here.

[c] Identify the type of diabetes. Coders cannot assume.

[d] The type of diabetes is documented in a way that can be used by the coder.

Coding

According to the *2008 Risk Adjustment Data Technical Assistance for Medicare Advantage Organizations Participant Guide* (*2008 RA Participant Guide*), a "laboratory test showing one reading of high blood sugar is not considered sufficient 'clinical evidence' of diabetes—the medical record needs to document a clinician's diagnosis of diabetes during the data collection period."[5] Report acute metabolic encephalopathy secondary to hypoglycemia with a diabetes code ending in .641 or .649, for hypoglycemia with or without coma; and G93.41, *Metabolic encephalopathy,* according to AHA's *Coding Clinic* (Third Quarter, 2016). Never report E16.2, *Hypoglycemia, unspecified*, found in the Alphabetic Index under "encephalopathy, hypoglycemic," for diabetic encephalopathy.[6]

According to ICD-10-CM Guideline Section I(C.4.a.3), if the "documentation in a medical record does not indicate the type of diabetes but does indicate that the patient uses insulin, code E11-, Type 2 diabetes mellitus, should be assigned. An additional code should be assigned from category Z79 to identify the long-term (current) use of insulin or oral hypoglycemic drugs. If the patient is treated with both oral medications and insulin, only the code for long-term (current) use of insulin should be assigned. Code Z79.4 should not be assigned if insulin is given temporarily to bring a type 2 patient's blood sugar under control during an encounter ."[2] Because patients with type 1 diabetes require insulin injections or infusions multiple times daily to survive, there is no need to report code Z79.4, *Long term (current) use of insulin,* with type 1 diabetes. To do so is redundant.

Until 2018, ICD-10-CM did not provide codes for Type 2 with ketoacidosis (DKA), and coders were directed by AHA's *Coding Clinic* to report E13.1- codes for documented type 2 diabetes with DKA. Beginning in October 2017, type 2 diabetes with DKA is reported with new codes E11.10, *Type 2 diabetes with ketoacidosis without coma,* and E11.11, *Type 2 diabetes mellitus with ketoacidosis with coma.* If the type of diabetes is not stated, and the patient has diabetic ketoacidosis, the default is type 1. Ketoacidosis occurs almost exclusively in type 1 diabetes; however, it can occur in Type 2 diabetes.

CODING TIP Diabetic autonomic neuropathy encompasses a neuropathy affecting the sympathetic or parasympathetic nerves, and is reported with a diabetes code ending in ".43"; eg, code E11.43, *Type 2 diabetes mellitus with autonomic (poly) neuropathy.* Symptoms or conditions indicative of diabetic autonomic neuropathy are:

- Gastroparesis
- Diarrhea or constipation
- Erectile dysfunction (may also be vascular)
- Postural hypotension
- Neurogenic bladder
- Anhydrosis
- Hypogylcemia unawareness

The revision of the 2017 *ICD-10-CM Guidelines,* which defined any Alphabetic Index subterm following "with" as a manifestation, changes how coders look at causal relationships in diabetes. When diabetes is supported in the record, any diagnosis that is listed under "with" in the Alphabetic Index is now automatically caused by the diabetes.[2] The diagnoses are:

- arthropathy
- Autonomic (poly) neuropathy
- Cataract
- Charcot's joints
- Chronic kidney disease
- Circulatory complication
- Dermatitis
- Foot ulcer
- Gangrene
- Gastroparesis
- Glomerulonephrosis
- Glomerulosclerosis
- Kidney complications
- Kimmelstiel-Wilson disease
- Loss of protective sensation (LOPS)
- Mononeuropathy
- Myasthenia
- Necrobiosis lipoidica
- Nephropathy
- Neuralgia
- Neurologic complication NEC
- Neuropathic arthropathy
- Neuropathy
- Ophthalmic complication NEC
- Oral complication NEC
- Osteomyelitis

- Periodontal disease
- Peripheral angiopathy
- Polyneuropathy
- Renal complication NEC
- Renal tubular degeneration
- Retinopathy
- Skin complication NEC
- Skin ulcer NEC

This list is very helpful, but it is not as straightforward as it appears. The entries for "complication NEC" provide plenty of room for interpretation, and seemingly, any complication could be linked to diabetes in this way. AHA's *Coding Clinic* (Fourth Quarter, 2017) provides guidance on this issue, using the entry, Diabetes/skin complication, NEC, as an example:

> The "with" guideline does not apply to "not elsewhere classified (NEC)" index entries that cover broad categories of conditions. Specific conditions must be linked by the terms "with," "due to" or "associated with." In order to link diabetes and a specific skin complication, the provider would need to document the condition as a diabetic skin complication. Each case is patient specific, and the relationship between diabetes and the skin complication should be clearly documented. Therefore, query the provider about the linkage, and if diabetes caused the specific skin complication. Coding professionals should not assume a causal relationship when the diabetic complication is "NEC."[7]

When assigning a combination code for diabetes, remember that the diabetes and the manifestation are not required to be documented together in the record for the current encounter. The diagnoses could be separate in the assessment, or mentioned on separate pages of the record for the current encounter. For the combination code to be used, both the diabetes and its manifestation must be documented, but not necessarily together.

CODING TIP The assumed causal link between diabetes and its complications includes cataracts, even though coders have been trained for years that the conditions are not related. The newest medical research links diabetes to cataracts.

Multiple diabetes codes may be required to capture all the complications of the patient's diabetes. All codes should come from the same category. Do not report E10 and E11 codes in the same patient encounter. A type 1 diabetic patient with gas gangrene due to diabetic peripheral angiopathy is reported with E10.52, *Type 1 diabetes mellitus with diabetic peripheral angiopathy with gangrene,* and an additional code to specify the gas gangrene, A48.0, *Gas gangrene,* according to AHA's *Coding Clinic* (Fourth Quarter, 2017).[7]

Don't overlook documented hyperglycemia or hypoglycemia. While these conditions were once considered incidental to DM, if they are supported in the record, they should be reported. Diabetic gastroparesis is reported as autonomic polyneuropathy (E--.43). Because there are other forms of autonomic polyneuropathy, also report the gastroparesis with K31.84, *Gastroparesis.* This will clarify the type of autonomic neuropathy the patient is experiencing.

ABSTRACT & CODE IT!

Abstract and code the clinical coding example below. Check your answers against the answers in Appendix C.

Patient 1

Patient with type 2 diabetes noted to have chronic gingivitis and has been referred to a periodontist for evaluation. Patient is a smoker.

Patient 2

Patient has limited ambulation due to peripheral neuropathy and morbid obesity. His BMI is 46, and I told him I would give him a referral to the bariatric center once his sugars were better. The patient's diabetes is out of control, with today's A1C at 12.4.

Patient 3

Assessment/Plan:

1. Controlled hypertension. Blood pressure today 125/81. Keep on current medications since they seem to be doing the job.
2. Improved chronic systolic heart failure. Edema is down, and patient is no longer short of breath at rest. Significant improvement.
3. Stable CKD, stage 4. Most recent GFR 22; will retest next visit.
4. Controlled diabetes mellitus, type 2. Today's A1C was 7.1. Her BG was 105. Continue metformin. Basic metabolic panel and HGB A1C ordered.

CODING TIP The earliest clinical manifestation of diabetic nephropathy is the persistent presence of small but abnormal levels of albumin in the urine, called microalbuminuria. When both diabetes and persistent microalbuminuria are supported in the medical record, report E11.29, *Type 2 diabetes mellitus with other diabetic kidney complication,* and R80.1, *Persistent proteinuria, unspecified.* If it lasts over 90 days, consider querying the physician to determine if CKD is present and if so, at what stage.

Drug/Alcohol Use Disorders

Drug/alcohol psychosis
HCC 54 0.383

Drug/alcohol dependence
HCC 55 0.383

According to the NIH, the abuse of tobacco, alcohol, and illegal drugs costs the US more than $740 billion yearly in costs related to productivity, crime, and health care.[8] In drug or alcohol dependence, changes in the brain make it difficult for a person to resist the urge to abuse the drug, or, having resisted, make it easy to relapse, whether the drug is tobacco, alcohol, or an opioid. Addiction is a treatable chronic disease. Multiple relapses may occur before a person successfully stops using the drug. Susceptibility to addiction is based on genetics, environment, and when in a person's development use of the substance begins. Earlier use is more likely to lead to addiction, as is a family history of addiction and environmental factors, including abuse.

Physician Documentation

Substance abuse and dependence will affect the health and wellness of the patient, and determine the potential for compliance with a treatment plan for any other illness. Prevention and screening, and coordination of care with behavioral health specialists, help provide opportunities for earlier intervention and improved outcomes for patients with substance abuse and dependency.

ICD-10-CM divides substance codes into three categories for use, abuse, and dependence. For 2018, the ICD-10-CM Alphabetic Index correlated the DSM-5 nomenclature of "mild drug or alcohol use disorder" to drug or alcohol abuse and "moderate or severe drug or alcohol use disorder" to drug or alcohol dependence. Documentation of the term "drug or alcohol use disorder" without the terms of mild, moderate, or severe cannot be reported in ICD-10-CM without further clarification from the physician.

It is the responsibility of the physician or other acceptable healthcare provider to document the severity of the disorder by documenting use, abuse, or dependence or by stating mild, moderate, or severe drug or alcohol use disorder. In some cases, complications of substance use can only be reported with one of the levels. For example, alcohol withdrawal in ICD-10-CM can only be reported with dependence, not with use or abuse.

Recreational use of (as opposed to abuse or dependence on) a mood-altering drug (eg, cannabis, alcohol) as documented in the medical record is not abstracted by the coder, unless there is a medical concern linked to the recreational drug (eg, septal ulcer related to cocaine use or tachycardia in a patient using methamphetamines).

It is always best and eliminates ambiguities when the relationships between etiologies and manifestations are clearly stated as causal in documentation. However, the ICD-10-CM Alphabetic Index links many conditions to an underlying abuse or dependence of drugs. When these conditions are due to other etiologies, but coexist with a drug/alcohol abuse or dependency, the causal relationship should be clearly stated in documentation.

Conditions that may be automatically linked to abuse or dependence by the classification include:

- Anxiety
- Delusions
- Delirium
- Dementia
- Hallucinations
- Mood disorder
- Perceptual disturbance
- Persisting amnesia
- Psychotic disorder
- Sexual dysfunction
- Sleep disorders

Use caution in documenting a "history of dependence" in reference to a patient who is still dependent. The ICD-CM classifies "history of dependence" to any substance as substance dependence, in remission. Do not use the word "history" for a condition that is still active. In a similar vein, "history of abuse" will be coded as "drug or alcohol use in remission," even though the patient still abuses drugs or alcohol.

Many patients with previous alcohol or drug abuse or dependence, even those with 20 years of sobriety, will admit that they still crave the mood alteration that their chemical use gave them and that they are one drink or one scheduled drug prescription away from a relapse. ICD-10-CM classifies these patients as in early (3 months sober) or late (over 12 months sober) remission. Be aware that a documented "prolonged remission" of substance dependence or abuse will not be reported as an active substance dependence or abuse.

According to ICD-10-CM Guideline Section I(C.5.b.1), "[s]election of codes for 'in remission' for categories F10-F19, Mental and behavioral disorders due to psychoactive substance use (categories F10-F19 with -.21) requires the provider's clinical judgment. The appropriate codes for 'in remission' are assigned only on the basis of provider documentation.[2]

In addition, per Guideline Section I(C.5.b.2), "[w]hen the provider documentation refers to use, abuse and dependence of the same substance (e.g. alcohol, opioid, cannabis, etc.), only one code should be assigned to identify the pattern of use based on the following hierarchy:

- If both use and abuse are documented, assign only the code for abuse
- If both abuse and dependence are documented, assign only the code for dependence
- If use, abuse and dependence are all documented, assign only the code for dependence
- If both use and dependence are documented, assign only the code for dependence."[2]

Document the recurring nature of a disorder in each encounter. The medical record for each date of service must stand on its own. A diagnosis in the patient's problem list or past medical history (PMH) cannot be abstracted unless it is addressed in the current encounter. When assessing or treating substance disorders, document time when it is invested in counseling and coordination of care or when the time is excessive.

CLINICAL EXAMPLES

NONSPECIFIC DOCUMENTATION	SPECIFIC DOCUMENTATION
Example 1 Assessment: Alcohol use disorder[a]	**Example 1** Mild alcohol use disorder with alcohol-induced impotence[b]
Example 2 Patient is being admitted to the treatment center with a history of opioid dependence.[c]	**Example 2** Patient is being admitted to the treatment center for treatment of opioid dependence. He has been an IV heroin user for five years.[d]

[a] "Disorder" is not sufficient; the documentation must identify the type of disorder caused by the alcohol use (eg, anxiety, delusions, intoxication, liver disease).

[b] Specify the severity of the disorder with "abuse," and the manifestation as sexual disorder, specifically, impotence.

[c] If the patient is being admitted, it seems unlikely this patient is in remission, but that is what is documented. Patient has opioid dependence, not a history of opioid dependence.

[d] Here we have quantified the time the patient has been an opioid user without making the mistake of using "history of."

Coding

Drug and alcohol problems and behavioral disorders are increasingly diagnosed and treated by the patient's general practitioner and should be reported as often as they are supported in documentation. According to ICD-10-CM Guideline Section I(C.5.b.3), "[a]s with all other diagnoses, the codes for psychoactive substance use (F10.9-, F11.9-, F12.9-, F13.9-, F14.9-, F15.9-, F16.9-) should only be assigned based on provider documentation and when they meet the definition of a reportable diagnosis (see Section III, Reporting Additional Diagnoses). The codes are to be used only when the psychoactive substance use is associated with a mental or behavioral disorder, and such a relationship is documented by the provider."[2]

If documented drug use is not treated or noted as affecting the patient's health, **do not** code it. A patient's incidental use of drugs is only reported when the use affects the treatment or care of a patient (eg, other psychiatric conditions exacerbated by drug use or liver disease documented as affected by the use of recreational drugs).

Do not make assumptions regarding the documentation describing patient conditions. Look up the exact terminology from the medical record in the Alphabetic Index to properly abstract the diagnosis code. Never report a condition that is more complex than what is documented and indexed.

 **ADVICE/ALERT NOTE**

Per ICD-10-CM Guideline Section I(C.5.b.3), "[a]s with all other diagnoses, the codes for psychoactive substance use (F10.9-, F11.9-, F12.9-, F13.9-, F14.9-, F15.9-, F16.9-) should only be assigned based on provider documentation and when they meet the definition of a reportable diagnosis (see Section III, Reporting Additional Diagnoses). The codes are to be used only when the psychoactive substance use is associated with a mental or behavioral disorder, and such a relationship is documented by the provider."[2]

When the physician refers to use or abuse with dependence of the same substance, report only the dependence. If the physician reports use and abuse of the same substance, report only abuse. Diagnoses reported with codes F10-F19 include the legal substances alcohol and tobacco, but substances reported with codes for opioid, cannabis, sedative, stimulant, or other types of drugs may be legal as well. The source or legality of the drug is not pertinent to the coding; the patient's relationship to the drug and complications arising from its use are. A patient who is receiving a prescribed maintenance dose of methadone is reported with the same code as a patient who is addicted to hydrocodone due to a chronic injury, or the patient who is dependent on self-injected heroin: F11.20, *Opioid dependence, uncomplicated.*

CODING TIP History of drug dependence is reported as drug dependence, in remission, according to the ICD-10-CM Alphabetic Index. Report history of drug abuse with code Z87.898, *Personal history of other specified conditions.* Physicians or healthcare providers may wish to amend their documentation of "history of drug abuse" to "drug abuse in remission" to capture new codes created for 2018 for this diagnosis.

"Smoker" is sufficient documentation to abstract a code from category F17.21-, *Nicotine dependence, cigarettes.* If the smoker is using electronic cigarettes, report a code from category F17.29-, *Nicotine dependence, other tobacco product*, instead. If documentation links the patient's current or past status as a smoker to chronic obstructive pulmonary disease (COPD) or vascular disease, report a code for nicotine dependence with other nicotine-induced disorders.

CODING TIP Report codes for nicotine dependence, in remission, when a patient is using patches or oral medications during the initial period following nicotine dependence, or when remission is so stated in documentation. Report code Z87.891, *Personal history of nicotine dependence*, for the patient who is no longer being treated or monitored for a previous nicotine dependence, or when personal history of nicotine dependence is so stated in documentation.

Blood Alcohol Level and Content

The level of alcohol involvement can be documented and coded by means of blood alcohol level testing. Blood alcohol content (BAC) and blood alcohol level testing results report the same thing, however, BAC reports in gm/dL and blood alcohol level testing reports in mg/ml. Move the decimal point of the BAC to the right three digits to achieve the blood alcohol level. For example, a BAC of 0.10 mg/dL would be a blood alcohol testing level of 100 mg/ml, or reported with Y90.5, *Blood alcohol level of 100-119 mg/100 ml.*

The codes for reporting alcohol levels in the blood are:

Y90.0	Blood alcohol level of less than 20 mg/100 ml
Y90.1	Blood alcohol level of 20-39 mg/100 ml
Y90.2	Blood alcohol level of 40-59 mg/100 ml
Y90.3	Blood alcohol level of 60-79 mg/100 ml
Y90.4	Blood alcohol level of 80-99 mg/100 ml
Y90.5	Blood alcohol level of 100-119 mg/100 ml
Y90.6	Blood alcohol level of 120-199 mg/100 ml
Y90.7	Blood alcohol level of 200-239 mg/100 ml
Y90.8	Blood alcohol level of 240 mg/100 ml or more
Y90.9	Presence of alcohol in blood, level not specified

Only report these codes secondary to a code from category F10, *Alcohol related disorders,* and when the alcohol level is documented by the physician.

ABSTRACT & CODE IT!

Abstract and code the clinical coding example below. Check your answers against the answers in Appendix C.

Patient: Jennie LaGrange **DOB:** 8/17/1950 **Date of Consultation:** 6/16/2017

CC [chief complaint]: Insomnia.

HPI [history of present illness]: The patient is a 66-year-old female with alcohol dependence and depressive disorder who presents reporting that she would like something for her insomnia. Psychiatry was asked to evaluate for some bizarre behaviors. The patient self-reports depression and skin-picking behaviors. Excoriation sites are apparent on her arms and face, but do not seem to be infected. On interview, the patient reports that she has been dealing with both emotional and physical pain. She complains of back pain. Emotionally, she has been involved in a relationship and reports that for the past couple of days, that male has not wanted to speak with her and that is the source of stress for her. On interview, the patient appears linear, denies suicidal ideation, and has some mild cognitive impairment. The patient has decreased insight into her history.

Past Psychiatric History: The patient again has alcohol dependence, and a history of dependence on opioids.

Substance Use History: Patient refuses treatment for alcohol dependence, saying it is a coping mechanism for her depression. In the past, she was dependent on intravenous (IV) opioids, but hasn't used in years. No noted tremors or seizures or other withdrawal symptoms. The patient smokes two packs of cigarettes per day.

PMH [past medical history]: Pertinent for anterior wall myocardial infarction [AMI] in 2015.

Current Medications: The patient is unable to recall most recent medications.

Past Medications

1. Paroxetine
2. Amitriptyline
3. Bupropion Hcl
4. Trazodone
5. Carisoprodol
6. Escitalopram
7. Venlafaxine

Social History: The patient is unmarried, lives on her own.

Mental Status Examination: The patient appears disheveled. She makes good eye contact. Her speech is of normal rate, tone, and prosody. She displays no psychomotor agitation or slowing. Her mood appears euthymic, but her affect is constricted. The patient is at times tangential in her thought process. She denies any suicidal or homicidal ideations. No delusions detected. She denies any auditory or visual hallucinations or history of hallucinations. Her judgment and insight are fair. She has mild cognitive impairment.

Diagnostic Data: Sodium 140, potassium 3.3, chloride 103, CO_2 of 30, calcium 8.5. Glucose 92. Liver function tests within normal limits with the exception of a decreased albumin at 2.7. CBC showing slightly elevated white count at 13.1. The rest of the CBC and differential WNL [within normal limits].

Impression: The patient is a 66-year-old female with a recurrent major depression and alcohol dependence. She reports severe insomnia and has a history of IV drug use. Judging from the patient's current presentation, biological factors include history of chronic medical illness and the patient's history of current and past substance abuse/dependence. Psychologically, the patient seems to be intact with intact coping mechanism as the patient has been able to not require inpatient hospitalization for quite some time. The patient is living on her own, appears to have good resources. In terms of her decreased memory, there is a question of whether there is a component of dementia in her presentation. Socially, the patient appears to be linked with case management services and appears to have somewhat supportive social environment though there are some acute stressors present. The patient is able to live on her own.

continued

Diagnoses

Axis I: Major depressive disorder, recurrent, moderate. Alcohol dependence. Rule out dementia.

Axis II: Diagnosis deferred.

Axis III: Insomnia, history of AMI, and polysubstance abuse.

Axis IV: Problems with social environment and occupational functioning.

Axis V: 50.

Plan

The patient does not require inpatient treatment at this time in terms of acute stabilization. The patient appears to have no suicidal symptoms or acute symptomatology. She has had success with Zolpidem in the past, so she is receiving a 30-day prescription for 10 mg.

Electronically signed by Thelma Morris, MD at 2:45 p.m. 06/16/2017

Emphysema *see* Pulmonary Disorders: Chronic

Epilepsy *see* Seizure, Epilepsy

Esophageal Reflux

Esophageal reflux and other disorders of esophagus
RxHCC 68 0.076

Food must pass through the lower esophageal sphincter (LES) to enter the stomach, where it is mixed with stomach acids and digestive enzymes to dissolve the food and ready it for nutritional update. The environment in the stomach is very acidic, and if the LES is faulty, and there is backflow of stomach contents into the esophagus, the acids can cause esophageal burning. Because this burning sensation is felt in the central chest, this feeling is called heartburn. When heartburn becomes chronic, it is called gastroesophageal reflux disease (GERD). GERD can be treated with antacid tablets that neutralize the stomach acid, or histamine-2 antagonists (eg, ranitidine) or proton pump inhibitors (PPIs) that slow production of acid by stomach cells. Surgery can strengthen the LES.

GERD is more common in patients who smoke, who are obese, or who use alcohol. It can be an adverse effect of some medications. GERD can cause chest pain, swallowing pain, respiratory problems, or erosion of tooth enamel. The chronic acid wash of the lower esophagus by GERD can lead to a worsening condition (eg, esophagitis or Barrett's esophagus). In Barrett's esophagus, chronic inflammatory damage to the esophagus leads to changes in its cells from a squamous to a columnar epithelium and increases a patient's risk for esophageal adenocarcinoma.

Physician Documentation

GERD is an exceedingly common condition, and for most patients, easily managed with low-risk oral prescription medications or over-the-counter drugs. For this reason, it is often overlooked in routine medical documentation, appearing only in the past medical record. Document any manifestations of GERD, its severity or mitigating factors, and any complications. Be sure to evaluate the patient's treatment and GERD regularly, and document the results. Identify any change in the condition with language compatible with ICD-10-CM, as:

- GERD with esophagitis
- Stenosis of esophagus
- Esophageal ulcer with or without bleeding
- Barrett's esophagus, without dysplasia, with low-grade dysplasia, or with high-grade dysplasia

Barrett's esophagus can occur without GERD. Document GERD when it coexists with Barrett's esophagus so that coders know to abstract both conditions. Link the patient's alcohol or tobacco status to the GERD as appropriate.

CLINICAL EXAMPLES

NONSPECIFIC DOCUMENTATION	SPECIFIC DOCUMENTATION
Example 1 EGD with biopsy confirms Barrett's esophagus.[a]	**Example 1** EGD with biopsy confirms gastroesophageal reflux disease and Barrett's esophagus with low-grade dysplasia.[b]
Example 2 Assessment: Heartburn. Treatment: pantoprazole 40 mg[c]	**Example 2** Assessment: Gastroesophageal reflux disease (GERD) Treatment: pantoprazole 40 mg daily[d]

[a] This is nonspecific. Identify without dysplasia, with low-grade or high-grade dysplasia in Barrett's esophagus.

[b] Document the GERD and the Barrett's esophagus, as we see here. The dysplasia has also been documented.

[c] Pantoprazole is a prescription proton pump inhibitor that is indicated for erosive esophagitis and GERD, not heartburn. This patient likely has a diagnosis of GERD. "Heartburn" is a symptom and does not risk-adjust.

[d] The physician documents the meaning of GERD, even though it is a common acronym and substantiates the need for pantoprazole by documenting GERD rather than heartburn.

Coding

When Barrett's esophagus and GERD are both documented, report both. Do not, however, assume GERD exists in a patient documented with Barrett's esophagus, as it can occur without GERD. Do not report esophagitis and GERD with two codes; instead report code K21.0, *Gastro-esophageal reflux disease with esophagitis*. If the Barrett's esophagus evolves into adenocarcinoma, do not report Barrett's. Instead report a neoplasm code (eg, code C15.5, *Malignant neoplasm of lower third of esophagus*).

Treatment for GERD or Barrett's esophagus may include medications, such as PPIs esomeprazole, lansoprazole, omeprazole, pantoprazole, rabeprazole, and dexlansoprazole; antacids, such as Maalox, Mylanta, Rolaids, or Tums; H-2 receptor blockers, including cimetidine, famotidine, nizatidine, and ranitidine; or Baclofen to enhance contractions of the LES. Other remedies for GERD include dietary changes, elevating the head of the bed, losing weight, and smoking cessation.

CODING TIP Reflux and acid reflux are classified to GERD in ICD-10-CM. Barrett's esophagus may be documented as LGD (low-grade dysplasia); HGD (high-grade dysplasia); or NDBE (non-dysplastic Barrett's esophagus).

ABSTRACT & CODE IT!

Abstract and code the clinical coding example below. Check your answers against the answers in Appendix C.

Patient: Martine Davis **DOB:** 03/23/1944 **DOS [date of service]:** 11/23/2017

CC: Itchy throat, runny nose

HPI: Ms. Davis is a 72-year-old woman who has been coughing for a month. She was treated with azithromycin last month which helped, but her cough never went away. She will occasionally hear wheezing mainly on her left chest when she lies down on the left. She complains of continued runny nose and itchy, scratchy throat. She did not take any medicine. Her mucus has been clear. No fevers or chills.

Systems Review: All indicated in HPI. Otherwise unremarkable.

Current Medications: Ranitidine HCl 150 mg; risedronate 35 mg; hydrocortisone 2.5% cream; Caltrate 600+D; Vitamin D 50,000 units, once weekly. (Last reviewed 11/23/2017)

Active Problems: Allergic rhinitis July 2012. Esophageal reflux December 2014. Generalized anxiety disorder December 2014. Vitamin D deficiency July 2016.

Surgical History: Tonsillectomy, appendectomy, thyroidectomy, and bladder surgery.

Social History: She was a smoker until the 1980s; 30 cigarettes a day for 20 years.

continued

Vitals: Recorded by Corky Jackson 11/23/2017. BP: 110/64, LUE, sitting; HR: 73 L radial; Resp: 18; Temp: 98.6°F, oral; Weight 172 lb; BMI: 29.4.

PE [physical examination]: General: Patient in no acute distress. HEENT: PERRLA, EOMI, conjunctiva normal. TMs normal, oropharynx clear, nasal turbinate pal and boggy. Lungs: good air movement, no chest retractions, exp wheezes bilateral L>R. Heart: RRR no murmurs. Extremities: No edema. Back: No TTP.

Labs Reviewed: CBC, Lipid panel, comprehensive metabolic panel ordered. Vitamin D ordered.

Assessment: Wheezing. History of smoking. Allergic rhinitis. GERD well controlled.

Orders: Renew Ranitidine HCl 150 MG tablet. Take twice daily for GERD heartburn, qty 60. Prednisone 20 mg tabs, take 3 tabs daily, qty 15. Tiotropium bromide 18 mcg capsule, qty 60. ProAir HFA 109 (90 base) mcg/act aerosol solution PRN cough, SOB, qty 1.

Plan: Moderate asthma with /history of smoking – Albuterol 2.5 mg with 3 cc NS via HHN given × 1 – still with wheezing so another treatment was given; only occasional wheezing and she was comfortable. Advised to start on tiotropium bromide daily and use the albuterol sulfate inhalation aerosol as needed and the prednisone as directed. For upper respiratory airway resistance, use the fluticasone nasal spray. Ordered full PFT [pulmonary function test] to be done by Full House Pulmonary. Follow-up within 1-2 weeks after the test is done.

Electronically signed by Wayne Souvern MD 20:14 11/23/2017

Heart Arrhythmias

Specified heart arrhythmias
HCC 96 0.268

Atrial arrhythmias
RxHCC 193 0.288

The heart contracts as a reaction to electrical pulses along its conduction system. These contractions are called heartbeats and function to push deoxygenated blood into the lungs from the right ventricle or re-oxygenated blood into the body from the left ventricle. The electrical pulses are conducted from the sinoatrial node in the right atrium along the atrioventricular node to the bundle of HIS and then into left and right bundles of fibers that extend into the heart muscle. Heart rhythm defects can often be traced to defects along the electrical conduction pathway.

The most common form of cardiac arrhythmia is atrial fibrillation (aFib), during which the atria of the heart contract chaotically, rapidly, and ineffectively. As a result the atria are not completely emptied of blood, and this residual blood is at risk for clotting. If a clot enters circulation, it may become lodged in the lung, brain, or coronary artery, causing life-threatening ischemia. The threat posed by clots is the main concern in atrial fibrillation because most of the heart's work is performed by the ventricles, not the atria. There are times, however, when a failing left ventricle needs the extra support that the atrium can give if it is in normal sinus rhythm, prompting physicians to maintain it if possible.

Ventricular fibrillation, by contrast, is a medical emergency, as the pumping of blood into the lungs and throughout the body becomes ineffectual and the patient dies. Ventricular fibrillation and flutter are reported with the same HCC as cardiac arrest (HCC 84).

AFib may be caused by defects along the electrical pathway of the heart, hyperthyroidism, hypertension, or previous myocardial infarction (MI). Sleep apnea may also contribute to aFib. AFib is diagnosed by electrocardiogram or through the use of a cardiac event recorder or Holter monitor. Treatment of atrial fibrillation may include electrical cardioversion, in which an electrical charge

Fibrillation
Chaotic irregular rhythms of heart chambers, most commonly occurring in the atria, but can occur in the ventricles, a terminal event.

Flutter
An electrical signal that moves along a pathway within the right atrium in an organized circular motion, or "circuit," causing the atria to beat faster than the ventricles.

to the heart restores the normal heart rhythm of a sedated patient, or ablation, in which damaged electrical conduits are destroyed along the electrical impulse pathway of the heart. Commonly, the patient will be prescribed blood thinners to prevent the development of clots, and in some cases, medication to regulate the rhythm and rate of the heartbeat. Pacemakers can also stabilize the heart of a patient with aFib. It is not uncommon that medications, such as amiodarone, flecanide, propofanone, sotalol, or other medications, are used to maintain sinus rhythm, in essence treating the aFib.

Another arrhythmia similar to aFib, atrial flutter (AFL), involves a circular rhythm in the right atrium that results in a tachycardia, albeit one that is regular as opposed to one that is irregular, as in aFib. Risk factors include heart failure, previous heart attack, valve abnormalities or congenital defects, hypertension, recent surgery, hyperthyroidism, alcoholism, and others. AFL may degenerate into aFib. AFL is harder to convert to normal sinus rhythm with medications, thus often requires electrical cardioversion. Like aFib, it may require chronic medications or ablation of cardiac tissue to suppress AFL.

Another form of arrhythmia is sick sinus syndrome (SSS), also known as sinoatrial node disease (SND) or sinus dysfunction. Symptoms of SSS vary by patient, but may include syncope, weakness, dyspnea, bradycardia, tachycardia, or bradycardia-tachycardia. The condition is often treated with a pacemaker. Atrioventricular block occurs when the electrical pathway of the heart is interrupted, and signals are slowed as they travel from the sinoatrial node through the atrioventricular node. Heart blocks are defined by degree. First degree is the mildest form and may cause no symptoms. Second degree affects the heart pumping because the contractions are strong but less frequent to a disruption in electrical conduction. Third-degree heart block is a total block in the normal route of conduction. The complete block usually requires a pacemaker.

Tachycardia
A resting heartbeat of more than 100 beats per minute.

Bradycardia
A heartbeat of less than 60 beats per minute.

Heart block
The interruption of electrical impulses in the heart's conduction system, resulting in abnormal rhythms (arrhythmias).

Physician Documentation

Identify the type of aFib diagnosed in the patient. The types of aFib and their ICD-10-CM codes are listed in Table 4-2.3.

TABLE 4-2.3 Types of Atrial Fibrillation and ICD-10-CM Codes[9]

ATRIAL FIBRILLATION	
I48.0	**Paroxysmal**—intermittent, stopping, starting by itself within 7 days.
I48.1	**Persistent**—lasts more than 7 days and subject to a rhythm control strategy (eg, plan to cardiovert; maintain on anti-arrhythmic medication), even if currently in normal sinus rhythm as a result.
I48.2	**Chronic**—physician and patient agree to leave the patient in atrial fibrillation (permanent) and focus management on rate control and clot prevention.
I48.91	**Unspecified**—physician doesn't know or doesn't state type (common with new onset atrial fibrillation).

The nature of these distinctive types of aFib may create confusion in documentation. For example, if the physician is not clear about the current status of the aFib, a patient with paroxysmal aFib may have a regular heart rhythm and rate during an encounter because by definition, paroxysmal aFib is intermittent. Report "history of aFib" only if the patient's aFib is resolved and not being treated. For example, in some cases, aFib may resolve for years, or never recur, without drugs or with a single cardioversion. This would be an example of "history of aFib." However, the patient whose heart rate and rhythm continues to be normal because the aFib is controlled with heart-regulating medication still has aFib, because the aFib would be present without the treatment.

Many physicians document atrial fibrillation as AF. However, AF may also be an abbreviation for atrial flutter, aortofemoral, and numerous other word combinations. Best practices would be to use the term and abbreviation atrial fibrillation (AF, aFib) for the first reference, and then AF or aFib for subsequent references. This must be repeated for documented encounter in the medical record.

If the patient is experiencing any symptoms of aFib (lightheadedness, shortness of breath, chest pain, fatigue, palpitations), document these symptoms and link them to the aFib, as appropriate.

For current aFib, identify the patient's condition, for example, as controlled, or by identifying the rate and rhythm irregularities. Do not rely on an electronic health record (EHR) medication list to capture long-term use of medications. Actively document long-term use of anticoagulants, antithrombolitics, antiplatelets, NSAIDs, aspirin, or any other pertinent pharmaceuticals in the medical record, and link the medication(s) to the aFib as appropriate.

In addition to atrial fibrillation, some heart blocks risk-adjust. Identify a block as first, second, or third degree, and for second degree, specify if Mobitz type 1 or type 2. Note the site of the block as left anterior or posterior fascicular, as appropriate. Bradycardia, tachycardia, and palpitations are nonspecific symptoms that do not risk-adjust, which should not be reported if a more definitive diagnosis is available. EKGs and telemetry strips are not permitted to be interpreted by coding staff. Diagnoses must be documented by the physician.

CLINICAL EXAMPLES

NONSPECIFIC DOCUMENTATION	SPECIFIC DOCUMENTATION
Example 1 HPI: Patient is being seen today for his history of atrial fibrillation. He continues digoxin therapy and is also taking dabigatran as prophylaxis. Current exam reveals regular rate and rhythm.[a]	**Example 1** HPI: Patient is being seen today for paroxysmal atrial fibrillation. He continues digoxin therapy and is also taking dabigatran as prophylaxis. Current exam reveals regular rate and rhythm.[b]
Example 2 The patient will undergo insertion of a pacemaker for atrioventricular and right bundle branch blocks.[c]	**Example 2** The patient will undergo insertion of a leadless pacemaker for a third-degree atrioventricular block and a right bundle branch block.[d]

[a] The patient does not have "history of" atrial fibrillation, as the patient is still actively taking medications to treat his atrial fibrillation. Avoid "history of" for active conditions and identify the type of atrial fibrillation the patient has.

[b] The type of atrial fibrillation is noted and the medications are clearly linked to the diagnosis.

[c] Only a third-degree block maps for RA. Always identify the degree of block, and for second degree, note if it is a Mobitz type 1 or type 2.

[d] Documenting the degree of the atrioventricular block ensures the HCC is captured.

Coding

If the patient's heart arrhythmia is resolved by placement of a pacemaker, do not report the resolved condition. Instead, report the pacemaker status code. If the pacemaker is the sole treatment for the SSS, or other arrhythmia, report only Z95.0, *Presence of cardiac pacemaker,* or Z95.810, *Presence of automatic (implantable) cardiac defibrillator,* and **not** the condition it corrects. However, if the patient has a pacemaker but also is prescribed other medications to treat the arrhythmia, report the arrhythmia in addition to the pacemaker code. Third-degree heart blocks affect cardiac output significantly and map for RA. A third-degree block may be documented as a complete heart block, AV dissociation, AV block III, or AV block 3.

ABSTRACT & CODE IT!

Abstract and code the clinical coding example below. Check your answers against the answers in Appendix C.

Patient 1

Procedure: Implant of a single-lead cardiac pacemaker

Preoperative diagnosis: Sick sinus syndrome

Postoperative diagnosis: Sick sinus syndrome

Patient 2

Chief complaint: One-year check for pacemaker in patient with permanent atrial fibrillation and bradycardia. Patient is asymptomatic since the pacemaker was implanted.

Patient 3

Chief complaint: One-year check for pacemaker in patient with permanent atrial fibrillation and bradycardia. Patient is asymptomatic since the pacemaker was implanted. Clopidogrel prescription renewed for prophylaxis of aFib-related thrombi.

Hemiplegia *see* Paralysis

Hepatitis *see* Liver Disease

Hip Fracture *see* Trauma: Hip

HIV and Opportunistic Infections

HIV/AIDS
HCC 1 **0.312**
RXHCC 1 **3.192**

Opportunistic infections
HCC 6 **0.435**
RxHCC 5 **0.261**

Human immunodeficiency virus (HIV) is a blood-borne retrovirus transmitted through the exchange of bodily fluids during sexual intercourse, needle sharing, or from mother to child in pregnancy, childbirth, or breastfeeding. HIV attacks the immune system of the host. While there is no cure for HIV, its effect on the immune system can be slowed or stopped with medications at any stage. If diagnosis and treatment begin early, a patient with HIV infection may have a normal lifespan.

HIV has three stages: acute infection (which may or may not be symptomatic), asymptomatic infection, and symptomatic disease. The acute infection occurs within weeks of exposure to the HIV virus. During this phase, the patient is highly infective and may have flu-like symptoms, which, if symptoms occur, is labeled as the acute HIV infection syndrome. Upon recovery, an asymptomatic phase follows. During this phase, a patient is "HIV positive." In the third phase, an HIV positive patient experiences symptoms, which may include lymphadenopathy, certain cancers, or opportunistic infections. Without treatment, late symptomatic patients survive approximately three years. Antiretroviral therapy is prescribed to extend the asymptomatic and symptomatic stages of HIV infection.

HIV positive status and HIV disease status both map to the same HCC and RxHCC. Opportunistic diseases associated with HCC 6 and RxHCC 5 may be commonly linked to HIV or may be seen in other patients with immunosuppressed states. See Table 4-2.4 for the diseases included in HCC 6 and RxHCC 5. Other disorders commonly linked to HIV disease or immunosuppressed states may be classified to HCCs and RxHCCs for malignant neoplasms, pneumonias, or other infections.

TABLE 4-2.4 Diseases Included in HCC 6 and RxHCC 5

CODE	DESCRIPTION
A31.0	Pulmonary mycobacterial infection
A31.2	Disseminated mycobacterium avium-intracellulare complex (DMAC)
B25.-	Cytomegaloviral infection
B37.1	Pulmonary candidiasis
B37.7	Candidal sepsis
B37.81	Candidal esophagitis
B44.0	Invasive pulmonary aspergillosis
B44.1	Other pulmonary aspergillosis
B44.2	Tonsillar aspergillosis
B44.7	Disseminated aspergillosis
B44.89	Other forms of aspergillosis
B44.9	Aspergillosis, unspecified
B45.-	Cryptococcosis
B46.-	Zygomycosis/mucormycosis
B48.4	Penicillosis
B48.8	Other specified mycoses
B58.2	Toxoplasma meningoencephalitis
B58.3	Pulmonary toxoplasmosis
B59	Pneumocystosis

Physician Documentation

Physicians must clearly document whether a patient with a true positive HIV infection has or has not ever had a symptom or disease related to the HIV infection. Patients who have had any HIV-related symptoms, diseases, or illness, which includes the early acute HIV syndrome, should always be coded with ICD-10-CM code B20, *Human immunodeficiency virus [HIV] disease*, even if the patient's disease is currently asymptomatic with or without drug treatment. Those who have never had a symptom related to their HIV infection should be reported with ICD-10-CM code Z21, *Asymptomatic human immunodeficiency virus [HIV] infection status*, except in jurisdictions where the reporting of Z21 is prohibited (eg, California). Documentation does not always reflect coding guidelines, which can lead to erroneous abstraction. According to ICD-10-CM Guideline Section I(C.1.a.2.f):

Previously diagnosed HIV-related illness
Patients with any known prior diagnosis of an HIV-related illness should be coded to B20, Human immunodeficiency virus [HIV] disease. Once a patient has developed an HIV-related illness, the patient should always be assigned code B20 on every subsequent admission/encounter. Patients previously diagnosed with any HIV illness (B20) should never be assigned to R75, Inconclusive laboratory evidence of human immunodeficiency virus [HIV], or Z21, Asymptomatic human immunodeficiency virus [HIV] infection status.[2]

Physicians must remember that coders are not permitted to review previous encounters when they have questions regarding the current encounter. If the physician does not make the distinction that the patient is asymptomatic and stable on highly active antiretroviral therapy (HAART) but has had symptoms, diseases, or illnesses related to HIV in the past on every encounter, the coder could mistakenly report code Z21, *Asymptomatic human immunodeficiency virus [HIV] infection status,* when, according to ICD-10-CM guidelines, the correct diagnosis is code B20, *Human immunodeficiency virus [HIV] disease.* Therefore, physicians should note in the record if a patient has a history of HIV-related symptoms, diseases, or illnesses rather than HIV-positive status in every encounter to capture the HIV-related disease because coders cannot reference previous encounters to determine the patient's HIV history. Do not rely on PMH to inform the coding.

Language aligning with symptomatic HIV disease reported with code B20, includes:

- HIV disease
- Acquired immunodeficiency syndrome (AIDS)
- AIDS-related complex (ARC)
- Current symptomatic HIV infection

Language aligning with asymptomatic HIV infection in ICD-10 (optimally documented as without a past or current history of symptoms) reported with code Z21, includes:

- HIV infection
- HIV-positive status
- Known HIV
- HIV status
- HIV virus
- Asymptomatic HIV infection

Be sure to clearly document any clinical relationship between a comorbidity and HIV infections.

CLINICAL EXAMPLES

NONSPECIFIC DOCUMENTATION	SPECIFIC DOCUMENTATION
Example 1 HIV positive with new onset candidiasis of lungs, bilateral.[a]	**Example 1** HIV disease resulting in the new onset candidiasis of lungs, bilateral.[b]
Example 2 History of HIV; responding well to HAART.[c]	**Example 2** HIV disease, asymptomatic in response to HAART.[d]
Example 3 HIV positive with CD4 count of 100. Start on HAART.[e]	**Example 3** HIV disease, based on CD4 count of 100. Starting on HAART.[f]

[a] This information is ambiguous to the coder, since an HIV-positive patient with a noted opportunistic diagnosis (candidiasis of the lung) should be reported as AIDS, according to the Centers for Disease Control and Prevention's (CDC's) list of opportunistic diagnoses.

[b] In this case, the use of AIDS clearly defines the patient's condition and aligns with the diagnosis of candidiasis of the lungs.

[c] There is no such thing as a past "history of" AIDS. It is a current condition. Do not use ambiguous language.

[d] HIV disease identifies this disorder as classifying to B20. The patient is asymptomatic and on medication, providing good support for the diagnosis.

[e] Based on the clinical definition of HIV disease, this patient has HIV disease, not HIV-positive status. The coder cannot base coding on lab values, and so would report HIV-positive when the patient actually has HIV disease.

[f] Here, documentation identifies the HIV status as disease, and provides ample support for the diagnosis.

Coding

The diagnosis code for an HIV-positive patient who has never had a Centers for Disease Control and Prevention (CDC)–defined opportunistic infection or a symptom related to their HIV infection is Z21, *Asymptomatic human immunodeficiency virus [HIV] infection status.* A patient who is HIV positive and has had depressed T-cell counts (CD4 count less than 200) or a past or present opportunistic infection is said to have AIDS, which is reported with code B20, *Human immunodeficiency virus [HIV] disease.* Problems arise when documentation states the patient is HIV positive, but the documentation notes past or current HIV-related symptoms, illnesses, or diseases. When this happens, query the physician to see if code B20 should be reported instead of code Z21, *Asymptomatic human immunodeficiency virus [HIV] infection*. If a query is not possible, refer to your internal coding policies for guidance. Per ICD-10-CM Guideline Section I(C.1.a.2.f):

> Patients with any known prior diagnosis of an HIV-related illness should be coded to B20. Once a patient has developed an HIV-related illness the patient should always be assigned code B20 on every subsequent admission/encounter. Patients previously diagnosed with any HIV illness (B20) should never be assigned to R75 or Z21, Asymptomatic human immunodeficiency virus [HIV] infection status.[2]

Once a patient is diagnosed with B20, the diagnosis should never revert to Z21; however, since coding is based only on what is documented in the current encounter, each note must be clear as to whether or not the patient currently has or in the past has had HIV-related symptoms, diseases, or illnesses. Internal policies may be necessary to determine how coders will approach cloned PMH that shows evidence of HIV disease when the current encounter only supports HIV-positive status.

CODING TIP Any symptom or disease that is attributed in the current medical record to HIV would result in the coding of B20, *Human immunodeficiency virus (HIV) disease.*

The infant of an HIV-infected mother usually tests positive for HIV serologies, but these results may be a false positive due to a mixing of fetal and maternal blood before birth. It may take more than a year to determine if the infant is infected. Until a determination is made, the infant's condition is reported with R75, *Inconclusive laboratory evidence of human immunodeficiency virus [HIV].*

According to ICD-10-CM Guideline Section I(C.1.a.2d), "Z21, Asymptomatic human immunodeficiency virus [HIV] infection status, is to be applied when the patient without any documentation of current or past HIV-related symptoms is listed as being 'HIV positive,' 'known HIV,' 'HIV test positive,' or similar terminology. Do not use this code if the term 'AIDS', 'history of AIDS', 'symptomatic HIV', or "past history of symptomatic HIV" is used, if the patient is currently or in the past treated for any HIV-related illness or is described as having any condition(s) resulting from his/her HIV positive status; use B20 in these cases."[2]

In addition, Guideline Section I(C.1.a.2.f) states "[p]atients with any known prior diagnosis of an HIV-related illness should be coded to B20. Once a patient has developed an HIV-related illness, the patient should always be assigned code B20 on every subsequent admission/encounter. Patients previously diagnosed with any HIV illness (B20) should never be assigned to R75 or Z21, *Asymptomatic human immunodeficiency virus [HIV] infection status.*"[2]

ABSTRACT & CODE IT!

Abstract and code the clinical coding example below. Check your answers against the answers in Appendix C.

Patient 1

Assessment: The HIV-positive patient is experiencing noninfectious HIV-associated colitis, an adverse effect of the antiretroviral therapy. I am prescribing crofelemer, 125 mg po b.i.d.

Patient 2

HIV-positive patient is admitted with bilateral *Pneumocystis jiroveci* pneumonia due to HIV. The patient has been on antiretroviral medications since his initial diagnosis in 1998.

Patient 3

HIV status; his CD4 is 522 and states he adheres to his daily HIV regimen.

Huntington's Disease – *see* Systemic Atrophy of CNS

Hyperlipidemia

Disorders of lipoid metabolism
RxHCC 45 0.038

Hyperlipidemia describes elevated levels of any of the lipids or lipoproteins found in blood. It is classified as familial (eg, caused by specific genetic markers); acquired (eg, resulting from an underlying disorder); or idiopathic (eg, of unknown origin). High levels of lipids in the bloodstream double a person's chances of coronary artery disease, according to the NIH.[10] That's because over time, the fats in the bloodstream are deposited on the walls of the artery and combine with other substances to form plaque. The plaque hardens, narrowing and stiffening the walls of the arteries. This is called atherosclerosis, or coronary artery disease. Plaque is an irritant, and may rupture, causing a blood clot to form, leading to an acute MI or, if it occurs in the brain, ischemic stroke.

There are three basic types of cholesterol in the bloodstream: high-density lipoproteins (HDL), low-density lipoproteins (LDL), and triglycerides. The HDL is considered "good" cholesterol, not leading to atherosclerosis, and LDL is considered "bad" cholesterol. Triglycerides also increase a person's risk for plaque development in arteries. The NIH reports that 71 million adult Americans have high LDL, but only one of every three adults has the condition under control, and less than half get treatment. Hyperlipidemia responds well to medication to lower LDL, and for some, to dietary change.[10]

Familial hypercholesterolemia (FH) is an uncommon autosomal dominant genetic disorder that disrupts the body's ability to eliminate LDL. FH causes lipids to be deposited beneath the skin, and along the tendons. The condition is confirmed through genetic testing. Treatment for FH patients includes cholesterol-lowering medication, LDL apheresis, extracorporeal removal of LDL cholesterol, and in severe cases, liver transplant.

Physician Documentation

Do not let the ICD-10-CM Alphabetic Index "choose" a cholesterol-related diagnosis for your patient. Documentation of "high cholesterol" will classify to code E78.00, *Pure hypercholesterolemia, unspecified*, while "hyperlipidemia" classifies to code E78.5, *Hyperlipidemia, unspecified.* Choose language that aligns with the patient's laboratory results and the language of ICD-10-CM codes. See Table 4-2.5 for RxHCC codes for risk-adjusting lipid disorders.

TABLE 4-2.5 Risk-adjusting Lipid Disorders RxHCC Codes

CODE	DESCRIPTION
E71.30	Disorder of fatty-acid metabolism, unspecified
E75.5	Other lipid storage disorders
E75.6	Lipid storage disorder, unspecified
E78.00	Pure hypercholesterolemia, unspecified
E78.01	Familial hypercholesterolemia
E78.1	Pure hyperglyceridemia
E78.2	Mixed hyperlipidemia
E78.3	Hyperchylomicronemia
E78.4	Other hyperlipidemia
E78.5	Hyperlipidemia, unspecified
E78.6	Lipoprotein deficiency
E78.70	Disorder of bile acid and cholesterol metabolism, unspecified
E78.79	Other disorders of bile acid and cholesterol metabolism
E78.81	Lipoid dermatoarthritis
E78.89	Other lipoprotein metabolism disorders
E78.9	Disorder of lipoprotein metabolism, unspecified
E88.2	Lipomatosis, not elsewhere classified

CLINICAL EXAMPLES

NONSPECIFIC DOCUMENTATION	SPECIFIC DOCUMENTATION
Example 1 Patient's LDL is 265 and HDL is 45.[a]	**Example 1** Pure hyperglyceridemia. Patient's LDL is 265 and HDL is 45.[b]
Example 2 High cholesterol.[c]	**Example 2** Hyperlipidemia, group B; patient is responding well to ezetimibe 10 mg daily.[d]

[a] Coders cannot abstract diagnoses from lab values.

[b] Pure hyperglyceridemia echoes the language of ICD-10-CM, so it is precise and makes accurate code abstraction easy.

[c] Physicians should keep in mind that high cholesterol is classified to unspecified pure hypercholesteremia. If that isn't what is intended, more specific documentation should be employed.

[d] Hyperlipidemia group B is an inclusion term under E78.1, *Pure hyperglyceridemia.* Discussion of the patient's response to the medication strengthens documentation.

Coding

Coders should become familiar with the inclusion terms under each code for high cholesterol and pay attention to the details in the language. For example, code E78.2 reports mixed hyperlipidemia (high level of fats in the blood), but code E78.3, *Hyperchylomicronemia,* reports a more specific diagnosis of mixed hyperglyceridemia (high triglycerides). Triglycerides are associated with atherosclerosis and increase a patient's risk for heart disease.

Report code Z83.42, *Family history of familial hypercholesterolemia (FH),* for patients being tested for the disorder. There is no need to report code Z83.42 if a patient is diagnosed with FH. Instead, report the FH with code E78.01, *Familial hypercholesterolemia.*

ABSTRACT & CODE IT!

Abstract and code the clinical coding example below. Check your answers against the answers in Appendix C.

Patient 1
Elevated cholesterol with high triglycerides, treated with ezetimibe.

Patient 2
High cholesterol controlled with atorvastatin.

Patient 3
LDL type hyperlipoproteinemia; patient noncompliant with medication.

Hypertension

Hypertension
RxHCC 187 0.123

Approximately one-third of adult Americans have a diagnosis of hypertension, according to the CDC, and another third have blood pressure that is higher than normal, but not yet hypertensive (prehypertension). Hypertension describes the force of blood pushing against the arteries, and if the blood pressure is too high, it causes damage to these vessels and to the heart. Hypertension is a major risk factor for stroke, MI, vascular disease, and chronic kidney disease. Only half of people who have hypertension have their blood pressure under control. As a result, hypertension is a primary contributing cause of death of more than 1,100 people every day. Risk factors for hypertension include diabetes, smoking dependence, high-sodium diet, inactivity, obesity, alcohol consumption, and prehypertension.

Hypertension is defined by measuring the patient's blood pressure during a heartbeat (systolic) and during rest (diastolic). A reading of 120/80 mmHg identifies a blood pressure that is 120 mmHg when the heart is contracting, and 80 mmHg when the heart is at rest. Generally speaking, systolic blood pressures between 120 and 139 mmHg *or* diastolic blood pressures between 80 and 89 mmHg are considered to be prehypertension. Any systolic blood pressure at *or* above 140 mmHg or diastolic blood pressure at or above 90 mmHg is hypertension. Hypertensive crisis, a serious elevation of blood pressure with impending or actual end-organ damage, is diagnosed when the systolic blood pressure is at or above 180 mmHg or the diastolic blood pressure is at or above 120 mmHg. Hypertension usually responds well to medication. See Table 4-2.6 for the diagnoses included in RxHCC 187.

TABLE 4-2.6 Risk-adjusting Codes for RxHCC 187

CODE	DESCRIPTION
I10	Essential (primary) hypertension
I11.9	Hypertensive heart disease without heart failure
I12.0	Hypertensive chronic kidney disease with stage 5 chronic kidney disease or end stage renal disease
I12.9	Hypertensive chronic kidney disease with stage 1 through stage 4 chronic kidney disease, or unspecified chronic kidney disease
I13.10	Hypertensive heart and chronic kidney disease without heart failure, with stage 1 through stage 4 chronic kidney disease, or unspecified chronic kidney disease
I13.11	Hypertensive heart and chronic kidney disease without heart failure, with stage 5 chronic kidney disease, or end stage renal disease
I15.-	Secondary hypertension
I16.-	Hypertensive crisis
I67.4	Hypertensive encephalopathy
N26.2	Page kidney

Physician Documentation

Blood pressure and efficacy of pharmacologic therapy should be assessed at every encounter involving a hypertensive patient. Clarity is important in documenting hypertension. "High blood pressure" may be incidental and transient; hypertension is a chronic condition. Document chronic elevations of blood pressure using the terminology "hypertension" to avoid ambiguity. A patient on medication for hypertension who has normal blood pressure readings still has hypertension, not history of hypertension, since it is being treated. Ensure the diagnosis is captured by noting it in the documentation. Coders cannot abstract diagnoses from PMH without support.

An isolated instance of elevated blood pressure should be documented and will be reported with R03.0, *Elevated blood pressure reading without a diagnosis of hypertension.* Prehypertension does not have a listing in the ICD-10-CM Alphabetic Index or Tabular List. Borderline hypertension, a term that should be considered as an alternative to prehypertension, is reported with R03.0, and R03.0 does not risk-adjust.

The guidelines state that a causal relationship can be assumed for hypertension when it occurs with heart failure, cardiomegaly, unspecified myocarditis, unspecified myocardial degeneration, Takotsubo syndrome, or chronic kidney disease unless the physician explicitly documents another cause. Be sure to document when these conditions coexist and are **not** related to hypertension, as diabetes and hypertension are not automatically linked. It is common for a diabetic patient to be diagnosed with both hypertension and chronic kidney disease. Identify the causal relationship of the hypertension, if known, to avoid confusion in abstraction.

Coders cannot abstract diagnoses from numbers, therefore, a blood pressure reading of 180/110 cannot be coded at all. Coders can only abstract what the physicians diagnose. If a patient has secondary hypertension, identify the source (eg, renovascular, other renal, or endocrine) and link the specific underlying condition to the hypertension in documentation. Specify a pregnant patient with hypertension as having a pre-existing, gestational, pre-eclampsic, or eclampsic hypertension.

Document the smoking status of a patient with hypertension as current smoker, personal history of tobacco dependence, tobacco use, or exposure to environmental tobacco smoke. Document any causal relationship between hypertension and background retinopathy, or other condition in which the hypertension caused vascular changes and organ damage.

Hypertensive Crisis

A hypertensive crisis occurs when blood pressure rises fast enough and high enough that it has the potential to damage organs. It may be caused by medication noncompliance or interaction, stroke, MI, renal failure, abdominal aorta rupture, or pre-eclampsia/eclampsia in pregnancy.

The American Heart Association defines **hypertensive urgency** as a systolic blood pressure exceeding 180, or diastolic exceeding 110, without progressive organ dysfunction.[11] **Hypertensive emergency** occurs when levels exceed 180 systolic or 120 diastolic, with impending or progressive organ damage.[11] **Hypertensive crisis** is reported when neither urgency nor emergency is specified.

Accelerated, malignant, and uncontrolled are not terms associated with hypertensive crisis in ICD-10. Rather, they are associated with I10, *Essential (primary) hypertension.*

Also document any consequences of the uncontrolled blood pressure:

- Hypertensive urgency (I16.0)
- Hypertensive emergency (I16.1)
- Hypertensive crisis, unspecified (I16.9)

According to ICD-10-CM Guideline Section I(C.9.a), the "classification presumes a causal relationship between hypertension and heart involvement and between hypertension and kidney involvement, as the two conditions are linked by the term 'with' in the Alphabetic Index. These conditions should be coded as related even in the absence of physician documentation explicitly linking them, unless the documentation clearly states the conditions are unrelated. For hypertension and conditions not specifically linked by relational terms such as 'with,' 'associated with' or 'due to' in the classification, provider documentation must link the conditions in order to code them as related."[2]

CLINICAL EXAMPLES

NONSPECIFIC DOCUMENTATION	SPECIFIC DOCUMENTATION
Example 1 ESRD, HTN, GFR 10.[a]	**Example 1** End-stage renal disease (ESRD) and hypertension. Patient's glomerular filtration rate is stable at 10. Continue dialysis three times a week. Patient's hypertension[b] is well controlled with antihypertensives noted on today's updated medication list.
Example 2 Hypertension and hyperthyroidism.[c] We will increase her methimazole from 5 mg to 10 mg before considering surgery. She will keep a blood pressure log at home and return in 1 week.	**Example 2** Hypertension due to thyrotoxicosis with Grave's disease. We will increase her methimazole from 5 mg to 10 mg before considering surgery. She will keep a blood pressure log at home and return in 1 week.[d]

[a] Avoid acronyms. Here, the physician states the patient has end-stage renal disease, but there is no mention of dialysis.

[b] This note identifies the patient's end-stage renal disease (ESRD), hypertension, and renal dialysis status and provides details for all three diagnoses. No causal link is required to be documented for the ESRD and the hypertension.

[c] Both of these are nonspecific diagnoses and there is no link between them.

[d] A clear link between the hyperthyroidism and the hypertension is established.

Coding

The guidelines tell us to assume a causal link between hypertension and chronic kidney disease and heart disorders reported with codes I51.4-I51.9, or from I50.-, *Heart failure*. Although only codes I51.4-I51.9 are listed in the inclusion note under I11, *Hypertensive heart disease*, this note is not intended to be all inclusive. Code I11.0, *Hypertensive heart disease with heart failure*, for example, requires a heart failure diagnosis. See Table 4-2.7 for codes other than heart failure with assumed causal links to hypertensive heart disease.

TABLE 4-2.7 Codes Other than Heart Failure with Assumed Causal Links to Hypertensive Heart Disease

CODE	DESCRIPTION
I51.4	Myocarditis, unspecified
I51.5	Myocardial degeneration
I51.7	Cardiomegaly
I51.81	Takotsubo syndrome
I51.89	Other ill-defined heart diseases
I51.9	Heart disease, unspecified

RA coders commonly code as they go, capturing a hypertension diagnosis as code I10, *Essential (primary) hypertension,* before reaching the part of the chart in which chronic kidney disease or heart failure is introduced as a diagnosis. Always double-check the coding when a chart is completed. Never report code I10 with a code from category I50.-, *Heart failure*, with codes I51.4-I51.9, or with code I10, or with a code for chronic kidney disease.

These causal relationship combinations are very specific. Do not automatically link an unspecified or acute kidney disease with kidney disease in hypertension. The link only exists for chronic kidney disease. The codes in categories I12, *Hypertensive chronic kidney disease,* and I13, *Hypertensive heart and chronic kidney disease,* require that a condition reported with codes N18.1-N18.6 also be documented and coded for the patient. Similarly, the hypertensive heart disease codes require a heart condition reportable with a code from category I50.- or I51.4-I51.9.

According to ICD-10-CM Guidelines Section I(C.9.a.1 and C.9.a.2), "[h]ypertension with heart conditions classified to I50.- or I51.4-I51.9, are assigned to a code from category I11, Hypertensive heart disease. Use an additional code from category I50, Heart failure, to identify the type of heart failure in those patients with heart failure.

Assign codes from category I12, Hypertensive chronic kidney disease, when both hypertension and a condition classifiable to category N18, Chronic kidney disease (CKD), are present. CKD should not be coded as hypertensive if the physician has specifically documented a different cause. The appropriate code from category N18 should be used as a secondary code with a code from category I12 to identify the stage of chronic kidney disease. If a patient has hypertensive chronic kidney disease and acute renal failure, an additional code for the acute renal failure is required."[2]

In addition, ICD-10-CM Guideline Section I(C.9.a.7) states to "[a]ssign code R03.0, Elevated blood pressure reading without diagnosis of hypertension, unless patient has an established diagnosis of hypertension. Assign code O13.-, Gestational [pregnancy-induced] hypertension without significant proteinuria, or O14.-, Pre-eclampsia, for transient hypertension of pregnancy."[2] While, Guideline Section I(C.9.a.10) states to "[a]ssign a code from category I16, Hypertensive crisis, for documented hypertensive urgency, hypertensive emergency or unspecified hypertensive crisis. Code also any identified hypertensive disease (I10-I15)."[2]

CODING TIP Report two codes, at a minimum, for hypertension crisis. The crisis code is reported in addition to the underlying hypertension code.

ABSTRACT & CODE IT!

Abstract and code the clinical coding example below. Check your answers against the answers in Appendix C.

Patient 1

Patient with long-standing hypertension diagnosis has been noncompliant with her antihypertensives and now presents to the emergency department in a hypertensive urgency, with a blood pressure reading of 180/110.

Patient 2

End-stage renal disease (ESRD) and hypertension. Patient's glomerular filtration rate is stable at 14. Continue dialysis three times a week. Patient's hypertension is well controlled with antihypertensives noted on today's updated medication list.

Patient 3

Hypertension due to thyrotoxicosis with Grave's disease. We will increase her methimazole from 5 mg to 10 mg before considering surgery. She will keep a blood pressure log at home and return in 1 week.

Intellectual Disabilities – *see* Chromosomal Abnormalities, Intellectual Disabilities, and Other Development Disorders

Intestinal Disorders

Intestinal obstruction/perforation
HCC 33 0.246

Inflammatory bowel disease
HCC 35 0.294
RxHCC 67 0.527

The digestive system is comprised of the alimentary canal, a single tube that begins in the mouth and continues to the anus, and digestive organs that connect to the alimentary canal via ducts. Digestion involves both mechanical and chemical processes. Peristalsis describes the involuntary muscle contractions that move nutrients along the alimentary canal. Valves provide stops and reduce backflow along the route. The liver produces bile, which is stored in the gallbladder and released into the duodenum in reaction to fatty nutrients detected there. The pancreas releases enzymes that contribute to digestion, and the mouth and stomach each release chemicals that also aid in the breakdown of food. At the beginning of the digestive cycle, fluid is added to food to create a slurry: in the mouth, the stomach, and small intestine. In the large intestine, this fluid is reabsorbed before defecation.

Patency of the alimentary canal is essential to its operation. Obstruction can occur if the lumen has been damaged or in mechanical problems like adhesions, intussusception, or volvulus. In obstruction, the normal flow through the lumen is disrupted. Fecal impaction may cause obstruction, or be the consequence of obstruction.

Perforation may occur for a variety of reasons, including secondary to stomach and duodenal ulcers as well as from intestinal causes. This exposes the peritoneum to acidic or potentially infective digestive or fecal matter. Most ulcers are duodenal, as the duodenum is where the hepatopancreatic duct delivers bile and pancreatic enzymes for digestion. Peptic ulcer describes a digestive ulcer with an unknown site. Gastrojejunal ulcers occur in the jejunum that is exposed to higher concentrations of bile acids and enzymes following gastric bypass or duodenal resection.

Crohn's disease and ulcerative colitis are forms of inflammatory bowel disease. Crohn's disease may affect any part of the alimentary canal and causes inflammatory changes to the full-thickness of the intestinal wall, while ulcerative colitis is limited to the large intestine and involves only the mucosal lining of the colon. Both conditions lead to intestinal bleeding, diarrhea, abdominal pain, and cramps. Both Crohn's disease and ulcerative colitis are risk factors for intestinal cancers.

Physician Documentation

Crohn's disease and ulcerative colitis may have periods in which the symptoms are dormant, with or without medication. Symptomatic remission doesn't mean the disease is not present. Typically, these patients are still monitored and still undergo an accelerated colonoscopy schedule to monitor the condition. Document these inflammatory diseases, even when inactive, if they are discussed or monitored during a patient encounter as part of the history of present illness (HPI), laboratory result review, or physical examination.

Irritable bowel syndrome (IBS) and inflammatory bowel disease (IBD) are conditions that should be carefully documented so that the correct codes can be abstracted. Documented "irritable bowel" classifies as unspecified IBS. Documentation for IBS should state with constipation, diarrhea, mix of both, or other complication. IBS is considered a diagnosis of exclusion, ie, the patient has tested negative for diverticular, gallbladder, and celiac diseases, and does not risk-adjust. In contrast, IBD is a nonspecific diagnosis grouping that includes Crohn's disease and ulcerative colitis, which risk-adjust. Physicians and other healthcare providers should document the specific condition they are treating. "Inflammatory bowel disease" classifies to code K52.9, *Noninfective gastroenteritis and colitis, unspecified*. Crohn's and ulcerative colitis are inflammatory conditions that can be definitively diagnosed via colonoscopy and upper gastrointestinal endoscopy, computed tomography (CT) scans, or barium enema studies.

For Crohn's disease or ulcerative colitis, the site(s) affected should be identified, along with any complication (eg, bleeding, obstruction, abscess, fistula). For patients with either form of IBD, document the etiology of any anemia as nutritional (iron or vitamin B12 deficiency), due to chronic or acute blood loss, or due to medications treating the inflammatory condition. Document the presence of any ostomy in a patient with Crohn's disease or ulcerative colitis as ostomy status risk-adjusts separately.

Peptic is a nonspecific description of a gastrointestinal ulcer. Identify an ulcer as gastric, duodenal, or gastrojejunal. Identify the patient's condition as chronic or acute, and document any complications of ulcer, including hemorrhage or perforation. Document the results of *Helicobacter pylori* testing. Also link any long-term use of NSAIDs to the ulcer, as appropriate.

CLINICAL EXAMPLES

NONSPECIFIC DOCUMENTATION	SPECIFIC DOCUMENTATION
Example 1 The anemia is caused by the patient's peptic ulcer.[a]	**Example 1** The patient's chronic blood-loss anemia is caused by the patient's chronic gastric ulcer with hemorrhage. We are going to test for *H. pylori* and start her on proton pump inhibitors as well as a two-week course of tetracycline.[b]
Example 2 IBD. We will treat the current flare-up with a short course of prednisone.[c]	**Example 2** Crohn's disease of the large and small intestine, with an acute flare-up causing limited rectal bleeding. We will start him on a short course of prednisone.[d]

[a] Connect the dots: State that the ulcer is bleeding. Also, identify the ulcer type. "Peptic" is an unspecified term. Identify whether the ulcer and the bleeding are acute or chronic conditions.

[b] Here, the site of the ulcer and the cause of the bleeding is noted, as well as the duration of the conditions (chronic).

[c] Identify the type of inflammatory bowel disease (eg, Crohn's disease or irritable bowel syndrome) and identify the site(s) affected. Specify the complication, if known.

[d] The type of IBD has been identified, the site specified, and the complication described here.

Coding

Gastrointestinal bleeding may be documented in association with intestinal disorders. Combination codes exist to capture both the bleeding and its etiology, and these combination codes should be used rather than separate codes if a causal relationship is established.

Gastrointestinal (GI) bleeding may be associated with Crohn's disease, ulcerative colitis, peptic ulcers, diverticulosis, angiodysplasia, or any number of other GI conditions. Often, when the physician performs an endoscopy to determine the cause of bleeding, a condition may be diagnosed, but no active bleeding noted at the site. Coders cannot assume a causal link between bleeding and a GI condition unless the link is established in the ICD-10-CM Alphabetic Index or by the physician. If there is no link, report the patient's GI condition, and the type of bleeding as hematemesis, melena, occult bleeding or hematochezia. If there is a causal link from the documentation or from the index, a combination code for the GI condition and bleeding is reported instead of two codes. Causal links in the Alphabetic Index are found when the word "with" links two terms, for example:

Ulcer, ulcerated, ulcerating, ulceration, ulcerative
duodenum, duodenal (eroded) (peptic) K26.9
with
hemorrhage K26.4
and perforation K26.6
perforation K26.5

According to ICD-10-CM Guideline Section 1(A.15), the Alphabetic Index establishes a causal relationship when two terms are linked with the word "with."[2] In this example, "with" establishes a link between a duodenal ulcer and hemorrhage. The same "with" linkage exists for stomach and peptic ulcers, regional enteritis (Crohn's disease), and ulcerative colitis. Look up individual diagnoses to see whether the Alphabetic Index establishes a causal relationship between bleeding or other complications (eg, fistula, obstruction, or abscess, and the GI disorder).

IBS and IBD are not the same, and are an example in which the language of the physician or other acceptable provider must be followed exactly. IBS does not cause inflammation or ulcers and does not increase the patient's risk for cancer. IBS is sometimes called a spastic colon. IBD is a name for autoimmune bowel disorders. IBD is the name given to Crohn's disease and ulcerative colitis, both conditions that cause inflammation and ulcerations in the bowel. A significant number of patients with ulcerative colitis undergo colectomy for their condition. Though ulcerative colitis is not considered a curable disease, it only affects the colon, and colectomy does eliminate the condition. Colectomy is performed for patients with severe symptoms, extensive bleeding, if the patient is diagnosed with toxic megacolon, or if traditional medications are contraindicated.

When a patient presents with a gastrointestinal ulcer with hemorrhage, and the hemorrhage is attributed to the patient's anticoagulant therapy, report a code specific to the GI ulcer with hemorrhage, D68.32, *Hemorrhagic disorder due to extrinsic circulating anticoagulant*, and a code for the adverse effect of the anticoagulant, according to AHA's *Coding Clinic* (First Quarter, 2016).[12] The physician does not need to document "hemorrhagic disorder," but must link the bleeding to the therapeutic anticoagulant in order to abstract code D68.32.

Hematemesis
Vomiting of blood indicative of an upper gastrointestinal source.

Melena
Passing of stool laced with darkened (old) blood, indicating an upper or lower gastrointestinal source.

Occult bleeding
Blood indicating microscopic evidence of gastrointestinal bleeding of unknown source.

Hematochezia
Passing of bright red blood, indicating a lower intestinal source.

Toxic megacolon
Toxic megacolon can be a complication of Crohn's disease or ulcerative colitis that causes a dilation of a segment or the entire colon. Inflammation in the colon's mucosa migrates into the muscles and serosa of the colon, causing it to expand. This causes pain and tenderness, and may lead to perforation of the colon.

ABSTRACT & CODE IT!

Abstract and code the clinical coding example below. Check your answers against the answers in Appendix C.

Patient 1
The patient will be admitted for cecal volvulus, with gangrene and perforation. She is being prepped for emergency surgery.

Patient 2
The patient's chronic blood-loss anemia is caused by the patient's chronic gastric ulcer with hemorrhage. We are going to test for *H. pylori* and start her on omeprazole, amoxicillin, and clarithromycin.

Patient 3
Crohn's disease of the large and small intestine, with an acute flare-up causing limited rectal bleeding. We will start him on a short course of prednisone.

Ischemic Heart Disease

Acute myocardial infarction
HCC 86 0.233

Unstable angina and other acute ischemic heart disease
HCC 87 0.218

Angina pectoris
HCC 88 0.140

Coronary artery disease
RxHCC 188 0.125

Ischemic heart disease occurs when the flow of blood nourishing and oxygenating the heart muscle is reduced. Ischemia can result in muscle pain in reaction to the reduced oxygen flow, or infarction, the death of muscle tissue.

The chief causes of reduced blood flow to the heart are atherosclerosis and blood clots. Atherosclerosis describes deposits of cholesterol-rich plaque on the interior lining of the arteries, known as coronary artery disease (CAD). CAD itself can cause vessels to occlude, but can also narrow the vessels so that they are more susceptible to be blocked by debris in the blood, such as with a blood or fat embolus, air bubble, or other substance. Blood clots can be formed on site in a vein (thrombus) and then be carried through the bloodstream elsewhere until they reach an artery too small to pass. Sudden stress can cause vessels to constrict, also leading to ischemia, and less commonly, patients experience involuntary spasms of their coronary arteries, affecting blood flow.

A myocardial infarction (MI) occurs when an artery oxygenating the muscle of the heart is occluded or when the heart's demand for oxygen outstrips its supply, resulting in the death of a portion of muscle tissue due to lack of oxygen and nutrients. While other parts of the heart muscle may take over the work of the dead tissue, the dead tissue will never regenerate.

An MI is usually an emergent condition treated as an inpatient encounter, with follow-up and ongoing care often provided in the physician office. Signs and symptoms vary from mild indigestion and shortness of breath to severe chest pain, nausea, and loss of consciousness at the time of the acute event. The site and size of the MI affect symptoms and outcomes. MI can be diagnosed by interpreting blood markers (eg, serum troponin values) in light of typical symptoms, abnormal electrocardiography or echocardiography, or demonstration of a clot within the coronary artery.

More than 15 million people have coronary heart disease, according to the 2016 Heart Disease and Stroke Statistics update of the American Heart Association.[13] Heart disease remains the leading cause of death in the US. Chief risk factors for heart disease include high blood pressure, total cholesterol, diabetes, smoking, and inactivity.

Physician Documentation

Heart health treatments may include pharmacologic, nonpharmacologic, and surgical approaches. Details are important when documenting cardiac conditions, as treatment approaches and outcomes vary, depending on the exact etiology. ICD-10-CM subdivides

Embolus
Thrombus that breaks free and is carried antegrade from the site at which it is formed; pleural is emboli.

Thrombus
Intravascular clot of blood that remains in the location where it was formed; plural is thrombi.

Myocardial infarction (MI)
Death of heart muscle; colloquially known as a heart attack.

many heart ailments that were once bundled into a single code, so specificity in the medical record also contributes to accurate coding and risk scores.

Identify angina pectoris as stable or unstable (eg, accelerated, spasmodic, or progressive), link it to its underlying cause (eg, coronary atherosclerosis, coronary artery bypass graft [CABG] atherosclerosis, coronary spasm) and its relationship to any complication of a CABG or intracoronary stent. If a patient's angina is controlled with medications but would recur if taken off their medication (eg, a beta blocker, nitrates, ranolazine), the angina is stable. If symptoms break through their current treatment, the angina may be unstable.

When an MI occurs, document if it is an ST-elevation MI (STEMI) or non-ST-elevation MI (NSTEMI), its underlying mechanism (eg, type 1, 2, 3, 4, or 5), its location (eg, anterior, inferior, lateral) and/or vessel involvement (eg, left main, right coronary artery), and any immediate or prolonged consequences (eg, papillary muscle dysfunction, ventricular septal defects, left ventricular systolic heart failure, Dressler's syndrome).

Always note the date of the MI in the record. If more than one MI occurs within a four-week period, the dates of both MIs should be documented. ICD-10-CM differentiates between an MI in its acute phase (eg, within 28 days of occurrence) and encounters for that same infarction occurring at a later time. Subsequent MIs occurring within 28 days of a previous MI are classified differently than those occurring at a time more distant to an initial infarction. Be very specific in documenting the timeline of infarctions in a patient's chart so that the appropriate codes can be captured.

A patient who experiences a second acute type 1 MI within 28 days of a previous MI requires two codes to capture the condition: a code from category I21, STEMI and NSTEMI, and a code from category I22, Subsequent STEMI and NSTEMI. Document both infarctions, so that these conditions can be abstracted accurately. Be sure to note specifically the site and date of each infarction.

One the other hand, subsequent type 2 MIs are reported with code I21.A1, *Myocardial infarction type 2,* and subsequent type 4 or 5 MIs are reported with code I21.A9, *Other myocardial infarction type,* and not a code from category I22. ICD-10-CM guidelines require that I22 codes be used only for new type 1 or unspecified MIs within 28 days of a previous MIs, not type 2, 3, 4, or 5 MIs. Any MI not documented otherwise will be coded as a type 1 MI, as this is the default in the ICD-10-CM Alphabetic Index. The presence of any MI older than 28 days is classified as I25.2, *Old myocardial infarction.* Old MIs risk-adjust to RxHCC 188, and therefore, it should be documented at least annually for all patients with a history of MI.

In CAD, document any lipid-rich plaque or chronic total occlusion. Note if the diseased vessels are native vessels or grafts, and in a heart transplant patient, whether the vessels are native or grafts. Note whether the CAD is accompanied by angina pectoris, with or without spasm or instability.

Do not report the acronyms CAD, MI, AMI, STEMI, or NSTEMI as a first reference. Instead, spell out the first reference (eg, non-ST-elevation myocardial infarction [NSTEMI]). Document any history of coronary artery bypass surgery, cardiac pacemaker, or heart valve replacement. Document heart transplant status or if the patient is awaiting transplant. Note any current or past nicotine dependence or use. See Table 4-2.8 for a list of the common tobacco use and history codes.

TABLE 4-2.8 Common Tobacco Use and History Codes

CODE	DESCRIPTION
F17.210	Nicotine dependence, cigarettes, uncomplicated
F17.211	Nicotine dependence, cigarettes, in remission
F17.218	Nicotine dependence, cigarettes, with other nicotine-induced disorder
Z72.0	Tobacco use
Z77.22	Exposure to environmental tobacco smoke (acute) (chronic)
Z87.891	Personal history of tobacco dependence

Do not rely on EHR medication lists to capture long-term use of medications. Actively document long-term use of anticoagulants, antithrombolitics, antiplatelets, NSAIDs, aspirin, or any other pertinent pharmaceuticals in the medical record.

An old MI that has no current symptoms is a diagnosis that risk-adjusts for RxHCCs. If the old MI is assessed or its presence is considered in treatment care for a current illness, note it. It is not sufficient to simply have it listed in the PMH. The old MI should be documented somewhere in the active medical record (eg, as part of the HPI or physical examination).

CLINICAL EXAMPLES

NONSPECIFIC DOCUMENTATION	SPECIFIC DOCUMENTATION
Example 1 Assessment/Plan: 1. Hypercholesterolemia 2. Old MI 3. CAD 4. DM[a] 5. PAD	**Example 1** Assessment/Plan: 1. Pure hypercholesterolemia. Stable on ezetimibe. 2. Old MI, apical-lateral transmural, stable and asymptomatic. 3. Coronary artery disease of native vessels, with angina pectoris; ezetimibe and atorvastatin. Schedule another stress test in six months. 4. Diabetes mellitus, type 2, well controlled with insulin. 5. Bilateral atherosclerosis of lower extremities and bilateral intermittent claudication. Patient is not a candidate for bypass.[b]
2. Chief complaint: Patient being seen for follow-up on the AMI for which he was hospitalized recently.[c]	2. Chief complaint: Patient being seen for follow-up on ST-elevation myocardial infarction (STEMI) involving the oblique marginal coronary artery, for which he was hospitalized two weeks ago. The STEMI occurred 4/15/2017.[d]

[a] While this states it is an assessment and plan, no plans for the conditions are noted. Identify the type of hypercholesterolemia if known, and describe the symptoms and findings related to the old myocardial infarction. Always spell out acronyms on first reference. Provide information on the vessels affected by coronary artery disease, and document any presence of angina. For diabetes, identify the type and how it is treated. Provide manifestation details for the PAD [peripheral artery disease] and discuss treatment options.

[b] These notes provide a clearer view of the patient's conditions, their severity, and treatments.

[c] Spell out acute myocardial infarction, and identify as STEMI/NSTEMI. Also document the site, which should be available in hospital records. Time is an important element in code selection for AMIs; state how long ago, and provide a date of the AMI when possible.

[d] The critical elements of the AMI are all presented here: STEMI vs NSTEMI; site of infarction; date of infarction.

Coding

According to ICD-10-CM Guideline Section I(C.9.b):

> ICD-10-CM has combination codes for atherosclerotic heart disease with angina pectoris. The subcategories for these codes are I25.11, Atherosclerotic heart disease of native coronary artery with angina pectoris and I25.7, Atherosclerosis of coronary artery bypass graft(s) and coronary artery of transplanted heart with angina pectoris.
>
> When using one of these combination codes it is not necessary to use an additional code for angina pectoris. A causal relationship can be assumed in a patient with both atherosclerosis and angina pectoris, unless the documentation indicates the angina is due to something other than the atherosclerosis.[2]

In addition, ICD-10-CM Guideline Section I(C.9.e.1) states:

> The ICD-10-CM codes for type 1 acute myocardial infarction (AMI) identify the site, such as anterolateral wall or true posterior wall. Subcategories I21.0-I21.2 and code I21.3 are used for type 1 ST elevation myocardial infarction (STEMI). Code I21.4, Non-ST elevation (NSTEMI) myocardial infarction, is used for type 1 non-ST elevation myocardial infarction (NSTEMI) and nontransmural MIs.
>
> If a type 1 NSTEMI evolves to STEMI, assign the STEMI code. If a type 1 STEMI converts to NSTEMI due to thrombolytic therapy, it is still coded as STEMI.
>
> For encounters occurring while the myocardial infarction is equal to, or less than, 28 days old, including transfers to another acute setting or a postacute setting, and the myocardial infarction meets the definition for "other diagnoses" (see Section III, Reporting Additional Diagnoses), codes from category I21 may continue to be reported. For encounters after the 4 week time frame and the patient is still receiving care related to the myocardial infarction, the appropriate aftercare code should be assigned, rather than a code from category I21. For old or healed myocardial infarctions not requiring further care, code I25.2, Old myocardial infarction, may be assigned.[2]

The addition of codes reporting types of MIs in 2018 changed how coders must approach these diagnoses in the future. According to ICD-10-CM Guideline Section I(C.9.e.5):

> The ICD-10-CM provides codes for different types of myocardial infarction. Type 1 myocardial infarctions are assigned to codes I21.0-I21.4.
>
> Type 2 myocardial infarction, and myocardial infarction due to demand ischemia or secondary to ischemic balance, is assigned to code I21.A1, Myocardial infarction type 2 with a code for the underlying cause. Do not assign code I24.8, Other forms of acute ischemic heart disease for the demand ischemia. Sequencing of type 2 AMI or the underlying cause is dependent on the circumstances of admission. When a type 2 AMI code is described as NSTEMI or STEMI, only assign code I21.A1. Codes I21.01-I21.4 should only be assigned for type 1 AMIs.
>
> Acute myocardial infarctions type 3, 4a, 4b, 4c and 5 are assigned to code I21.A9, Other myocardial infarction type.
>
> The "Code also" and "Code first" notes should be followed related to complications, and for coding of postprocedural myocardial infarctions during or following cardiac surgery.[2]

CODING TIP A type 2 myocardial infarction (T2MI) due to demand ischemia should be reported with code I21.A1. Codes from I21.0-I21.4 should not be used for a T2MI, even if the physician documents STEMI, NSTEMI, or a location (eg, anterior). The I21.0-I21.4 codes are reserved for Type 1 MIs.

According to AHA's *Coding Clinic* (Second Quarter, 2017), category I23, *Certain complications following ST elevation (STEMI) and non-ST elevation (NSTEMI) myocardial infarction (within the 28-day period),* also reports complications of an MI diagnosed beyond the 28-day period associated as the acute phase of an MI. Therefore, an additional code is not required for the previous NSTEMI.[14] Per ICD-10-CM Guideline Section 1(C.9.e.2), "[c]ode I21.9, Acute myocardial infarction, unspecified, is the default for unspecified acute myocardial infarction or unspecified type. If only type 1 STEMI or transmural MI without the site is documented, assign code I21.3, ST elevation (STEMI) myocardial infarction of unspecified site."[2]

In addition, per ICD-10-CM Guideline Section I(C.9.e.4), a "code from category I22, Subsequent ST elevation (STEMI) and non-ST elevation (NSTEMI) myocardial infarction, is to be used when a patient who has suffered a type 1 or unspecified AMI has a new AMI within the 4 week time frame of the initial AMI. A code from category I22 must be used in conjunction with a code from category I21. The sequencing of the I22 and I21 codes depends on the circumstances of the encounter.

Do not assign code I22 for subsequent myocardial infarctions other than type 1 or unspecified. For subsequent type 2 AMI assign only code I21.A1. For subsequent type 4 or type 5 AMI, assign only code I21.A9."[2]

Cardiology is a complex specialty with its own nomenclature. Care must be taken to use the documented language in the ICD-10-CM Alphabetic Index and in abstraction. Refer to anatomy references or search online to understand unfamiliar diagnoses. The American Heart Association maintains an encyclopedia of heart disease terminology, which can be accessed at http://www.heart.org/HEARTORG/Conditions/HeartAttack/HeartAttackToolsResources/Cardiac-Glossary_UCM_303945_Article.jsp#m.

Signs and symptoms that can be used as support for a patient diagnosed with MI or ischemia include chest pain; pain that radiates down the arm, back, or jaw; indigestion; abdominal pain; shortness of breath; fatigue; sweating; anxiety; or nausea. While these signs and symptoms support a diagnosis of MI, they are considered intrinsic to the MI and are not separately reported, nor do they risk-adjust. Tests may include an electrocardiogram, chest X ray, CT scan, or coronary angiography.

Type 1 MIs are the default in the ICD-10-CM Alphabetic Index. For type 1 MIs, the vessel causing the infarction is pertinent to code selection, as is the timeline from the initial MI to the current encounter. If the vessel is noted, but the documentation states the infarction was nontransmural, report code I21.4, *Non-ST elevation (NSTEMI) myocardial infarction,* rather than the vessel site for an initial infarction, or code I22.2, *Subsequent non-ST elevation (NSTEMI) myocardial infarction,* for a subsequent event. The words "myocardial infarction" are essential to coding from categories I21, I22, and I23. An MI cannot be reported based on documented "ST elevation" or "non-ST elevation" alone. Report any old MI (I25.2), heart transplant status (Z94.1), heart valve replacement status, and any long-term use of blood-thinners or aspirin.

In CAD, assume the affected vessels are native arteries if not otherwise documented. Autologous graft is a graft using a vessel removed from the patient for a bypass. Use additional codes to report calcified coronary lesion (I25.84), lipid rich plaque (I25.83), or chronic total occlusion (I25.82).

CODING TIP In CAD, assume the affected vessels are native arteries if not otherwise documented. Use additional codes to report calcified coronary lesion (I25.84), lipid-rich plaque (I25.83), or chronic total occlusion (I25.82).

If a patient has a second MI more than 28 days after a previous MI, the new infarction is reported as an initial MI with a code from category I21.-. If a patient has a second MI within 28 days of a previous MI, the new infarction is reported as a subsequent MI and is reported with a code from category I22.-. The initial MI would be reported secondarily. An acute MI that is identified as subendocardial or nontransmural is reported as an NSTEMI (I21.4), regardless of the documented site of the MI.

CODING TIP Autologous graft is a graft using a vessel removed from the patient for a bypass. Nonautologous biological graft is usually composed of processed vessels from cadavers (allografts [same species]) or animals (xenografts [different species, ie, pigs or cows]).

ABSTRACT & CODE IT!

Abstract and code the clinical coding example below. Check your answers against the answers in Appendix C.

Patient 1

Patient is being seen today for new onset angina of effort. She states the chest pain begins after climbing the flight of stairs to her bedroom, and she must sit until it dissipates, usually a few minutes. I have scheduled her for coronary angiography on Tuesday.

Patient 2

Assessment/Plan:

1. Pure hypercholesterolemia. Stable on ezetimbe.
2. Old MI, apical-lateral transmural, stable and asymptomatic.
3. Coronary artery disease of native vessels, with angina pectoris; ezetimbe and atorvastatin. Schedule another stress test in six months.
4. Diabetes mellitus, type 2, well controlled with insulin.
5. Bilateral atherosclerosis of lower extremities and bilateral intermittent claudication. Patient is not a candidate for bypass.

Patient 3

Chief complaint: Patient being seen for follow-up on ST-elevation myocardial infarction (STEMI) involving the oblique marginal coronary artery, for which he was hospitalized two weeks ago. The STEMI occurred 4/15/2017.

Leukemia *see* Neoplasms

Lewy Body Disease *see* Dementia

Liver Disease

End-stage liver disease
HCC 27 0.962

Cirrhosis of liver
HCC 28 0.390

Chronic viral hepatitis C
HCC 29 0.165
RxHCC 54 3.202

Chronic hepatitis, except C
RxHCC 55 0.521

The liver is crucial to life: It is responsible for nutrient management, producing the bile that emulsifies fats in digestion, and regulating blood glucose for energy supply. It filters damaged blood cells, bacteria, and other foreign substances from the blood, and performs biotransformation of toxins, hormones, and drugs. It synthesizes albumin, globulin, and clotting factors. It stores minerals and vitamins. Common diseases of the liver include cirrhosis, hepatitis, alcoholic liver disease, and fatty liver disease.

Chronic liver disease and cirrhosis can be caused by many conditions, but the majority of cases can be linked to hepatitis C or alcoholic liver disease. The CDC reports that there are 3.5 million persons in the US currently infected with hepatitis C,[15] and that it kills 20,000 Americans a year—more than any other infectious disease reported to the CDC. While there is no cure for cirrhosis or chronic liver disease, there is medication to treat and cure chronic hepatitis C.

The third largest cause of liver disease is obesity, which can lead to non-alcoholic fatty liver, which in turn may cause the fibrosis that leads to cirrhosis. Most chronic forms of hepatitis risk-adjust; acute forms of hepatitis do not. As an inflammatory condition, hepatitis is often curable.

Physician Documentation

Key to proper documentation of liver disease is identifying the etiology of the disease in every encounter. The coder is not permitted to look at other encounters to determine if the hepatitis is caused by infection, obesity, toxicity, or alcohol use. The cause must be specific: for alcoholic fatty liver, identify whether the patient is diagnosed with alcohol dependence, abuse, or use. In viral hepatitis, identify the infective agent in addition to whether the condition is chronic or acute. Manifestations of the liver disease must be noted: coma, ascites, necrosis, failure.

For viral hepatitis, ensure all data elements necessary for coding are captured by documenting the following:

- **Type:** Hepatitis A, B, C, E, delta (super) infection of B carrier
  - For type B, with or without delta agent
- **Chronicity:** acute or chronic
- **Severity:** with or without coma

Often, in chronic liver disease, there is a series of diagnoses that are linked. Each diagnosis must be in the medical record and must be linked to its causal elements. While the link between cirrhosis and esophageal hemorrhage may be inferred by the physician, the coder is not permitted to code what isn't in the record. All elements must be documented so that all codes can be captured and the severity of the patient's condition accurately reported.

Cirrhosis
Liver tissue is replaced by fibrous tissue that cannot perform liver functions effectively.

Hepatitis
Inflammation by viruses, toxins, or an autoimmune response. Hepatitis may resolve, may cause permanent damage, or may cause liver failure.

Alcoholic liver disease
Hepatic dysfunction associated with alcohol consumption and resulting in fatty liver, cirrhosis, and scarring.

Fatty liver disease
Usually in obesity and/or alcohol abuse, fat accumulates in liver cells in this reversible condition.

Physicians cannot assume that coders can make the logical leap from an etiology to a manifestation (eg, from esophageal varices to cirrhosis of the liver or alcoholism). All diagnoses must be documented and causal relationships established in order for the coder to properly abstract, per Figure 4-2.1.

F10.288 Alcohol dependence with other alcohol-induced disorder

K70.30 Alcoholic cirrhosis of liver without ascites

K76.6 Portal hypertension

I85.11 Secondary esophageal varices with bleeding

D62 Acute posthemorrhagic anemia

DOCUMENTATION TIP Hepatitis C begins as an acute condition within six months of exposure to the virus. Between 75% and 85% of patients with acute hepatitis C will develop chronic hepatitis C, which can lead to more serious liver disease, according to the CDC. Always document hepatitis as "chronic" or "acute," as appropriate, so that an unspecified code is avoided. Only chronic hepatitis risk adjusts.[15]

FIGURE 4-2.1 Elements of Chronic Liver Disease

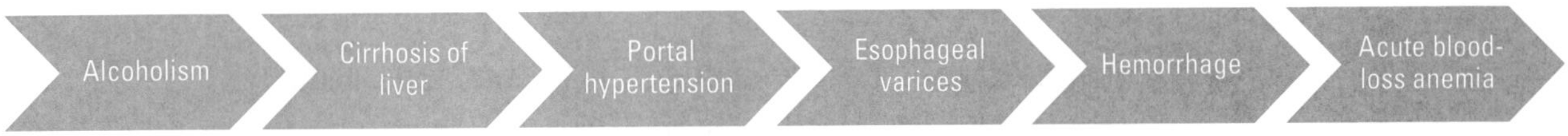

CDC Morbidity and Mortality Weekly Report

This excerpt is from the CDC's *Morbidity and Mortality Weekly Report*, August 17, 2012[16]:

CDC estimates that although persons born during 1945–1965 comprise an estimated 27% of the population, they account for approximately three fourths of all HCV infections in the United States, 73% of HCV-associated mortality, and are at greatest risk for hepatocellular carcinoma and other HCV-related liver disease. With the advent of new therapies that can halt disease progression and provide a virologic cure (i.e., sustained viral clearance following completion of treatment) in most persons, targeted testing and linkage to care for infected persons in this birth cohort is expected to reduce HCV-related morbidity and mortality. CDC is augmenting previous recommendations for HCV testing (CDC. Recommendations for prevention and control of hepatitis C virus (HCV) infection and HCV-related chronic disease. MMWR 1998; 47 [No. RR–19]) to recommend one-time testing without prior ascertainment of HCV risk for persons born during 1945–1965, a population with a disproportionately high prevalence of HCV infection and related disease. Persons identified as having HCV infection should receive a brief screening for alcohol use and intervention as clinically indicated, followed by referral to appropriate care for HCV infection and related conditions.

Cirrhosis describes a more severe liver disease with formation of scars and fibrous tissue that represents irreversible damage to the liver. Cirrhosis may be caused by hepatitis or by alcoholic liver disease. All cirrhosis diagnoses risk-adjust.

Cirrhosis may cause portal hypertension, an increase in the blood pressure of the veins in the portal venous system leading into the liver from digestive organs. Scarring in the liver compresses the veins within it, causing congestion in venous blood. Portal hypertension is sometimes diagnosed when a patient is seen emergently for treatment of hemorrhaging esophageal varices. The varices are a common complication of portal hypertension.

In liver failure, the liver can no longer perform its normal functions adequately to meet the demands of the body. As its function worsens, some patients develop hepatic encephalopathy. Liver failure may be an acute condition or a chronic condition that lasts for years.

CLINICAL EXAMPLES

NONSPECIFIC DOCUMENTATION	SPECIFIC DOCUMENTATION
Example 1 Ascites 2/2 ESLD 2/2 ETOH & HCV.[a]	**Example 1** Ascites secondary to end-stage liver disease, secondary to alcoholic hepatitis with chronic hepatitis C.[b]
Example 2 Alcoholic fatty liver.[c]	**Example 2** Alcoholic fatty liver in patient with alcoholism, in remission.[d]

[a] Spell out acronyms on first reference. "ETOH" is not a diagnosis; it is chemistry. Avoid ETOH. The acronym shorthand misses identifying whether the patient has a chronic or acute form of hepatitis.

[b] In this case, we have identified the cause of the ascites, and spelled out acronyms that may have been confusing. We have identified the hepatitis as chronic.

[c] Diagnoses in ICD-10 with "alcoholic" in the title require a second code to identify the status of the alcohol use of the patient, but coders need the conditions documented in order to abstract them.

[d] Documentation appropriately uses the language "in remission" to describe the patient with alcohol dependence who is no longer drinking. "History of alcohol dependence" would also be acceptable. Both the alcohol dependence code and the liver disease code are necessary to describe the patient's status, but only the alcohol dependence in remission code risk-adjusts.

Coding

Codes for hepatitis are found in the infectious disease, digestive, and perinatal chapters of ICD-10-CM. Viral forms of the disease are reported according to type of virus, whether chronic or acute, and with or without coma. Only chronic forms of hepatitis risk-adjust. If possible, query the physician regarding the type of hepatitis C the patient has, if not documented. The most common type of hepatitis C is chronic. The default in ICD-10-CM is to an unspecified hepatitis C. The viral hepatitis codes are as follows:

B15.0 Hepatitis A with hepatic coma

B15.9 Hepatitis A without hepatic coma

B16.0 Acute hepatitis B with delta-agent with hepatic coma

B16.1 Acute hepatitis B with delta-agent without hepatic coma

B16.2 Acute hepatitis B without delta-agent with hepatic coma

B16.9 Acute hepatitis B without delta-agent and without hepatic coma

B17.0 Acute delta-(super) infection of hepatitis B carrier

B17.10 Acute hepatitis C without hepatic coma

B17.11 Acute hepatitis C with hepatic coma

B17.2 Acute hepatitis E

B17.8 Other specified acute viral hepatitis

B17.9 Acute viral hepatitis, unspecified

B18.0 Chronic viral hepatitis B with delta-agent

B18.1 Chronic viral hepatitis B without delta-agent

B18.2 Chronic viral hepatitis C

B18.8 Other chronic viral hepatitis

B18.9 Chronic viral hepatitis, unspecified

B19.0 Unspecified viral hepatitis with hepatic coma

B19.10 Unspecified viral hepatitis B without hepatic coma

B19.11 Unspecified viral hepatitis B with hepatic coma

B19.20 Unspecified viral hepatitis C without hepatic coma

B19.21 Unspecified viral hepatitis C with hepatic coma

B19.9 Unspecified viral hepatitis without hepatic coma

End-stage liver disease (ESLD) is reported with codes from category K72, *Hepatic failure, not elsewhere classified,* or subcategory K70.4-, *Alcoholic hepatic failure.* For toxic liver failure, report a code from K71.1, *Toxic liver disease with hepatic necrosis.* A fifth digit reports with or without coma for these types of failure. Only K71.11, *Toxic liver disease with hepatic necrosis, with coma,* risk-adjusts. With ESLD, also report the underlying cause (eg, a specific form of hepatitis and/or cirrhosis) so that the patient's condition is captured completely.

If a patient is documented with toxic liver disease due to a drug, at least three codes are required: Code first the external cause of poisoning due to a drug or toxin; report the liver disease with a code from K71, *Toxic liver disease*; and report a code identifying the adverse effect of a drug from codes T36-T50.

Model for End-Stage Liver Disease (MELD)

Patients with liver disease or failure are often given a Model for End-Stage Liver Disease (MELD) score, a system for evaluating liver function, predicting liver failure, and prioritizing patients on a waiting list for liver transplant. The score may range from 6, indicating a patient who is less ill, to 40, indicating a patient who is gravely ill.

The calculation is based on the patient's date of birth, bilirubin (mg/dl), serum sodium (mEq/L), international normalized ratio (INR), and serum creatinine (mg/dl). The creatinine result will default to 4 mg/dl if the patient has had dialysis twice, or 24 hours of continuous venovenous hemodialysis within a week prior to the creatinine test. A MELD score supports a liver disease diagnosis. To view a MELD calculator, go to https://optn.transplant.hrsa.gov/resources/allocation-calculators/meld-calculator/

Hepatic encephalopathy is not a synonym for hepatic coma; however, it is an indication of hepatic failure. According to AHA's *Coding Clinic* (First Quarter, 2017), a patient with chronic hepatitis C and hepatic encephalopathy is assigned B18.2, *Chronic viral hepatitis C,* and K72.10, *Chronic hepatic failure without coma.*[3]

Malnutrition
Insufficient nutrition or undernutrition due to lack of availability of all foods or lack of the right foods, or due to an inability or unwillingness to eat, which does not meet the metabolic demands of the body. Criteria differ between patients with acute illness, chronic diseases, and environmental circumstances (eg, hunger strike, anorexia nervosa).[18]

Cachexia
Excessive weight loss in the setting of ongoing disease, usually with disproportionate muscle wasting, which is not amendable to nutritional therapy.[19]

Sarcopenia
Muscle atrophy due to a disease or age-related state.

ABSTRACT & CODE IT!

Abstract and code the clinical coding example below. Check your answers against the answers in Appendix C.

Patient 1
Patient with alcoholic liver failure is diagnosed with hepatic encephalopathy and admitted through the emergency department. The patient's blood alcohol was 30 mg/100 ml, and was also diagnosed with alcohol abuse.

Patient 2
Ascites secondary to end-stage liver disease, secondary to alcoholic hepatitis with chronic hepatitis C. Patient's alcoholism is in remission.

Patient 3
Alcoholic fatty liver in patient who drinks regularly despite warnings to cease alcohol consumption due to hepatic status.

Lymphoma *see* Neoplasms

Malnutrition

Protein-calorie malnutrition
HCC 21 0.545

The Medicare population in the US is at risk for malnutrition due to the vagaries of aging: decreased sense of taste and smell also reduces the desire for food; poor oral health makes eating less enjoyable; limited income can mean the cupboards have little to offer; and a decline in physical and mental health may make an aging patient forget about food altogether.[17] The cumulative effect can be insidious. The patient eats less due to symptoms, and the symptoms increase because the patient eats less. Eventually, diminished mobility and cognitive functions affect activities of daily living.

Malnutrition, whether mild, moderate, or severe, risk-adjusts. It is considered such a liability that it risk-adjusts at twice the value as morbid obesity. Cachexia also risk-adjusts. Cachexia is severe weight loss associated with chronic disease. In cachexia, the body cannot process nutrients and fat. In sarcopenia, muscles waste away. It may be seen in end-stage COPD, cancer, AIDS, or dementia.

Physician Documentation

Malnutrition and cachexia are diagnoses that are often not documented by physicians who are evaluating patients with more serious conditions including AIDS, cancer, or dementia. However, malnutrition or cachexia is almost always going to affect the health of the patient and is a predictor of risk. These conditions should be documented and addressed in any encounter in which the condition is observed.

Body mass index (BMI) is a valuable screening tool for weight and nutrition status; however, one can have malnutrition with a normal or elevated BMI. Ensure the patient's BMI is calculated at least once or twice annually. When the BMI is less than 18.5, or when the patient's BMI is steadily declining, it reflects a risk physicians should note and act upon.

Also be sure to document the discussion, any care plan, and any diagnosis associated with the weight loss as well as any cause for it. Low BMIs associated with malnutrition or cachexia do not of themselves risk-adjust and are insufficient for reporting the patient's condition without a weight-related malnutrition diagnosis. The physician must document the diagnosis and care plan.

DOCUMENTATION TIP Malnutrition diagnostic medical decision making (MDM) requires a thorough evaluation of the patient's circumstances, dietary intake, pattern and rapidity of weight loss, an assessment of muscle and fat loss, and other clinical indicators, not just a simple reporting based solely on the BMI, clear documentation of its presence in the medical record, and detailed plans to address it when present. The Academy of Nutrition and Dietetics published their consensus statement on malnutrition in 2012 (available at http://www.tinyurl.com/2012malnutrition), which should be considered by treating physicians or healthcare providers. The federal Office of Inspector General and the Department of Justice regularly audit malnutrition codes for clinical validity, particularly if these codes affect RA and/or reimbursement.

Choose clear and concise language. State "malnutrition," a diagnosis, rather than "malnourished," an adjective describing the patient's appearance. State "cachexia," not "cachectic" for the same reason. Differentiate between cachexia and sarcopenia. If a patient's weight is causing other health issues (eg, anemia or falls), document the health issues and link them to the weight diagnosis. Similarly, if cachexia is caused by an underlying disease (eg, COPD, AIDS, dementia, or malignant neoplasm), document the underlying cause.

CLINICAL EXAMPLES

NONSPECIFIC DOCUMENTATION	SPECIFIC DOCUMENTATION
Example 1 Patient's pancreatic cancer has advanced. I have suggested parenteral feeding, but she declines.[a]	**Example 1** Patient's pancreatic cancer has metastasized to the peritoneum and liver. I have suggested parenteral feeding to address her severe malnutrition, but she declines.[b]
Patient 2 She has developed wasting disease.[c]	**Patient 2** She has developed wasting disease with a current BMI of 15.8. The main goal is to keep her hydrated and comfortable in her end-stage COPD.[d] She is receiving morphine for her dyspnea.

[a] A coder may be able to infer from this documentation that the patient has a nutritional deficit, but without a diagnosis, it cannot be abstracted. Only pancreatic cancer, NOS, can be coded from this note.

[b] The cover understands the patient has severe malnutrition, and that the pancreatic cancer has metastasized to other locations. In this case, the coder would be able to abstract the pancreatic cancer NOS, the secondary cancers, and the severe malnutrition.

[c] While wasting disease is not clinical language, it is classified to cachexia in the ICD-10-CM Alphabetic Index. However, there is no etiology identifying why the patient has cachexia. More information is needed.

[d] The addition of a BMI supports the cachexia, which is documented as being caused by the end-stage COPD.

Coding

According to ICD-10-CM Guideline Section I(B.14):

> For the Body Mass Index (BMI), depth of non-pressure chronic ulcers, pressure ulcer stage, coma scale, and NIH stroke scale (NIHSS) codes, code assignment may be based on medical record documentation from clinicians who are not the patient's provider (i.e., physician or other qualified healthcare practitioner

legally accountable for establishing the patient's diagnosis), because this information is typically documented by other clinicians involved in the care of the patient (e.g., a dietitian often documents the BMI, a nurse often documents the pressure ulcer stages, and an emergency medical technician often documents the coma scale). However, the associated diagnosis (such as overweight, obesity, acute stroke, or pressure ulcer) must be documented by the patient's provider. If there is conflicting medical record documentation, either from the same clinician or different clinicians, the patient's attending provider should be queried for clarification. If that is not possible, abstract the provider's diagnosis and the BMI.

The BMI, coma scale, and NIHSS codes should only be reported as secondary diagnoses.[2]

CODING TIP For 2018, ICD-10-CM refined the code description of code Z68.1, *Body mass index (BMI) 19.9 or less, adult.* Previously, the descriptor identified a BMI of "19 or less, adult."

Malnutrition is always going to affect the health of the patient and should be reported as often as it is documented and addressed by the physician. BMI is an important quality measure tool and should be coded whenever documented. Abstract the BMI with any encounter in which it is documented. BMIs documented by medical assistants or other support staff are acceptable and may be abstracted from a medical record signed by the treating physician. Abnormally low BMIs do not risk-adjust; look for a diagnosis in the record.

Use caution in reporting kwashiorkor, a risk-adjusting diagnosis, as this disease usually is limited to newly weaned children in impoverished countries. Query the physician if kwashiorkor appears in the chart of an elderly patient. Use the ICD-10-CM Alphabetic Index to find the exact language of the documentation (eg, abnormal weight loss, underweight).

When documentation for an adult includes the diagnosis, "emaciation," report code R64, *Cachexia*, according to AHA's *Coding Clinic* (Third Quarter, 2017).[20] Emaciation classifies to E41, *Nutritional marasmus,* in the Alphabetic Index, but marasmus is defined as a type of malnutrition occurring in the very young, caused by severe protein-energy deficiency. It is inappropriate to report E41, *Nutritional marasmus*, in adults. Further, "emaciated" is not codeable.

CODING TIP "Cachexia" is a diagnosis, "cachectic" is not. When a physician documents that a patient is "cachectic," this is an adjective describing the patient, but it is not a diagnosis of cachexia. A rule of thumb is to look at the main terms in the Alphabetic Index to determine if the adjectival form of a word can be used as a diagnosis. Main terms are **the bolded, unindented** terms in the Alphabetic Index:

• Cachexia	the adjectival form is not present
• Hernia, hernial	the adjectival form is present and acceptable
• Nephritis, nephritic	the adjectival form is present and acceptable
• Malnutrition	the adjectival form is not present

ABSTRACT & CODE IT!

Abstract and code the clinical coding example below. Check your answers against the answers in Appendix C.

Patient 1
Patient has Alzheimer's disease, anorexia, and a BMI of 16.5. Her daughter stated that Mary forgets to eat, even when meals are prepared and set before her. She has lost 19 lbs since the beginning of the year.

Patient 2
She weighs 89 lbs now with a BMI of 17.41. She is down 4 lbs in six weeks. We discussed that she doesn't have weight to lose. She states she has no appetite, and that her major depression has returned since her husband's death in June. She is seeing her therapist again, weekly, and reports she has been back on Zoloft for two weeks. Her affect is still flat, and she states her energy level is very low. I will contact her therapist to consult on how we can best approach her mild malnutrition and recurrent depression.

Patient 3
Martin's emphysema has worsened, and although he is cachexic, he refuses parenteral nutritional support.

Metabolic, Immune and Endocrine Disorders

Other significant endocrine and metabolic disorders
HCC 23 0.228

Specified hereditary metabolic/immune disorders
RxHCC 40 2.990

Pituitary, adrenal, and other endocrine and metabolic disorders
RxHCC 41 0.100

Most of the diagnoses described in this grouping are less common disorders caused by endocrine and metabolic defects. Some of the more common diagnoses are hemochromatosis, diabetes insipidus, Cushing's disease, and Addison's disease.

Migraine

Migraine headaches
RxHCC 166 0.138

A migraine is a disorder characterized by recurrent severe headache, often unilateral, with visual or sensory disturbances, and often with nausea and vomiting. About 70% of patients with migraines have other family members with migraines. The chance of having a migraine increases exponentially if a family member experiences auras with migraines. More than 37 million people in the US suffers from migrainess.[21] About 85% of chronic migraine sufferers are women.[22]A migraine headache often intensifies with physical movement and may last as little as four hours to as long as three days. The International Headache Society[23] requires a diagnosis of migraine in a patient to include at least five headache events without another possible cause, with at least two of the following characteristics:

- Unilateral location
- Pulsatile pain
- Moderate to severe pain
- Worsened by physical activity

The following precipitants have been linked to migraine events:

- Hormonal change in the female reproductive cycle or pregnancy
- Stress
- Sleep disturbances
- Strong odors (eg, perfumes or petroleum distillates)
- Head trauma
- Weather changes
- Exposure to red wine, caffeine, chocolate, artificial sweeteners, MSG, nitrites in meats, or tyamine (aged cheese). Each patient with migraine determines which foods to avoid to reduce the incidence of attacks.

People who suffer from migraine headaches are more likely to have cardiovascular or cerebrovascular disease (ie, stroke, MI).[24] The Women's Health Study found that "migraine with aura raised the risk of MI by 91% and ischemic stroke by 108% and that migraine without aura raised both risks by approximately 25%."[25] The etiology of migraines is not fully understood, and there is no cure, according to the NIH. Treatment involves preventing migraines or reducing their frequency, and mitigating the symptoms during a migraine.[22]

Physician Documentation

DOCUMENTATION TIP ICD-10 defines an "intractable" migraine as one that is pharmacoresistant, treatment resistant, poorly controlled, or refractory.

Migraines are a chronic condition that should be regularly evaluated in patients with migraines. If a patient has an active prescription for medication to prevent or treat symptoms of migraine, do not document "history of migraine," as history indicates a resolved condition. For most patients, migraines are a lifelong disorder, although some women see their migraines diminish or disappear after menopause.

When reporting migraine, be specific as to its manifestations:

- With aura, without aura
- With status migrainosus, without status migrainosus
- Intractable, not intractable
- Hemiplegic
- Perisistent, with cerebral infarction (document site of infarction)
- Chronic
- Cyclical vomiting
- Ophthalmoplegic
- Menstrual (document also any premenstrual tension syndrome)

If migraine appears in a PMH or problem list, address the diagnosis with the patient and document the current status and frequency of migraines. For all headaches, document the etiology, acuity, duration, severity, laterality, and modifying factors associated with the headache, and the efficacy of current prescriptions. For example:

> A 32-year-old established patient presents with an acute, right-sided migraine with aura, intractable. It began 36 hours ago and is not responding to self-administered rizatriptan benzoate. Her migraines are menses-related, and she also had a glass of red wine three days ago, which can sometimes be a trigger. Her last migraine was four weeks ago.
>
> - Etiology: menses-related
> - Acuity: acute
> - Duration: 36 hours
> - Severity: intractable
> - Laterality: right-sided
> - Modifying factors: red wine consumption

CLINICAL EXAMPLES

NONSPECIFIC DOCUMENTATION	SPECIFIC DOCUMENTATION
Example 1 PMH: Tonsillectomy, migraines HPI: Maria is here today to discuss the possibility of a botox injection because the frequency and severity of her headaches has increased.[a] She has developed auras as a new symptom.	**Example 1** PMH: Tonsillectomy, migraines HPI: Maria is here today to discuss the possibility of a botox injection because the frequency and severity of her migraines[b] has increased. She has developed auras as a new symptom.
Example 2 MWOA, intractable.[c]	**Example 2** Migraine without aura (MWOA), intractable. We are going to try IV dihydroergotamine (DHE 45) 1 mg combined with intravenous (IV) metoclopramide 10 mg.[d]

[a] Here we have information necessary to report a migraine with aura, not intractable, without status migrainosus.

[b] The diagnosis of migraine is found only in the PMH here. It should be brought into the description of today's encounter.

[c] Always spell out the first reference, and document the treatment plan.

[d] The migraine is specified as without aura and intractable. The treatment plan is carefully outlined. The acronym is spelled out.

CODING TIP "Menstrual" or "premenstrual" headache classifies to menstrual migraine (G43.82-) from the ICD-10-CM Alphabetic Index, under the entry for "Headache."

All migraine codes in ICD-10-CM appear under category G43, *Migraine*. The codes are self-explanatory, and selection is based upon the medical record. When there is an underlying cause or factor associated with the migraine (eg, premenstrual syndrome, cerebral infarct, or seizure), report those conditions secondarily. Most other headache diagnoses are found in category G44, *Other headache syndromes.*

A diagnosis of migraine is based on the patient's personal and family history. There are no definitive tests for determining a migraine diagnosis. Therefore, when the physician determines the patient is experiencing migraine, and migraine is documented without further explanation, the correct code would be G43.909, *Migraine, unspecified, not intractable, without status migrainosus.*

ABSTRACT & CODE IT!

Abstract and code the clinical coding example below. Check your answers against the answers in Appendix C.

Patient 1

Cyclical vomiting without refractory migraine. Patient is in obvious discomfort and exhausted.

Patient 2

PMH: Tonsillectomy, migraines

HPI: Maria is here today to discuss the possibility of a botox injection because the frequency and severity of her migraines has increased. She has developed auras as a new symptom.

Patient 3

Migraine without aura (MWOA), intractable. We are going to try IV dihydroergotamine (DHE 45) 1 mg combined with intravenous (IV) metoclopramide 10 mg.

Motor Neuron and Myoneural Junction Disease and Inflammatory Polyneuropathies

Amyotrophic lateral sclerosis and other motor neuron disease
HCC 73 0.970

Myasthenia gravis/myoneural disorders and Guillain-Barre syndrome/inflammatory and toxic neuropathy
HCC 75 0.457

Myasthenia gravis, amyotrophic lateral sclerosis and other motor neuron disease
HCC 156 0.361

Inflammatory and toxic neuropathy
RxHCC 159 0.171

Motor neuron diseases (MNDs) are irreversible disorders that progressively destroy nerve cells controlling voluntary and involuntary muscle function. Motor neurons are so called because these nerve cells bring messages of activation from the brain to a muscle or gland. In contrast, sensory neurons perceive stimuli from central and peripheral sites and transmit information about those stimuli to the brain.

Amyotrophic lateral sclerosis (ALS), also known as Lou Gehrig's Disease, is the most common motor neuron disease. The CDC estimated there were between 14,000 and 15,000 Americans with ALS in 2016. It is more common in people in the 55 to 75 age range, and men are slightly more likely to have ALS than women. A small percentage of people with ALS have a familial variety. Although the reason is unclear, military veterans have an increased risk of ALS. As a result, ALS is considered by the US Department of Veteran Affairs to be a service-related illness.[26]

Amyotrophic lateral sclerosis (ALS)
Progressive, idiopathic, neurodegenerative disease of the brain and spinal cord. ALS usually is fatal within 3 to 5 years from the onset of symptoms, although some patients live 10 years or more.

Myoneural junction diseases are different in that the muscle weakness is due to a defect in the translation of a nerve signal (eg, acetylcholine) at the muscle receptor. The most common myoneural junction disease in the US is myasthenia gravis (MG), an autoimmune condition that causes antibodies to interfere with the chemical receptors involved in nerve signals to muscles. Many patients with MG have oversized thymus glands, which have functions in immunity that are not fully understood. Myasthenia gravis usually affects women under 40 but men over 60.[27] Up to 20% of patients with MG will have a myasthenic crisis, a condition in which their respiratory muscles are so weakened that mechanical ventilation is required. Approximately 60,000 people in the US have been diagnosed with MG.[27]

Guillain-Barre syndrome (GBS) is another autoimmune disorder affecting motor neuron function, but usually a transient one occurring following a viral infection or surgery. Weakness usually peaks three weeks after symptoms begin, as the immune system destroys the myelin sheath that surrounds peripheral nerves. In addition to motor nerves, sensory nerves are affected by this condition. Some patients require ventilator support. Recovery from the late effects of GBS usually requires significant physical therapy.[28]

HCC 75 and RxHCC 159 also capture secondary neuropathies of certain diseases, such as diabetes, paraneoplastic syndromes, sarcoidosis, and rheumatoid arthritis, and those caused by critical illness, toxic drugs, alcohol, or radiation. In secondary neuropathy, the peripheral nerves are permanently damaged by the disease process or toxin.

Note that other neuropathies are found in other HCCs. For example, diabetic autonomic neuropathies, a common cause of erectile dysfunction and constipation in diabetics, are classified as HCC 18, *Diabetes with Chronic Complications.* Systemic sclerosis and rheumatoid arthritis neuropathies are classified in HCC 40, *Rheumatoid Arthritis and Inflammatory Connective Tissue Disease.*

Myasthenia gravis (MG)
Chronic autoimmune neuromuscular junction disease causing muscle weakness that worsens with activity and improves with rest. Some patients may have permanent remission, while for others, it is a lifelong disorder.

Guillain-Barre syndrome (GBS)
Acute and usually transient inflammatory polyneuropathy causing muscle weakness and sensory loss; thought to have an autoimmune etiology.

Physician Documentation

DOCUMENTATION TIP The CDC and AHA's *Coding Clinic* have not quantified whether quadriplegia originating with a motor neuron disease would be defined as a "functional quadriplegia" or as "neurological quadriplegia." Physicians must determine which diagnosis to document in these cases. The exact term "functional quadriplegia" is optimally documented for abstraction of code R53.2, *Functional quadriplegia;* however, documentation of the term "complete immobility due to severe physical disability or frailty" may suffice, given this is a subterm under code R53.2. Functional quadriplegia may be seen in advanced cases of motor neuron disease, dementia, severe cases of rheumatoid arthritis, or severe physical deconditioning. It is acceptable to document functional quadriplegia for patients with quadriplegia due to ALS or GBS, if the patient's physical impairment is so severe that the patient is completely immobile and all activities of daily living are performed by someone else. Both neurological quadriplegia and functional quadriplegia map to HCC 70, *Quadriplegia.*

Note also that in the ICD-10-CM Alphabetic Index to Diseases, the term "quadriparesis," which is indicative of neurological weakness of all four extremities, is equivalent to "quadriplegia," a neurological paralysis of all four extremities. Many physicians are hesitant to assign a quadriplegia code if the patient is not paralyzed, missing the opportunity to adequately report the severity of their patient's condition. Physicians must be encouraged to use terminology and coding for monoplegia, hemiplegia, paraplegia, or quadriplegia when corresponding paretic conditions are present, given that ICD-10-CM equates "plegia" with "paresis."

Motor neuron diseases are chronic disorders that will almost certainly contribute to MDM, and so these conditions should be pulled from PMH into the current HPI during every encounter. Document all manifestations of ALS, GBS, MG, or associated disorders (eg, monoparesis, hemiparesis, quadriparesis) that are evaluated or treated during an encounter. These diagnoses have gradations that can only be understood if the manifestations are reported in addition to the underlying disease. A newly diagnosed ALS patient, for example, may be experiencing foot drop and occasional falls. A patient with more advanced ALS may have quadriplegia, dysphagia, dysphasia, and ventilator dependence. The two ALS patients would not consume the same medical resources due to the difference in the severity of their disease.

DOCUMENTATION TIP New codes specific to motor neuron disease were added to 2018 ICD-10-CM and documentation should specify these conditions when they occur. The new codes are:

G12.23	Primary lateral sclerosis
G12.24	Familial motor neuron disease
G12.25	Progressive spinal muscle atrophy
G12.29	Other motor neuron disease

In addition to code G12.21, *Amyotrophic lateral sclerosis*, each manifestation evaluated or treated should be documented and coded in order to capture the patient's medical status accurately. Many of the more severe manifestations of ALS, GBS, and MG risk-adjust. Because of the duration of GBS, documentation should specify when the patient's recovery is complete, and whether any impairment is due to the active condition, or is a sequela. ICD-10-CM differentiates between the ongoing condition and sequelae of GBS.

CLINICAL EXAMPLES

NONSPECIFIC DOCUMENTATION	SPECIFIC DOCUMENTATION
Example 1 Under fluoroscopy, we placed a nasogastric feeding tube to address Mr. Dinkle's ALS.[a]	**Example 1** Under fluoroscopy, we placed a nasal feeding tube into the stomach to address Mr. Dinkle's moderate malnutrition, a direct result of his dysphagia due to amyotrophic lateral sclerosis (ALS). His weight is currently 105 and his BMI is 16.4. His wife will be able to manage his feedings at home. On good days, Mr. Dinkle is still able to ambulate short distances with his walker.[b]
Example 2 Patient with AIDP is admitted to ICU with respiratory failure, neurogenic bladder, and renal failure.[c]	**Example 2** Patient with acute demyelinating poylyradiculoneuropathy (AIDP) is admitted to the ICU with acute respiratory failure. She underwent tracheostomy and is dependent on a mechanical ventilator. She is also in acute renal failure, secondary to urinary retention due to a neurogenic bladder. This can be attributed to the AIDP.[d]

[a] The nasal feeding tube is addressing the patient's feeding problems, which are due to dysphagia secondary to ALS. It is important to connect the dots in documentation. Any conditions that resulted from the dysphagia (eg, malnutrition) should also be captured. Malnutrition risk-adjusts in addition to the ALS.

[b] The moderate malnutrition is described sufficiently here, and the dysphagia brought about by the ALS. BMI is always useful when documenting a weight-related diagnosis, although low BMIs do not risk-adjust. Malnutrition does risk-adjust.

[c] Identify any link between the system failures and the AIDP. Specify whether the respiratory and renal failures are acute or chronic. Document how the AIDP led to renal failure (eg, due to urinary retention).

[d] Obviously documentation of a patient needing long-term advanced life support measures would be more expansive than noted here. The point here is to demonstrate how the manifestations must be tied back to the principal diagnosis, and include every step (eg, identify the cause of the renal failure as urinary retention and the cause of the urinary retention as neurogenic bladder due to AIDP).

Coding

According to ICD-10-CM Guideline Section I(B.5), "[s]igns and symptoms that are associated routinely with a disease process should not be assigned as additional codes, unless otherwise instructed by the classification. Additional signs and symptoms that may not be associated routinely with a disease process should be coded when present."[2]

ADVICE/ALERT NOTE

Per ICD-10-CM Guideline Section I(B.5), "[s]igns and symptoms that are associated routinely with a disease process should not be assigned as additional codes, unless otherwise instructed by the classification. Additional signs and symptoms that may not be associated routinely with a disease process should be coded when present."[2]

For GBS, ALS, MG, and associated disorders, report the code for the disorder and report the codes for any documented manifestations of the disorder (eg, quadriplegia, malnutrition, acute or chronic respiratory failure, and/or dependence on ventilator). Each of these disorders has a range of symptoms from mild to life-threatening, and the codes for the disorders themselves do not capture the severity of each individual's case.

CODING TIP Acute demyelinating poylyradiculoneuropathy (AIDP) is a synonym for GBS, which is reported with code G61.0 *Guillain-Barre syndrome*. Report AIDP or GBS for the duration of the patient's active treatment and recovery. If symptoms are documented as sequelae of AIDP/GBS, report the documented sequelae first followed by code G65.0, *Sequelae of Guillain-Barre syndrome*.

GBS is a temporary paralytic event that can last for months. Any manifestations occurring during the active paralysis phase of GBS are reported in addition to the code for the condition itself. Some patients have residual disorders that continue after the acute phase of this disease (eg, muscle weakness, sensory loss, or nerve pain). Report these residuals with code G65.0, *Sequelae of Guillain-Barre syndrome*, rather than code G61.0, *Guillain-Barre syndrome*. Motor neuron disease can lead to paralysis, which should be coded when documented. Paralysis is not considered a sign or symptom of ALS, GBS, or any of the motor neuron diseases. The paralysis may be documented as a paresis or a plegia, and the Alphabetic Index should be consulted to align the specific nomenclature in the medical record with the appropriate code. Functional paralysis is a form of paralysis that is due to frailty or physical debility. The Alphabetic Index classifies complete immobility due to severe physical disability or frailty to code R53.2, *Functional quadriplegia*.

CODING TIP Motor neuron disease puts a patient at risk for paralysis, which can lead to pressure ulcers. The Braden Scale for Predicting Pressure Sore Risk is a preventive tool for clinicians that allows them to document a patient's risk of developing pressure ulcers from being wheelchair-bound or bedridden. It assesses the sensory perception, skin moisture, activity, nutrition, friction and shear, and mobility of the patient. The Braden Scale has several elements and one of them is the mobility element. A Braden Scale mobility score of 1 indicates a patient is "[c]ompletely immobile. Does not make even slight changes in body or extremity position without assistance."[29] Coders must never abstract from Braden Scale scores, as coders cannot report test findings, and Braden Scale scores are usually documented by nurses, whose documentation is unacceptable for ICD-10-CM code assignment and RA. However, a Braden Scale mobility score of 1 would be a cause to query the physician regarding the patient's mobility status and its underlying causes. A Braden Scale score may also be used as support for a paralysis-related diagnosis. A copy of the Braden Scale scoring table can be viewed or downloaded at www.bradenscale.com/images/bradenscale.pdf

ABSTRACT & CODE IT!

Abstract and code the clinical coding example below. Check your answers against the answers in Appendix C.

Patient 1

Polyneuropathy in hands and feet, secondary to etoposide, administered two years ago when the patient was being treated for lung cancer. Gabapentin has been helping with symptoms.

Patient 2

Under fluoroscopy, we placed a nasogastric feeding tube to addressed Mr. Dinkle's moderate malnutrition, a direct result of his dysphagia due to amyotrophic lateral sclerosis (ALS). His weight is currently 105 and his BMI is 16.4. His wife will be able to manage his feedings at home. On good days, Mr. Dinkle is still able to ambulate short distances with his walker.

Patient 3

Patient with acute demyelinating poylyradiculoneuropathy (AIDP) is admitted to the ICU with acute respiratory failure. She underwent tracheostomy and is dependent on a mechanical ventilator. She also is in acute renal failure, secondary to urinary retention due to a neurogenic bladder. This can be attributed to AIDP.

Multiple Sclerosis

Multiple sclerosis
HCC 77 0.441
RxHCC 160 12.350

The myelin sheath is a protective layer surrounding each nerve fiber. Demyelinating diseases strip this protection from the nerve fibers, causing inflammation, scarring, and a disruption in nerve impulses that can lead to nerve pain, weakness, or paralysis. Multiple sclerosis (MS) is a demyelinating disease of the brain and spinal cord, affecting 400,000 Americans, according to the NIH.[30] The spectrum of severity of MS symptoms is broad: some patients have blurred or double vision; others experience paralysis, cognitive impairment, and nerve pain. Symptoms and severity depend on the location of the damaged central nervous system (CNS) nerve fibers. Many MS patients also experience dysthymia or major depression in the course of their illness. The most common form of MS is relapsing-remitting, with patients experiencing periods of good health followed by exacerbations. A less common type is primary progressive MS, in which there is a steady and gradual worsening of symptoms. MS is considered an immune-mediated inflammatory disorder. There is no single treatment for MS, although some cases respond to beta interferon, immunosuppressants, ocrelizumab, steroids, or a synthetic form of myelin basic protein called copolymer. Patients with MS may use orthotics like braces to support their feet or legs, or may use canes, walkers, or wheelchairs during exacerbations. In addition, they are advised to avoid heat and excessive physical activity to prevent fatigue.[31] Women are at two- to three-times the risk of developing MS than men. MS most commonly is diagnosed in patients between the ages of 20-40,[31] and is a chronic, incurable disease.

Multiple sclerosis (MS)
A central nervous system disease that affects the brain and spinal cord, which damages the myelin sheath, the material that surrounds and protects the nerve cells, and it causes weakness, numbness, a loss of muscle coordination, and problems with vision, speech, and bladder control.

Physician Documentation

Document all manifestations of MS that are evaluated or treated during an encounter. Manifestations of MS have gradations that can only be understood if the manifestations are reported in addition to the underlying disease. Because MS is an incurable disease, it should never be documented as "history of MS." ICD-10-CM classifies "history of MS" as MS that is cured. Instead, note "A 25-year history of relapsing-remitting multiple sclerosis, which is currently stable," or in some way indicate that the condition is long established and currently present. Always spell out the first time MS is noted in an encounter (eg, multiple sclerosis [MS]). MS is an acronym for many conditions, including morning stiffness and mitral stenosis.

DOCUMENTATION TIP A diagnosis of MS usually requires two or more clinically distinct episodes of CNS dysfunction with some level of resolution between episodes. As a result, the initial medical encounter for a patient with suspected MS is often documented "probable" or "suspected" multiple sclerosis. If it has been ascertained that the patient is experiencing manifestations of a demyelinating disease of the central nervous system, "unspecified demyelinating CNS disorder" should be documented in addition to "probable" or "suspected" MS. Coders cannot abstract probable or suspected conditions in an outpatient setting. Documentation of the unspecified demyelinating CNS disorder allows them to report code G37.9, *Demyelinating disease of central nervous system, unspecified,* until the MS diagnosis can be confirmed. Code G37.9 risk-adjusts.

CLINICAL EXAMPLES

NONSPECIFIC DOCUMENTATION	SPECIFIC DOCUMENTATION
Example 1 Probable MS.[a]	**Example 1** Radiographic evidence of demyelinating central nervous system disorder, probable multiple sclerosis.[b]
Example 2 Multiple sclerosis?[c] progressive versus relapsing/remitting, based on symptoms and history. The MRI shows numerous T2 hyperintense lesions in the periventricular and subcortical white matter of the brain and at least one lesion is in the corpus callosum. There appears to be Dawson's fingers.	**Example 2** Multiple sclerosis but unknown whether progressive versus relapsing/remitting, based on symptoms and history. The MRI shows numerous T2 hyperintense lesions in the periventricular and subcortical white matter of the brain and at least one lesion is in the corpus callosum. There appears to be Dawson's fingers.[d]

[a] A probable diagnosis cannot be reported in physician or outpatient billing, but only in an inpatient discharge summary. Instead, identify the signs and symptoms that led to the probable diagnosis. Spell out the first reference of the diagnosis rather than using an acronym.

[b] Identifying the demyelinating CNS system disorder adds specificity. Identifying the contributor to the diagnosis (eg, the radiographic evidence) strengthens the documentation.

[c] Question marks are very difficult to interpret. Is this documentation suggesting the MS is uncertain, or that the uncertainty lies with whether it is progressive or relapsing/remitting? The coder will not be able to determine this without querying the physician.

[d] Good support for the diagnosis of MS is presented here.

Coding

Although the name of the HCC is "Multiple Sclerosis," other diagnoses are grouped into this HCC:

- G36.0 Neuromyelitis optica [Devic]
- G36.1 Acute and subacute hemorrhagic leukoencephalitis [Hurst]
- G36.8 Other specified acute disseminated demyelination
- G36.9 Acute disseminated demyelination, unspecified
- G37.0 Diffuse sclerosis of central nervous system
- G37.1 Central demyelination of corpus callosum
- G37.2 Central pontine myelinolysis
- G37.5 Concentric sclerosis [Balo] of central nervous system
- G37.8 Other specified demyelinating diseases of central nervous system
- G37.9 Demyelinating disease of central nervous system, unspecified

For MS, report code G35, *Multiple sclerosis,* and codes for any manifestations of the disorder (eg, functional or neurological quadriplegia, polyneuropathies, weakness, diplopia, central pain syndrome). MS has a range of symptoms from mild to life-threatening, and the MS code does not capture of the severity of each individual's case.

Dawson's fingers
Radiographic evidence of demyelinating plaques in the corpus callosum along the medullary veins around the ventricles of the brain as commonly seen in MS patients.

Kurtzke Expanded Disability Status Scale

The Kurtzke Expanded Disability Status Scale (EDSS) measures the disability status of people with MS and can be useful in crafting queries or to support an MS diagnosis. Levels 1.0 to 4.5 describe patients with a high level of ambulatory ability, and levels 5.0 to 9.5 describe increasingly limited ability. The scoring combines gait and ambulatory status with function scores for eight systems:

LEVEL	LEVEL DESCRIPTION
0.0	Normal neurological exam (all grade 0 in all Functional System (FS) scores*).
1.0	No disability, minimal signs in one FS* (ie, grade 1).
1.5	No disability, minimal signs in more than one FS* (more than one FS grade 1).
2.0	Minimal disability in one FS (one FS grade 2, others 0 or 1).
2.5	Minimal disability in two FS (two FS grade 2, others 0 or 1).
3.0	Moderate disability in one FS (one FS grade 3, others 0 or 1) or mild disability in three or four FS (three or four FS grade 2, others 0 or 1) though fully ambulatory.
3.5	Fully ambulatory but with moderate disability in one FS (one grade 3) and one or two FS grade 2; or two FS grade 3 (others 0 or 1) or five grade 2 (others 0 or 1).
4.0	Fully ambulatory without aid, self-sufficient, up and about some 12 hours a day despite relatively severe disability consisting of one FS grade 4 (others 0 or 1), or combination of lesser grades exceeding limits of previous steps; able to walk without aid or rest some 500 meters.
4.5	Fully ambulatory without aid, up and about much of the day, able to work a full day, may otherwise have some limitation of full activity or require minimal assistance; characterized by relatively severe disability usually consisting of one FS grade 4 (others or 1) or combinations of lesser grades exceeding limits of previous steps; able to walk without aid or rest some 300 meters.
5.0	Ambulatory without aid or rest for about 200 meters; disability severe enough to impair full daily activities (eg, to work a full day without special provisions); (Usual FS equivalents are one grade 5 alone, others 0 or 1; or combinations of lesser grades usually exceeding specifications for step 4.0).
5.5	Ambulatory without aid for about 100 meters; disability severe enough to preclude full daily activities; (Usual FS equivalents are one grade 5 alone, others 0 or 1; or combination of lesser grades usually exceeding those for step 4.0).
6.0	Intermittent or unilateral constant assistance (cane, crutch, brace) required to walk about 100 meters with or without resting; (Usual FS equivalents are combinations with more than two FS grade 3+).
6.5	Constant bilateral assistance (canes, crutches, braces) required to walk about 20 meters without resting; (Usual FS equivalents are combinations with more than two FS grade 3+).
7.0	Unable to walk beyond approximately 5 meters even with aid, essentially restricted to wheelchair; wheels self in standard wheelchair and transfers alone; up and about in wheelchair some 12 hours a day; (Usual FS equivalents are combinations with more than one FS grade 4+; very rarely pyramidal grade 5 alone).
7.5	Unable to take more than a few steps; restricted to wheelchair; may need aid in transfer; wheels self but cannot carry on in standard wheelchair a full day; May require motorized wheelchair; (Usual FS equivalents are combinations with more than one FS grade 4+).
8.0	Essentially restricted to bed or chair or perambulated in wheelchair, but may be out of bed itself much of the day; retains many self-care functions; generally has effective use of arms; (Usual FS equivalents are combinations, generally grade 4+ in several systems).
8.5	Essentially restricted to bed much of day; has some effective use of arm(s); retains some self-care functions; (Usual FS equivalents are combinations, generally 4+ in several systems).
9.0	Helpless bed patient; can communicate and eat; (Usual FS equivalents are combinations, mostly grade 4+).
9.5	Totally helpless bed patient; unable to communicate effectively or eat/swallow; (Usual FS equivalents are combinations, almost all grade 4+).
10.0	Death due to MS.

* Excludes cerebral function grade 1.

The functional system scores use a scale of 0 (low level of problem) to 5 (high level of problem) to reflect clinically observed disability. The systems are pyramidal motor function; cerebellar; brainstem; sensory, bowel and bladder; visual; cerebral or mental; and other. For details of the functional-systems scores, download the Kurtzke form at http://www.nationalmssociety.org/NationalMSSociety/media/MSNationalFiles/Brochures/10-2-3-30-Functional_Systems_Kurtzke_Form.pdf While coders cannot abstract diagnoses from the EDSS, they can use the documented scores to query the physician about the patient's functional status.

ABSTRACT & CODE IT!

Abstract and code the clinical coding example below. Check your answers against the answers in Appendix C.

Patient 1
Encephalitis periaxialis causing right hemiplegia.

Patient 2
Radiographic evidence of demyelinating central nervous system disorder, probable multiple sclerosis.

Patient 3
Multiple sclerosis but unknown whether progressive versus relapsing/remitting, based on symptoms and history. The MRI shows numerous T2 hyperintense lesions in the periventricular and subcortical white matter of the brain and at least one lesion is in the corpus callosum. There appears to be Dawson's fingers.

Muscular Dystrophy

Muscular dystrophy
HCC 76 0.505

Muscular dystrophy (MD) describes a group of genetic disorders usually diagnosed in childhood that lead to progressive weakness and loss of muscle mass. Almost all MD patients are male. Weakness causes poor posture and resultant spinal deformities, affecting the patient's ability to walk, and potentially affecting cardiopulmonary function. Contractures of joints in the hands and feet interfere with mobility and dexterity.

There is no cure for MD. Treatment's goal is to help the patient retain independent living for as long as possible and to maintain the patient's quality of life. MD in its mildest form progresses very slowly, and patients have a normal life expectancy. MD may manifest itself at birth, or as late as the fourth decade of life. More than half of the cases of MD are diagnosed before a child reaches school age. Life expectancy for patients with MD is tied to the degree of muscle weakness and the severity of complications.

Physician Documentation

The codes for MD do not identify the severity of the patient's manifestations, but these can be reported in addition to the code for MD. Document all manifestations of MD when they occur, and identify causal effects as required. For example, prednisone may be prescribed on a long-term basis to MD patients, which can result in adverse effects of osteoporosis or hypertension. Document the osteoporosis or hypertension and, if appropriate, its link to the steroid use. Describe orthopedic symptoms, such as toe-walking, contractures, or scoliosis, and any respiratory complications, developmental delay, wheelchair dependence, dysphagia, dysphasia, or cardiomyopathy. Denote any intellectual disability as mild, moderate, or severe. For late-stage MD, document any functional quadriplegia or dependence on a respirator.

The following forms of dystrophy risk-adjust:

- Muscular dystrophy (G71.0)
- Myotonic muscular dystrophy (G71.11)
- Congenital myopathies (G71.2)

For contractures in MD, specify whether the contracture is a muscle contracture or a joint contracture and identify the site. There are specific codes in ICD-10-CM for joint contracture (M24.5-) and for muscle contractures (M62.4-). Acronym use with muscular dystrophy should be avoided on first references. Myotonic dystrophy type 1 and myotonic dystrophy type 2 are often abbreviated as DM1 and DM2, common acronyms for type 1 and type 2 diabetes mellitus. Spell out the first reference to avoid misinterpretation of the medical record.

CLINICAL EXAMPLES

NONSPECIFIC DOCUMENTATION	SPECIFIC DOCUMENTATION
Example 1 DMD[a]	**Example 1** Duchenne muscular dystrophy[b]
Example 2 Patient with MD is here for arthrodesis with tendon lengthening to treat planovalgus deformity.[c]	**Example 2** Patient with myotonic muscular dystrophy is here for bilateral arthrodesis with tendon lengthening to treat painful, acquired bilateral planovalgus deformity.[d]

[a] Spell out Duchenne muscular dystrophy.

[b] DMD is spelled out here.

[c] The patient's muscular dystrophy was not identified by type, and the laterality of the deformity were not addressed.

[d] The medical necessity of the procedure (pain) was addressed in addition to the defect's laterality and the specific form of muscular dystrophy.

Coding

Most manifestations of MD are reported in addition to the MD (eg, pressure ulcer in a wheelchair-dependent patient, torticollis, dysphagia, or dysarthria). Some patients with MD require assisted oxygenation or ventilation, in which supplemental oxygen is delivered through a mask or a tube that is threaded into the lungs. Assisted ventilation is not the equivalent of ventilator dependence. Some patients are ventilator dependent only at night. Read the medical record carefully so that the patient's respiratory status can be accurately abstracted.

Joint contraction is a limitation in the passive range of motion of a joint and are common in MD. There are specific codes in ICD-10-CM for joint contracture (M24.5-) and for muscle contractures (M62.4-). Joint contracture can be caused by muscle, but when the joint movement is inhibited by pain or by spasticity, it is a joint contracture. In muscle contracture, there is a permanent shortening of the muscle. Query the physician if "contracture" is documented without reference to joint or muscle. Joint contracture can lead to ankylosis of a joint, which can lead to loss of mobility or dexterity.

CODING TIP Planovalgus deformity or pes planovalgus in myotonic MD refers to an acquired flat foot. It may also be documented as pes planus. This condition can be painful to the patient and may require surgery or physical therapy. Planovalgus deformity is difficult to abstract in ICD-10-CM because the only Alphabetic Index entry for planovalgus is for "Talipes/planovalgus," a form of clubfoot. The correct codes are found at category M21.4-, *Flat foot [pes planus] (acquired)*. For bilateral planovalgus deformity, two codes would be required: M21.41, *Flat foot [pes planus] (acquired), right foot*, and M21.42, *Flat foot [pes planus] (acquired), left foot*.

ABSTRACT & CODE IT!

Abstract and code the clinical coding example below. Check your answers against the answers in Appendix C.

Patient 1
Audiologist's examination revealed severe bilateral hearing loss in patient with facioscapulohumeral muscular dystrophy (FSHD).

Patient 2
Duchenne muscular dystrophy.

Patient 3
Patient with myotonic muscular dystrophy is here for bilateral arthrodesis with tendon lengthening to treat painful, acquired bilateral planovalgus deformity.

Myocardial Infarction *see* Ischemic Heart Disease

Torticollis
A symptom of defective muscle control resulting in the head and neck being persistently asymmetrical, tilted, and rotated to one side. Torticollis is synonymous with cervical dystonia and is a symptom seen with many neurologic or muscular disorders.

Dysphagia
Difficulty swallowing.

Dysarthria
A speech disorder caused by impaired muscle movement in the lips, tongue, and diaphragm.

Joint contraction
Limitation in the passive range of motion of a joint.

References

1. National Institute on Aging. *Alzheimer's Disease & Related Dementias.* https://www.nia.nih.gov/health/alzheimers/related-dementias. Accessed Nov 21, 2017.
2. Centers for Disease Control and Prevention. *ICD-10-CM Official Guidelines for Coding and Reporting* (FY 2018). https://www.cdc.gov/nchs/data/icd/10cmguidelines_fy2018_final.pdf. Accessed Oct 30, 2017.
3. American Hospital Association. *Coding Clinic® for ICD-10-CM and ICD-10-PCS Q1.* 2017;4(1):43.
4. Centers for Disease Control and Prevention. *National Diabetes Statistics Report, 2017: Estimates of Diabetes and Its Burden in the United States.* https://www.cdc.gov/diabetes/pdfs/data/statistics/national-diabetes-statistics-report.pdf. Accessed Nov 21, 2017.
5. Centers for Medicare & Medicaid Services. *2008 Risk Adjustment Data Technical Assistance for Medicare Advantage Organizations Participant Guide.* https://www.csscoperations.com/mwg-internal/de5fs23hu73ds/progress?id=04WTUGzH8NVu7krDOTYPeYjddO9VvdH6yE8I9-B9MLA. Accessed Nov 1, 2017.
6. American Hospital Association. *Coding Clinic® for ICD-10-CM and ICD-10-PCS Q3.* 2016;3(3):42.
7. American Hospital Association. *Coding Clinic® for ICD-10-CM and ICD-10-PCS Q4.* 2017;4(4):100-102.
8. National Institute on Drug Abuse. Trends & Statistics. https://www.drugabuse.gov/related-topics/trends-statistics#supplemental-references-for-economic-costs. Accessed Nov 21, 2017.
9. American College of Cardiology; American Heart Association Task Force on Practice Guidelines; Heart Rhythm Society; Society of Thoracic Surgeons. 2014 AHA/ACC/HRS Guideline for the Management of Patients with Atrial Fibrillation. *J Am Coll Cardiol.* 2014;64(21):1-76. http://www.hrsonline.org/content/download/18916/838794/file/2014%20Guideline%20for%20the%20Management%20of%20Patients%20With%20AFib.pdf. Accessed Nov 21, 2017.
10. Centers for Disease Control and Prevention. Cholesterol Fact Sheet. https://www.cdc.gov/dhdsp/data_statistics/fact_sheets/fs_cholesterol.htm. Accessed Nov 21, 2017.
11. American Heart Association. The Facts About High Blood Pressure. http://www.heart.org/HEARTORG/Conditions/HighBloodPressure/GettheFactsAboutHighBloodPressure/The-Facts-About-High-Blood-Pressure_UCM_002050_Article.jsp#.Wh8WIEqnEdU. Accessed Nov 21, 2017.
12. American Hospital Association. *Coding Clinic® for ICD-10-CM and ICD-10-PCS Q1.* 2016;3(1):14.
13. Sanchis-Gomar F, Perez-Quilis C, Leischik R, Alejandro L. Epidemiology of Coronary Heart Disease and Acute Coronary Syndrome. *Ann Transl Med.* 2016;4(13); 256. doi: 10.21037/atm.2016.06.33. Accessed Nov 21, 2017.
14. American Hospital Association. *Coding Clinic® for ICD-10-CM and ICD-10-PCS Q2.* 2017;4(2):11.
15. Centers for Disease Control and Prevention. *Surveillance for Viral Hepatitis—United States, 2015.* https://www.cdc.gov/hepatitis/statistics/2015surveillance/commentary.htm. Accessed Nov 21, 2017.
16. Centers for Disease Control and Prevention. *Morbidity and Mortality Weekly Report,* August 17, 2012. https://www.cdc.gov/mmwr/pdf/rr/rr6104.pdf. Accessed Nov 21, 2017.
17. Mogensen KM, DiMaria-Ghalili. RA Malnutrition in Older Adults. *Today's Dietitian.* 2016;17(9):56. http://www.todaysdietitian.com/newarchives/090115p56.shtml. Accessed Dec 4, 2017.
18. White JV, Guenter P, Jensen G, Malone A, et al. Characteristics Recommended for the Identification and Documentation of Adult Malnutrition (Undernutrition), *J Parenter Enteral Nutr.* 2012;36(3). http://journals.sagepub.com/doi/full/10.1177/0148607112440285. Accessed Nov 21, 2017.
19. Morley JE, Thomas DR, Wilson M-M G. Cachexia: Pathophysiology and Clinical Relevance. *Am J Clin Nutr.* 2006;83(4):735-743. http://ajcn.nutrition.org/content/83/4/735.full. Accessed Nov 21, 2017.
20. American Hospital Association. *Coding Clinic® for ICD-10-CM and ICD-10-PCS Q3.* 2017;4(3):24-25.
21. Migraine.com. Migraine Statistics. https://migraine.com/migraine-statistics/. Accessed Nov 21, 2017.
22. National Institute of Neurological Disorders and Stroke. Migraine Information Page. https://www.ninds.nih.gov/Disorders/All-Disorders/Migraine-Information-Page. Accessed Nov 21, 2017.

23. International Headache Society. *The International Classification of Headache Disorders*. 3rd ed (beta version). London: Sage Publications; 2013:644-645. http://www.ihs-headache.org/binary_data/1437_ichd-iii-beta-cephalalgia-issue-9-2013.pdf. Accessed Nov 21, 2017.

24. Klein E, Spencer D. Migraine frequency and risk of cardiovascular disease in women. *Neurology*. 2009;73(8):e42-3. In: Chawla J. Migraine Headache. Medscape. http://misc.medscape.com/pi/iphone/medscapeapp/html/A1142556-business.html. Accessed Dec 4, 2017.

25. Woodward M. Migraine and the risk of coronary heart disease and ischemic stroke in women. *Womens Health (Lond)*. 2009;5(1):69-77. In: Chawla J. *Migraine Headache*. Medscape. http://misc.medscape.com/pi/iphone/medscapeapp/html/A1142556-business.html. Accessed Dec 4, 2017.

26. VA Office of Public and Intergovernmental Affairs. VA Secretary Establishes ALS as a Presumptive Compensable Illness. Sept 23, 2008. https://www.va.gov/opa/pressrel/pressrelease.cfm?id=1583. Accessed Dec 4, 2017.

27. National Institute of Neurological Disorders and Stroke. Myasthenia Gravis Fact Sheet. https://www.ninds.nih.gov/Disorders/Patient-Caregiver-Education/Fact-Sheets/Myasthenia-Gravis-Fact-Sheet. Accessed Dec 4, 2017.

28. National Institute of Neurological Disorders and Stroke. Guillain-Barré Syndrome Fact Sheet. https://www.ninds.nih.gov/Disorders/Patient-Caregiver-Education/Fact-Sheets/Guillain-Barr%C3%A9-Syndrome-Fact-Sheet. Accessed Nov 22, 2017.

29. Braden Scale. Braden Scale for Predicting Pressure Sore Risk. http://www.bradenscale.com/images/bradenscale.pdf. Accessed Nov 22, 2017.

30. National Institute of Neurological Disorders and Stroke. Multiple Sclerosis: Hope Through Research. https://www.ninds.nih.gov/Disorders/Patient-Caregiver-Education/Hope-Through-Research/Multiple-Sclerosis-Hope-Through-Research. Accessed Nov 22, 2017.

31. National Institute of Neurological Disorders and Stroke. Multiple Sclerosis Information Page. https://www.ninds.nih.gov/Disorders/All-Disorders/Multiple-Sclerosis-Information-Page. Accessed Nov 22, 2017.

CHAPTER 4

Clinical Documentation Integrity and Coding

PART 3: TOPICS N–P

Narcolepsy and Cataplexy

Narcolepsy and cataplexy
RxHCC 355 0.806

The National Institutes of Health (NIH) estimates that between 135,000 and 200,000 people in the United States (US) have narcolepsy, a chronic, lifelong sleep-wake disorder.[1] All patients with narcolepsy experience excessive daytime sleepiness (EDS) and some experience sudden loss of muscle tone, cataplexy.

Type 1 narcolepsy occurs in a patient with cataplexy or in patients who may not have cataplexy, but have cerebrospinal fluid (CFS) hypocretin-1 concentration, measured by immunoreactivity, either ≤110 pg/mL or <1/3 of mean values obtained in normal subjects with the same standardized assay. Type 2 narcolepsy occurs in a patient without cataplexy or without a positive CSF hypocretin-1 test result. Other symptoms of narcolepsy include hallucinations and sleep paralysis, a temporary inability to speak or move before or after sleeping.

Most patients with narcolepsy have extremely low levels of hypocretin (also known as orexin), a chemical that promotes appropriate wake-sleep cycles. Narcolepsy may be linked to a familial trait, brain injury, or autoimmune disorder. Most cases are diagnosed between the ages of 15 and 25.[2]

Physician Documentation

Code choices for narcolepsy are limited, but some differentiation in documentation is required. If the patient has narcolepsy because of another condition (eg, multiple sclerosis [MS]or hypothalamus injury), the link should be established in documentation so that the correct code can be selected, and the underlying condition must also be documented (see Table 4-3.1). It is not enough to simply document "narcolepsy in conditions classified elsewhere."

Narcolepsy
Chronic neurological disorder in which the wake-sleep cycles are not well controlled, and patients are chronically tired and have a propensity to fall asleep without warning.

Cataplexy
Abrupt loss of voluntary muscle tone, hypotonia, and sometimes collapse usually triggered by emotion; occurs as a symptom of narcolepsy.

TABLE 4-3.1 Narcolepsy Codes

CODE	DESCRIPTION
G47.411	Narcolepsy with cataplexy
G47.419	Narcolepsy without cataplexy
G47.421	Narcolepsy in conditions classified elsewhere with cataplexy
G47.429	Narcolepsy in conditions classified elsewhere without cataplexy

Carefully note symptoms associated with the patient's narcolepsy. Many patients' conditions are debilitating to the point that employment suffers, and the patient may need several years of documentation to support a disability claim.

DOCUMENTATION TIP Document cataplexy when it occurs. Type 1 narcolepsy is a new term that identifies narcolepsy with cataplexy or depressed hypocretin-1 levels, and type 2 narcolepsy is a new term that identifies narcolepsy without cataplexy. Unfortunately, these new designations are absent from the ICD-10-CM Tabular List and Alphabetic Index, and so, if documented, "type 1 narcolepsy" would be coded to G47.419, *Narcolepsy without cataplexy*, as cataplexy in this case is not documented. Cataplexy must be documented separately to be captured. In ICD-10-CM, documented cataplexy classifies to narcolepsy with cataplexy.

CLINICAL EXAMPLES

NONSPECIFIC DOCUMENTATION	SPECIFIC DOCUMENTATION
Example 1 Patient has been experiencing symptoms of narcolepsy and cataplexy[a] for 5 years, and has been unable to work for 2 years. She had a multiple sleep latency test last year and her symptoms have been somewhat diminished by methylphenidate.	**Example 1** Patient has been experiencing symptoms of narcolepsy and cataplexy for 5 years, and has been unable to work for 2 years. She had a multiple sleep latency test last year positive for narcolepsy,[b] and her narcolepsy and cataplexy have been somewhat diminished by methylphenidate.
Example 2 Type 1 narcolepsy.[c] It runs in Ruth's family and is resistant to medications.	**Example 2** Narcolepsy and cataplexy.[d] It runs in Ruth's family and is resistant to medications.

[a] There is no diagnosis of narcolepsy or cataplexy here. "Symptoms of" indicate the patient's condition appears similar to a disorder. It is not a diagnosis of the disorder.

[b] Here, both the narcolepsy and cataplexy diagnoses are confirmed.

[c] Type 1 narcolepsy is narcolepsy and may include cataplexy, but there is no way for the coder to code both conditions without documentation of both, as ICD-10-CM does not recognize type 1 and type 2 narcolepsy.

[d] The only way to capture cataplexy is to document it in the medical record.

Coding

The most common documentation support for narcolepsy is a discussion of the effect it has on the patient's activities of daily living, work or school accommodations, or disability status. A sleep study (polysomnogram) or multiple sleep latency test may be performed to assess the sleep patterns of a patient who is suspected of having, or who has, narcolepsy. Hypocretin levels can be measured in CFS aspirated in a lumbar puncture. Medications that may be prescribed to treat narcolepsy include modafinil, methylphenidate, and antidepressants. Cataplexy is sometimes treated with sodium oxybate, or gamma hydroxybutyrate (GHB). Patients may be counseled to take naps, maintain a regular sleep schedule, avoid tobacco, caffeine, alcohol, and heavy meals near bedtime, and to exercise regularly.

CODING TIP The ICD-10-CM Alphabetic Index presumes a causal link between any documented narcolepsy and cataplexy based on the word "with" in the code title. Coders should report code G47.411, *Narcolepsy with cataplexy,* or G47.421, *Narcolepsy in conditions classified elsewhere with cataplexy,* if both narcolepsy and cataplexy are documented. Cataplexy is not diagnosed absent narcolepsy, and coders can report G47.411 or G47.421 if only cataplexy is documented. This is based on the Alphabetic Index entry, "Cataplexy (idiopathic), *see* Narcolepsy."

Narcolepsy can be secondary to other conditions. Look for causal links in the documentation before reporting code G47.421, *Narcolepsy in conditions classified elsewhere with cataplexy,* or G47.429, *Narcolepsy in conditions classified elsewhere without cataplexy.*

Epworth Sleepiness Scale

A physician may record an Epworth sleepiness scale (ESS) for the patient with suspected or existing narcolepsy. An ESS score cannot be coded because it is used as a diagnostic tool. The results of an ESS can, however, provide an opportunity for the coder to query the physician regarding the results, or be used to support a diagnosis of narcolepsy or cataplexy.

In general, ESS scores are interpreted as follows:

0-5	Lower normal daytime sleepiness
6-10	Higher normal daytime sleepiness
11-12	Mild excessive daytime sleepiness
13-15	Moderate excessive daytime sleepiness
16-24	Severe excessive daytime sleepiness

Learn more about ESS at http://epworthsleepinessscale.com/about-the-ess/.

CODING TIP Do not confuse cataplexy with catalepsy. Cataplexy occurs only in patients with narcolepsy and is a weakness or involuntary immobility. Catalepsy is a trance or seizure with loss of consciousness that may be due to a dissociative event, or occur in schizophrenia.

ABSTRACT & CODE IT!

Abstract and code the clinical coding example below. Check your answers against the answers in Appendix C.

Patient 1

The patient is experiencing narcolepsy with cataplexy as a result of changes in her brain due to the cerebral infarction she experienced last March.

Patient 2

Patient has been experiencing symptoms of narcolepsy and cataplexy for 5 years, and has been unable to work for 2 years. She had a multiple sleep latency test last year positive for narcolepsy, and her narcolepsy and cataplexy have been somewhat diminished by methylphenidate.

Patient 3

Assessment: Narcolepsy. It runs in Ruth's family and is resistant to medications.

Neoplasms

Metastatic cancer and acute leukemia
HCC 8 2.625

Lung and other severe cancers
HCC 9 0.970

Lymphoma and other cancers
HCC 10 0.677

Colorectal, bladder, and other cancers
HCC 11 0.301

Breast, prostate, and other cancers and tumors
HCC 12 0.146

Chronic myeloid leukemia
RxHCC 15 7.383

Multiple myeloma and other neoplastic disorders
RxHCC 16 3.4946

Secondary cancers of bone, lung, brain and other specified sites; liver cancer
RxHCC 17 1.771

Lung, kidney and other cancers
RxHCC 18 0.294

Breast and other cancers and tumors
RxHCC 19 0.096

A neoplasm is an abnormal growth, classified by the type of growth and its site. In ICD-10-CM, neoplasms are primarily classified by site (location, including extension into other tissues), behavior (eg, in situ, benign, malignant, uncertain), and morphology (eg, lymphoma, melanoma, adenoma). Malignant neoplasms represent uncontrolled growth. Most malignant neoplasms risk-adjust, and all spreading cancers (ie, metastatic cancers) that have invaded adjacent or distant organs risk-adjust. Benign or in situ neoplasms associated with the brain and spine may risk-adjust, as their presence may cause pressure or displacement of critical structures. A few uncertain and unspecified neoplasms also risk-adjust.

Malignant neoplasms in the ICD-10-CM Tabular List can be divided into two broad categories: (1) solid tumors defined by their histology and/or locations (eg, primary breast cancer or colon cancer that metastasized to the liver) and (2) "liquid" tumors.

Solid tumors originate at a specific site and may spread to adjacent or remote sites. Liquid tumors (eg, multiple myeloma myeloma and hematopoietic cancers, such as leukemia, which have no locations) can develop simultaneously from multiple sites, with cancer cells circulating in the blood stream or lymphatic system. While solid tumors can metastasize from the primary site to other sites, leukemia and multiple myeloma are, by their very nature, systemic. There are no "secondary sites" for leukemia or for liquid tumors, lymphoma, or certain skin cancers (eg, basal cell carcinomas).

The American Cancer Society estimated that approximately 1.7 million new cases of cancer were diagnosed in 2017 (excluding basal cell and squamous cell skin cancers and *in situ* cancers, except urinary bladder).[3] More than 600,000 patients died of cancer in 2017, making it the second most common cause of death in the US after heart disease.[3] Almost 90% of cancers diagnosed in the US are diagnosed in patients who are 50 years of age or older.[3] The most common causes of cancer in men are lung/bronchus, prostate, colon/rectum/pancreas, and liver cancer. For women, the most common causes are lung/bronchus, breast, colon/rectum, pancreas, and uterus. Statistics on US cancer cases and mortality for 2017 are available at https://www.cancer.org/research/cancer-facts-statistics/all-cancer-facts-figures/cancer-facts-figures-2017.html.

Documentation and coding of neoplasms has proved over time to be a source of many errors in risk-adjustment (RA) coding. This is in part due to errors in correctly assigning the behavior classification, or morphology, to a diagnosis: primary malignant, secondary malignant, in situ carcinoma; uncertain behavior; or unspecified. However, the biggest issue with coding neoplasms in RA is correctly assigning codes for active cancer versus codes for a history of cancer.

If a physician documents the histology of a tumor, the ICD-10-CM Tabular List instructs coders to first look up the histology in the ICD-10-CM Alphabetic Index and follow its direction. If no histology is documented, the coder may refer to the ICD-10-CM Table of Neoplasms to determine what code in the ICD-10-CM Tabular List should be referenced. Additional instructions in the Tabular List, such as Excludes1, Excludes2, Code First, and Code Also, should be followed.

Physician Documentation

Neoplasms are classified in ICD-10-CM by anatomical location and morphology. Essential to proper coding and documentation is noting the specific site including any laterality. Avoid words like "mass," "lump," "tumor," "neoplasm," "lesion," or "growth," if more specific language is available. Specify the histology and/or behavior of the neoplasm, if known, as benign, primary malignant, secondary malignant, in situ, or uncertain. Do not confuse *uncertain* neoplasm with *unspecified* neoplasm. An uncertain neoplasm has been examined microscopically and its nature (eg, benign, malignant) cannot be ascertained. An unspecified neoplasm is of unknown histology because no microscopic examination has yet occurred.

Hematopoietic
Of or relating to the production of blood cells, occurring in the bone marrow.

Morphology
In oncology, the study of the form and structure of aberrant cells to determine the nature of their origin and potential for growth.

Histology
The study of microscopically visible changes in cells or tissue to determine morphology. Examples include adenocarcinoma, large cell carcinoma, melanoma, lymphoma, adenomas, and carcinoid tumors.

How ICD-10-CM classifies malignancy is different from how physicians perceive cancer and its treatment, and this can be a significant source of error in RA audits. ICD-10-CM codes for solid tumors are classified according to site. Although breast cancer may be the etiology of the secondary bone cancer in a patient, the patient may have had the breast removed and completed treatment for breast cancer, and therefore, would correctly be reported to have a history of breast cancer. On the other hand, the patient would still have an active secondary malignancy of the bone. If only a lumpectomy of the breast was performed, the diagnosis, once treatment is completed, would still be reported as a history of breast cancer when metastases are discovered. Document the active bone cancer (which codes to a secondary malignancy of the bone) and a history of breast cancer in this case.

DOCUMENTATION TIP Physicians should use language that allows the coder to abstract the appropriate diagnosis for the patient. In ICD-10-CM, the only malignant conditions that can be categorized as "in remission" are multiple myeloma and leukemia. Other cancers are identified as "active" or "current" disease, meaning the condition is still present or still being treated, or "history of" disease, meaning the condition has been excised or eradicated and all treatment completed.

In a history of cancer of a primary site (eg, a colon cancer that was removed), a secondary site (eg, metastasis of the colon cancer to the liver) may still be undergoing treatment.

Conversely, do not document "history of malignant neoplasm" or "no evidence of disease" (NED) if the neoplasm is still being actively treated. Instead, document the continuum of care, noting what has been done and what is left to do. "History of" and "no evidence of disease" indicate an eradicated condition and a complete cure, according to coding rules, and would result in a history of malignant neoplasm code (eg, Z85.-) instead of an active malignant neoplasm code. According to ICD-10-CM Guideline Section I(C.2.d), "[w]hen a primary malignancy has been previously excised or eradicated from its site and there is no further treatment directed to that site and there is no evidence of any existing primary malignancy, a code from category Z85, Personal history of malignant neoplasm, should be used to indicate the former site of the malignancy. Any mention of extension, invasion, or metastasis to another site is coded as a secondary malignant neoplasm to that site. The secondary site may be the principal or first-listed diagnosis with the Z85 code used as a secondary code."[4]

 **ADVICE/ALERT NOTE**

Per ICD-10-CM Guideline Section I(C.2.d), "[w]hen a primary malignancy has been previously excised or eradicated from its site and there is no further treatment directed to that site and there is no evidence of any existing primary malignancy, a code from category Z85, Personal history of malignant neoplasm, should be used to indicate the former site of the malignancy. Any mention of extension, invasion, or metastasis to another site is coded as a secondary malignant neoplasm to that site. The secondary site may be the principal or first-listed with the Z85 code used as a secondary code."[4]

If a selective estrogen receptor modulatory (SERM) like tamoxifen is prescribed, document whether the medication is treatment for active cancer or for prophylaxis against the cancer's return. Active treatment warrants a code for the presence of the malignant neoplasm; prophylaxis warrants a code for a "history of malignant neoplasm" code.

DOCUMENTATION TIP Documentation of metastatic disease requires special care, as "metastatic" and "metastasis" can be ambiguous in describing the primary and secondary sites. Use of the words "to" and "from" in notes will clarify the origin of the neoplasm; for example, "breast cancer with metastases to the lung," or "metastatic lung cancer from the breast." Or, simply use the descriptors "secondary" and "primary." With use of "secondary," however, remember to document what it is secondary "to."

ICD-10-CM defines metastasis as a spread of malignancy to a distant site **or** an extension into an adjacent site. Document metastatic cancer when a tumor invades neighboring sites (eg, a bladder cancer invading the seminal vesicle is metastatic bladder cancer to the seminal vesicle). For multiple metastatic sites, identify each site. Be specific.

If the staging of the cancer is known, enter it into the medical record. This helps the coder understand the severity of the patient's condition. The American Hospital Association's (AHA's) *Coding Clinic for ICD-10-CM and ICD-10-PCS* (*Coding Clinic*) (First Quarter, 2014) states that it is "appropriate to use the completed cancer staging form for coding purposes when it is authenticated by the attending physician."[5]

Clearly link complications caused by the neoplasm. For example, document anemia as caused by the cancer versus anemia as caused by the cancer treatment. Document diabetes due to pancreatic carcinoma, or pathologic fracture due to breast cancer metastasizing to the radius. Always document etiology and manifestation.

Leukemia and multiple myeloma should be noted by histology, and as one of the following:

- Not having achieved remission
- In remission
- In relapse
- History of—if considered completely cured (which, while uncommon when the onset of leukemia is in adults, may be considered when its onset is in childhood)

Leukemia and multiple myeloma are the only cancers classified in ICD-10-CM with "in remission" or "in relapse" designation. Documentation of "minimal residual disease," a term used after treatment when leukemia cells cannot be found in the bone marrow using standard laboratory tests (such as looking at cells under a microscope), but can still be detected with more sensitive tests (such as flow cytometry), requires physician documentation of whether remission has been achieved.

For other cancers, state "active" or "history of." Do not report, for example, "sigmoid colon cancer in remission"; instead, report "history of sigmoid colon cancer" if the cancer is completely resolved **and** is not being treated, or "sigmoid colon cancer responding well to bevacizumab" if the patient is still undergoing active treatment.

DOCUMENTATION TIP New codes specific to the following malignant mast cell neoplasms were created for the 2018 ICD-10-CM code set, and these conditions should be specified when they exist:

C96.20	Malignant mast cell neoplasm, unspecified
C96.21	Aggressive systemic mastocytosis
C96.22	Mast cell sarcoma
C96.29	Other malignant mast cell neoplasm
D47.01	Cutaneous mastocytosis
D47.02	Systemic mastocytosis
D47.09	Other mast cell neoplasms of uncertain behavior

CLINICAL EXAMPLES

NONSPECIFIC DOCUMENTATION	SPECIFIC DOCUMENTATION
Example 1 Patient with history of prostate cancer is being seen today for his quarterly leuprolide injection.[a]	**Example 1** Patient with prostate cancer is being seen today for his quarterly 22.5 mg leuprolide injection.[b]
Example 2 Extradural spinal tumor.[c]	**Example 2** Extradural spine metastasis at L4-L5, with symptoms of sciatica and intermittent urinary incontinence.[d] Primary is a history of lung cancer, treatment completed 18 months ago, NED.

[a] Leuprolide treats advanced prostate cancer. This patient does not have a history of prostate cancer, although based on this documentation, a history is what could be reported.

[b] Patient accurately reported with active prostate cancer.

[c] While spinal cancers can be assumed to be secondary cancers, in this case it is documented as "tumor" and the Alphabetic Index takes the coder to neoplasm of unspecified behavior. Use specific language. Identify the morphology of the neoplasm, the site on the spine, and any symptoms related to the growth. If a secondary cancer, identify the primary cancer.

[d] Documentation provides a clear view of the patient's symptoms as well as the site of the secondary neoplasm and the site of the resolved primary neoplasm.

Coding

Neoplasms can be documented in many ways. Ideally, the physician will document with specificity the neoplasm's site and nature, or provide histology that is further explained in the ICD-10-CM Alphabetic Index (eg, "Adenoma—*see also* Neoplasm, benign, by site"). From the Alphabetic Index entry, the coder can look up the information in the ICD-10-CM Neoplasm Table. Keep in mind that a note at the beginning of the ICD-10-CM Neoplasm Table states that if documentation conflicts with the Alphabetic Index advice (eg, the physician has documented "malignant adenoma"), the documented diagnosis takes precedence over the Alphabetic Index entry and a malignant condition would be abstracted.

According to ICD-10-CM Guideline Section I(C.2), "[c]ertain benign neoplasms, such as prostatic adenomas, may be found in the specific body system chapters. To properly code a neoplasm it is necessary to determine from the record if the neoplasm is benign, in situ, malignant, or of uncertain histologic behavior. If malignant, any secondary (metastatic) sites should also be determined."[4]

> **ADVICE/ALERT NOTE**
>
> Per ICD-10-CM Guideline Section I(C.2), "[c]ertain benign neoplasms, such as prostatic adenomas, may be found in the specific body system chapters. To properly code a neoplasm it is necessary to determine from the record if the neoplasm is benign, in situ, malignant, or of uncertain histologic behavior. If malignant, any secondary (metastatic) sites should also be determined."[4]

Do not make assumptions about coding "mass," "growth," "tumor," "polyp," or other terms found in the medical record as benign or malignant neoplasms. Be sure to start in the Alphabetic Index and look up the exact words from documentation. For example, a "polyp" may be indexed to a benign neoplasm, a neoplasm of uncertain behavior, an "other or unspecified disorder," and for some sites will classify to a unique polyp code. If a coder regularly jumps into the Table of Neoplasms without first consulting the Alphabetic Index, errors will be made. From the Alphabetic Index, go to the ICD-10-CM Neoplasm Table, and then to the Tabular List of the ICD-10-CM.

Do not confuse "uncertain" with "unspecified" neoplasms. An uncertain neoplasm has been examined microscopically but its nature, whether benign or malignant, could not be ascertained. A note at the beginning of the section on neoplasms of unspecified behavior in ICD-10-CM states that "[c]ategories D37-D44 , and D48 classify by site neoplasms of uncertain behavior, i.e., histologic confirmation whether the neoplasm is malignant or benign cannot be made."[4]

By definition, "histologic confirmation" indicates the tissue specimen was examined under a microscope by the treating physician or by a pathologist. A physician who documents that patient has "two neoplasms of uncertain behavior on her right shoulder and should undergo skin biopsy" is clearly not identifying a lesion that is of "uncertain behavior" by ICD-10-CM definition, and should be queried. A physician who documents the patient as having two "lesions of uncertain behavior" is an easier puzzle, since what is documented is "lesions," not "neoplasms." The skin lesion would be classified in the Alphabetic Index to code L98.9, *Disorder of the skin and subcutaneous tissue, unspecified.* In a limited number of instances, specific diagnoses may classify to a neoplasm of uncertain behavior without those words being documented (eg, bladder polyp indexes to code D41.4, *Neoplasm of uncertain behavior of bladder*).

An unspecified neoplasm is completely different from an uncertain neoplasm. The note at the beginning of the section for neoplasms of unspecified behavior in ICD-10-CM states that "[c]ategory D49 classifies by site neoplasms of unspecified morphology and behavior. The term 'mass,' unless otherwise stated, is not to be regarded as a neoplastic growth. Includes: 'growth,' NOS; 'neoplasm,' NOS; 'new growth,' NOS; 'tumor,' NOS."[4]

A neoplasm of unspecified behavior has not been examined by a pathologist and is of unknown etiology because no microscopic examination has been performed or documented. Alternately, the neoplasm is determined to be of unspecified behavior because the documentation was not detailed enough for a more specific diagnosis to be abstracted.

> **CODING TIP** According to the AHA's *ICD-10-CM and ICD-10-PCS Coding Handbook*, if the primary/secondary status is not stated in documentation, the following sites should be considered secondary sites of malignancy[6]:
>
> | | | |
> |---|---|---|
> | Bone | Heart | Lymph nodes |
> | Pleura | Brain | Mediastinum |
> | Spinal cord | Diaphragm | Meninges |
> | Retroperitoneum | Peritoneum | |
>
> Sites classified to C76 (other and ill-defined sites). Consider all other sites primary, if primary/secondary is not stated, with the exception of the liver.[6] The liver has a specific code for use in these cases, C22.9, *Malignant neoplasm of liver, not specified as primary or secondary.*

"Metastatic from . . ." indicates a primary malignancy: the original site of the cancer. "Metastatic to . . ." indicates a secondary malignancy: a new site for cancer that has grown from seeds from the original, primary site. The primary site may be coded as an active cancer, or if treatment is complete, the primary site for metastatic disease may be coded as history of cancer. Query the physician if the documentation is unclear whether a site is primary or secondary.

According to ICD-10-CM Guidelines Section I(C.2.j) and I(C.2.k), "[c]ode C80.0, Disseminated malignant neoplasm, unspecified, is for use only in those cases where the patient has advanced metastatic disease and no known primary or secondary sites are specified. It should not be used in place of assigning codes for the primary site and all known secondary sites.

Code C80.1, Malignant (primary) neoplasm, unspecified, equates to cancer, unspecified.This code should only be used when no determination can be made as to the primary site of a malignancy."[4]

> **ADVICE/ALERT NOTE**
>
> Per ICD-10-CM Guidelines Section I(C.2.j) and I(C.2.k), "[c]ode C80.0, Disseminated malignant neoplasm, unspecified, is for use only in those cases where the patient has advanced metastatic disease and no known primary or secondary sites are specified. It should not be used in place of assigning codes for the primary site and all known secondary sites.
>
> Code C80.1, Malignant (primary) neoplasm, unspecified, equates to Cancer, unspecified. This code should only be used when no determination can be made as to the primary site of a malignancy. This code should rarely be used in the inpatient setting."[4]

Comorbidities are sometimes caused by a neoplasm. Look for linking language in documentation and report related conditions when they are associated with the neoplasm (eg, hyperthyroidism due to thyroid malignancy or diabetes caused by pancreatic cancer).

Melanoma and Merkel cell carcinoma are aggressive forms of skin cancer that can spread to internal organs. Both are linked to increased sun exposure, but while melanoma can occur at any age, Merkel cell is much more prevalent in the senior population. As skin cancers, melanoma and Merkel cell carcinoma have unique codes, selected by site. Do not use other malignant skin neoplasm codes to report these two conditions. Melanoma and Merkel cell carcinoma risk-adjust, while other forms of skin cancers do not.

Contiguous sites are sites within the same organ that are adjacent to each other. In ICD-10-CM, contiguous sites are reported with codes for "overlapping sites," using a code ending in ".8." Do not report each specific site; instead, report "overlapping sites" with the specific ".8" code. Review anatomy references if unsure whether sites are contiguous (eg, if the splenic flexure and transverse colon are adjacent sites in the colon [they are]). Codes for overlapping sites will always be reported for the same organ, ie, while the cecum and ileum are adjacent, there is no single code for these overlapping sites as the cecum is large intestine and the ileum is small intestine. Each would be separately coded.

As instructed in ICD-10-CM's Chapter 2 on Neoplasms (C00-D49), a "primary malignant neoplasm that overlaps two or more contiguous (next to each other) sites should be classified to the subcategory/code .8 ('overlapping lesion'), unless the combination is specifically indexed elsewhere. For multiple neoplasms of the same site that are not contiguous, such as tumors in different quadrants of the same breast, codes for each site should be assigned."[4]

> **ADVICE/ALERT NOTE**
>
> As instructed in ICD-10-CM's Chapter 2 on Neoplasms (C00-D49), a "primary malignant neoplasm that overlaps two or more contiguous (next to each other) sites should be classified to the subcategory/code .8 ('overlapping lesion'), unless the combination is specifically indexed elsewhere. For multiple neoplasms of the same site that are not contiguous, such as tumors in different quadrants of the same breast, codes for each site should be assigned."[4]

It is important to differentiate if a malignant neoplasm is advancing deeper into the site, advancing from its site of origin to a contiguous site, or a malignant neoplasm metastasizing:

- A malignant neoplasm of the ascending colon extends and advances, but growth remains within the ascending colon. Report code C18.2, *Malignant neoplasm of ascending colon.*
- A malignant neoplasm of the ascending colon extends and advances into the cecum. Report code C18.8, *Malignant neoplasm of overlapping sites of the colon.*
- A malignant neoplasm of the ascending colon and cecum (eg, the large intestine extends and invades the adjacent ileum [eg, the small intestine]). Report codes C18.8, *Malignant neoplasm of overlapping sites of the colon,* and C78.4, *Secondary malignant neoplasm of small intestine.* This may be called invasive cancer to an adjacent site.
- A malignant neoplasm of the ascending colon and cecum sends cells through the

bloodstream to the liver, where another growth has been discovered. Report codes C18.8, *Malignant neoplasm of overlapping sites of the colon,* and C78.7, *Secondary malignant neoplasm of liver and intrahepatic bile duct.* This may be called a distant metastasis.

If a specific code cannot be found in the ICD-10-CM Table of Neoplasms for a blood vessel, bursa, fascia, ligament, muscle, peripheral nerve, sympathetic and parasympathetic nerve and ganglion, synovia, or tendon, refer to the entry for "connective tissue" in the table, by site.

Cancer Staging Form[5]

Cancer staging has its own classification system. Completed cancer staging forms can be used for abstracting diagnoses from the medical record if the forms are authenticated by the attending physician, according to AHA's *Coding* Clinic (First Quarter, 2014).[5] Coders can use the completed cancer staging form to abstract diagnoses when the form is authenticated by the attending physician.

Cancer Staging Form

Stage 0: Carcinoma in situ

Stage I, II, III: Identify incrementally the size and extent of the malignancy

Stage IV: Distant metastases

Another form of staging is the TNM Staging System:

T indicates the size and extent of the primary tumor

N indicates the number of lymph nodes near the primary tumor that are positive for malignancy (primary tumor metastasized to lymph nodes)

M indicates whether the primary malignancy has metastasized to other organs in the body

Key for T

TX: Main malignancy cannot be measured

T0: Main malignancy cannot be found

T1-T4: Identifies incrementally the size and extent of the malignancy. Ts may be further divided to provide more information about the maligancy (eg, T3a or T3b)

Key for N

NX: Malignancy in regional lymph nodes cannot be measured

N0: No malignancy in regional lymph nodes found

N1-N3: Identifies incrementally the number and location of malignant lymph nodes

Key for M

MX: Metastasis cannot be measured

M0: No metastases found

M1: Metastases to other parts of the body

For example, if a patient's TNM stage for ovarian cancer were T3N2M0, report the ovarian cancer (T3) and secondary cancer of the lymph nodes (N2). The physician would not have to specifically document "metastatic to lymph nodes," in order for it to be captured because this is documented, albeit in an abbreviated format, in the authenticated cancer staging form.

CODING TIP Only leukemia and multiple myeloma have "remission" or "relapse" codes in ICD-10-CM cancer coding. If your physician documents another form of cancer as "in remission," query to see if the patient has a history of malignancy, or active disease.

Lymphoma is a malignancy of the lymphatic system. Secondary lymph cancer codes are only reported when a solid tumor from another site metastasizes to the lymph node (eg, breast, metastasizes to lymph nodes [eg, axillary nodes]). Not all lymphomas are malignant. If benign, a lymphoma is reported with code D36.0, *Benign neoplasm of lymph nodes.* If the specific type of lymphoma is not noted as a variety of Hodgkin, follicular, non-follicular lymphoblastic, etc, query the physician. The default code for documented lymphoma is C85.90, *Non-Hodgkin lymphoma, unspecified, unspecified site.*

Multiple myeloma is cancer in the plasma cells produced in the bone marrow, while leukemia is cancer in the white cell or platelet progenitor cells (eg, promyelocytes, megakaryoblasts) produced in the bone marrow.

CODING TIP A cancer becomes history of cancer when it is no longer present and treatment is completed (eg, excision, radiotherapy, chemotherapy is completed), according to the ICD-10-CM guidelines. For example, following lobectomy and chemotherapy, a patient is diagnosed with metastatic brain cancer, secondary to lung cancer. The patient's diagnosis is reported with codes C79.31, *Secondary malignant neoplasm of brain,* and Z85.118, *Personal history of other malignant neoplasm of bronchus and lung.*

While coders may become overwhelmed with the variety and complexity of the "liquid" malignancies posed by myelomas, lymphomas, and leukemias, the real source of consternation for coding neoplasms comes from the confusing use of the phrase "history of" in medical records. Physicians often document history of cancer in cases of active cancer, or active cancers as histories. As noted in earlier chapters, the definition of "history" as used or understood in clinical practice differs from the ICD-10-CM coding requirements. It is the coder's responsibility to read the documentation thoroughly and query the physician if the documentation seems ambiguous or contradictory regarding the nature of the patient's neoplasm diagnosis. If a query is not possible, the coders should read the documentation, look for medications that support active cancer treatment, and follow the internal policies of their organization. If the physician documents active cancer but the record obviously supports a history of cancer, (eg, right breast cancer, right mastectomy eight years ago, clear PET scan six months ago, NED today), report a personal history of breast cancer.

CODING TIP If primary pulmonary malignancy is causing pericardial effusion, do not code this diagnosis of malignant pericardial effusion as a secondary malignant neoplasm. Refer to the Alphabetic Index entry, "Pericarditis (with decompensation) (with effusion)/neoplastic," and choose between chronic and acute. For chronic or unspecified, select code I31.8, *Disease of pericardium, unspecified,* and for acute, select code I30.9, *Acute pericarditis, unspecified.* Code the pericarditis in addition to the code for the primary malignancy. If the physician documents that a malignancy has spread to the pericardium, then code C79.89, *Secondary malignant neoplasm of other specified sites*, may be reported.

ABSTRACT & CODE IT!

Abstract and code the clinical coding example below. Check your answers against the answers in Appendix C.

Patient 1

The patient presented to the emergency department with abdominal pain and distension that was due to a bowel obstruction caused by peritoneal carcinomatosis, secondary to right ovarian malignancy.

Patient 2

Patient with history of prostate cancer is being seen today for his quarterly 22.5 mg leuprolide injection. Upon physical examination, no increase in the size of his tumor was noted.

Patient 3

Extradural spine metastasis at L4-L5, with symptoms of right-sided sciatica and intermittent urinary incontinence. Primary is a history of lung cancer, treatment completed 18 months ago, NED.

Neuralgia

Trigeminal and postherpetic neuralgias
RxHCC 168 0.134

Neuralgia describes pain occurring along the course of a nerve caused by damage or inflammation of the nerve and unrelated to sensory input. Postherpetic neuralgia (PHN) is a common sequela to a herpes zoster (shingles) infection in a peripheral nerve and can persist for months or years after the shingles has resolved. Peripheral nerves are derived from nerve roots on the right or left of the spinal cord. Due to the anatomy of nerve distribution, PHN is by definition a unilateral condition affecting only one side of the body.

The herpes zoster infection, also called shingles, often manifests along a dermatome of the torso but may also affect facial nerves. Sometimes, more than one dermatome is infected. The incidence of shingles increases with age. One in three people develops shingles in their lifetime, with the risk increasing after age 50. There are 1 million cases of herpes zoster in the US each year.[7]

Trigeminal neuralgia (TN) is similar in pain and intensity to PHN, but affects the trigeminal nerve. The trigeminal nerve, the fifth cranial nerve, is a large network of nerves that gathers at the temple and spread throughout the face. It has three main branches: ophthalmic, maxillary, and mandibular. Any or all branches of the trigeminal nerve can be affected in TN, which is also unilateral. In some rare cases, both nerves may be affected simultaneously. TN can occur due to tumors, injury, or idiopathically, in people with MS, or following nerve injury.

Physician Documentation

When documenting PHN and TN, use language that reflects the contents of ICD-10-CM (see Table 4-3.2).

TABLE 4-3.2 PHN AND TN CODES

CODE	DESCRIPTION
B02.21	Postherpetic geniculate ganglionitis
B02.22	Postherpetic trigeminal neuralgia
B02.23	Postherpetic polyneuropathy
B02.29	Other postherpetic nervous system involvement
G50.0	Trigeminal neuralgia
G50.1	Atypical facial pain
G50.8	Other disorders of trigeminal nerve
G50.9	Disorder of trigeminal nerve, unspecified

Identify the cause of any neuralgia, if known. If reporting TN, state the cause. If due to sequela of herpes zoster, it will be reported with code B02.22, *Postherpetic trigeminal neuralgia*. Otherwise, it will be reported with code G50.0, *Trigeminal neuralgia*. Identify any current traumatic injury or sequela as the cause for TN. Always spell out the first reference, as TN can also be interpreted as normal intraocular tension. Instead, document trigeminal neuralgia (TN).

DOCUMENTATION TIP Differentiate in documentation the nerve pain associated with an active herpes zoster (shingles) infection versus postherpetic neuropathy.

Postherpetic neuralgia (PHN)
Pain persisting or recurring in an area after a shingles infection has resolved; usually due to fibrosis, scarring, or persistent inflammation of the nerve following the shingles outbreak.

Herpes zoster
Infection from reactivation of the varicella-zoster virus (chickenpox) in a nerve ganglion; also known as shingles. The unilateral disorder results in a painful, blistering rash along the course of the nerve.

Dermatome
A contiguous area of skin flowing from the spinal column associated by a nerve from a specific spinal root.

Trigeminal neuralgia
Pain and other neuropathic symptoms in the lips, eyes, nose, scalp, forehead, or jaw often caused by a blood vessel pressing on the fifth cranial nerve as it exits the brain stem, or from other causes. The trigeminal nerve is the fifth cranial nerve.

Coding

For current herpes zoster infection and pain, do not report a code from B02.2, *Zoster with other nervous system involvement.* Codes from B02.2 are reserved for pain that remains or develops after the herpes zoster infection has resolved, identified as "postherpetic" in the code descriptions. For current herpes zoster infection, report a code from B02.3-B02.8, selecting a code based on the site of the infection as a specified ocular site (cornea, conjunctiva, iris, sclera, etc), ear, other site, or disseminated herpes zoster. "Disseminated" generally refers to a concurrent herpes zoster infection of three or more dermatomes according to the Centers for Disease Control and Prevention (CDC),[8] and is reported with code B02.7, *Disseminated zoster.*

TN is commonly called tic douloureux; however, the Alphabetic Index classifies tic douloureux to code B02.22, *Postherpetic trigeminal neuralgia,* if caused by herpes zoster. Look for the causal agent in tic douloureux. The Alphabetic Index default for tic douloureux is code G50.0, *Trigeminal neuralgia.* If TN is due to a current traumatic injury, report a code from category S04.3-, *Injury of trigeminal nerve*. PHN codes are determined by site (see Table 4-3.3).

TABLE 4-3.3 PHN Codes and Sites

CODE	DESCRIPTION	SITE
B02.21	Postherpetic geniculate ganglionitis	PHN where the motor and sensory nerve mains meet in the facial nerve, causing severe ear pain and vertigo.
B02.22	Postherpetic trigeminal neuralgia	PHN anywhere else along the trigeminal nerve.
B02.23	Postherpetic polyneuropathy	PHN that affects nerves that were not part of the original zoster infection site.
B02.29	Other postherpetic nervous system involvement	PHN along the dermatome that was affected by the original zoster infection (PHN radiculopathy).

ABSTRACT & CODE IT!

Abstract and code the clinical coding example below. Check your answers against the answers in Appendix C.

Patient: Karina Martinez **DOB:** 3/27/1947 **DOS:** 11/17/2017

Subjective: Mrs. Martinez comes in today due to severe pain in her back. The site of the pain is the same site as the herpes zoster infection the patient experienced three months ago. The zoster was treated with acyclovir and naproxen.

The skin is healed, with pink scarring. She identified an area approximately 4 cm by 18 cm as the site of the pain. This area corresponds to the site of the previous zoster infection. She describes the pain as relentless, and 7.5 on a scale of 1 to 10, sometimes spiking to 10. She states she cannot wear normal clothes and must wear loose shirts belonging to her husband. She has been homebound since the shingles began. She has been waiting for the pain to recede, but the blisters from the rash have all healed, and the pain persists.

Objective

PMH [past medical history]
Shingles
Diabetes
Neuropathy in feet
Osteoporosis with frailty fracture of L hip May 2016
CAD [coronary artery disease]

Medications
nateglinide 120 mg with meals
gabapentin 300 mg 3x day

Vitals

Ht: 5"1"	Wt: 192.5	BMI: 36.4	Temp: 98.5	BP: 129/89	Heart: 78 BPM	Resp: 21 BPM

PE [physical examination]
Constitutional: General appearance: healthy appearing, well-nourished, and well-developed. Level of Distress: moderate

Ambulation: Ambulating normally.

Psychiatric: Insight: good judgment. Mental status: depressed mood related to pain level and sleeplessness. Orientation: to time, place, and person. Memory: recent memory normal and remote memory normal.

Head: normocephalic and atraumatic.

Neck: Supple, FROM [full range of motion], trachea midline, and no masses. Lymph nodes: no cervical, supraclavicular, axillary, or inguinal lymphadenopathy. Thyroid: no enlargement or nodules and non-tender.

Lungs: Respiratory effort: no dyspnea. Percussion: no dullness, flatness, or hyperresonance. Auscultation: no wheezing, rales/crackles, or rhonchi.

Cardiovascular: Apical impulse: not displaced. Heart auscultation: normal S1 and S2; no murmurs, rubs, or gallops; and RRR [regular rate and rhythm]. Neck vessels: no carotid bruits. Pulses including femoral/pedal: normal throughout.

Abdomen: Obese abdomen. Bowel sounds: normal. Inspection and palpation: no tenderness, guarding, masses, rebound tenderness.

Musculoskeletal: Motor strength and tone: normal tone and motor strength. Joints, bones, and muscles: no contractures, malalignment, tenderness, or bony abnormalities and normal movement of all extremities.

Neurologic: Gait and station: normal. Cranial nerves: grossly intact. Sensation: significant for chronic, severe pain along L1 dermatome, at site of recent herpes zoster infection and scarring.

Assessment
Postherpetic neuralgia

Plan
Increase gabapentin prescribed for diabetic neuropathy pain, to up to double the current dose as needed for PHN if topical 5% lidocaine patches applied directly to PHN site do not sufficiently reduce the pain.

Electronically signed by Herman Manowitz MD 6:45PM 11/17/2017

Obesity

Morbid obesity

HCC 22	**0.273**
RxHCC 43	**0.056**

The CDC reports that more than 72 million American adults are obese, meaning they have too much body fat.[8] Excess weight is always going to affect the health of the patient. Obesity and overweight are conditions that occur when the patient has an underlying condition causing weight gain, or more commonly, when a patient consumes more calories daily than he or she expends. Obesity and overweight are measured based on a person's weight in relation to height, by a body mass index (BMI). Any BMI over 25 is considered high and should be documented for any encounter in which the condition is observed. BMI is a valuable screening tool for weight and nutrition status.[9]

Obesity and morbid obesity are contributing factors to heart disease, stroke, diabetes, and some forms of cancer. Obesity can cause sleep apnea, mobility issues, and joint problems, all contributing to a higher cost of medical care.

Physician Documentation

Codes for extreme (morbid) obesity or a BMI of 40 or greater risk-adjust. Patients are considered extremely obese when they have a BMI of 40 or greater, according to the CDC. Extreme obesity, also called class 3 obesity, greatly increases a patient's risks for other disorders, and risk-adjusts for both medical and pharmaceutical interventions. Note that ICD-10-CM uses the nomenclature "overweight," "obesity," and "morbid obesity," rather than class 1, 2, or 3 BMI scores adopted by the CDC. Overweight corresponds with class-1 BMI, and obese corresponds with class-2 BMI. Class-3 BMI corresponds to extreme or severe obesity, and is the equivalent of morbid obesity in ICD-10-CM.

Ensure the patient's BMI is calculated at least once or twice annually, and when abnormal, documented and coded along with a corresponding disease state (eg, overweight, obesity, morbid [extreme] obesity). Identify the cause of the weight issue as excess calorie intake (hyperalimentation), adverse effect of a medication (document drug), or other cause. Document a weight-related diagnosis for any patient with an abnormal BMI according to standards published by the American Heart Association in conjunction with the American College of Cardiology (see Table 4-3.4).

TABLE 4-3.4 American Heart Association/American College of Cardiology BMI Standards and Associated Conditions

BMI	ASSOCIATED CONDITION
18.5-24.99	Normal
25.00-29.9	Overweight
30 to less than 39.9	Obese (Classes 1 and 2)
40 or greater	Morbidly obese (extreme, severe, Class 3)

If a patient's weight is causing other health issues (eg, hypertension, diabetes, osteoarthritis of the knees), document the health issues and link them to the weight diagnosis. Similarly, if the weight issue is caused by an underlying cause (eg, hypothyroidism or Cushing's syndrome), document the underlying cause. Ensure that both the weight diagnosis and patient's BMI appear in the record, and link to any weight-related comorbidities.

DOCUMENTATION TIP A BMI alone is not a weight diagnosis; it is a tool for determining a weight diagnosis. Review the BMI when assigning a weight diagnosis to ensure the BMI and diagnosis are compatible (eg, do not state that a person with a BMI of 30 as "morbidly obese," when the patient would best be described clinically as "obese," according to national standards). The contradiction may affect the outcome of an audit, since obesity does not risk-adjust, but morbid obesity does.

Always consider and document obesity diagnoses in relation to other conditions present in the patient. For example, document obesity or morbid obesity in a pregnant patient during each encounter in which the patient's weight is addressed. Her morbid obesity affects the management of the pregnancy, her health, and the health of her fetus and affects HCC RA. ICD-10-CM Guideline Section I(C.15.a.1) instructs that "[i]t is the physician's responsibility to state that the condition being treated is not affecting the pregnancy."[4] A documented weight condition in a pregnant patient is going to be a complication of pregnancy, according to the defaults set up in ICD-10-CM, and requires reporting code O99.21-, *Obesity complicating pregnancy, childbirth, and the puerperium,* and a separate code for the morbid obesity (see Table 4-3.5). Note that the weight condition does not affect the pregnancy, if that is the case.

TABLE 4-3.5 Adult BMI Code and BMI Description

ADULT BMI CODE	BMI DESCRIPTION
Z68.1	19.9 or less, adult
Z68.2- and Z68.3-	Append first two digits of BMI to create codes for all adult BMIs from 20.0 through 39.9. For example, a BMI of 34.5 would be reported as Z68.34.
Z68.41	40.9-44.9, adult
Z68.42	45.0-49.9, adult
Z68.43	50.0-59.9, adult
Z68.44	60.0-69.9, adult
Z68.45	70.0 or greater, adult

Document a treatment plan for the patient's obesity or morbid obesity. If a patient undergoes bariatric surgery, report the patient's postsurgical status because gastric bypass or other weight-reduction surgeries may or will cause future health issues for the patient. Report any sequelae of hyperalimentation in a patient who remains obese, or who has successfully undergone bariatric surgery (eg, bilateral osteoarthritis of the knees as sequelae of morbid obesity).

CLINICAL EXAMPLES

NONSPECIFIC DOCUMENTATION	SPECIFIC DOCUMENTATION
Example 1 **Vitals** Height: 6′1″ Weight: 322 lb BMI: 42.5 Temp: 98.65 BP: 138/90 Heart: 64 BPM Resp: 20 BPM Mickey is an obese[a] man who is here today as a follow-up to his COPD and hypertension, and to discuss a weight-loss referral.	**Example 1** **Vitals** Height: 6′1″ Weight: 322 lb BMI: 42.5 Temp: 98.65 BP: 138/90 Heart: 64 BPM Resp: 20 BPM Mickey is a morbidly[b] obese man who is here today as a follow-up to his COPD and his controlled hypertension, and to discuss a weight-loss referral.
Example 2 The patient is being seen today for weight-loss counseling. The patient has a BMI of 36[c] and is morbidly obese, with comorbidities relating to obesity.	**Example 2** The patient is being seen today for weight-loss counseling. The patient has a BMI of 36[d] and is morbidly obese, with comorbidities relating to obesity, which are new-onset type 2 diabetes mellitus, hypertension, and obstructive sleep apnea. The patient's diabetes is stable and the hypertension is regulated with lisinopril and a salt-restricted diet. He started using a sleep apnea machine 2 years ago.

[a] The patient's BMI of 42.5 is a BMI that aligns with the definition of morbidly obese but documentation states obese. Physician should ensure that the BMI in a diagnosis aligns with the documentation of a weight-related condition.

[b] In reviewing the vitals, the physician noted that the patient's BMI qualifies as morbidly obese and documents his weight condition accordingly.

[c] In this instance, the physician has documented comorbidities of obesity and tied them to the obesity but has not itemized the specific complications, which essentially nullifies complications from a coding standpoint.

[d] There are provisions for a patient with a BMI of 35 or greater to be diagnosed with morbid obesity if the patient has comorbidities associated with obesity. However, the comorbidities must be named and must be linked to the obesity.

Coding

Excess weight is always going to affect the health of the patient and should be reported as often as it is documented and addressed by the physician. BMI is an important quality measure tool. Coders are not allowed to calculate the BMI from the patient's weight and height for coding purposes. Code the BMI whenever it is documented.

There is no mechanism for a coder to change a weight diagnosis as documented by a physician. If a BMI seems inappropriate to the diagnosis, the coder may query the physician. If a query is not possible, the coder should report what is documented, even if it is contradictory (eg, report an overweight diagnosis with a BMI reflecting morbid obesity based on documentation). It is not the coder's role to align a conflicting diagnosis and BMI.

CODING TIP Use the Alphabetic Index to find the exact language of the documentation (abnormal weight loss, underweight). Obese abdomen or abdominal obesity describes localized fat, not obesity. A person with a normal BMI may have abdominal obesity. It is clinically significant because it hinders the physical examination. Report localized adiposity for any "apron of fat" or abdominal obesity documented by the physician. An apron of fat condition can lead to integumentary complications.

BMI codes cannot be reported without an accompanying weight-related diagnosis. Some organizations worry that not coding the BMI will affect quality ratings because BMI is a component of some quality measures. There are Healthcare Common Procedure Coding System (HCPCS) Level II codes for reporting compliance with BMI quality measures, and these can be reported in physician offices when a weight diagnosis is not present. Some electronic medical records (EMRs) automatically generate the HCPCS Level II BMI codes; in other systems, coders have to abstract them.

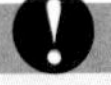 **ADVICE/ALERT NOTE**

Per ICD-10-CM Guideline I(C.15.a.1), it is the "physician's responsibility to state that the condition being treated is not affecting the pregnancy."[4]

Obesity affects the health of a patient and influences any comorbidities. For example, a pregnant patient who is obese or morbidly obese is at a higher risk for gestational diabetes and other complications of pregnancy. According to ICD-10-CM guidelines, a pregnant patient being treated or assessed for a comorbidity has a complication of pregnancy, even if the physician does not state the comorbidity is a complication of pregnancy. Obesity is, therefore, considered a complication of pregnancy. Two codes are reported: one for the complication of pregnancy and one for the condition. The pregnancy and obesity diagnosis would not be linked only if the physician specifically documents that the obesity is not affecting the pregnancy.

ABSTRACT & CODE IT!

Abstract and code the clinical coding example below. Check your answers against the answers in Appendix C.

Patient 1

The patient's abdominal fat interfered with the ultrasound of her ovaries.

Patient 2

Vitals

Height: 6′1″

Weight: 322 lb

BMI: 42.5

Temp: 98.65

BP: 138/90

Heart: 64 BPM

Resp: 20 BPM

Mickey is a morbidly obese man who is here today as a follow-up to his COPD and controlled hypertension, and to discuss a weight-loss referral.

Patient 3

The patient is being seen today for weight-loss counseling. The patient has a BMI of 36 and is morbidly obese, with comorbidities relating to obesity, which are new onset type 2 diabetes mellitus, hypertension, and obstructive sleep apnea. The patient's diabetes is stable and the hypertension is regulated with lisinopril and a salt-restricted diet. He started using a sleep apnea machine 2 years ago.

Ophthalmic Disorders

Exudative macular degeneration
HCC 124 0.499

Open-angle glaucoma
RxHCC 243 0.280

The macula is the most sensitive segment of the retina and is responsible for central vision and visual sharpness and detail. Age-related macular degeneration (AMD or ARMD) is a common cause of vision loss among people 50 years of age and older, according to the National Eye Institute (NEI).[10] Vision is blurred, and objects do not appear as bright as they once did.

AMD can be characterized as exudative or nonexudative. In nonexudative or dry AMD, the macula thins and small deposits of protein form. These are called drusen. Dry AMD causes gradual vision loss and progression may be slowed with vitamin and mineral supplements in some patients.

Exudative AMD, or wet AMD, is characterized by abnormal blood vessel growth under the macula. This form progressive rapidly and may cause severe vision loss.

AMD cannot be reversed. AMD risk factors include smoking, family history of AMD, and race. Caucasians are more susceptible to AMD than other races. NEI estimates that 1.75 million Americans have AMD, and that the number will increase to almost 3 million by the year 2020.[10]

Glaucoma is a condition in which high ocular pressure in the eye damages the optic nerve. The eye is constantly generating and recycling fluid, and if there is a blockage in the outflow of fluid, congestion in the eye can lead to high ocular pressure. Sometimes the blockage occurs because the patient has an abnormal narrowing of the angle through which the outflow of fluid exits, or an acute closing of the angle causing a medical emergency called acute angle-closure glaucoma. The most common form of glaucoma, however, is primary open-angle glaucoma (POAG), in which the anatomy is normal, but fluid drains from the eye at a slower pace than new fluid enters. Treatment for open-angle glaucoma often includes eyedrops, which improve the circulation of fluid in the eye. According to NIH, 2.2 million Americans have been diagnosed with glaucoma, and POAG is the most common.[10]

Physician Documentation

According to the new guideline regarding visual loss in the ICD-10-CM Guideline Section I(C.7.b), "[i]f 'blindness' or 'low vision' of both eyes is documented but the visual impairment category is not documented, assign code H54.3, Unqualified visual loss, both eyes. If 'blindness' or 'low vision' in one eye is documented but the visual impairment category is not documented, assign a code from H54.6-, Unqualified visual loss, one eye. If 'blindness' or 'visual loss' is documented without any information about whether one or both eyes are affected, assign code H54.7, Unspecified visual loss."[4]

Consider these coding requirements when documenting AMD:

- Code the laterality (right, left, bilateral)
- For nonexudative AMD, a 7th character is assigned to designate the stage:

  0 = stage unspecified

  1 = early dry stage

  2 = intermediate dry stage

  3 = advanced atrophic without subfoveal involvement

  4 = advanced atrophic with subfoveal involvement

- For exudative AMD, a 7th character is assigned to designate the stage:

  0 = stage unspecified

  1 = with active choroidal neovascularization

  2 = with inactive choroidal neovascularization with involuted or regressed neovascularization

  3 = with inactive scar

Coding

ADVICE/ALERT NOTE

Per the new ICD-10-CM Guideline Section I(C.7.b) regarding visual loss, "[i]f 'blindness' or 'low vision' of both eyes is documented but the visual impairment category is not documented, assign code H54.3, Unqualified visual loss, both eyes. If 'blindness' or 'low vision' in one eye is documented but the visual impairment category is not documented, assign a code from H54.6-, Unqualified visual loss, one eye. If 'blindness' or 'visual loss' is documented without any information about whether one or both eyes are affected, assign code H54.7, Unspecified visual loss."[4]

Ophthalmologists use documentation techniques and language that are a bit different from other physicians. Principally, coders need to understand laterality abbreviations:

OD = oculus dexter, the right eye

OS = oculus sinister, the left eye

OU = oculus uterque, or both eyes

A common screening tool for AMD is the Amsler grid, an enlarged sheet that looks like graph paper. Patients are asked to identify portions of the chart that appear to have wavy lines, dark patches, or blurred spots. The American Academy of Ophthalmologists provides a list of other ophthalmology acronyms, which is available at https://www.aao.org/young-ophthalmologists/yo-info/article/learning-lingo-ophthalmic-abbreviations.

ABSTRACT & CODE IT!

Abstract and code the clinical coding example below. Check your answers against the answers in Appendix C.

Patient: Sharon Peyson **DOB:** 2/21/1941 **DOS:** 2/1/2018

HPI: Retired schoolteacher reports she has noticed the onset of decreased vision in her left eye associated with a "dark spot" close to the center of her vision, whether reading or driving. Her vision has been slightly blurred in that eye for a while. She denies any recent trauma, eye pain, or discharge. Peripheral vision is normal. She has not had an eye exam in eight years.

Past Ocular History: No prior history of eye surgery, trauma, or childhood eye disorders.

Ocular Medications: None.

PMH: Significant for hypertension, hypercholesterolemia, CAD, history of DVTs [deep vein thrombosis].

Surgical History: Tonsillectomy, cesarean section x2.

Social History: History of 1-pack a day smoking. Stopped 10 years ago. No alcohol. Lives with husband.

Medications: Baby aspirin, lisinopril, metroprolol, atorvastatin.

ROS [review of systems]: Denies any other recent symptoms or illnesses.

Ocular Exam

Visual Acuity: OD: 20/30 OS: 20/100

IOP [intraocular pressure]: OD: 16 mmHg OS: 17 mmHg

Pupils: Equal, round, and reactive to light, no APD [afferent pupillary defect] OU

Extraocular Movements: Full OU. No nystagmus.

Confrontational Visual Fields:

Full to finger counting OU.

External: Normal, both sides.

Slip lamp: Lids, lashes, conjunctiva, sclera, cornea, anterior chamber, iris, lens, anterior vitreous, all normal OU.

Amsler Grid:

OD: Normal

OS: Blurry spot near the center of the grid with wavy lines

Dilated Fundus Exam:

OD: Clear view, CDR 0.5 with sharp optic disc margins, flat macula, scattered large soft drusen within the arcades, normal vessels and peripheral retina.

OS: Clear view, CDR 0.6 with sharp optic disc margins, flat macula, scattered soft drusen within the arcades, 1 disc area of subretinal hemorrhage in macular area near fovea.

Assessment

Wet age-related macular degeneration OU with choroidal neovascularization OS.

Plan

I am referring Mrs. Peyson to Retinal Associates for further evaluation and treatment with antivascular endothelial growth factor agents.

Osteomyelitis, Aseptic Necrosis and Joint Infection

Bone/joint/muscle infection/necrosis
HCC 39 0.425

Aseptic necrosis of bone
RxHCC 80 0.177

Any joint or bone with an underlying pathology, such as osteoarthritis, rheumatoid arthritis, or presence of a prosthesis, has a higher risk of developing infection. Nearly all codes in HCC 39 and RxHCC 80 address infection or necrosis of the bone or joint with one significant exception, necrotizing fasciitis, a bacterial infection that destroys skin, fat, fascia, muscle, and other soft tissue.

Osteomyelitis is infection or inflammation of the bone. Injury can predispose a bone or joint to infection. The injury need not be directly to the bone or joint (eg, an injury in the skin overlying the joint or bone could lead to infection). Similarly, bone infection may be caused when a pathogen enters the bloodstream and becomes established in the bone or joint, such as Salmonella, which is seen with sickle cell anemia. Traumatic injury can also cause direct infection of a joint or bone. Infection is more likely to occur in immunocompromised patients or those with impaired circulation (eg, in diabetes).

Osteomyelitis in the diabetic foot can be a complication of a chronic skin ulcer. The patient's circulation is compromised, the bone is near the surface of the skin, and the tissue erodes until the bone is affected. Introduction of an infective agent (eg, Staphylococcus) causes further destruction of soft tissue and bone in the patient, leading to necrosis (gangrene) and bone sequestration (segmental chips of bone breaking away from the blood supply). Osteomyelitis can lead to a major osseous defect that significantly weakens the bone. The major osseous defect is reported with a second code. Septic arthritis can permanently alter the structure of a joint and lead to chronic pain or disability. The inflammatory process that follows colonization of an infective agent can lead to destruction of tissue and permanent changes in the bone or joint.

Physician Documentation

For patients with joint infection, physicians should document:

- The site of the infection
- Laterality
- Organism responsible for the infection
- Whether direct joint infection or an indirect joint infection as described in ICD-10-CM
- For indirect join infection, whether postinfective or reactive arthropathy
- Any bone changes related to diabetes mellitus

Without further documentation on the infective agent in pyogenic arthritis, the disorder is reported with code M00.9, *Pyogenic arthritis, unspecified*, even if the joint site is known. For patients with bone infection, physicians should document:

- Site of the infection
- Laterality
- Organism responsible for the direct or indirection arthritis
- For chronic infections, whether acute, subacute, or other osteomyelitis
- Whether hematogenous
- Existence of any draining sinus
- Any major osseous defect
- Underlying diseases (eg diabetes), or associated injuries (eg, a previous fracture or trauma); provide information on the type of diabetes or injury that caused the osteomyelitis

Direct infection of joint
ICD-10-CM terminology described as organisms that invade synovial tissue and microbial antigen is present in the joint. Most physicians label this as "septic arthritis."

Indirect joint infection
ICD-10-CM terminology that may be of two types: a reactive arthropathy, where microbial infection of the body is established but neither organisms nor antigens can be identified in the joint, and a postinfective arthropathy in which microbial antigen is present but recovery of an organism is inconstant and evidence of local multiplication is lacking. Examples in ICD-10-CM include arthropathy following intestinal bypass surgery, dysenteric infection (eg, Yersinia, Salmonella, or Shigella), or immunization.

CDC Definitions of Osteomyelitis and Joint Infection

While physicians may use different criteria or standards in establishing the following diagnosis, the CDC National Healthcare Safety Network issued the following surveillance definitions for osteomyelitis and joint infection in January 2017:

Bone – Osteomyelitis

Osteomyelitis must meet at least ***one*** of the following criteria:

1. Patient has organism(s) identified from bone by culture or non-culture based microbiologic testing method, which is performed for purposes of clinical diagnosis and treatment (e.g., not Active Surveillance Culture/Testing [ASC/AST].
2. Patient has evidence of osteomyelitis on gross anatomic or histopathologic exam.
3. Patient has at least ***two*** of the following localized signs or symptoms: fever (>38.0°C), swelling,* pain or tenderness,* heat,* or drainage.*

And at least *one* of the following:

a. organism(s) identified from blood by culture or non-culture based microbiologic testing method which is performed for purposes of clinical diagnosis and treatment (e.g., not Active Surveillance Culture/Testing [ASC/AST].
and
imaging test evidence suggestive of infection (e.g., x-ray, CT scan, MRI, radiolabel scan [gallium, technetium, etc.]), which if equivocal is supported by clinical correlation (i.e., physician documentation of antimicrobial treatment for osteomyelitis).

b. imaging test evidence suggestive of infection (e.g., x-ray, CT scan, MRI, radiolabel scan [gallium, technetium, etc.]), which if equivocal is supported by clinical correlation (i.e., physician documentation of antimicrobial treatment for osteomyelitis).

Reporting instruction

Report mediastinitis following cardiac surgery that is accompanied by osteomyelitis as SSI-MED rather than SSI-BONE**

JNT – Joint or bursa infection

Joint or bursa infections must meet at least ***one*** of the following criteria:

1. Patient has organism(s) identified from joint fluid or synovial biopsy by culture or non-culture based microbiologic testing method which is performed for purposes of clinical diagnosis and treatment (e.g., not Active Surveillance Culture/Testing [ASC/AST].
2. Patient has evidence of joint or bursa infection on gross anatomic or histopathologic exam.
3. Patient has at least ***two*** of the following: swelling,* pain,* or tenderness,* heat,* evidence of effusion,* or limitation of motion.*

And at least *one* of the following:

a. elevated joint fluid white blood cell count (per reporting laboratory's reference range) OR positive leukocyte esterase test strip of joint fluid
b. organism(s) and white blood cells seen on Gram stain of joint fluid
c. organism(s) identified from blood by culture or non-culture based microbiologic testing method which is performed for purposes of clinical diagnosis and treatment (e.g., not Active Surveillance Culture/Testing [ASC/AST].
d. imaging test evidence suggestive of infection (e.g., x-ray, CT scan, MRI, radiolabel scan [gallium, technetium, etc.]), which if equivocal is supported by clinical correlation (i.e., physician documentation of antimicrobial treatment for joint or bursa infection).

* With no other recognized cause

(***Author's note:*** While this is true for the CDC NHSN, if both mediastinitis and sternal osteomyelitis are documented, both are coded in ICD-10-CM. In addition, ICD-10-CM requires that the physician explicitly document that it is a complication of surgery.)

The entire CDC document can be accessed at https://www.cdc.gov/nhsn/pdfs/pscmanual/17pscnosinfdef_current.pdf.

Coding

Causal links in osteomyelitis are important to report, as noted in the instruction at the beginning of the osteomyelitis section of ICD-10-CM: "Use additional code (B95-B97) to identify infectious agent."[4] There are, however, other causal links to consider when coding osteomyelitis. Coders should link osteomyelitis and diabetes mellitus, unless another cause for osteomyelitis (eg, a pressure ulcer, trauma) is documented, as osteomyelitis falls under the "with" rule in the ICD-10-CM Alphabetic Index. In diabetes with osteomyelitis, the infectious agent (eg, staphylococcus), is not a "causal agent" in this case, per se. The diabetic status of the patient precipitates the situation in which the infection can become established. Code the diabetes mellitus as the cause of osteomyelitis (eg, E11.69, *Type 2 diabetes mellitus with other specified complication*). Instructions state "Use additional code to identify complication," so identify the osteomyelitis with a code from category M86, *Osteomyelitis*. An instruction at category M86 states, "Use additional code (B95-B97) to identify infectious agent."[4] Code also the specific infection code (eg, B95.7, *Other staphylococcus as a cause of diseases classified elsewhere*). Another note directs coders to "Use addition code to identify any major osseous defect, if applicable (M89.7)."[4]

Although AHA's *Coding Clinic* (First Quarter, 2016) stated that ICD-10-CM does not presume a causal relationship between osteomyelitis and diabetes mellitus, this guidance was superseded by changes to the Alphabetic Index and to the ICD-10-CM Guideline Section I(A.15) that was published in October 2016.[11] Current guidance is to link the osteomyelitis and diabetes mellitus, unless the physician documents another cause.

CODING TIP ICD-10-CM classifies joint infections according to whether direct, indirect, or postinfective or reactive, except when the joint is prosthetic. For prosthetic joint infections, refer to the Alphabetic Index entry, "Complication/joint prosthesis/infection or inflammation."

Without further documentation on the infective agent in pyogenic arthritis, the disorder is reported with code M00.9 *Pyogenic arthritis, unspecified*, even if the joint site is known.

ABSTRACT & CODE IT!

Abstract and code the clinical coding example below. Check your answers against the answers in Appendix C.

Preoperative Diagnosis: Gangrene in chronic osteomyelitis, R second toe

Postoperative Diagnosis: Same

Patient is a 48-year-old gentleman with a 42-year history of type 1 diabetes and severe peripheral angiopathy and loss of protective sensation (LOPS). Patient has a previous history of right foot infection due to poor circulation and neuropathy. This led to a first ray resection 18 months ago. He returned last month with an ulceration on right second toe at the proximal interphalangeal joint, with *Staphylococcus aureus* invading his second phalangeal shaft. He has failed to respond to outpatient IV antibiotics, and both the soft tissue and bone of his R second digit have developed necrotic areas. He presents today for disarticulation of the second toe down to the level of the metatarsophalangeal (MTP) joint. His most recent A1C test was 7.1 and his BG [blood glucose] is currently 118, so we are going ahead with the surgery.

Operative Report: After an IV was started by Dr. Martindale, the patient was taken back to the operating room and placed on the operative table in the supine position. An ankle pneumatic tourniquet was placed around the patient's right leg. After adequate amounts of sedation had been given to the patient, we administered a block of 10 cc of 0.5% Marcaine plain in proximal digital block around the 2nd digit. The area was then prepared in the normal sterile manner. An Esmarch bandage applied to exsanguinate the foot. The tourniquet was then inflated to 250. The second toe identified. With a fresh #10 blade, skin incision was made circumferentially in the racket-shaped manner around the second toe. A #15 blade was used to deepen the incision and take it down to the second MTP joint. Care was taken to identify bleeders and cautery was used as necessary for hemostasis. After cleaning up all the soft tissue attachments, the second toe was disarticulated down to the level of the MTP joint. All remaining tissue was noted to be healthy and granular in appearance with no necrotic tissue evident. Areas of subcutaneous tissue were then removed through a sharp dissection in order to allow better approximation of the skin edges. After copious amounts of irrigation using sterile saline, deep vertical mattress sutures were used to reapproximate the skin edges and bring the plantar flap of skin up to the dorsal skin using #2-0 nylon suture. The

continued

remaining exposed tissue from the wound was covered using gauze. The wound was dressed using gauze then Kling and Kerlix dressings and an ACE bandage to provide compression. The tourniquet was deflated at 42 minutes' time and hemostasis was achieved. The ACE bandage was extended up to just below the knee and no bleeding was appreciated. The patient tolerated the procedure well with vital signs stable and vascular status intact, as was evidenced by capillary bleeding, which was present during the procedure. The patient was given postoperative introductions, and was warned to remain non-weight-bearing on his right foot. The patient was instructed to keep the foot elevated and to apply ice behind his knee as necessary, no more than 20 minutes each hour. The patient was to continue an IV antibiotic course. The patient was instructed as to signs and symptoms of infection. The excised toe was sent to pathology for examination.

Osteoporosis, Vertebral, and Pathological Fractures

Vertebral fractures without spinal cord injury
HCC 169 0.495

Osteoporosis, vertebral and pathological fractures
RxHCC 87 0.052

Osteoporosis is a reduction in the bone mineral density of the matrix structure of bone that makes a patient more susceptible to fracture. Osteoporosis affects the vertebrae by making them prone to collapse and compression, so that a patient with osteoporosis may lose several inches in height as the disease progresses. This compression may affect the nerves entering the spinal column and therefore, osteoporosis also causes significant pain and disability. Many hip fractures in the older population are caused by osteoporosis, as the head of the neck of the femur is a relative narrow part of the femur that undergoes significant stresses during ambulation. Learn more about hip fractures in the entry in Chapter 4, Part 4 under the topic, Trauma: Hip.

Risks for osteoporosis increase with age. According to the CDC, 5.1% of men eligible for Medicare (65 years or older) have osteoporosis of the femur neck or lumbar spine, compared to 24.5% of women of the same age.[12] This is in part due to the naturally denser bones of men and partially due to hormonal changes that women undergo at menopause. Poor diet and lack of weight-bearing exercise can also contribute to osteoporosis, and some medications have an adverse effect of causing osteoporosis.

To diagnose osteoporosis, the physician usually orders an X-ray bone density scan called dual-energy X-ray absorbtiometry (DEXA or DXA). The DEXA scan measures bone mineral density (BMD). Medications are available to stop the loss of, or slowly improve, bone density. NIH reports that more than 53 million people in the US either have been diagnosed with osteoporosis or are at high risk due to low bone mass.[13]

Pathological fracture describes a fracture that is the result of a medical condition rather than trauma. Pathological fractures may be caused by osteoporosis, neoplastic disease, overuse, or some other condition. Vertebrae are common sites for fracture in the elderly, and these vertebral fractures may be caused by trauma, osteoporosis, or some other bone-weakening disease. These fractures may be acute or chronic conditions.

Physician Documentation

While the ICD-10-CM Alphabetic Index considers a fracture due to osteoporosis as a pathological fracture, many physicians consider osteoporotic fractures to be traumatic fractures when selecting their diagnoses in the problem lists or billing software until they are reminded that osteoporosis is a disease, just like cancer, infection, inherited bone disorders, or bone cysts that causes pathological fractures. In addition, any documentation of the term "fragility fracture" with (as well as "due to") osteoporosis is classified in the ICD-10-CM Tabular List subcategory as M80, *Osteoporosis with current pathological fracture.* A fragility fracture is a type of

Pathological fracture
A break in a bone due to disease weakening the bone structure, occurring without any traumatic precipitating event or following only minor trauma; sometimes called an insufficiency fracture.

Traumatic fractures
Breaks in bone due to traumatic stressors upon the bone.

pathologic fracture that occurs as result of normal activities, such as a fall from standing height or less, that would not occur in normal bone under the same circumstances. Given that ICD-10-CM assumes a causal relationship between two conditions linked by the word "with" or "in" in the Alphabetic Index or Tabular List of ICD-10-CM, any fragility fracture that occurs with osteoporosis should be assigned a code for a pathological fracture. This automatic linkage of fragility fractures and osteoporosis as a pathological fracture, unfortunately, does not apply to other diseases, such as malignancies, multiple myeloma, Paget's disease, osteomalacia, and bone cysts. In those cases, the physician must use linking language (eg, pathological fracture due to secondary bone cancer).

If a fracture is traumatic, describe the circumstances. If pathological, identify the underlying pathology, such as osteoporosis or neoplastic disease. For osteoporosis, identify any causal agent (eg, long-term use of prednisone, menopause, or Cushing's syndrome).

Absent documented etiology of the fracture, coders cannot abstract the patient's condition correctly. There is no default in the Alphabetic Index for fracture, since there are separate main terms for Fracture/traumatic, Fracture/pathological, and Fracture/nontraumatic, not elsewhere classified (NEC). As such, the physician must document the underlying cause of the fracture, being aware of the options of pathological, nontraumatic, and traumatic fracture. Complete documentation eliminates the need for coder assumptions regarding the nature of the patient's fracture.

When no causal link exists between osteoporosis and a fracture in documentation, coders may turn to ICD-10-CM Guideline Section I(C.13.d.2), which states that a "code from category M80, not a traumatic fracture code, should be used for any patient with known osteoporosis who suffers a fracture, even if the patient had a minor fall or trauma, if that fall or trauma would not usually break a normal, healthy bone."[4] This gives the coder the responsibility to interpret the medical record, and creates an opportunity for error. Complete documentation eliminates the need for assumptions.

Also be very clear in documenting an episode of care, noting whether the fracture is a new diagnosis or receiving active treatment (initial encounter) or is in the healing phase (subsequent encounter). Pathological fractures only risk-adjust during the active treatment (initial encounter) phase; subsequent encounters (healing phase) do not risk-adjust. The same is true for some traumatic vertebral fractures. It is critical to capture accurately the treatment phase of the fracture (eg, active–initial encounter, healing–subsequent encounter). The ICD-10-CM guidelines provide some direction:

- Code all documented conditions that coexist at the time of the encounter/visit, and require or affect patient care treatment or management. Do not code conditions that were previously treated and no longer exist. [Section IV(J)]
- 7th character "A," initial encounter, is used for each encounter where the patient is receiving active treatment for the condition. [Section I(C.19.a.)]
- The appropriate 7th character for initial encounter should also be assigned for a patient who delayed seeking treatment for the fracture or nonunion. [Section I(C.19.c.1)][4]

DOCUMENTATION TIP Identify the episode of care for the pathological fracture as:

- **A**, initial encounter for fracture
- **D**, subsequent encounter for fracture with routine healing
- **G**, subsequent encounter for fracture with delayed healing
- **K**, subsequent encounter for fracture with nonunion
- **P**, subsequent encounter for fracture with malunion
- **S**, sequela

Identify the pathological fracture by site and laterality, as appropriate, and specify its cause as due to:

- Osteoporosis
- Neoplastic disease
- Other disease (identify disease)

Describe the fracture using the language of ICD-10-CM, eg:

- Acute/chronic
- Displaced/nondisplaced (**note:** nondisplaced is default)
- Open/closed (**note:** closed is default)
- Stable burst/unstable burst
- Pathological compression/traumatic compression
- Pathological wedge/traumatic wedge

For traumatic vertebral fractures, identify by specific site on the spine (eg, T6).

If the physician is still treating the compression fracture, it should be documented as an active fracture (initial encounter) or as follow-up when active treatment is completed and the patient is receiving routine care during healing (subsequent encounter). For follow-up after active treatment is completed, note if the fracture is resolving with routine healing or nonhealing, or with nonunion or malunion. If the fracture is resolved, document history of compression fracture. If a patient with hip pain is first diagnosed with a long-standing hip fracture, it is reported as an initial encounter, because this is when the fracture was first diagnosed, even though the patient delayed initial treatment.

CLINICAL EXAMPLES

NONSPECIFIC DOCUMENTATION	SPECIFIC DOCUMENTATION
Example 1 Compression fractures, T8-T10.[a]	**Example 1** Traumatic wedge compression fractures, T8-T10.[b]
Example 2 Fracture due to neoplastic disease.[c]	**Example 2** X ray revealed pathological fracture of the left ulna, which we determined to be metastatic cancer from the breast to the ulna. The patient underwent a right mastectomy six months ago and has completed radiation and chemotherapy.[d]

[a] A compression fracture can be traumatic, pathological, or nontraumatic, NOS. There is no default in the ICD-10-CM Alphabetic Index, so absent more information, the coder cannot report this diagnosis.

[b] Identifying the fracture as traumatic and adding that it is a wedge compression fracture will supply sufficient information for coding.

[c] Identify the site and laterality of the fracture. State if the bone cancer is primary or secondary. If secondary, identify the primary site, if known. Identify whether the primary site is still active, or if treatment has been completed.

[d] The site and laterality of the fracture, the etiology of the bone cancer, and the status of the primary cancer are captured here. The use of "from" and "to" make clear which cancer is primary.

Coding

Chapter 13 (Diseases of the Musculoskeletal System and Connective Tissue) in ICD-10-CM, explains the classification and coding of osteoporosis as "[o]steoporosis is a systemic condition, meaning that all bones of the musculoskeletal system are affected. Therefore, site is not a component of the codes under category M81, Osteoporosis without current pathological fracture. The site codes under M80, Osteoporosis with current pathological fracture, identify the site of the fracture, not the osteoporosis."[4]

If the physician does not link a fracture to documented osteoporosis, is not available for query, and it is unclear whether the fracture is due to osteoporosis or a traumatic fracture, consider these issues when determining which codes to report:

- Was there a precipitating event to the fracture (eg, a fall down stairs or from a height, an automobile accident) or other circumstance that would explain a fracture? If so, assigning the fracture as traumatic can be defended, even though it was not properly documented.
- Is there evidence in the HPI that the patient was performing normal weight-bearing activities when the fracture occurred (eg, the hip fractured when she took a step or wrist bones fracture when she lifted her purse or pushed open a door)? If so, assigning the fracture as pathological can be defended; however, assigning it as traumatic can also be defended. The organization should have a policy on how to code this type of occurrence. ICD-10-CM Guideline Section I(C.13.d.2) states that a "code from category M80, not a traumatic fracture code, should be used for any patient with known osteoporosis who suffers a fracture, even if the patient had a minor fall or trauma, if that fall or trauma would not usually break a normal, healthy bone."[4] However, it is not necessarily within a coder's anatomy knowledge to understand when what type of fall or trauma would constitute a "minor" event that should not break a bone.

Also consider that the most common sites for fragility fractures are the neck of the femur, vertebral fractures, and Colles fractures of the wrist.

 **ADVICE/ALERT NOTE**

Per ICD-10-CM Guidelines Section I(C.13.d.1) and I(C.13.d.2), "[c]ategory M81, Osteoporosis without current pathological fracture, is reported for patients with osteoporosis who do not currently have a pathologic fracture due to the osteoporosis, even if they have had a fracture in the past. For patients with a history of osteoporosis fractures, status code Z87.310, Personal history of (healed) osteoporosis fracture, should follow the code from M81.

Category M80, Osteoporosis with current pathological fracture, is for patients who have a current pathologic fracture at the time of an encounter. The codes under M80 identify the site of the fracture. A code from category M80, not a traumatic fracture code, should be used for any patient with known osteoporosis who suffers a fracture, even if the patient had a minor fall or trauma, if that fall or trauma would not usually break a normal, healthy bone."[4]

All codes from category M80, *Osteoporosis with current pathological fracture*, require seven characters. The 7th character is selected based on the character of the encounter as:

A = Initial encounter for fracture

D = Subsequent encounter for fracture with routine healing

G, = Subsequent encounter for fracture with delayed healing

K = Subsequent encounter for fracture with nonunion

P = Subsequent encounter for fracture with malunion

S = Sequela

In some cases, a 6th character "X" must be added to the code as a placeholder to ensure the code has seven characters. This rule applies to fracture codes M84.3-, *Stress fracture*; M84.4-, *Pathological fracture, not elsewhere classified*; M84.5-, *Pathological fracture in neoplastic disease*; and M84.6-, *Pathological fracture in other disease.* For compression fractures of the vertebra, report with codes from M48.5, *Collapsed vertebra, not elsewhere classified,* and 7th characters "K" and "P" do not apply.

Vertebral compression fractures may have issues with chronicity in documentation. Carefully review the documentation of a vertebral fracture to determine if the vertebral fracture is receiving active treatment, and therefore, can be reported as "initial encounter;" if the fracture is in a healed state; or if the vertebral fracture is a chronic fracture that is receiving subsequent care during routine healing. Only initial encounters or those receiving active treatment for pathological vertebral fractures risk-adjust.

In ICD-10-CM, "chronic fracture" classifies as pathological fractures, as indicated in the Alphabetic Index entry under "Chronic." Insufficiency fractures also classify as pathological fractures. "Collapsed vertebra" has its own subcategory, M48.5, *Collapsed vertebra, not elsewhere classified*, but pathological, stress, and traumatic fractures are excluded from that subcategory. Before October 1, 2017, a new vertebral collapse in the presence of osteoporosis could not be assumed to be a pathological fracture. This changed on October 1, 2017, when the *ICD-10-CM Guidelines* were changed to allow the term "in" within a term in the Alphabetic Index or Tabular List to be automatically linked unless the physician explicitly documents another cause.

Compression fractures
Bone fractures causing collapse, usually vertebral; may be traumatic or pathological. In vertebral compression fractures, the bone collapses into itself, flattening, causing loss of height and, in in some cases, pain from spinal nerve compression. Compression fractures of the vertebral column occur most commonly in patients with osteoporosis.

Collapse R55
vertebra M48.50-
in (due to)
metastasis -*see* Collapse, vertebra, in, specified disease NEC
osteoporosis -*see also* Osteoporosis M80.88
cervical region M80.88
cervicothoracic region M80.88
lumbar region M80.88
lumbosacral region M80.88
multiple sites M80.88
occipito-atlanto-axial region M80.88
sacrococcygeal region M80.88
thoracic region M80.88
thoracolumbar region M80.88
specified disease NEC M48.50-
cervical region M48.52-
cervicothoracic region M48.53-
lumbar region M48.56-
lumbosacral region M48.57-
occipito-atlanto-axial region M48.51-
sacrococcygeal region M48.58-
thoracic region M48.54-
thoracolumbar region M48.55-

Notice how collapsed vertebrae "in" osteoporosis are classified as a pathological fracture (M80), whereas those "in" other specified diseases are not (M48). "Compression," however, can indicate a traumatic fracture, as reported with wedge compression codes from S22, *Fracture of thoracic vertebra,* and S32, *Fracture of lumbar spine and pelvis.*

A pathological compression fracture of the spine may be documented as OVCF (osteoporotic vertebral compression fracture) or VCF (vertebral compression fracture); the first term is coded as a pathological fracture, whereas the second term is not. Documented compression fracture or wedging of the vertebra is reported with a code from M48.5, *Collapsed vertebra, not elsewhere classified,* if no pathological, stress, or traumatic etiology is documented. The codes in M48.5 for an initial encounter also risk-adjust. Traumatic vertebral fractures risk-adjust to the same HCCs and RxHCCs in some cases as pathological fractures.

DEXA Scores

Coders cannot abstract diagnoses from DEXA scores, but the scores do offer a glimpse of the patient's bone health and can be used as support for the physician's diagnosis:

- BMD reports the bone mineral density. Any number of +1.0 or higher is considered normal.
- T score compares the patient's BMD to the average bone density during peak years for women.
  - Score of -1.0 and -2.5 standard deviation (SD) is suggestive of osteopenia.
  - Score of less than -2.5 SD indicates osteoporosis.
  - Score of less than -2.5 SD with fragility fracture indicates severe osteoporosis.

Documentation about osteoporosis and pathological fractures is often found in descriptions in the physical exam (dowager hump, loss of height), in discussion of DEXA tests or BMD, and a plan including increasing calcium and vitamin D intake and exercise. Common medications to treat osteoporosis include alendronate, risedronate, zoledronic acid, and denosumab.

ABSTRACT & CODE IT!

Abstract and code the clinical coding example below. Check your answers against the answers in Appendix C.

Patient 1
A 78-year-old female reports she heard a crack and felt severe pain in her lower back while emptying the dishwasher. She is diagnosed with a new compression fracture of the L-3 vertebra. She has chronic compression fractures secondary to osteoporosis at T-7 and T-8. She is on alendronate and supplemental vitamin D for the osteoporosis.

Patient 2
Kyphosis due to multiple collapsed vertebra in the patient's thoracic spine, secondary to osteoporosis. New full-body bone densitometry has been ordered. We are fitting her for a brace to help reduce back pain.

Patient 3
MRI reveals a stable burst fracture of T-3. We will treat him conservatively with NSAIDs for now, and see if his symptoms improve.

Pancreatic Disorders

Chronic pancreatitis
HCC 34 0.276
RxHCC 65 0.265

Pancreatic disorders and intestinal malabsorption, except pancreatitis
RxHCC 66 0.105

The pancreas is a large gland in the abdomen that contains both endocrine and exocrine components, meaning it secretes hormones directly into the blood (endocrine function; insulin and glucagon hormones) and excretes enzymes into localized ducts (exocrine function; digestive enzymes). To facilitate digestion, the head of the pancreas communicates with the duodenum through the pancreatic duct and common bile duct just prior to the ampulla of Vater. Digestive enzymes flow through this duct to aid in the breakdown of proteins, lipids, and carbohydrates in food. More than 90% of pancreatic tissue is devoted to exocrine activities. The pancreas also houses the islets of Langerhans, which manufacture insulin used to metabolize sugars in the bloodstream, and glucagon, stored in the liver and released to regulate blood glucose levels to prevent hypoglycemia.

Pancreatitis is a painful inflammation of the pancreas that can disrupt the functions of the pancreas, and in severe cases, lead to permanent damage. Acute pancreatitis often occurs with the presence of gallstones or with heavy alcohol use, and usually requires hospitalization. While acute pancreatitis does not risk-adjust, a systemic inflammatory response syndrome (two out of the following: tachycardia, tachypnea, elevated white count, fever) or an acute organ failure (eg, acute kidney injury, distributive shock) that occurs in reaction to the pancreatitis does risk-adjust.

Chronic pancreatitis (CP) is a continual inflammation of the pancreas that usually gets worse over time. Heavy alcohol use is the most common cause of CP, although it can also be caused by hyperlipidemia, cystic fibrosis, or certain autoimmune conditions. With fibrosis and scarring, the ducts carrying enzymes from the pancreas may become stenosed, and its own digestive fluids can inflame or destroy pancreatic tissue. Patients with CP lose weight because they are not able to digest food properly. Scarring and damage to the pancreas can lead to irreversible changes and secondary diabetes mellitus, requiring insulin injections. The risk of pancreatic cancer increases in patients with CP.

Numerous digestive disorders are captured in RxHCC 66, most of which have to do with pancreatic conditions. Notably, celiac disease risk-adjusts for RxHCCs. Celiac disease is an autoimmune disease that carries with it an intolerance for gluten, a protein found in wheat, rye, and barley. Individuals with celiac disease have an inflammation of the proximal small intestinal mucosa. They avoid gluten to prevent gastrointestinal disturbances.

Physician Documentation

Pancreatitis is classified in ICD-10-CM as either an acute form or a chronic form. There are various etiologies for each type, and the two can coexist in a patient with an acute exacerbation of a CP. Only chronic pancreatitis risk-adjusts for HCCs (see Table 4-3.6), although some varieties of pancreatic disorders risk-adjust for RxHCCs (see Table 4-3.7).

TABLE 4-3.6 Risk-adjusting Pancreatitis Codes (HCC)

CODE	DESCRIPTION
K86.0	Alcohol-induced chronic pancreatitis
K86.1	Other chronic pancreatitis

Alcohol-induced CP should be documented with an alcohol status diagnosis (eg, alcohol dependence in remission or current alcohol abuse or dependence). Also note any exocrine pancreatic insufficiency as a result of the pancreatitis.

TABLE 4-3.7 Risk-Adjusting Pancreatic Disorder Codes (RxHCC)

CODE	DESCRIPTION
E16.3	Increased secretion of glucagon
E16.4	Increased secretion of gastrin
E16.8	Other specified disorders of pancreatic internal secretion
E16.9	Disorder of pancreatic internal secretion, unspecified
K86.2	Cyst of pancreas
K86.3	Pseudocyst of pancreas
K86.81	Exocrine pancreatic insufficiency
K86.89	Other specified diseases of pancreas
K86.9	Disease of pancreas, unspecified
K87	Disorders of gallbladder, biliary tract and pancreas in diseases classified elsewhere
K90.0	Celiac disease
K90.1	Tropical sprue
K90.2	Blind loop syndrome, not elsewhere classified
K90.3	Pancreatic steatorrhea
K90.49	Malabsorption due to intolerance, not elsewhere classified
K90.81	Whipple's disease
K90.89	Other intestinal malabsorption
K90.9	Intestinal malabsorption, unspecified
K91.2	Postsurgical malabsorption, not elsewhere classified

For code K87, *Disorders of gallbladder, biliary tract and pancreas in diseases classified elsewhere,* also document the disease (eg, cytomegaloviral pancreatitis or tuberculosis of gallbladder). Codes with a description stating "in diseases classified elsewhere" always require a second diagnosis to identify the disease causing the condition.

Diabetes mellitus is a common complication of CP. Document any link between the pancreatitis and the diabetes mellitus so that the correct secondary diabetes code may be abstracted.

Because celiac disease is a chronic and incurable disease that is managed almost exclusively by the patient with dietary control (eg, gluten-free diet), it is often underdocumented, appearing only in the patient's problem list or PMH. Discuss and document with the celiac patient his or her symptoms, dietary habits, and nutritional requirements and monitor the patient for malnutrition at least annually. Document any symptoms associated with the malabsorption that accompanies celiac disease, whether gastrointestinal or related to dental or bone disorders, joint pain, or mouth sores. For patients with newly diagnosed celiac disease, document any order for dietetic counseling.

CLINICAL EXAMPLES

NONSPECIFIC DOCUMENTATION	SPECIFIC DOCUMENTATION
Example 1 ERCP confirmed pancreatitis.[a]	**Example 1** Endoscopic retrograde cholangiopancreatography (ERCP) confirmed chronic pancreatitis due to alcohol dependence, in remission.[b]
Example 2 Acute[c] on chronic pancreatitis.	**Example 2** Pancreatitis with necrosis on chronic pancreatitis due to cystic fibrosis,[d] with exocrine pancreatic insufficiency.

[a] Spell out acronym on first use. Identify type of pancreatitis and its cause.

[b] Physician correctly documents alcohol status in the patient with alcoholic pancreatitis.

[c] There are numerous subclassifications for acute pancreatitis. Specify the type.

[d] The acute pancreatitis has been specified due to cystic fibrosis, and other manifestations named.

Coding

According to ICD-10-CM Guideline Section I(B.8), "[i]f the same condition is described as both acute (subacute) and chronic, and separate subentries exist in the Alphabetic Index at the same indentation level, code both and sequence the acute (subacute) code first."[4] If a physician documents acute on chronic pancreatitis, code both conditions according to the guidelines, as each subentry (acute and chronic) is at the same indentation level in the Alphabetic Index under "Pancreatitis." In addition, code both if the physician documents an acute exacerbation of CP. The ICD-10-CM default for pancreatitis without documentation specifying acute or chronic is K85.90, *Acute pancreatitis without necrosis or infection, unspecified.* Documented "gallstone pancreatitis" is classified by ICD-10-CM to biliary pancreatitis.

Typically, acute pancreatitis is treated inpatient, but CP may not be. CP generally gets worse over time and leads to permanent damage of the pancreas.

For patients with celiac disease, report code K90.0, *Celiac disease*, as well as any specific manifestations of the disease (eg, dermatitis, gluten ataxia, malabsorption or malnutrition, or exocrine pancreatic insufficiency). Gastrointestinal symptoms are not reported separately with celiac disease.

ADVICE/ALERT NOTE

Per ICD-10-CM Guideline Section I(B.8), "[i]f the same condition is described as both acute (subacute) and chronic, and separate subentries exist in the Alphabetic Index at the same indentation level, code both and sequence the acute (subacute) code first."[4]

ABSTRACT & CODE IT!

Abstract and code the clinical coding example below. Check your answers against the answers in Appendix C.

Patient 1

Acute pancreatitis due to adverse effect of sitagliptin, initial encounter.

Patient 2

Endoscopic retrograde cholangiopancreatography (ERCP) confirmed chronic pancreatitis due to alcohol dependence, in remission.

Patient 3

Acute biliary pancreatitis with necrosis on chronic pancreatitis due to cystic fibrosis, with exocrine pancreatic insufficiency.

Paralysis, Malformation of Brain/Spinal Cord

Quadriplegia
HCC 70 **1.314**

Paraplegia
HCC 71 **1.007**

Spinal cord disorders/injuries
HCC 72 **0.528**
RxHCC 157 **0.114**

Hemiplegia/hemiparesis
HCC 103 **0.538**

Monoplegia, other paralytic syndromes
HCC 104 **0.395**

Spastic hemiplegia
RxHCC 207 **0.191**

Paralysis or neurological weakness may be caused by a brain injury or a spinal cord injury (SCI) or a peripheral nerve injury. Hemiplegia or hemiparesis, a unilateral paralysis or weakness, is associated with traumatic brain injury (TBI) or cerebrovascular accident. In hemiplegia, paralysis affects only the right or left side of the body and involves both the upper and lower extremity. Bilateral strokes may cause quadriparesis, which is reported as quadriplegia. In monoplegia or monoparesis, only one extremity is affected. In many cases, therapies can restore some or all functions lost due to hemiplegia or monoplegia following stroke or TBI.

According to the National Spinal Cord Injury Association, as many as 450,000 people in the US are living with a SCI, however, other organizations conservatively estimate this figure to be about 250,000.[14] Approximately 11,000 new SCIs occur each year in the US, and 51.3% of the new injuries occur in persons between 16 and 30 years of age and of this, 81.2% are males.[14]

The spinal cord is a bundled cord of nerves that travels through the vertebral canal in the center of the spine. Motor nerve roots exit the anterior (ventral) spinal cord bilaterally at each level, sending signals to the brain from the peripheral nervous system (PNS). Sensory serve roots enter the posterior (dorsal) spinal cord bilaterally at each level, sending signals to the PNS from the brain. There are 8 cervical, 12 thoracic, 5 lumbar, 5 sacral, and 1 coccygeal spinal cord levels.

The scope of an SCI depends on the spinal cord site and level affected. Spinal nerve roots are identified according to the site of their insertion or emergence along the vertebral canal.

Because nerves branch off from the spinal cord at each vertebral level beginning in the neck, the number of nerves in the spinal cord decreases the more distal from the brain. As a result, the further down the spine an SCI occurs, the lesser number of nerves affected by an SCI. A significant cervical injury may cause quadriplegia; a lumbar injury may cause paraplegia.

In a complete SCI, the full thickness of the cord is damaged, so that all nerves distal to the site are damaged. Almost half of all SCIs are complete. In an incomplete SCI, some nerve pathways distal to the SCI are preserved and some function remains (eg, loss may be sensory, motor, unilateral, or a mix). For more information on SCI, see http://www.aans.org/Patients/Neurosurgical-Conditions-and-Treatments/Spinal-Cord-Injury.

While the vertebral column provides significant protection to the spinal cord, during times of injury, the bony pathway can contribute to injury. Pressure from swelling or hemorrhage following injury can pinch the nerve and cause temporary paralysis or other symptoms and may lead to permanent damage if blood supply is compromised and ischemia and tissue death occur.

Dermatomes have been mapped for each of 31 pairs of spinal nerve roots. A dermatome represents an specific skin area tied to 1 of the 31 pairs of bilateral spinal nerve roots. Because dermatomes map only to one nerve root level, it may be possible to derive from the site of a skin sensory abnormality the level of a spinal nerve root defect.

Physician Documentation

When documenting the condition of a patient with longstanding paralysis, document the cause (eg, sequela from motor vehicle accident), and also identify the following:

- For paralysis or weakness of both lower extremities, document paraplegia as complete or incomplete.
- For quadriplegia, document C1-C4 or C5-C7 as the level of injury, and document complete or incomplete.
- Specify functional quadriplegia as appropriate if the patient's complete immobility is due to severe physical disability or frailty.
- For monoplegia or monoparesis, identify upper or lower extremity, laterality, and dominant side and its underlying cause.
- Document any paralytic syndrome as locked-in state, Brown-Sequard syndrome, anterior cord syndrome, posterior cord syndrome, or Todd's paralysis.
- Identify any monoplegia, monoparesis, hemiplegia, or hemiparesis by site and as due to TBI, nontraumatic subarachnoid hemorrhage, nontraumatic intracerebral hemorrhage, cerebral infarct, or other cerebrovascular disease.

DOCUMENTATION TIP The exact term "functional quadriplegia" is optimally documented for abstraction of code R53.2, *Functional quadriplegia*; however, documentation of the term "complete immobility due to a severe physical disability or severe frailty" may suffice, given this is a subterm under R53.2. Functional quadriplegia may be seen in advanced cases of motor neuron disease, dementia, severe cases of rheumatoid arthritis, or severe physical deconditioning. It is acceptable to document functional quadriplegia for patients with quadriplegia due to amyotrophic lateral sclerosis (ALS) or Guillain-Barre syndrome (GBS), if the patient's physical impairment is so severe that the patient is completely immobile and all activities of daily living are performed by someone else. Both neurological quadriplegia and functional quadriplegia map to HCC 70, *Quadriplegia*.

Note also that in the ICD-10-CM Alphabetic Index, the term "quadriparesis," indicative of neurological weakness of all four extremities, is equivalent to "quadriplegia," a neurological paralysis of all four extremities. Many physicians are hesitant to assign a quadriplegia code if the patient is not paralyzed, missing the opportunity to adequately report the severity of the patient's condition. Physicians must be encouraged to use terminology and coding for monoplegia, hemiplegia, paraplegia, or quadriplegia when corresponding paretic conditions are present, given that ICD-10-CM equates "plegia" with "paresis."

For patients with traumatic injury, document the site of the cord lesion including:

- Episode of care as initial, subsequent care, or sequela
- Level at which the injury occurred (eg, C6-C7)
- Whether the injury was:
  - Complete
  - Incomplete

- Central cord syndrome
- Anterior cord syndrome
- Brown-Sequard syndrome
- Other specified cord syndromes that the physician may desire to describe

For patients with hemiplegia (hemiparesis) or monoplegia (monoparesis) following stroke, link the hemiplegia to the stroke and identify the laterality. Specify the type of stroke as nontraumatic intracerebral hemorrhage, nontraumatic intracranial hemorrhage, nontraumatic subarachnoid hemorrhage, or cerebral infarction. Also identify the patient's dominant side so that the severity of the paralysis is captured.

One of the most devastating consequences of a neurodegenerative illness is the loss of one's mobility, resulting in frequent falls and trauma and requiring total care that is quite expensive. Some patients with dementia or other debilitating illness become so incapacitated that they become bedridden, chair-ridden, or wheelchair-confined. They cannot move from one place to another without total assistance.

To address this, ICD-10-CM introduced the term "functional quadriplegia" in 2008, which, when queried on http://www.pubmed.gov, has no clinical literature to define it. As such, only the ICD-10-CM Alphabetic Index, the *ICD-10-CM Official Guidelines for Coding and Reporting*, or the AHA's *Coding Clinic for ICD-9-CM* has supplied the clinical indicators supporting this diagnosis. These include:

1. **ICD-10-CM Alphabetic Index:** Complete immobility due to severe physical disability or frailty.
2. ***ICD-10-CM Official Guidelines for Coding and Reporting* (2017):** Functional quadriplegia (R53.2) is the lack of ability to use one's limbs or to ambulate due to extreme debility. It is not associated with neurologic deficit or injury, and code R53.2 should not be used for cases of neurologic quadriplegia. It should only be assigned if functional quadriplegia is specifically documented in the medical record.
3. **AHA's *Coding Clinic for ICD-9-CM* (Fourth Quarter, 2008):** The inability to move due to another condition (eg, dementia, severe contractures, arthritis, etc). The patient is immobile because of a severe physical disability or frailty. There is usually some underlying cause, which most often will involve severe dementia. The individual does not have the mental ability to ambulate and functionally is the same as a paralyzed person.

The guidance on functional quadriplegia was deleted from the 2018 *ICD-10-CM Guidelines*. Therefore, as of October 1, 2017, the only definition of functional quadriplegia that exists is the listing in the ICD-10-CM Alphabetic Index, which is a complete immobility due to severe physical disability or frailty, or that of the AHA's *Coding Clinic* cited earlier.

To meet the ICD-10-CM definition of functional quadriplegia, the patient must meet all of the following criteria:

1. The patient must be completely immobile, which means that he or she is bedbound or, perhaps in some cases, chair-bound, requiring total care. Envision what the mobility of an individual with a spinal cord injury would look like: the mobility of a patient with functional quadriplegia would resemble this. Can this patient feed himself or herself? If patients with a spinal cord injury can feed themselves, then those with functional quadriplegia can, too. They just cannot move themselves to go get the food, thus they require total care.
2. The patient's immobility must be *due to* a severe physical disability or frailty, not just *with* a severe physical disability or frailty. For example, an individual with a severe alcohol use disorder upon which cirrhosis, ascites, extreme sarcopenia, and severe malnutrition ensued. Upon arrival to the hospital, she could not ambulate because of her extreme frailty. The physician documented that she had functional quadriplegia, given that she was completely immobile due to extreme frailty. Another case can be one with severe contractures that make the patient bedbound or a patient with an end-stage dementing illness who would immediately fall if he or she were to try and ambulate.
3. The patient cannot have a significant neurological quadriparesis or quadriplegia that would explain the immobility, given that there is an Excludes1 note for functional quadriplegia and neurological quadriplegia.

CLINICAL EXAMPLES

NONSPECIFIC DOCUMENTATION	SPECIFIC DOCUMENTATION
Example 1 The patient is bedridden.[a]	**Example 1** The patient has full-time caregivers due to her functional quadriplegia brought on by advanced progressive multiple sclerosis.[b]
Example 2 Martin was referred to Mountain View Physical Therapy for his persisting monoplegia.[c]	**Example 2** Martin was referred to Mountain View Physical Therapy for persisting weakness in his right arm, related to the cerebral infarction he experienced in May. He is right-handed.[d]

[a] This is not a diagnosis at all and covers a spectrum of illness severities.

[b] The extent of the patient's physical limitations is well defined, and its etiology is explained.

[c] The site and cause of the monoplegia should be documented.

[d] The site and cause are documented, as well as the specific type of stroke the patient had and the patient's right-handedness.

Coding

Codes from category G82, *Paraplegia (paraparesis) and quadriplegia (quadriparesis),* are reported alone only when the condition is not further specified in the record or is longstanding but of unspecified cause. If the cause is known and unrelated to stroke, report a code from category G82 to identify the paralysis, and a code identifying the circumstance that led to the paralysis (eg, S34.115S, *Complete lesion of L5 level of lumbar spinal cord, sequela*). A code for the external cause of the injury is also appropriate (eg, W11.XXXS, *Fall on and from ladder, sequela*), although it is seldom documented in long-standing conditions.

According to ICD-10-CM Guideline Section I(B.10), "[a] sequela is the residual effect (condition produced) after the acute phase of an illness or injury has terminated. There is no time limit on when a sequela code can be used. The residual may be apparent early, such as in cerebral infarction, or it may occur months or years later, such as that due to a previous injury. Examples of sequela include: scar formation resulting from a burn, deviated septum due to a nasal fracture, and infertility due to tubal occlusion from old tuberculosis. Coding of sequela generally requires two codes sequenced in the following order: the condition or nature of the sequela is sequenced first. The sequela code is sequenced second."[4]

ADVICE/ALERT NOTE

Per ICD-10-CM Guideline Section I(B.10), a "sequela is the residual effect (condition produced) after the acute phase of an illness or injury has terminated. There is no time limit on when a sequela code can be used. The residual may be apparent early, such as in cerebral infarction, or it may occur months or years later, such as that due to a previous injury. Examples of sequela include: scar formation resulting from a burn, deviated septum due to a nasal fracture, and infertility due to tubal occlusion from old tuberculosis. Coding of sequela generally requires two codes sequenced in the following order: the condition or nature of the sequela is sequenced first. The sequela code is sequenced second."[4]

According to ICD-10-CM Guideline Section I(C.6.a):

> Codes from category G81, Hemiplegia and hemiparesis, and subcategories G83.1, Monoplegia of lower limb, G83.2, Monoplegia of upper limb, and G83.3, Monoplegia, unspecified, identify whether the dominant or nondominant side is affected. Should the affected side be documented, but not specified as dominant or nondominant, and the classification system does not indicate a default, code selection is as follows:
>
> - For ambidextrous patients, the default should be dominant.
> - If the left side is affected, the default is non-dominant.
> - If the right side is affected, the default is dominant.
>
> When coding a traumatic spinal cord injury affecting more than one site along the cord, code to the highest level for that segment of spine, e.g., one code to identify the highest level injured for each site: cervical, thoracic, lumbar, or sacral spine. Also report any concurrent fractures, open wounds, or transient paralysis."[4]

Clinical Documentation Integrity and Coding

ADVICE/ALERT NOTE

Per ICD-10-CM Guideline Section I(C.6.a), "[c]odes from category G81, Hemiplegia and hemiparesis, and subcategories G83.1, Monoplegia of lower limb, G83.2, Monoplegia of upper limb, and G83.3, Monoplegia, unspecified, identify whether the dominant or nondominant side is affected. Should the affected side be documented, but not specified as dominant or nondominant, and the classification system does not indicate a default, code selection is as follows:

- For ambidextrous patients, the default should be dominant.
- If the left side is affected, the default is non-dominant.
- If the right side is affected, the default is dominant."[4]

Query the physician if monoplegia (monoparesis) or hemiplegia (hemiparesis) is noted in a patient with a history of stroke to determine the cause of the paralysis. Select the appropriate code based on the paralysis and its stroke etiology: nontraumatic subarachnoid, intracerebral, intracranial hemorrhage, or cerebral infarction. If documentation links a cerebrovascular accident to hemiplegia or monoplegia, AHA's *Coding Clinic* (First Quarter, 2017) says to report the condition as sequela of a stroke with a code from category I69, *Sequela of cardiovascular disease.*[15]

CODING TIP The immobility that accompanies paralysis can lead to pressure ulcers. The Braden Scale for Predicting Pressure Sore Risk is a preventive tool for clinicians, which allows them to document a patient's risk of developing pressure ulcers from being immobile or having limited mobility. It assesses the sensory perception, skin moisture, activity, nutrition, friction and shear, and mobility of the patient. Coders must never abstract from Braden Scale scores, as coders cannot report test findings and Braden Scale scores are usually documented by nurses, whose documentation is unacceptable for ICD-10-CM code assignment and RA. However, low Braden Scale scores for mobility would be a cause to query the physician regarding the patient's mobility status and its underlying causes. A Braden Scale score may also be used as support for a paralysis-related diagnosis. A copy of the Braden Scale scoring table can be viewed or downloaded at http://www.bradenscale.com/images/bradenscale.pdf.

Functional quadriplegia is a form of quadriplegia in which the patient's spinal column has not been injured, but the patient is unable to move independently due to severe weakness or debility, as seen in patients with advanced stages of MS, Alzheimer's, or ALS. Functional quadriplegia risk-adjusts and may be documented as "complete immobility," which is found in the Alphabetic Index under "Immobile, immobility/complete, due to severe physical disability or frailty," and classifies to code R53.2, *Functional quadriplegia.*

ABSTRACT & CODE IT!

Abstract and code the clinical coding example below. Check your answers against the answers in Appendix C.

Patient 1

The patient is a 27-year-old wheelchair-bound paraplegic, due to an accident 10 years ago with a complete spinal cord lesion at T10. He is here today for evaluation of inflammation at his colostomy site, which is clearly *Candida albicans*. The patient was prescribed miconazole, and he and his wife were counseled on stoma hygiene to prevent recurrence.

Patient 2

The patient has full-time care due to her functional quadriplegia brought on by advanced progressive multiple sclerosis.

Patient 3

Martin was referred to Mountain View Physical Therapy for persisting weakness in his right arm related to the cerebral infarction he experienced in May. He is right-handed.

Parkinson's and Huntington's Disease

Parkinson disease and Huntington disease

HCC 78 0.674
RxHCC 161 0.505

Parkinson disease (PD) and Huntington disease (HD) are both disorders in which symptoms arise as brain cells are destroyed. Both disorders are progressive, but while HD is a genetic disorder that usually manifests itself between the ages of 30 and 50,[16] researchers believe PD has both genetic and environmental factors, and usually is first diagnosed in people who are older than 50.[17] Symptoms in PD include tremor in extremities, stiffness of limbs, and impaired balance. About 20% of PD patients have dementia.[18] In PD, production of the neurotransmitter dopamine is defective. The symptoms are progressive and may eventually interfere with activities of daily living. Most cases of PD are primary and idiopathic. Secondary PD may be caused by medications, hydrocephalus, or some toxins.

Offspring of parents with HD have a 50-50 chance of inheriting the HD gene and developing HD later in life.[16] It can affect either sex. People with HD usually live for 15 or 20 years after becoming symptomatic.[16] Symptoms include problems with muscle control and coordination, which can lead to slurred speech, difficulty swallowing, and unsteadiness. Psychiatric symptoms occur as the symptoms worsen. According to the CDC, more than 30,000 people in the US have HD.[16] The American Parkinson Disease Association estimates there are 1 million Americans in the US with PD.[19]

Physician Documentation

Patients who test positive for the HD gene may do so without clinical symptoms or a clinical diagnosis of HD, usually in the context of an encounter for genetic counseling related to procreation. There is no mechanism in the Alphabetic Index of ICD-10-CM to guide coders as to how to report a diagnosis for a patient who has tested positive for the HD gene but has not yet developed HD. The closest code is Z91.89, *Other specified personal risk factors, not elsewhere classified.* Take care to document if the patient does not yet have a diagnosis of HD, but only a positive genetic test, and direct in documentation how this should be coded. Similarly, if clinical changes have been detected, document HD clearly, even if the symptoms are as yet minor. All symptoms of HD at all stages should be documented clearly, whether movement, cognitive, or psychiatric disorders.

Patients with PD have motor symptoms in the early stages of the disease that are largely considered signs and symptoms that would not be separately reported. Nonmotor symptoms of PD are also common, and similar to those of HD. Nonmotor symptoms of HD and PD should be documented and addressed, and may include:

- Cognitive impairment, including dementia
- Constipation, spastic bladder, loss of libido, or incontinence
- Major depression, anxiety, psychosis, delirium, and other significant behavioral disorders
- Dysphagia, with potential for malnutrition or gastrostomy tube placement

Clarify whether these symptoms are complications of the PD or HD, or in the case of PD, adverse effects of medication. Identify issues that may affect activities of daily living, including mobility, bathing, and psychiatric challenges. PD and HD are not the only disorders that involve systemic atrophy of the central nervous system that risk-adjust (see Table 4-3.8).

TABLE 4-3.8 Risk-Adjusting Codes for Parkinson's and Huntington's Diseases

CODE	DESCRIPTION
G10	Huntington's disease
G20	Parkinson's disease
G21.11	Neuroleptic induced parkinsonism
G21.19	Other drug induced secondary parkinsonism
G21.2	Secondary parkinsonism due to other external agents
G21.3	Postencephalitic parkinsonism
G21.4	Vascular parkinsonism
G21.8	Other secondary parkinsonism
G21.9	Secondary parkinsonism, unspecified
G23.0	Hallervorden-Spatz disease
G23.1	Progressive supranuclear ophthalmoplegia [Steele-Richardson-Olszewski]
G23.2	Striatonigral degeneration
G23.8	Other specified degenerative diseases of basal ganglia
G23.9	Degenerative disease of basal ganglia, unspecified
G90.3	Multi-system degeneration of the autonomic nervous system

Coding

HD and PD are both irreversible, progressive diseases of the central nervous system. Query the physician if either condition is noted as a "history of" disorder or appears in PMH in documentation.

Carefully read the documentation of patients with a new diagnosis of HD. Patients with a family history of HD are often tested to determine if they carry the gene, and if they carry the gene, they will develop HD. Often, this testing occurs when the patient is considering procreation, because the patient may want to ensure offspring will not be at risk for inheriting the disease. A patient who tests positive for HD will develop HD, but the test result itself is not a diagnosis of HD. This is similar to HIV-positive status not being the same as AIDS, the difference being that in the case of HD, every patient who is HD-positive will develop the disease. The earliest symptoms of HD are usually cognitive. The physician will make the clinical decision of when a diagnosis of HD is appropriate. There is no code for reporting the risk associated with a positive HD test. The best choice in ICD-10-CM would be code Z91.89, *Other specified personal risk factors, not elsewhere classified.*

Patients with a diagnosis of PD or HD have a wide range of symptoms and complications, from a slight tremor to functional quadriplegia. For patients with PD or HD, report all manifestations of the disorder, with the exception of motor nerve dysfunctions like bradykinesia and tremor or chorea.

CODING TIP The ICD-10-CM Alphabetic Index entry, "Parkinson's disease syndrome or tremor – *see* Parkinsonism," can be misleading. Parkinsonism is defined as tremor and abnormalities in movement. Patients with PD, a specific neurological disorder, have parkinsonism, but not all patients with parkinsonism have PD. It is best to ignore this PD entry in the Alphabetic Index, and make a note there to go to G20, *Parkinson's disease.*

Code PD or parkinsonism with dementia without behavioral disturbance as follows:

Dementia due to PD:

G20	Parkinson's disease
F02.80	Dementia in diseases classified elsewhere without behavioral disturbance

Dementia due to parkinsonism:

G31.83	Dementia with Lewy bodies
F20.80	Dementia in diseases classified elsewhere without behavioral disturbance

Bradykinesia
Hesitation in initiating movement, and slowed movements once initiated.

Parkinsonism
Tremor and slowness of movement as a symptom.

Akinesia
Impairment of voluntary motor controls affecting movement, creating difficulty in movement.

Symptoms of PD and HD include bradykinesia, tremor, akinesia, poor balance, impaired speech, and rigid muscles. Not all symptoms are motor symptoms, as the disorders can also cause significant neuropsychiatric and autonomic symptoms, including depression, dementia, psychosis, sleep disorders, urinary complications, and constipation. While bradykinesia, tremor, akinesia, balance, and muscle problems are normal in PD and HD, other manifestations would be reported secondarily if addressed in the encounter.

The most common treatment for PD is a prescription to levodopa, which can temporarily reduce tremors in patients. In some patients, brain surgeries are performed to treat PD, including the implantation of deep brain stimulators. There are no medications or surgeries effective in treating HD, but documentation should address issues like psychiatric and cognitive function, activities of daily living, and pressure ulcer prevention.

ABSTRACT & CODE IT!

Abstract and code the clinical coding example below. Check your answers against the answers in Appendix C.

Code the following operative report:

Preoperative Diagnosis: 1. Moderate protein calorie malnutrition. 2. Huntington disease.

Postoperative Diagnosis: 1. Moderate protein calorie malnutrition. 2. Huntington disease.

Procedure: EGD with PEG tube placement.

Indications: This 47-year-old man has severe dysphagia as a result of his Huntington disease, and this has caused decreased p.o. intake and significant weight loss. He currently weighs 126 pounds with a BMI of 16.6 and is here today for placement of a gastrostomy tube so that he can take supplemental nutrition.

Procedure: The patient was taken to the operating room and placed in the supine position. The area was prepped and draped in the sterile fashion. After adequate IV sedation was obtained, esophagogastroduodenoscopy was performed. The esophagus, stomach, and duodenum were visualized without difficulty. There was no gross evidence of any disease process. The appropriate location was noted on the anterior wall of the stomach. This area was localized externally with 1% lidocaine. Large-gauge needle was used to enter the lumen of the stomach under

continued

endoscopic visualization. A guidewire was then passed again under visualization and the needle was subsequently removed. A scalpel was used to make a small incision down through the fascia next to the guidewire. A dilator with break-away sheath was then inserted over the guidewire and under direct visualization was seen to enter the lumen of the stomach. The guidewire and dilator were removed again and the PEG tube was placed through the sheath and endoscopically visualized within the stomach. The balloon was then insufflated and the sheath was pulled away. Proper placement of the tube was confirmed through the endoscope. The tube was then sutured into place using nylon suture. The endoscope was removed. Appropriate sterile dressing was applied.

Disposition: The patient was transferred to the recovery room in stable condition.

Pathological Fracture – *see* Osteoporosis, Vertebral and Pathological Fracture

Pemphigus

Pemphigus
RxHCC 314 0.356

Pemphigus is a chronic autoimmune disease that causes blistering on the skin of the patient. Pemphigus vulgaris causes fragile blisters to break out on the skin, and these blisters rupture to produce painful open lesions that can be fatal without treatment with corticosteroids; pemphigus foliaceous attacks more superficial tissue and its prognosis is better. It is seen almost exclusively in adults, with a mean onset between 50 and 60 years of age. The autoimmune defect causes the body to attack skin cells that produce keratin. Blisters form and can lead to significant fluid loss and vulnerability to infection in large, superficial skin lesions. Diagnosis of pemphigus usually requires a shave or punch biopsy of a suspected lesion. It is estimated that there are between 30,000 and 40,000 cases of pemphigus in the US.[20]

Physician Documentation

Up to 80% of pemphigus cases are pemphigus vulgarus,[20] but the ICD-10-CM default for pemphigus is an unspecified pemphigus code. Be sure to identify the type of pemphigus, when known, and document mucous membrane involvement when the patient has oral lesions (see Table 4-3.9).

TABLE 4-3.9 Pemphigus Codes

CODE	DESCRIPTION
L10.0	Pemphigus vulgaris
L10.1	Pemphigus vegetans
L10.2	Pemphigus foliaceous
L10.3	Brazilian pemphigus [fogo selvagem]
L10.4	Pemphigus erythematosus
L10.5	Drug-induced pemphigus
L10.81	Paraneoplastic pemphigus
L10.89	Other pemphigus
L10.9	Pemphigus, unspecified

Document any dysphagia resulting from oral or esophageal lesions, and any other functional disorders that may be limiting the patient's activities of daily living. For drug-induced pemphigus, note the drug responsible.

Coding

Pemphigoid and pemphigus are not the same condition. Pemphigoid lesions are subepidermal, while pemphigus lesions are superficial. Be sure to refer to the Alphabetic Index for coding guidance related to either term in documentation. Complications of pemphigus (eg, cellulitis, secondary infection, sepsis, or dehydration) should be reported in addition to the pemphigus. For drug-induced pemphigus, identify the drug using an adverse effect code. Pemphigus can develop secondary to underlying neoplasms. This is reported with code L10.81, *Paraneoplastic pemphigus.*

Support for pemphigus may be prescriptions for corticosteroids, rituximab, methotrexate, or other immunosuppressants. Pemphigus neonatorum is a form of impetigo and not a true pemphigus autoimmune disorder, despite its name. Report pemphigus neonatorum with code L01.03, *Bullous impetigo.*

CODING TIP Other terms used for pemphigus, and their classifications:

- Cazenave's disease, L10.2
- Dermatitis vegetans, L10.1
- Neumann's disease/syndrome, L10.1

ABSTRACT & CODE IT!

Abstract and code the clinical coding example below. Check your answers against the answers in Appendix C.

Patient: Suzanne Burlman **DOB:** 11/12/1948
DOS: October 1, 2017

Chief Complaint [CC]: Cankers in mouth.

HPI: A 51-year-old female patient presents to the clinic today with a complaint of cankers, saying she has a burning sensation and tenderness in the gums, which worsened on intake of spicy food. She originally thought she had cold sores, but the pain has continued for three months, with periods of blisters on her gums, and periods when they would heal without medical intervention.

Her medical history is non-contributory.

There are no associated ocular, cutaneous, or genital lesions. Oral examination reveals an acutely erythematous and inflamed labial gingiva with some areas of normal gingiva. The marginal gingiva was scalloped in outline. There was a diffuse area of desquamation and erythema involving the buccal and gingival mucosa anteriorly. Multiple areas of erosion were present.

Manipulation of the normal mucosa induced a positive Nikolsky's sign. An incisional biopsy was taken from the buccal aspect of left maxillary gingival region (adjacent to the bullae region) for histopathologic and immunofluorescent studies. Presence of eroded and sloughed bullae are positive for pemphigus vulgaris. The patient was prescribed topical application of clobetasol propionate three times daily for one month and vitamin supplements (zincovit capsules) once daily for one month. She will return in two weeks; earlier if her symptoms worsen.

Peripheral Vascular Disease – *see* Vascular Disease

Pick's Disease *see* Dementia

Pneumonia *see* Pulmonary Disorders: Acute

Psoriasis – *see* Arthritis

Pulmonary Disorders: Acute

Aspiration and specified bacterial pneumonias
HCC 114 0.599

Pneumococcal pneumonia, empyema, lung abscess
HCC 115 0.221

Pneumonia is an infection affecting one or more lobes of the lung tissue, not just the bronchi. In pneumonia, the site of infection displaces air within the alveoli with fluid or pus, interfering with oxygen exchange and breathing. The patient's age, health status, and the infective agent all contribute to the severity of disease. According to the CDC, pneumonia claims more than 50,600 lives each year. The American Lung Association reports that 85% of pneumonia deaths in 2013 occurred in persons who were 65 years of age or older.[21] That rate has been fairly constant for the past 20 years. More than 1 million patients are hospitalized for pneumonia yearly.[21]

Physician Documentation

When documenting pneumonia, note the clinical signs and symptoms (eg, dyspnea, fever, chest pain, etc). Refer to radiological and laboratory findings in your notes, and if a causal agent is known, document it, even if it suspected (eg, pneumonia probably due to MRSA requiring vancomycin). Most patients with pneumonia have a positive

Nikolsky's sign
A positive result in a skin test; the outer epidermis separates easily from the basal layer when a finger presents sliding manual pressure; seen in skin conditions like pemphigus vulgaris or toxic epidermal necrolysis.

X ray; however, if one was not done or was found to be negative, a clear and convincing physical examination (eg, bronchial breath sounds, dullness to percussion) can support the clinical validity of the documented diagnosis.

Unspecified pneumonia (eg, healthcare- or nursing home–associated pneumonia) does not risk-adjust, but many specified bacterial (not viral) pneumonias do. If all that is known is that it is viral or bacterial, document at least that much information. While it is permissible to document "probable" when describing pneumonia or its etiology if it is not known, uncertain diagnoses may not be coded for outpatient or physician billing. Only an inpatient facility may code uncertain diagnoses when documented in the discharge summary, which is why it is important for inpatient physicians to document the likely viral, bacterial, or other suspected causes of pneumonia in their inpatient discharge summary. If the inpatient facility can report the uncertain diagnosis as if it was established, it can then be coded and affect RA.

Aspiration pneumonia provides particular challenges for documentation and coding integrity. If only documented as aspiration pneumonia, ICD-10-CM classifies this as J69.0, *Pneumonitis due to inhalation of food and vomit.* If the physician documents that the patient aspirated bacteria or viruses, the ICD-10-CM Alphabetic Index recommends J15.9, *Unspecified bacterial pneumonia,* or J12.9, *Viral pneumonia, unspecified,* respectively. To see how the Centers for Medicare & Medicaid Services (CMS) has classified pneumonia HCCs, see Table 4-3.10.

Most physicians treat community-acquired pneumonia empirically with a lower respiratory broader spectrum antibiotic covering pneumococcus and atypical organisms (eg, mycoplasma, chlamydia), such as moxifloxacin, gemifloxacin, or levofloxacin, or a combination of a beta-lactam antibiotic (eg, ceftriaxone) that covers pneumococcus with the option of adding a macrolide (eg, azithromycin) to cover atypical organisms. While studies have demonstrated that only around 10% of community-acquired pneumonia is due to pneumococcus and that the rest are likely due to viral agents (eg, rhinovirus, human metapneumovirus) or other unknown causes, many physicians still provide treatment of community-acquired pneumonia with bacterial agents covering pneumococcus for a full course. If the physician only states "pneumonia," "healthcare-acquired pneumonia," or other descriptions that do not mention the name of a bacterium, the assigned ICD-10-CM code does not risk-adjust. For more information, see the Infectious Diseases Society of America (IDSA) 2007 Guideline on Community-Acquired Pneumonia in Adults: Guidelines for Management at http://tinyurl.com/yarfktqg.

Hospital-acquired or healthcare-acquired pneumonia or pneumonia that occurs in an immunocompromised state has a different bacteriology and treatment strategy. These patients require broader spectrum antibiotics that address anaerobic infections (eg, piperacillin/taxobactam, clindamycin), *Staphylococcus aureus* (eg, vancomycin), or gram-negative rods (eg, cefepime, an aminoglycoside and/or carbapenem antibiotic). Most of these patients are treated in an inpatient environment. While the cultures may be negative, the physician should document the suspected organism of these pneumonias at the time of the inpatient discharge, justifying the care plan and treatment (eg, pneumonia probably due to MRSA justifying vancomycin; pneumonia suspected to be due to a gram-negative rod requiring piperacillin/tazobactam or imipenem). IDSA's discussion of healthcare-associated pneumonia is available at http://tinyurl.com/y7ac5p4g.

Interestingly, the term "lobar pneumonia" risk-adjusts without a specified organism to HCC 115, whereas documentation of pneumonia or bacterial pneumonia without a specified infectious agent does not. In ICD-9-CM, applicable prior to October 1, 2015, the term "lobar pneumonia" was classified as pneumonia due to pneumococcus, whereas in ICD-10-CM, the term "lobar pneumonia" does not classify as a specified organism unless one is separately documented by the physician and coded. AHA's *Coding Clinic for ICD-9-CM* (Third Quarter, 2009) discouraged use of the phrase "lobar pneumonia." In ICD-10-CM, the term "lobar pneumonia" is not classified as pneumonia due to pneumococcus, but has a unique code, J18.1, *Lobar pneumonia.* In some cases, a patient with influenza will develop a secondary infection as pneumonia. Specify the causal agent of the pneumonia in influenza, ie, when it is due to the influenza and when it is due to a second infectious organism.

TABLE 4-3.10 Pneumonia HCCs

NO HCC/NO RELATIVE WEIGHT	HCC 115/RELATIVE WEIGHT 0.221	HCC 114/RELATIVE WEIGHT 0.559
Pneumonia, unspecified Community-acquired pneumonia HCAP Healthcare-associated pneumonia Nursing home–associated pneumonia Bacterial pneumonia Viral pneumonia Congenital pneumonia	Amebic lung abscess Pneumonic plague Pulmonary tularemia Pulmonary anthrax Pulmonary actinomycosis Pulmonary nocardiosis Acute pulmonary coccidioidomycosis Chronic pulmonary coccidioidomycosis Pulmonary coccidioidomycosis, unspecified Acute pulmonary histoplasmosis capsulati Chronic pulmonary histoplasmosis capsulati Pulmonary histoplasmosis capsulati, unspecified Acute pulmonary blastomycosis Chronic pulmonary blastomycosis Pulmonary blastomycosis, unspecified Pulmonary paracoccidioidomycosis Paragonimiasis Echinococcus granulosus infection of lung Pneumonia due to: • *Streptococcus pneumonia* • *Hemophilus influenzae* • Streptococcus, group B • Other streptococci • Salmonella • Typhoid • Gonoccus Gangrene and necrosis of lung Lobar pneumonia, unspecified organism Abscess of lung with pneumonia Abscess of mediastinum Pyothorax with fistula Pyothorax without fistula Abscess of lung without pneumonia	Pneumonia due to: • *Klebsiella pneumoniae* • Pseudomonas • Legionnaires' disease • Staphylococcus, unspecified • Methicillin susceptible *Staphylococcus aureus* • Methicillin resistant *Staphylococcus aureus* • Other staphylococcus • *Escherichia coli* • Other aerobic Gram-negative bacteria • Other specified bacteria (**Note:** These are specific bacteria that do not have unique codes, such as Corynebacterium or anaerobes.) • Inhalation of food and vomit • Inhalation of oils and essences • Inhalation of other solids and liquids Ventilator associated pneumonia

DOCUMENTATION TIP Identification of an infective organism by describing the antibiotic chosen to treat the infective agent (eg, "coverage for *Streptococcus pneumoniae*") is not sufficient documentation of the infective agent; the organism must be stated directly as the causal agent (eg, pneumonia due to *Streptococcus pneumoniae*). While outpatient and physician billing does not allow for the coding of uncertain diagnoses, inpatient admission does allow for the coding of likely, possible, probable, and suspected diagnoses so stated in the hospital discharge summary.

Manifestations and consequences of the pneumonia should be clearly documented, including any sepsis, severe sepsis, acute respiratory failure, hypoxia without acute respiratory failure, hemoptysis, pleural effusions, or empyema.

According to ICD-10-CM Guideline Section I(C.10.d.1), "[a]s with all procedural or postprocedural complications, code assignment is based on the provider's documentation of the relationship between the condition and the procedure. Code J95.851, Ventilator associated pneumonia, should be assigned only when the provider has documented ventilator associated pneumonia (VAP). An additional code to identify the organism (e.g., Pseudomonas aeruginosa, code B96.5) should also be assigned. Code J95.851 should not be assigned for cases where the patient has pneumonia and is on a mechanical ventilator and the provider has not specifically stated that the pneumonia is ventilator-associated pneumonia."[4]

ADVICE/ALERT NOTE

Per ICD-10-CM Guideline Section I(C.10.d.1), "[a]s with all procedural or postprocedural complications, code assignment is based on the provider's documentation of the relationship between the condition and the procedure. Code J95.851, Ventilator associated pneumonia, should be assigned only when the provider has documented ventilator associated pneumonia (VAP). An additional code to identify the organism (e.g., Pseudomonas aeruginosa, code B96.5) should also be assigned. Code J95.851 should not be assigned for cases where the patient has pneumonia and is on a mechanical ventilator and the provider has not specifically stated that the pneumonia is ventilator-associated pneumonia."[4]

In aspiration pneumonia, document the specific substance inhaled, and note any foreign body in the respiratory tract. If a full course of antibiotics is prescribed, document which type of organism is being treated (eg, anaerobes, gram-negative rods, MRSA). Document the aspiration pneumonia as postprocedural, if associated with anesthesia or surgery, and whether it was a complication of surgery or due to another cause (eg, anesthesia, a drug overdose, or the late effect of a stroke). A patient's tobacco dependence, exposure, or history should always be noted when a patient has a respiratory condition.

CLINICAL EXAMPLES

NONSPECIFIC DOCUMENTATION	SPECIFIC DOCUMENTATION
Example 1 Bronchopneumonia due to Streptococcus.[a]	**Example 1** Bronchopneumonia due to Streptococcus pneumoniae.[b]
Example 2 Patient admitted for dehydration after four-day history of nausea and vomiting. Chest X ray showed RLL pneumonia.[c] Clindamycin ordered.	**Example 2** Patient admitted for dehydration after a four-day history of nausea and vomiting. Chest X ray showed RLL pneumonia, certainly due to aspiration of vomit.[d] Clindamycin ordered to treat anaerobes as the cause of the pneumonia since the patient is allergic to penicillin.

[a] Streptococcus alone is classified as an unspecified streptococcal pneumonia and does not map for RA.

[b] Specific streptococcal pneumonias including group B and *Streptococcus pneumoniae* map for RA. Provide as much information in the documentation as possible to ensure proper coding and proper RA.

[c] The cause of the pneumonia should be documented.

[d] In this case, the cause of the pneumonia is established, and the substance aspirated is documented.

Coding

In ICD-10-CM, codes for pneumonia do not consider laterality or lobe involvement; the code selection is based on causal agent and complication (eg, empyema, respiratory failure, or abscess). Pneumonia can also be caused by inhaling fluid into the lungs (eg, food, vomit, or blood). It may be a component of influenza.

Many pneumonia codes are found in Chapter 1 of ICD-10-CM, which outlines infectious diseases; others are found throughout the respiratory chapter (Chapter 10). Coders must begin their code look-up in the Alphabetic Index, or they may choose a code in error. Most pneumonia codes are combination codes, capturing the infective agent and the site of the infection in a single code (eg, B06.81, *Rubella pneumonia,* or J14, *Pneumonia due to Hemophilus influenzae*). In some cases, J17, *Pneumonia in diseases classified elsewhere,* is reported in combination with another code, as directed in the Alphabetic Index or in the "Code first" notes in the Tabular List. Do not use a nonspecific pneumonia code in combination with a code from B95-B97 if a combination code exists.

Coders must always abstract a diagnosis of pneumonia to the highest level of specificity possible based on physician documentation. Not only is this a guideline requirement, but also unspecified pneumonia does not risk-adjust, while many other forms of bacterial or aspiration pneumonia do risk-adjust. The specificity helps clarify the severity of the illness, as well as providing epidemiological information. When the physician documents only "pneumonia," but a laboratory report provides the infective agent, the coder cannot abstract the infective agent from the report. All acceptable diagnoses must come from a physician, and laboratory results are often performed by automated machinery or by laboratory technicians or technologists. Conversely, a pathology report signed by a pathologist may be used to further specify a diagnosis from a treating physician, because a pathologist is a physician.

Hemoptysis, a symptom of pneumonia, is not considered integral to pneumonia in ICD-10-CM. It should be documented and coded when hemoptysis occurs in a patient with pneumonia, according to AHA's *Coding Clinic for ICD-9-CM* (Fourth Quarter, 2013).[22] This is a change from ICD-9-CM, when hemoptysis was a nonessential modifier of pneumonia in the Alphabetic Index and would not have been separately reported.

When the patient has bronchitis and pneumonia, report only the pneumonia. A note at the beginning of the respiratory chapter (Chapter 10) of ICD-10-CM states, "[w]hen a respiratory condition is described as occurring in more than one site and is not specifically indexed, it should be classified to the lower anatomical site (eg, tracheobronchitis to bronchitis in J40)."[4]

According to ICD-10-CM Guideline Section I(C.10.d. 2), a "patient may be admitted with one type of pneumonia (e.g., code J13, Pneumonia due to Streptococcus pneumonia) and subsequently develop VAP. In this instance, the principal diagnosis would be the appropriate code from categories J12-J18 for the pneumonia diagnosed at the time of admission. Code J95.851, Ventilator associated pneumonia, would be assigned as an additional diagnosis when the physician has also documented the presence of ventilator associated pneumonia."[4]

ADVICE/ALERT NOTE

Per ICD-10-CM Guideline Section I(C.10.d.2), a "patient may be admitted with one type of pneumonia (e.g., code J13, Pneumonia due to Streptococcus pneumonia) and subsequently develop VAP. In this instance, the principal diagnosis would be the appropriate code from categories J12-J18 for the pneumonia diagnosed at the time of admission. Code J95.851, Ventilator associated pneumonia, would be assigned as an additional diagnosis when the physician has also documented the presence of ventilator associated pneumonia."[4]

Empyema
Accumulation of pus in the pleural cavity, usually the result of bacterial pneumonia; also called pyothorax or purulent pleuritis.

Hemoptysis
Expectoration of blood or blood-stained mucus that originates in the lung or bronchial tube, as seen in cancer, tuberculosis, or pneumonia.

A patient who is dependent on a ventilator and who develops pneumonia does not necessarily have ventilator-associated pneumonia (VAP). J95.851, *Ventilator associated pneumonia,* is only assigned when the physician has documented VAP. It is not assigned, unless the physician has attributed the pneumonia to VAP.

Aspiration pneumonia occurs when food, saliva, vomit, or some other liquid is inhaled into the lungs. This is a common occurrence in infirm, frail, or elderly patients. Although aspiration pneumonia is usually accompanied by infection, ICD-10-CM does not recognize aspiration pneumonia as an infectious process, unless it is explicitly documented by a physician. Instead, it is classified as a lung disease due to external agents. If an infective agent is identified in the aspiration pneumonia, the Alphabetic Index requires that a J12-J18 code be reported rather than code J69.0, *Pneumonitis due to inhalation of food and vomit.* This is supported by the ICD-10-CM Alphabetic Index listings as follows:

Pneumonia
  aspiration J69.0
    due to
      aspiration of microorganisms
        bacterial J15.9
        viral J12.9
      food (regurgitated) J69.0
      gastric secretions J69.0
      milk (regurgitated) J69.0
      oils, essences J69.1
      solids, liquids NEC J69.8
      vomitus J69.0

Code Y95, *Nosocomial condition,* should be reported in addition to the pneumonia code when the infection is documented as a healthcare-acquired condition. This code can be found in the ICD-10-CM Index to External Causes. Nosocomial pneumonia may be documented as hospital acquired pneumonia (HAP).

Nosocomial
Referring to a disease or condition that has its origins in the healthcare setting, ie, a hospital, nursing home, or ambulatory setting.

ABSTRACT & CODE IT!

Abstract and code the clinical coding example below. Check your answers against the answers in Appendix C.

Patient 1
Assessment: Streptococcal empyema.

Plan: Infusion of tPA via chest tube; dilute empyema so that it can be drained.

Patient 2
Bronchopneumonia due to *E. coli.* Patient on 2 liters of oxygen and IV cefoxitin.

Patient 3
Patient's COPD is exacerbated by her *Pseudomonas pneumoniae,* and she will be admitted until her condition stabilizes. Her pO_2 is currently 82 on room air, and we have started her on portable oxygen with a nasal cannula until she gets to her room. This improved her hypoxemia and brought her pO_2 up to 89.

Pulmonary Disorders: Chronic

Chronic obstructive pulmonary disease
HCC 111 0.328

Chronic obstructive pulmonary disease and asthma
RxHCC 226 0.334

Fibrosis of lung and other chronic lung disorders
HCC 112 0.209
RxHCC 227 0.334

Chronic obstructive pulmonary disease (COPD) is the third leading cause of death in the US, and more than 11 million Americans have a COPD diagnosis, according to the American Lung Association. About 75% of people with COPD are current or past smokers, but COPD can also be caused by environmental factors including air pollution, second-hand smoke, dust, or fumes, according to NIH.[23] Alpha-1-antitrypsin, a protein that protects the lungs, can be absent in some people, and though rare, Alpha-1-antitrypsin deficiency also causes COPD. Alpha-1-antritrypsin deficiency is a genetic condition.

Chronic obstructive bronchitis and emphysema are the two forms of COPD. In chronic obstructive bronchitis, persistent and irreversible bronchial airway obstruction is due to inflammation with chronic expectoration and shortness of breath. Systemic steroids and bronchodilators can be useful in reducing inflammation and opening up the airways to reverse or mitigate the symptoms of chronic obstructive bronchitis. Most patients with chronic obstructive bronchitis have frequent infections and exacerbations and exhibit rhonchi and wheezes.

In emphysema, some of the alveoli responsible for oxygen exchange are destroyed and there is no way to recover their function. Patients are short of breath, but a cough or mucous production are usually absent, unlike other forms of COPD. In emphysema, chests are usually without rhonchi and wheezes. Both chronic bronchitis and emphysema risk-adjust for HCCs and RxHCCs.

Asthma is another common chronic lower respiratory disease that risk-adjusts, though only for RxHCCs. In asthma, spasms in the bronchial tubes are caused by allergies or hypersensitivities and result in restricted airways with extra mucous production. Typically, asthma patients have variations in airway obstruction depending on the exposure to triggers, while COPD patients have a more constant airway restriction with a slow decline in functionality and exacerbations during respiratory infections. There is some overlap in COPD and asthma, and the conditions can occur together. Asthma and COPD patients are typically treated with inhaled steroids and bronchodilators.

Physician Documentation

COPD and asthma can have a tremendous impact upon the quality of life and activities of daily living for patients. Ensure all aspects of COPD and asthma are tracked in the medical record. Acute bronchitis is usually infectious in origin and does not risk-adjust. Chronic bronchitis, even if not obstructive, does risk-adjust. Without further information, documented "bronchitis" is classified to code J40, *Bronchitis, not specified as acute or chronic*. For bronchitis, document acute or chronic.

Alveoli

Tiny orbs forming grape-like clusters at the distal end of the bronchial system. Alveoli have walls that are only one-cell thick and are surrounded by small vessels through which the exchange of oxygen for carbon dioxide occurs with each breath.

Identify chronic bronchitis as obstructive, if appropriate, and specify emphysema if it is present.

ICD-10-CM differentiates between COPD with acute exacerbation and COPD with lower respiratory infection. It is appropriate to code both the COPD with acute exacerbation and COPD with a lower respiratory infection, so document both as such, when they occur. Be specific in documentation, including the type of infection (eg, bronchitis or pneumonia), as well as the infective agent. Record results of pulmonary function tests (PFTs) to document airway limitations and document results of any chest radiography results. See Table 4-3.11 for COPD and emphysema codes.

TABLE 4-3.11 COPD and Emphysema Codes with HCCs

CODE	DESCRIPTION
J41.0	Simple chronic bronchitis
J41.1	Mucopurulent chronic bronchitis
J41.8	Mixed simple and mucopurulent chronic bronchitis
J42	Unspecified chronic bronchitis
J44.0	COPD with acute lower respiratory infection
J44.1	COPD with (acute) exacerbation
J44.9	COPD, unspecified
J43.0	Unilateral pulmonary emphysema [MacLeod's syndrome]
J43.1	Panlobular emphysema
J43.2	Centrilobular emphysema
J43.8	Other emphysema
J43.9	Emphysema, unspecified
J98.2	Interstitial emphysema
J98.3	Compensatory emphysema

DOCUMENTATION TIP The Global Initiative for Chronic Obstructive Lung Disease (GOLD) staging of COPD as published by the Global Strategy for the Diagnosis, Management and Prevention of COPD, http://goldcopd.org/gold-2017-global-strategy-diagnosis-management-prevention-copd/, does not align with ICD-10-CM for accurate coding. If GOLD staging is documented, also document the acuity of the COPD using the language of ICD-10-CM.

For COPD, document severity (eg, mild, moderate, or severe). According to ICD-10-CM, COPD can occur with or without acute or chronic respiratory failure, so any respiratory failure should be separately noted. Coders cannot abstract from lab values or PFT scores, so specificity is necessary. Document acute respiratory failure when it occurs, even when it does not require intubation. Document chronic respiratory failure for any encounter in which it exists (eg, oxygen saturation less than 90% or pO_2 less than 60 mm Hg for hypoxia or pCO_2 over 50 mm Hg for hypercapnia) and affects the encounter. Document hypoxia or hypercapnia in respiratory failure, as appropriate.

In some COPD cases, the pulmonary artery blood pressure may rise in the setting of a normally functioning left heart. Cor pulmonale is enlargement of the right heart due to pulmonary hypertension in the setting of a normally functioning left heart, which may result in isolated right (without left) heart failure. Clinical symptoms include pedal edema and jugular venous distention and, in some cases, anasarca. Treatment is with low-flow oxygen, diuretics, and salt restriction. Documenting that the pulmonary hypertension is due to COPD and hypoxia is essential to capturing the underlying cause of cor pulmonale.

While intrinsic vs extrinsic were important components of code selection in asthma for ICD-9-CM, this distinction is missing from ICD-10-CM. For asthma, use language aligning with the following choices: mild severity and intermittent, mild severity and persistent, moderate severity and persistent, or severe severity and persistent. Document uncomplicated, with exacerbation, or with status asthmaticus. See Table 4-3.12 for asthma codes.

TABLE 4-3.12 Asthma Codes with RxHCCs

CODE	DESCRIPTION
J45.20	Mild intermittent asthma, uncomplicated
J45.21	Mild intermittent asthma with (acute) exacerbation
J45.22	Mild intermittent asthma with status asthmaticus
J45.30	Mild persistent asthma, uncomplicated
J45.31	Mild persistent asthma with (acute) exacerbation
J45.32	Mild persistent asthma with status asthmaticus
J45.40	Moderate persistent asthma, uncomplicated
J45.41	Moderate persistent asthma with (acute) exacerbation
J45.42	Moderate persistent asthma with status asthmaticus
J45.50	Severe persistent asthma, uncomplicated
J45.51	Severe persistent asthma with (acute) exacerbation
J45.52	Severe persistent asthma with status asthmaticus
J45.901	Unspecified asthma with (acute) exacerbation
J45.902	Unspecified asthma with status asthmaticus
J45.909	Unspecified asthma, uncomplicated
J45.990	Exercise induced bronchospasm
J45.991	Cough variant asthma
J45.998	Other asthma

DOCUMENTATION TIP In ICD-10-CM, there is no specific code for "end-stage COPD with continuous home oxygen." This diagnosis would be abstracted as J44.9, *Chronic obstructive pulmonary disease, unspecified,* and Z99.81, *Dependence on supplemental oxygen.* Document any acute exacerbation or acute/chronic respiratory failure with hypercapnia/hypoxia as appropriate to capture the morbidity of the patient's end-stage.

Signs and symptoms of COPD or asthma that are separately reported when they occur include hypercapnia, hypoxemia, polycythemia, and acute or chronic respiratory failure. Document any dependence on ventilator or supplemental oxygen. The HPI should describe the development of the patient's present illness, as noted in the 1995 Documentation Guidelines for Evaluation and Management Services, and include the following elements: location, quality, severity, duration, timing, modifying factors, and associated signs and symptoms.

Tobacco use or dependence, personal history of tobacco dependence, or exposure to secondary smoke (workplace, environment, perinatal), is pertinent to all respiratory conditions and should be noted. Document the type of tobacco in current use (chewing tobacco, electronic cigarettes, cigarettes, etc). Document any tobacco counseling, treatment, or intervention. Codes for reporting exposure to tobacco smoke versus exposure to electronic cigarette emissions are different, so specify in documentation the source of secondary smoke.

CLINICAL EXAMPLES

NONSPECIFIC DOCUMENTATION	SPECIFIC DOCUMENTATION
Example 1 End stage COPD. Patient is on continuous home oxygen and currently has chronic hypercapnia.[a] He is on the maximum dose of steroids. We have referred him to hospice.	**Example 1** End stage COPD. Patient is on continuous home oxygen and currently has acute on chronic respiratory failure with hypercapnia.[b] He is on the maximum dose of steroids. We have referred him to hospice.
Example 2 Asthma[c] exacerbation responding well to albuterol nebulizer.	**Example 2** Moderate persistent asthma[d] exacerbation responding well to albuterol nebulizer.

[a] This patient appears to be in respiratory failure. This condition should be reported in addition to the COPD.

[b] Here, the severity of the patient's COPD is captured with the acute on chronic respiratory failure with hypercapnia noted.

[c] Identify the type of asthma, if known.

[d] The type of asthma has been documented sufficiently.

Coding

In COPD or asthma, documentation of a worsening condition or decompensation is, by definition, documentation of an exacerbation. Acute respiratory failure in a patient with COPD would be a sudden worsening in respiratory symptoms and by definition would be an exacerbation. Exacerbation of COPD cannot be assumed, however, when a patient with COPD has a lower respiratory tract infection. Patients can have a lower respiratory infection and not experience an exacerbation of COPD. Exacerbation, worsening, decompensation, or failure must be stated in order for the exacerbation to be reported. When the patient has a lower respiratory infection and an exacerbation of COPD, report codes J44.0, *Chronic obstructive pulmonary disease with acute lower respiratory infection,* and J44.1, *Chronic obstructive pulmonary disease with (acute) exacerbation,* and a code for the bronchitis or pneumonia.

According to ICD-10-CM Guideline Section I(C.10.a.1), the "codes in categories J44 and J45 distinguish between uncomplicated cases and those in acute exacerbation. An acute exacerbation is a worsening or a decompensation of a chronic condition. An acute exacerbation is not equivalent to an infection superimposed on a chronic condition, though an exacerbation may be triggered by an infection."[4] AHA's *Coding Clinic* (Third Quarter, 2016 and First Quarter, 2017) advised that code J44.0, *Chronic obstructive pulmonary disease with acute lower respiratory infection,* should not be reported in cases in which the infection is caused by influenza, by a ventilator, or in cases of aspiration pneumonia.[24,25] Instead, report codes J44.9, *Chronic obstructive pulmonary disease, unspecified,* with J69.0, *Pneumonitis due to inhalation of food and vomit,* J95.851, *Ventilator associated pneumonia,* or the appropriate influenza code.[25] However, if a bacterial infection is superimposed over the influenza in a patient with COPD, report the influenza code, bacterial pneumonia code, and code J44.0, *Chronic obstructive pulmonary disease with lower respiratory infection,* according to AHA's *Coding Clinic* (Fourth Quarter, 2017).[26]

ADVICE/ALERT NOTE

Per ICD-10-CM Guideline Section I(C.10.a.1), the "codes in categories J44 and J45 distinguish between uncomplicated cases and those in acute exacerbation. An acute exacerbation is a worsening or a decompensation of a chronic condition. An acute exacerbation is not equivalent to an infection superimposed on a chronic condition, though an exacerbation may be triggered by an infection."[4]

When a patient has both COPD and asthma, report both conditions. Refer to documentation to determine if a documented exacerbation is describing the COPD or the asthma. According to AHA's *Coding Clinic* (First Quarter, 2017), "an exacerbation of COPD does not automatically make the asthma exacerbated."[25] In COPD or asthma, the patient's symptoms may be well controlled by medications and other treatments. The patient still has lung disease, and the disease would still be reported if supported in the medical record.

CODING TIP AHA's *Coding Clinic* (Third Quarter, 2016 and First Quarter, 2017) advised that code J44.0, *Chronic obstructive pulmonary disease with acute lower respiratory infection,* should not be reported in cases in which the infection is caused by influenza, by a ventilator, or in cases of aspiration pneumonia.[24,25] Instead, report codes J44.9, *Chronic obstructive pulmonary disease, unspecified,* with J69.0, *Pneumonitis due to inhalation of food and vomit,* J95.851, *Ventilator associated pneumonia,* or the appropriate influenza code.[25] However, if a bacterial infection is superimposed over the influenza in a patient with COPD, report the influenza code, the bacterial pneumonia code, and J44.0, *Chronic obstructive pulmonary disease with lower respiratory infection*, according to AHA's *Coding Clinic* (Fourth Quarter, 2017).[26]

Most important in abstracting bronchitis is the determination of whether it is chronic, and whether it is obstructive. Both of those conditions are components of COPD. All chronic forms of bronchitis risk-adjust (see Figure 4-3.1).

Support for any form of COPD may be found in the PE. Look for notations regarding any of the following, keeping in mind that negative findings still support that the condition was evaluated:

- Diminished breath sounds
- Crackles, rhonchi, rales, wheezing ("adventitious" sounds)
- Barrel chest
- Active use of neck/chest muscles to breathe
- Flared nostrils
- Clubbing of fingers

Prescriptions can also be used to support a diagnosis of COPD or asthma. Common medications associated with COPD and asthma include short-acting bronchodilators including albuterol, levalbuterol, and ipratropium; long-acting bronchodilators including aclidinium, arformoterol, formoterol, glycopyrrolate, indacaterol, olodaterol, salmeterol, tiotropium, and umeclidinium; and there are many combination bronchodilators. Other drugs include corticosteroids including fluticasone, budesonide, and prednisolone; theophylline; and roflumilast.

CODING TIP When a patient has both COPD and emphysema, report only the COPD code for 2017 diagnoses, but report only the emphysema code for 2018 diagnoses or beyond. The ICD-10-CM Alphabetic Index was amended for 2018, effecting this change, as issued in the official 2018 Addenda:

No change	*Disease, diseased* – see also Syndrome
No change	lung J98.4
No change	obstructive (chronic) J44.9
No change	with
Revise from	emphysema J44.9
Revise to	emphysema J43.9

This is in conflict with the note under code J44, *Other chronic obstructive pulmonary disease,* which states, "includes chronic bronchitis with emphysema," which may have been overlooked with the 2018 Alphabetic Index. As emphysema is a more specific diagnosis, report emphysema with COPD with code J43.9, unless further communication from AHA's *Coding Clinic* or the National Center for Health Statistics offers different guidance.

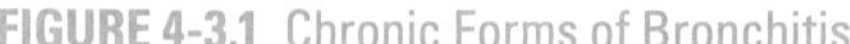

FIGURE 4-3.1 Chronic Forms of Bronchitis

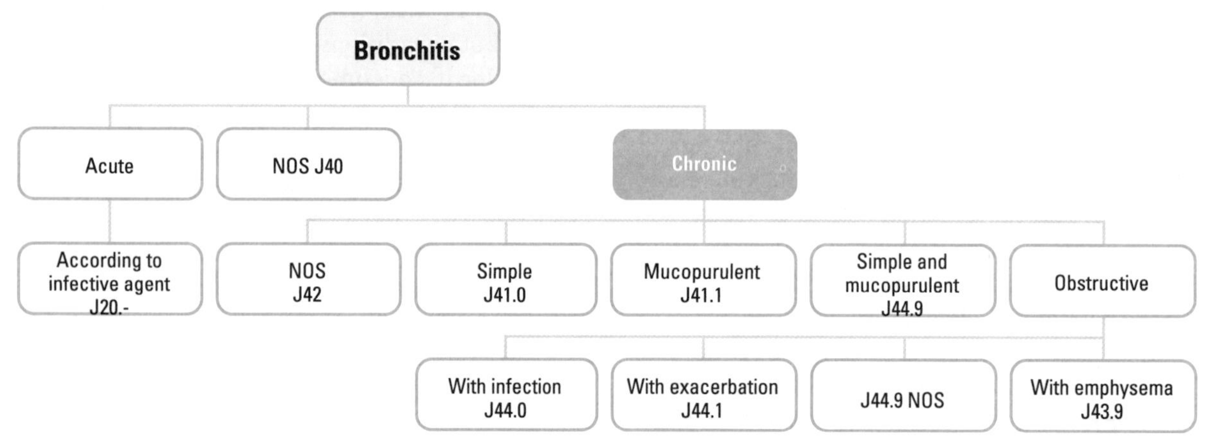

In emphysema, panlobular refers to a pattern of alveolar destruction in which entire clusters of alveoli are affected. It is usually associated with alpha-1-antitrypsin deficiency and is also called panacinar, diffuse, or generalized emphysema. Unilateral emphysema affects only one lung and occasionally occurs as a result of lung damage from a localized infection. Centrilobular emphysema is most commonly seen in smokers, and involves the upper cells in the proximal portion of the clusters of alveoli.

Any hypoxia, hypercapnia, hypoxemia, polycythemia, cor pulmonale, right heart failure, or respiratory failure in the patient with COPD or asthma is not integral to the lung disease, and should be separately reported when documented and present. If the patient's pulse oximeter reading is charted below 90% and the patient has respiratory symptoms noted in the chart, but no diagnosis of hypoxemia has been noted, query the physician as to whether the pulse oximetry reading is significant for any additional diagnoses.

Code Z99.11, *Dependence on respirator,* is reported for any dependence on a ventilator, including dependence on a continuous positive airway pressure (CPAP) or bilevel positive airway pressure (BiPAP) device when oxygen is delivered through tracheostomy. Report electronic cigarette dependence with code F17.21-, *Nicotine dependence, cigarettes.* Report code Z77.29, *Contact with and (suspected) exposure to other hazardous substances,* for adverse effects of second-hand smoke from electronic cigarettes, according to AHA's *Coding Clinic* (Second Quarter, 2016), as electronic cigarettes do not produce tobacco smoke.[27]

CODING TIP Report electronic cigarette dependence with code F17.21-, *Nicotine dependence, cigarettes.* Report code Z77.29, *Contact with and (suspected) exposure to other hazardous substances,* for adverse effects of second-hand smoke from electronic cigarettes, according to AHA's *Coding Clinic* (Second Quarter, 2016), as electronic cigarettes do not produce tobacco smoke.[27]

Abstract the patient's smoking status, if noted, when the patient has chronic lung disease. Do not link a current or past history of tobacco dependence with COPD or asthma unless the link is documented by the physician (see Table 4-3.13). If a link between smoking and the lung disease is documented, report the linkage (eg, code F17.218, *Nicotine dependence, cigarettes, with other nicotine-induced disorders*).

TABLE 4-3.13 Common Tobacco Use and History Codes

CODE	DESCRIPTION
F17.210	Nicotine dependence, cigarettes, uncomplicated
F17.218	Nicotine dependence, cigarettes, with other nicotine-induced disorders
F17.211	Nicotine dependence, cigarettes, in remission
Z72.0	Tobacco use
Z77.22	Contact with and (suspected) exposure to environmental tobacco smoke (acute) (chronic)
Z87.891	Personal history of nicotine dependence

Do not be confused by seemingly contradictory notes in ICD-10-CM regarding COPD and asthma. COPD and asthma represent clinically discrete conditions that are sometimes confusing to code together. In category J44, *Other chronic obstructive pulmonary disease,* an Includes note indicates that chronic obstructive asthma is included. However, under category J45, *Asthma,* an Excludes2 note indicates that asthma and chronic obstructive pulmonary disease (J44.9) can be reported in addition to the specific asthma code. Best practice is to abstract as much detail as possible from the record. Code both conditions.

ABSTRACT & CODE IT!

Abstract and code the clinical coding example below. Check your answers against the answers in Appendix C.

Patient 1
Asymptomatic former smoker with no airflow limitations is diagnosed with mild centrilobular emphysema on chest CT.

Patient 2
Acute end-stage COPD. Patient is on continuous home oxygen and currently has acute on chronic respiratory failure with hypercapnia. He is on the maximum dose of steroids. We have referred him to hospice.

Patient 3
Moderate persistent asthma exacerbation responding well to albuterol nebulizer.

References

1. National Institute of Neurological Disorders and Stroke. Narcolepsy Fact Sheet. https://www.ninds.nih.gov/Disorders/Patient-Caregiver-Education/Fact-Sheets/Narcolepsy-Fact-Sheet. Accessed Nov 22, 2017.
2. American Sleep Association. Narcolepsy. https://www.sleepassociation.org/sleep-disorders-n/narcolepsy/. Accessed Dec 5, 2017.
3. American Cancer Society. Cancer Facts & Figures 2017. https://www.cancer.org/research/cancer-facts-statistics/all-cancer-facts-figures/cancer-facts-figures-2017.html. Accessed Nov 22, 2017.
4. Centers for Disease Control and Prevention. *ICD-10-CM Official Guidelines for Coding and Reporting* (FY 2018). https://www.cdc.gov/nchs/data/icd/10cmguidelines_fy2018_final.pdf. Accessed Oct 30, 2017.
5. American Hospital Association. *Coding Clinic® for ICD-10-CM and ICD-10-PCS Q1.* 2014;1(1):12-13.
6. Leon-Chisen N. *ICD-10-CM and ICD-10-PCS Coding Handbook.* Chicago, IL: American Hospital Association: 2017.
7. Centers for Disease Control and Prevention. Shingles (Herpes Zoster). https://www.cdc.gov/shingles/hcp/clinical-overview.html. Accessed Nov 22, 2017.
8. Centers for Disease Control and Prevention. Adult Obesity. https://www.cdc.gov/vitalsigns/adultobesity/index.html. Accessed Nov 22, 2017.
9. Centers for Disease Control and Prevention. About Adult BMI. https://www.cdc.gov/healthyweight/assessing/bmi/adult_bmi/index.html. Accessed Nov 22, 2017.
10. National Eye Institute. Facts About Age-Related Macular Degeneration. https://nei.nih.gov/health/maculardegen/armd_facts. Accessed Nov 22, 2017.
11. American Hospital Association. *Coding Clinic® for ICD-10-CM and ICD-10-PCS Q1.* 2016;3(1):13.
12. Centers for Disease Control and Prevention. Percentage of Adults Aged 65 and Over With Osteoporosis or Low Bone Mass at the Femur Neck or Lumbar Spine: United States, 2005-2010. https://www.cdc.gov/nchs/data/hestat/osteoporsis/osteoporosis2005_2010.htm. Accessed Dec 7, 2017.
13. NIH Osteoporosis and Related Bone Diseases National Resource Center. Osteoporosis Overview. https://www.bones.nih.gov/health-info/bone/osteoporosis/overview. Accessed Dec 6, 2017.
14. American Association of Neurological Surgeons. Spinal Cord Injury. http://www.aans.org/Patients/Neurosurgical-Conditions-and-Treatments/Spinal-Cord-Injury. Accessed Dec 6, 2017.
15. American Hospital Association. *Coding Clinic® for ICD-10-CM and ICD-10-PCS Q1.* 2017;4(1):47-48.
16. National Institute of Neurological Disorders and Stroke. Huntington's Disease Information Page. https://www.ninds.nih.gov/Disorders/All-Disorders/Huntingtons-Disease-Information-Page. Accessed Nov 1, 2017.
17. National Institute of Neurological Disorders and Stroke. Parkinson's Disease Information Page. https://www.ninds.nih.gov/Disorders/All-Disorders/Parkinsons-Disease-Information-Page. Accessed Nov 1, 2017.
18. eMedicineHealth. Parkinson's Disease Dementia. https://www.emedicinehealth.com/parkinson_disease_dementia/article_em.htm. Accessed Nov 1, 2017.
19. American Parkinson Disease Association. Understanding the Basics of Parkinson's Disease. https://www.apdaparkinson.org/what-is-parkinsons/. Accessed Nov 1, 2017.
20. International Pemphigus & Pemphigoid Foundation. Pemphigus. http://www.pemphigus.org/research/clinically-speaking/pemphigus/. Accessed Dec 6, 2017.
21. American Lung Association. *Trends in Pneumonia and Influenza Morbidity and Mortality.* http://www.lung.org/assets/documents/research/pi-trend-report.pdf. Accessed Dec 6, 2017.
22. American Hospital Association. *Coding Clinic® for ICD-9-CM Q4.* 2013;30(4):118.
23. National Heart, Lung, and Blood Institute. COPD: Risk Factors. https://www.nhlbi.nih.gov/health/health-topics/topics/copd/atrisk. Accessed Dec 6, 2017.
24. American Hospital Association. *Coding Clinic® for ICD-10-CM and ICD-10-PCS Q3.* 2016;3(3):15-16.

25. American Hospital Association. *Coding Clinic® for ICD-10-CM and ICD-10-PCS Q3.* 2017;4(1):24-26.
26. American Hospital Association. *Coding Clinic® for ICD-10-CM and ICD-10-PCS Q4.* 2017;4(4):96.
27. American Hospital Association. *Coding Clinic® for ICD-10-CM and ICD-10-PCS Q2.* 2016;3(2):34.

CHAPTER 4

Clinical Documentation Integrity and Coding

PART 4: TOPICS Q-V

Quadriplegia *see* Paralysis

Renal Disorders

Dialysis status
HCC 134 0.422
RxHCC 261 0.246

Acute renal failure
HCC 135 0.422

Chronic kidney disease, stage 5
HCC 136 0.237
RxHCC 262 0.093

Chronic kidney disease, stage 4
HCC 137 0.237
RxHCC 263 0.093

The kidneys remove metabolic waste, excess fluid, ions, and chemicals from the bloodstream via a filtration system. The glomeruli filter the waste, which is collected and drained into the renal pelvis. From there, the ureters carry the waste (urine) to the bladder. The efficiency of glomerular filtration is called the glomerular filtration rate (GFR), which is the benchmark in the diagnosis and management of kidney disease.

In kidney disease, the kidney filtration is impaired. This can be due to underlying conditions like diabetes or hypertension. Kidney disease increases a patient's risk for other conditions including heart disease and stroke.

Chronic kidney disease (CKD) is defined as abnormalities of kidney structure or function present for greater than three months with implications for health. CKD is a nonspecific term that covers all degrees of chronic and irreversible decrease in renal function, representing conditions that range from mild to end-stage. CKD is reported based on the renal function of the patient as determined by the patient's physician, who considers the estimated or measured GFR. In contrast, acute renal failure (ARF) is a reduction of renal function that comes on rapidly, and may be reversible. ARF is usually due to an interruption of the blood supply to the kidney (prerenal), outflow tract obstruction (postrenal), or kidney pathologies (renal).

Some kidney conditions that cause CKD are congenital, such as polycystic kidney disease. Initially, CKD has no visible symptoms, but it can be detected with urinalysis identifying the level of protein (albumin) in the urine, microscopic hematuria, or a reduction of the eGFR to less than 60 ml/min/1.73m^2 with routine screening.

According to the National Institutes of Health (NIH), 14% of the United States (US) population has some form of CKD, and diabetes and hypertension are the principal causes.[1] More than 661,000 Americans have kidney failure, with nearly half a million people receiving dialysis, a process by which mechanical filters remove waste from the patient's blood.[1] Transplanted kidneys exist in about 193,000 Americans.[1] Medicare assigns patients with ESRD a separate status in risk-adjustment (RA) reimbursement models, making documentation and coding of ESRD essential to compliance.

Physician Documentation

Renal insufficiency is a generic term that covers a broad spectrum of illness and does not lend itself to precise coding or RA. "Renal insufficiency" is often documented in the medical record, and ICD-10-CM classifies it to code N28.9, *Disorder of the kidney and ureter, unspecified*, which does not risk-adjust. While chronic renal insufficiency is classified as CKD, acute kidney insufficiency is not classified as acute kidney injury or failure. Rather than simply documenting "renal insufficiency," describe the patient's condition by:

- **Functional status:** Acute kidney injury or CKD with an emphasis on staging (eg, CKD, Stage 3; end-stage renal disease requiring chronic dialysis).
- **Underlying cause:** Examples include acute renal hypoperfusion from hypovolemia or shock states, acute tubular necrosis, diabetic glomerulosclerosis, interstitial nephritis.
- **Consequences:** Examples include secondary hyperparathyroidism, fluid overload with or without exacerbation of underlying heart failure, hyperkalemia, or anemia (due to CKD itself or other causes).
- **Treatment:** Examples include acute or chronic peritoneal or hemodialysis, hemofiltration, transplant status and/or planning, and use of immunosuppressants to suppress transplant rejection.

ICD-10-CM classifies CKD based on five stages of severity, presuming that a qualifying pathology or an estimated GFR of less than 60 ml/min/1.73m^2 has been present for 90 days or more. These include:

- Stage 1, code N18.1
- Stage 2, code N18.2, equates to mild CKD
- Stage 3, code N18.3, equates to moderate CKD
- Stage 4, code N18.4, equates to severe CKD
- Stage 5, code N18.5

To see the criteria that support stages of CKD, visit http://kdigo.org/wp-content/uploads/2017/02/KDIGO_2012_CKD_GL.pdf. According to ICD-10-CM Guideline Section I(C.14.a.1), "if both a stage of CKD and ESRD are documented, assign code N18.6 only."[2] Code N18.6, *End stage renal disease (ESRD)*, indicates that the patient's chronic kidney disease is such that chronic dialysis or transplant is necessary to maintain life and is assigned when the physician has documented ESRD. ESRD patients qualify for the Medicare ESRD program. The term "ESRD" should not be applied to patients with acute kidney injury who require a short period of dialysis as they recovery from their illness.

ADVICE/ALERT NOTE

Per ICD-10-CM Guideline Section I(C.14.a.1), "if both a stage of CKD and ESRD are documented, assign code N18.6 only."[2]

Any patient suspected of having chronic kidney disease should have the stage of CKD determined and documented. Identify the specific stage in CKD as stage 1 through 5, or ESRD. A coder cannot abstract based on CKD noted as "mild" or "moderate," and likewise, cannot abstract a stage from a GFR result.

Make a note of a nephropathy as appropriate when a diabetic patient has persistent microalbuminuria but has not yet been diagnosed with CKD. A diagnosis of microalbuminuria without a note of nephropathy is reported as a symptom unrelated to the diabetes, while documenting mild nephropathy with microalbuminuria in a diabetic patient is reported as a complication of diabetes.

DOCUMENTATION TIP If present, CKD will always be pertinent in a patient with diabetes, heart failure, or hypertension. Always document those conditions when addressing a patient's kidney disease.

Document the underlying cause of CKD. ICD-10-CM assumes a causal relationship between CKD and hypertension, and between CKD and diabetes, unless the physician states otherwise in the medical record. If the patient has either diabetes or hypertension, and the patient's CKD is due to a different cause, clearly document that cause. Specify the type of glomerular disease or renal tubule interstitial disease, if known.

"Kidney injury" in ICD-10-CM defaults to a traumatic injury. "Acute kidney injury" defaults in ICD-10-CM to code N17.9, *Acute kidney failure*. If using "acute kidney injury" to describe a traumatic disorder, add "traumatic" to your documentation to prevent abstraction errors. Dependence on dialysis does not occur in a vacuum. Document the etiology and manifestations for the kidney disorder and the stage of CKD (in this circumstance, it will likely be ESRD) or the acute kidney failure and its cause. Document any presence of arteriovenous shunt for dialysis. Document any noncompliance. Note the etiology of anemia in the patient with CKD or ESRD as due to kidney disease, dialysis, or nutritional in nature. ICD-10-CM assumes that anemia in the presence of CKD or ESRD is due to these conditions unless the physician documents another cause (eg, iron or folate deficiency).

If there is a complication of dialysis (eg, infection, hypotension, catheter breakdown, leakage, etc), always link it to the dialysis or the appliances. Be very specific in documenting complications. When a patient has a complication related to dialysis, note whether the complication is with the dialysis catheter, the shunt, or skin adhesions. Note the type of complication (eg, breakdown, displacement, infection, adhesions) and the episode of care (initial, subsequent, sequela).

When a patient has a transplant complication, identify the type of complication (eg, failure, infection, or rejection). Specifically document a complication of a transplant as a complication of a transplant. For example, a patient may have CKD and a transplanted kidney, and the CKD may be a complication of the transplant, but unless it is documented as such, the patient's condition is reported as two unrelated diagnoses. Note if a patient is awaiting a kidney transplant, or has status as a transplant recipient. For hematuria, document whether gross, benign essential microscopic, or asymptomatic microscopic. Document kidney transplant status, dialysis status, or urinary stoma status (see Table 4-4.1 for an example of these codes).

TABLE 4-4.1 Risk-adjusting Kidney Status Codes

CODE	DESCRIPTION
Z43.5	Encounter for attention to cystostomy
Z76.82	Awaiting organ transplant status
Z90.5	Acquired absence of kidney
Z91.15	Patient's noncompliance with renal dialysis
Z93.50	Unspecified cystostomy status
Z93.51	Cutaneous-vesicostomy status
Z93.52	Appendico-vesicostomy status
Z93.59	Other cystostomy status
Z94.0	Kidney transplant status
Z97.8	Presence of other specified devices (for artificial kidney)
Z98.85	Transplanted organ removal status
Z99.2	Dependence on dialysis

ARF is an acronym for acute renal failure or acute respiratory failure. It is not an acceptable diagnosis. Spell out first reference to avoid documentation ambiguity and errors of abstraction.

CLINICAL EXAMPLES

NONSPECIFIC DOCUMENTATION	SPECIFIC DOCUMENTATION
Example 1 Assessment: 1. Type 1 diabetes mellitus. 2. Microalbuminuria based on today's laboratory results.[a]	**Example 1** Assessment: 1. Type 1 diabetes mellitus,[b] controlled well with insulin and diet. 2. Nephropathy with persistent microalbuminuria.
Example 2 The patient has a five-year history of CKD Stage 3,[c] but her GFR has been around 24. I am referring her to a nephrologist.	**Example 2** The patient has five-year history of CKD Stage 3, but based on trending GFRs, is now diagnosed with Stage 4 CKD.[d] I am referring her to a nephrologist.

[a] Note if the microalbuminuria is due to diabetic nephropathy, if appropriate.

[b] There is support here for the diabetes, and the microalbuminuria has been diagnosed as nephropathy. This allows a link to be made between the diabetes and the kidney symptoms.

[c] Coders cannot code from laboratory results. Identify the CKD Stage 4. Also "history of" should be avoided in language of documentation.

[d] Correctly identified the patient's advanced CKD.

Coding

According to ICD-10-CM Guideline Section I(C.9.a.1), "[h]ypertension in the presence (with) with heart conditions classified to I50.- or I51.4-I51.9, are assigned to a code from category I11, Hypertensive heart disease. Use an additional code(s) from category I50, Heart failure, to identify the type(s) of heart failure in those patients with heart failure."[2] In addition, Guideline Section I(C.9.a.2) states to "[a]ssign codes from category I12, Hypertensive chronic kidney disease, when both hypertension and a condition classifiable to category N18, Chronic kidney disease (CKD), are present. CKD should not be coded as hypertensive if the physician has specifically documented a different cause. The appropriate code from category N18 should be used as a secondary code with a code from category I12 to identify the stage of chronic kidney disease. If a patient has hypertensive chronic kidney disease and acute renal failure, an additional code for the acute renal failure is required."[2] CKD should not be coded as *due to hypertension* if the physician has specifically documented "secondary hypertension." Without more information, secondary hypertension is reported with code I15.9, *Secondary hypertension, unspecified.*

CODING TIP ICD-10-CM Guideline Section I(C.9.a.2) states that ICD-10 classifies hypertension *with* CKD as hypertensive chronic kidney disease (implying that the hypertension caused or contributed to the CKD). However, the American Hospital Association's (AHA's) *Coding Clinic for ICD-10-CM and ICD-10-PCS* (*Coding Clinic*) (Third Quarter, 2016) advised ignoring the presumed link for the hypertension causing the ESRD (a CKD), if a patient is documented with ESRD *due to* congenital polycystic kidney disease in the setting of hypertension *due to* the polycystic kidneys.[3] The appropriate codes to report would be code N18.6, *End stage renal disease*, Q61.3, *Polycystic kidney, unspecified*, and I15.1, *Hypertension secondary to other renal disorders*.[3]

A common coding error seen in CKD is reporting it in conjunction with code I10, *Essential (primary) hypertension*, for the same encounter. Instead, assign a hypertension code from I12, *Hypertensive chronic kidney disease*, or I13, *Hypertensive heart and chronic kidney disease*, for patients with hypertension and CKD, unless the physician documents that the hypertension is due to another cause, such as renovascular disease, which is an endocrine disease (eg, Cushing's syndrome), that will result in reporting a code from category N15, *Secondary hypertension*. Never assign a code from category N18, *Chronic kidney disease*, with code I10, *Essential (primary) hypertension*, for the same encounter.

Microalbumin is monitored in diabetic patients to watch for signs of kidney disease. Documentation of persistent microalbuminuria in a diabetic patient alone is insufficient to report it as a renal complication of diabetes, unless documentation includes a kidney diagnosis (eg, mild nephropathy).

Do not assign a CKD code based on GFR or on a notation of mild, moderate, or severe disease. Query the physician to assign the stage of CKD if it is not documented, or report unspecified CKD if a query is not possible. The presence of CKD in a patient with a transplanted kidney is not necessarily a complication of the transplant. The condition must be stated as a "complication" in order to be coded as such.

ARF is an acronym with several meanings. If "acute renal failure" is not stated or obvious from context, query the physician regarding the acronym. Assume a causal link between CKD and diabetes or hypertension, unless documentation states otherwise. If the patient has diabetes, hypertension, and CKD, query the physician to see if both conditions are responsible for the CKD, or only one should be linked to the hypertension. If a query is not possible, it would be acceptable to report both links. Always code documented kidney transplant status and dialysis status, or any of the status codes listed in Table 4-4.2, when they are documented.

TABLE 4-4.2 Status Codes Associated with Kidneys

CODE	DESCRIPTION
Z76.82	Awaiting organ transplant status
Z90.5	Acquired absence of kidney
Z91.15	Patient's noncompliance with renal dialysis
Z94.0	Kidney transplant status
Z97.8	Presence of other specified devices
Z98.85	Transplanted organ removal status
Z99.2	Dependence on dialysis

For a patient with erythropoietin-resistant anemia (EPO), resistant anemia, report code D63.1, *Anemia in chronic kidney disease*, along with the underlying CKD. Documented cardiorenal syndrome usually describes acute decompensated congestive heart failure resulting in acute kidney failure. There is no specific code for this syndrome, which the ICD-10-CM Alphabetic Index classifies to hypertension. Be sure to capture all elements of the syndrome by querying the physician if the elements are not documented completely.

Glomerular Filtration Rates

GFRs cannot be used to abstract a diagnosis of CKD, but they can be helpful in determining if a query to the physician regarding the diagnosis of a patient is appropriate, as a depressed GFR could be an indication that the patient has a diagnosis of CKD, but the physician did not document it.

CKD STAGE	LABORATORY VALUE OF eGFR	COMMENT
1	≥ 90	Do not assign a code for CKD for these eGFRs unless the physician explicitly documents that CKD is present.
2	60-90	
3	30-59	CKD is clinically valid based only on eGFR values less than 60 ml/min/1.73m^2 if present for three months or more.
4	15-29	
5	<15	Clinically defines kidney failure; however, the administrative term, ESRD, should be used if the patient requires chronic (not acute) dialysis or transplant.

If both ESRD and stage 5 CKD are documented, code only the ESRD.

According to the *2008 Risk Adjustment Data Technical Assistance for Medicare Advantage Organizations Participant Guide* (*2008 RA Participant Guide*), "[c]ertain combinations of coexisting diagnoses for an individual can increase their medical costs. The CMS-HCC model recognizes these higher costs through incorporating payments for disease interactions.

Examples of the disease interactions include a two-way combination of diabetes mellitus (DM) and congestive heart failure (CHF). In calculating this part of the risk score for an individual, the individual score for each HCC is added and then the disease interaction score is added."[4]

The *2008 RA Participant Guide* states that "[c]ertain combinations of coexisting diagnoses for an individual can increase their medical costs. The CMS-HCC model recognizes these higher costs through incorporating payments for disease interactions. Examples of the disease interactions include a two-way combination of diabetes mellitus (DM) and congestive heart failure (CHF). In calculating this part of the risk score for an individual, the individual score for each HCC is added and then the disease interaction score is added."[4]

ABSTRACT & CODE IT!

Abstract and code the clinical coding example below. Check your answers against the answers in Appendix C.

Patient 1

Assessment:

1. Type 1 diabetes mellitus, controlled well with insulin and diet.
2. Persistent microalbuminuria based on today's and March's laboratory results.

Patient 2

The patient has a five-year history of CKD Stage 3, but her GFR has been around 24. I am referring her to a nephrologist.

Patient 3

The patient has five-year history of CKD Stage 3, but based on trending GFRs, is now diagnosed with Stage 4 CKD. I am referring her to a nephrologist.

Rheumatoid Arthritis – *see* Arthritis

Rheumatoid Arthritis – *see* Arthritis

Schizophrenia – *see* Behavioral Disorders

Scleroderma – *see* Arthritis

Seizure and Epilepsy

Seizure disorders and convulsions
HCC 79 0.309

Epilepsy and other seizure disorders, except intractable epilepsy
RxHCC 164 0.121

Convulsions
RxHCC 165 0.053

Intractable epilepsy
RxHCC 163 0.293

Nerves are comprised of electrical signals, and the brain is the power transformer that converts electrical signals into sensory and motor messages. Seizures are uncontrolled electrical activity in the brain. Seizures may be caused by fever, hormonal changes, brain tumors, hypoglycemia, drugs, trauma, stroke, or other conditions. A seizure may be an isolated event or recurrent. Recurrent seizures are called epilepsy. Epilepsy is incurable but can often be controlled or limited with medications or surgical techniques.

Epilepsy manifests itself in a wide range of ways. For some patients with epilepsy, the symptoms of a seizure are mild and may include eye blinking, a blank stare, or confusion. More severe symptoms include unconsciousness accompanied by muscle spasms. In either case, most seizures only last a few seconds or minutes. Seizure may affect both sides of the brain or be localized to one area of the brain, in which case they are called focal or partial seizures.

According to the Centers for Disease Control and Prevention (CDC), approximately 1.2% of Americans have epilepsy, ie, 3 million adults and 470,000 children have the condition.[5] Most patients with epilepsy control their condition with medications that reduce or control the spread of seizure activity in the brain. Epilepsy that cannot be fully controlled with medication is called intractable. Status epilepticus is a condition in which the patient has serial seizures without recovery of consciousness between them. Insertion of a brain stimulator or excision of a brain lesion is successful in some cases in reducing or eliminating some of the symptoms of epilepsy.

Physician Documentation

Do not report "history of epilepsy" for a patient whose condition is controlled with medication. Epilepsy is incurable, so a history code would not be appropriate, especially if the patient is taking medication to reduce or eliminate symptoms. In documentation for a patient with seizures, the duration and quality of the seizures are important to note, as are any tests ordered or test results interpreted. Keep in mind, though, that seizure is a symptom; epilepsy is a disorder. Use the term "epilepsy" or "seizure disorder" when it is appropriate to ensure the correct diagnosis is abstracted.

For epilepsy, note if focal or generalized, and whether it is adequately controlled by medication (not intractable). This establishes the severity of the condition. Similarly, if the patient experiences a breakthrough seizure, note if the epilepsy is intractable or not intractable according to clinical judgment. In cases of intractable epilepsy, document any status epilepticus.

Absent an epilepsy diagnosis, seizures should be noted as to cause (eg, febrile, post-traumatic, autonomic, or related to alcohol withdrawal). Absent an epilepsy disorder, seizure-related diagnoses that risk-adjust include:

- Simple febrile convulsions (R56.00)
- Complex febrile convulsions (R56.01)
- Post-traumatic seizures (R56.1)
- Unspecified convulsions (R56.9)

CLINICAL EXAMPLES

NONSPECIFIC DOCUMENTATION	SPECIFIC DOCUMENTATION
Example 1 History of epilepsy. The patient has been seizure-free for 18 months, and came in today with paperwork to reinstate her driving privileges.[a]	**Example 1** Patient was originally diagnosed with absence epileptic syndrome when she was 19. The patient is now well-controlled with ethosuximide and has been seizure-free for 18 months. She came in today with paperwork to reinstate her driving privileges.[b]
Example 2 Assessment: 1. CP. 2. Worsening seizures; has been compliant with AEDs.[c]	**Example 2** Assessment: 1. Cerebral palsy with spastic diplegia. The patient uses a powered wheelchair for mobility. 2. Worsening symptoms related to complex partial seizure disorder heretofore controlled with phenobarbital.[d]

[a] "History of epilepsy" indicates a resolved condition. Because she has not had a seizure for 18 months, it cannot be reported as an active condition. All that can be reported for this encounter is code Z02.4, *Encounter for examination for driving license.*

[b] Evidence of the presence of epilepsy, plus ongoing medication, allow coders to abstract epilepsy. Here, the physician documented the specific type of epilepsy and how it is controlled.

[c] Spell out abbreviations on first reference. Type of cerebral palsy should be noted. Coders cannot abstract epilepsy from documented medication, ie, the AED (antiepileptic drug). Epilepsy must be so stated, preferably with specificity as to type.

[d] In this case, the CP and epilepsy are well documented.

Coding

While a documented "seizure disorder" or "recurrent seizure" is classified as epilepsy in the Alphabetic Index, simply documented "seizure" is not classified as epilepsy. Follow the language in documentation to look up the correct code in the Alphabetic Index for seizure, convulsion, or epilepsy. If a patient with epilepsy is documented as having a "breakthrough" seizure, query the physician regarding the patient's status as intractable/not intractable.

"Tonic-clonic" is a descriptor for seizure that involves loss of consciousness and intense muscle contractions, also called a grand mal seizure. Tonic-clonic is a symptom not separately reported in epilepsy. For a patient with dementia caused by epilepsy, report the appropriate epilepsy code with a code from category F02.8-, *Dementia in diseases classified elsewhere.*

CODING TIP Intractable epilepsy can be reported when documentation states poorly controlled, uncontrolled, treatment resistant, pharmacoresistant, or refractory epilepsy.

ABSTRACT & CODE IT!

Abstract and code the clinical coding example below. Check your answers against the answers in Appendix C.

Patient 1
Recurrent seizures are controlled well with carbamazepine.

Patient 2
Patient was originally diagnosed with absence epileptic syndrome when she was 19. The patient is now well controlled with ethosuximide and has been seizure-free for 18 months. She came in today with paperwork to reinstate her driving privileges.

Patient 3
Assessment:

1. Cerebral palsy with spastic diplegia. The patient uses a powered wheelchair for mobility.
2. Worsening symptoms related to complex partial seizure disorder heretofore controlled with phenobarbital.

Septicemia and SIRS

Septicemia, SIRS, shock
HCC 2 0.455

Sepsis is a clinical syndrome of physiologic, pathologic, and biochemical abnormalities brought about by infection, identified by signs and symptoms in a patient with a systemic infection. There is no single test to confirm or exclude sepsis. Sepsis is a life-threatening condition in which the body's response to infection is self-damaging.

Clinical understanding of the complexities of sepsis continues to evolve. Sepsis can be associated with an infection anywhere in the body (eg, pneumonia, urinary tract infection, gastrointestinal infection, or skin infection). More than 1.5 million people experience sepsis in the US each year, and sepsis is the leading cause of death in patients who die of infection (about 250,000 patients with sepsis die each year, according to the CDC).[6] Most diagnoses of sepsis are in the inpatient environment; however, it may be seen in skilled nursing facilities or other entities in which a decision not to transfer the patient to the inpatient environment has been made.

Physician Documentation

The definition of sepsis is controversial. Not all physicians agree on which clinical indictors support sepsis for a sepsis diagnosis. Given that coding is based solely on physician documentation, the AHA's *Coding Clinic* (Fourth Quarter, 2016) offers the following official advice:

> While physicians may use a particular clinical definition or set of clinical criteria to establish a diagnosis, the code is based on his/her documentation, not on a particular clinical definition or criteria. In other words, regardless of whether a physician uses the new clinical criteria for sepsis, the old criteria, his personal clinical judgment, or something else to decide a patient has sepsis (and document it as such), the code for sepsis is the same—as long as sepsis is documented, regardless of how the diagnosis was arrived at, the code for sepsis can be assigned. Coders should not be disregarding physician documentation and deciding on their own, based on clinical criteria, abnormal test results, etc., whether or not a condition should be coded. For example, if the physician documents sepsis and the coder assigns the code for sepsis, and a clinical validation reviewer later disagrees with the physician's diagnosis, that is a clinical issue, but it is not a coding error. By the same token, coders shouldn't be coding sepsis in the absence of physician documentation because they believe the patient meets sepsis clinical criteria. A facility or a payer may require that a physician use a particular clinical definition or set of criteria when establishing a diagnosis, but that is a clinical issue outside the coding system.[7]

The diagnosis of sepsis is dependent upon the definition assigned to the term documented by the physician, and the official clinical definition has been revised in recent years. This evolution of definitions is as follows:

- **Sepsis definition 1 (Sepsis-1)** (1992) – ICD-9-CM was based on this:
  - **Sepsis** – Infection plus 2 of 4 of the following systemic inflammatory response syndrome criteria:
    - Temperature above 100.4°F or less than 96°F
    - Tachycardia (pulse > 90)
    - Tachypnea (respiratory rate > 24)
    - White count abnormalities (less than 4,000, greater than 12,000, or 10% or more immature cells [bands]
  - **Severe sepsis** – Sepsis plus sepsis-induced organ dysfunction or failure
- **Sepsis definition 2 (Sepsis-2)** (2001) – ICD-10-CM is based on this:
  - Systemic inflammatory response syndrome – mentioned
  - **Sepsis** – same as Sepsis definition 1 but allowing for acute organ dysfunction or failure to substitute as a sepsis criteria. Patient must appear toxic or septic
  - **Severe sepsis** – same as Sepsis-1
- **Sepsis definition 3 (Sepsis-3)** (2016) – international consensus not consistent with ICD-10-CM:
  - Systemic inflammatory response syndrome – discarded in infectious processes
  - **Sepsis** – Same as severe sepsis in Sepsis-2, exhibited by a change in the Sepsis-related Organ Failure Assessment (SOFA) score of 2 or more
  - **Severe sepsis** – term discarded

As such, for a physician to represent sepsis in Sepsis-3, that same physician would have to document severe sepsis to represent sepsis that results in acute organ dysfunction, because it is this documentation that leads to the selection and assignment of ICD-10-CM code R65.20, *Severe sepsis without septic shock*. Furthermore, if a physician believes that a patient is systemically ill from an infection but does not have acute organ dysfunction, ICD-10-CM still allows the reporting of a sepsis code (eg, A40-A41) without code R65.20. However, the clinical validity of the documentation and coding may be challenged by a recovery auditor.

Sepsis
Definitions evolve as medical science advances. The *Journal of the American Medical Association* (*JAMA*) provides a detailed review of the international work toward consensus for definitions for sepsis, severe sepsis, and septic shock, along with numerous tables outlining the most recent clinical criteria for these diagnoses, in a February, 23, 2016 communication at http://jamanetwork.com/journals/jama/fullarticle/2492881#jsc160002t1.

Essentially, according to the new Sepsis-3 definition, documentation of "sepsis" requires an element of organ dysfunction or organ failure. However, sepsis with organ failure in ICD-10-CM is defined as "severe sepsis." Using the new Sepsis-3 definition, documenting "sepsis" is the equivalent of "severe sepsis" in ICD-10-CM. However, if a physician documents "sepsis," a code for sepsis without organ failure will be abstracted by the coder, unless the physician is very clear in documenting which organ system is failing, and clearly links it to the sepsis.

Some physicians do not embrace Sepsis-3, maintaining that a patient can be systemically ill due to an infection without having acute organ dysfunction. The AHA's *Coding Clinic* (Fourth Quarter, 2016) discussed the contradictory definitions of sepsis, and advised coders never to assign a code for sepsis based on clinical definition or criteria or clinical signs alone. In addition, code assignment should be based strictly on physician documentation (regardless of the clinical criteria the physician used to arrive at that diagnosis).[7] Therefore, it is imperative that physicians be familiar with the different sepsis classifications and document "severe sepsis," if the patient's diagnosis meets the ICD-10-CM definition.

According to the Introduction to *ICD-10-CM Guidelines*, a "joint effort between the healthcare provider and the coder is essential to achieve complete and accurate documentation, code assignment, and reporting of diagnoses and procedures."[2] ICD-10-CM Guideline Section I(C.1.d.1.a.ii) states that the "term urosepsis is a nonspecific term and does not have a code in ICD-10-CM. It is not to be considered synonymous with sepsis. It has no default code in the Alphabetic Index. Should a provider use this term, he/she must be queried for clarification."[2]

It is critical for physicians to ensure that the severity of illness is accurately reported, especially in cases of systemic infection. It is also critical for physicians to identify sepsis as the causal agent of any organ failure, as appropriate. Never report "urosepsis" as this is a term of ambiguity and cannot be abstracted without more information. The Alphabetic Index instructs the coder to "code to" the condition when classifying the term "urosepsis." When documenting sepsis, document the infective agent, if possible. Clearly specify any organ(s) in failure, and identify severe sepsis in cases of organ failure. Link the organ failure to the sepsis clearly. Document any septic shock.

ADVICE/ALERT NOTE

Per ICD-10-CM Guideline Section I(C.1.d.1.a.ii), the "term urosepsis is a nonspecific term and does not have a code in ICD-10-CM. It is not to be considered synonymous with sepsis. It has no default code in the Alphabetic Index. Should a provider use this term, he/she must be queried for clarification."[2]

DOCUMENTATION TIP According to the CDC, a "reliable sepsis surveillance definition based on objective clinical data is needed to more accurately track national sepsis trends and enable ongoing assessment of the impact of efforts to increase sepsis awareness and prevention."[6]

Recovery auditor
Reviewer charged with evaluating documentation and payment history of claims with the goal of recovering overpayments for the federal government.

CLINICAL EXAMPLES

NONSPECIFIC DOCUMENTATION	SPECIFIC DOCUMENTATION
Example 1 Assessment: 1. Sepsis due to MRSA[a]; vancomycin. 2. ARF. 3. Lower extremity cellulitis.	**Example 1** Assessment: 1. Severe sepsis due to methicillin resistant staphylococcus aureus (MRSA[b]); parenteral vancomycin. 2. Acute respiratory failure due to sepsis; tracheostomy and ventilator status. 3. Right ankle cellulitis due to MRSA.
Example 2 Urosepsis.[c]	**Example 2** *E. coli* urinary tract infection with gross hematuria.[d]

[a] Documentation fails to link the ARF to the sepsis and fails to identify the acronym ARF as of renal or respiratory origin. The cellulitis site is nonspecific and not linked to the MRSA.

[b] A clearer picture is presented here with information on the respiratory failure, tracheostomy, and ventilator status. The cellulitis site and infective agent are identified.

[c] A generic term that cannot be abstracted, urosepsis should be avoided in all documentation.

[d] A clear clinical picture of the patient's UTI including hematuria and infective agent.

Coding

The most important factor in the correct coding of sepsis is understanding the definitions of clinical and coding terms used in the documentation. In addition, physicians should ensure they are documenting using terminology that reflects ICD-10-CM definitions. Coding of septicemia, sepsis, and systemic inflammatory response syndrome (SIRS) has always been confusing, more so since the adoption of ICD-10-CM and the release of Sepsis-3. Read the preceding entry on physician documentation of sepsis carefully to better understand the problem.

The most important advice regarding sepsis coding for ICD-10-CM is to set aside everything thought to be known about sepsis coding, focus on the guidelines, and share this material with physicians so that they are aware of the problems inherent in using the new definition for sepsis in relation to the ICD-10-CM guidelines. Coders must abstract based on documentation, and physicians must align their documentation for sepsis with ICD-10-CM guidelines in order for the severity of illness to be effectively captured. According to AHA's *Coding Clinic* (Third Quarter, 2016), "[r]efer to the Official Guidelines for Coding and Reporting when assigning codes for sepsis, severe sepsis, and septic shock. The coding guidelines are based on the classification as it exists today. Therefore, continue to code sepsis, severe sepsis, and septic shock using the most current version of the ICD-10-CM classification and the ICD-10-CM Official Guidelines for Coding and Reporting, not clinical criteria."[3]

According to ICD-10-CM Guideline Section I(C.1.d.1.b), the "coding of severe sepsis requires a minimum of 2 codes: first a code for the underlying systemic infection, followed by a code from subcategory R65.2, Severe sepsis. If the causal organism is not documented, assign code A41.9, Sepsis, unspecified organism, for the infection. Additional code(s) for the associated acute organ dysfunction are also required." In addition, ICD-10-CM Guidelines Section I(C.1.d.1.a.iii) and I(C.1.d.1.a.iv) state that "[i]f a patient has sepsis and associated acute organ dysfunction or multiple organ dysfunction (MOD), follow the instructions for coding severe sepsis. If a patient has sepsis and an acute organ dysfunction, but the medical record documentation indicates that the acute organ dysfunction is related to a medical condition other than the sepsis, do not assign a code from subcategory R65.2, Severe sepsis without septic shock. An acute organ dysfunction must be associated with the sepsis in order to assign the severe sepsis code. If the documentation is not clear as to whether an acute organ dysfunction is related to the sepsis or another medical condition, query the provider."[2]

Furthermore, ICD-10-CM Guideline Section I(C.1.d.1.a) states that "[f]or a diagnosis of sepsis, assign the appropriate code for the underlying systemic infection. If the type of infection or causal organism is not further specified, assign code A41.9, Sepsis, unspecified organism. A code from subcategory R65.2, Severe sepsis, should not be assigned unless severe sepsis or an associated acute organ dysfunction is documented."[2]

If possible, meet with physicians to discuss the contradictory nature of sepsis documentation and coding, and develop a plan so that the severity of illness can be appropriately captured from the medical record. Sepsis is a topic that may be appropriate for a new entry in coding policy documents. The AHA's *Coding Clinic* (Fourth Quarter, 2017) issued guidance that "[p]rovider documentation must specifically link an acute organ dysfunction with sepsis in order to assign the severe sepsis code. The 'with' guidelines state that when another guideline exists that specifically requires a documented linkage between two conditions (e.g., sepsis guideline for 'acute organ dysfunction that is not clearly associated with the sepsis'), then provider documentation must link the conditions in order to code them as related. It is also appropriate to assign a code for severe sepsis when the provider documents 'severe sepsis,' or when the Index to Diseases directs to the code for 'severe sepsis.' Effective October 1, 2017, the 'with' guideline (Section I.A.15) has been revised to clarify 'When a guideline requires that a linkage between two conditions be explicitly documented, provider documentation must link the conditions in order to code them as related.' The sepsis guideline for 'acute organ dysfunction that is not clearly associated with sepsis' is an example of this exception, and the 'with' guideline would not apply since another guideline exists that specifically requires a documented linkage."[8]

ADVICE/ALERT NOTE

Per ICD-10-CM Guideline Section I(C.1.d.1.b), the "coding of severe sepsis requires a minimum of 2 codes: first a code for the underlying systemic infection, followed by a code from subcategory R65.2, Severe sepsis. If the causal organism is not documented, assign code A41.9, Sepsis, unspecified organism, for the infection. Additional code(s) for the associated acute organ dysfunction are also required."[2]

In some circumstances of sepsis reporting, coders can report diagnoses that have not been documented. For example, code severe sepsis when "severe sepsis" is not documented and reporting code:

- R65.20, *Severe sepsis,* when the physician documents "sepsis" and attributes one or more organ dysfunction(s) or failure(s) to the sepsis.
- R65.21, *Severe sepsis with septic shock,* when the physician documents "septic shock," which is acute circulatory failure due to systemic infection.

Report code A41.9, *Sepsis, unspecified organism,* if sepsis or severe sepsis is documented and there is no documentation of the infective agent.

According to ICD-10-CM Guideline Section I(C.1.d.2.a), "[s]eptic shock generally refers to circulatory failure associated with severe sepsis, and therefore, it represents a type of acute organ dysfunction. For cases of septic shock, the code for the systemic infection should be sequenced first, followed by code R65.21, Severe sepsis with septic shock, or code T81.12, Postprocedural septic shock. Any additional codes for the other acute organ dysfunctions should also be assigned. As noted in the sequencing instructions in the Tabular List, the code for septic shock cannot be assigned as a principal diagnosis."[2]

ADVICE/ALERT NOTE

Per ICD-10-CM Guideline Section I(C.1.d.2.a), "[s]eptic shock generally refers to circulatory failure associated with severe sepsis, and therefore, it represents a type of acute organ dysfunction. For cases of septic shock, the code for the systemic infection should be sequenced first, followed by code R65.21, Severe sepsis with septic shock, or code T81.12, Postprocedural septic shock. Any additional codes for the other acute organ dysfunctions should also be assigned. As noted in the sequencing instructions in the Tabular List, the code for septic shock cannot be assigned as a principal diagnosis."[2]

There is no ICD-10-CM code for sepsis due to a virus. The AHA's *Coding Clinic* (Third Quarter, 2016) states that code A41.89, *Other specified sepsis,* should be reported for viral sepsis, even though codes in categories A30-A49 classify bacterial illnesses.[9] In addition, a second code for the specific virus (eg, A41.89 for Lyme disease sepsis with A69.29, *Other conditions associated with Lyme disease*; for West Nile sepsis, A41.89, *Other specified sepsis*, and the appropriate West Nile disease code from category A92.3, *West Nile virus infection*) should be reported as well. Furthermore, metabolic changes from sepsis can lead to brain disorders; therefore, report code G93.41, *Metabolic encephalopathy,* for any documented sepsis-associated encephalopathy, according to AHA's *Coding Clinic* (Second Quarter, 2017).[10]

ABSTRACT & CODE IT!

Abstract and code the clinical coding example below. Check your answers against the answers in Appendix C.

Patient 1

Bacteremia due to PICC line, infective agent Enterococcus, in a patient undergoing chemotherapy for breast cancer.

Patient 2

Assessment:

1. Severe sepsis due to methicillin resistant staphylococcus aureus (MRSA); parenteral vancomycin.
2. Acute respiratory failure due to sepsis; tracheostomy and ventilator status.
3. Right ankle cellulitis due to MRSA.

Patient 3

Urosepsis.

Shock *see* Arrest, Shock, Ventilator Status

Skin Ulcers

Pressure ulcer of skin with necrosis through to muscle, tendon or bone
HCC 157 2.163

Pressure pre-ulcer skin changes or unspecified stage
HCC 160 (from 2018 list)

Chronic ulcer of skin, except pressure
HCC 161 0.535
RxHCC 311 0.162

Skin ulcers are open wounds that are slow to heal. Ischemia is the root cause of most skin ulcers, whether pressure (decubitus) ulcers or chronic skin ulcers. In pressure ulcers, the ischemia is caused by the weight of the patient's body upon a pressure point (eg, skin overlying bone at the sacrum, back of the head, or the heel of bedridden patients, or back of the knee, heel, or forearms of patients who are dependent on wheelchairs). Immobility causes chronic pressure on these points, and the skin tissue becomes inflamed and may break down.

Chronic skin ulcers can also develop in patients with compromised circulation. In venous stasis, for example, the lower extremities become congested with venous blood, damaging the small vessels in the leg. This causes skin to dry out, easily break down, and makes healing difficult. Alternatively, tissue ischemia can be caused by atherosclerosis of the distal arteries. In atherosclerosis, the arteries narrow, reducing the amount of blood flow. In the extremities, this can lead to ulcers, usually on bony prominences, the heel, or between the toes.

Patients with diabetes often develop lower extremity ulcers. In diabetic foot ulcers, the patient may have multiple problems:

- Changes to the bony structure of the foot
- Neuropathic changes to the feet that create mechanical stresses in the gait, leading to development of calluses that in turn lead to ulcerations
- Loss of protective sensation (LOPS) that allows a patient to continue to ambulate despite an injury to the foot (eg, a callus can become an ulcer without causing discomfort to the patient)
- Advanced peripheral atherosclerosis

The combination of these factors predisposes diabetic ulcers to ischemia and necrosis, which can lead to amputation.

Due to the compromised health status of these patients, chronic ulcers and pressure ulcers take longer to heal than regular wounds, and without intervention, spread to deeper tissues in ischemic, pressure, and diabetic foot ulcers, or to wider or multiple shallow ulcers in venous skin ulcers. Ulcers are classified according to the depth of the wound, as well as the site and the etiology.

Physician Documentation

There are more than 200 ulcer codes in the ICD-10-CM code set, but documentation and coding can be distilled to a few key data points:

- **Etiology;** choose from:
  - Venous stasis (link ulcer to varicose veins)
  - Atherosclerotic (ischemic)
    - Native arteries, autologous/nonautologous or nonbiological bypass grafts
    - Link ischemic ulcer and any gangrene to peripheral atherosclerosis
  - Others (such as a skin ulcer seen with chronic infections)

- Diabetic foot ulcer
  - Identify diabetes as type 1, type 2, or secondary, and etiology of secondary
- Pressure ulcer
  - Also document any contributing comorbidity (eg, functional quadriplegia, quadriplegia, paraplegia, multiple sclerosis, amyotrophic lateral sclerosis, etc)
- **Site and laterality**
- **Severity**
  - For pressure ulcers:
    - Stages 1-4
    - Deep tissue injury (code to unstageable)
    - Unstageable
  - For chronic ulcers (venous, diabetic foot, atherosclerotic [ischemic]):
    - Limited to breakdown of skin
    - With fat layer exposed
    - With necrosis of muscle
    - With necrosis of bone
    - With muscle involvement without evidence of necrosis
    - With bone involvement without evidence of necrosis
    - With other specified severity
    - Without staging

DOCUMENTATION TIP ICD-10-CM classifies foot ulcers in diabetic patients as due to diabetes unless the physician outlines another cause (eg, a pressure ulcer on the heel). Diabetic foot ulcer classification systems like the Wagner Diabetic Foot Ulcer Grade Classification System (Wagner Grade Classification) do not align with the ICD-10-CM classification for chronic wounds. For more information on the Wagner Grade Classification System, visit https://woundeducators.com/diabetic-foot-ulcer/. Be sure to use descriptive language in documenting the diabetic foot ulcer so that the correct diagnoses can be abstracted.

ICD-10-CM has conventions that will affect how documentation related to an ulcer is abstracted:

- A "wound" is classified as a traumatic injury in ICD-10-CM, so this term should not be documented in relation to chronic or pressure ulcers.
- "Skin ulcer" defaults in ICD-10-CM to a "chronic ulcer."
- "Deep tissue injury" is classified by ICD-10-CM as a "contusion" or "unstageable pressure ulcer," but without more information, the coder will not know which to choose. Document as "unstageable" if the intent is to have the condition classified as a pressure ulcer.

According to ICD-10-CM Guideline Section I(C.12.a.1), "[a]ssign as many codes from category L89 to identify all the pressure ulcers the patient has, if applicable."[2] ICD-10-CM does not provide much leeway in the classification of pressure ulcers; documentation must state the stage, or use clinical terms as found in the Alphabetic Index. Acceptable terms in parentheses following each stage here:

- **Stage 1** (changes limited to persistent focal edema)
- **Stage 2** (abrasion, blister, partial thickness skin loss involving epidermis and/or dermis)
- **Stage 3** (full-thickness skin loss involving damage or necrosis of subcutaneous tissue)
- **Stage 4** (soft tissues through to underlying muscle, tendon, or bone)

Other language to describe the ulcers cannot be used for staging the pressure ulcer, and the ulcer will be reported as unspecified.

 **ADVICE/ALERT NOTE**

Per ICD-10-CM Guideline Section I(C.12.a.1), "[a]ssign as many codes from category L89 to identify all the pressure ulcers the patient has, if applicable."[2]

Document pressure ulcers to the highest stage they reached, even when they are smaller due to epithelial growth and healing. The National Pressure Ulcer Advisory Panel (NPUAP) advises the staging of ulcers should always be to the highest level of stage the ulcer penetrated. Per the NPUAP, "[s]taging is an assessment system that classifies pressure ulcers based on anatomic depth of soft tissue damage.[11,12] Pressure ulcer staging is only appropriate for defining the maximum anatomic depth of tissue damage."[13] Do not "reverse stage" an ulcer by identifying a lesser stage as it begins to heal. NPUAP's position statement on reverse staging states, "Pressure ulcers heal to progressively more shallow depth, they do not replace lost muscle, subcutaneous fat, or dermis before they re-epithelialize. Instead, the ulcer is filled with granulation (scar) tissue composed primarily of endothelial cells, fibroblasts, collagen and extracellular matrix. A Stage IV pressure ulcer cannot become a Stage III, Stage II, and/or subsequently Stage I. When a Stage IV ulcer has healed it should be classified as a healed Stage IV pressure ulcer not a Stage 0 pressure ulcer."[14]

Document any necrosis identified in non-pressure ulcers. New codes for chronic ulcers were added to the ICD-10-CM classification for 2018 to allow for reporting of non-pressure ulcers to the depth of muscle or bone that do not have evidence of necrosis. Previous codes classified non-pressure ulcers to the level of bone or muscle as "with necrosis."

ICD-10-CM Guideline Section I(A.15) requires coders to link diabetes to most comorbidities when no other cause is documented (eg, a heel ulcer in a diabetic patient is automatically reported as a diabetic foot ulcer). Any other cause should be well documented. Note that in ICD-10-CM Guideline Section I(A.15), the "word 'with' or 'in' should be interpreted to mean 'associated with' or 'due to' when it appears in a code title, the Alphabetic Index, or an instructional note in the Tabular List. The classification presumes a causal relationship between the two conditions linked by these terms in the Alphabetic Index or Tabular List. These conditions should be coded as related even in the absence of provider documentation explicitly linking them, unless the documentation clearly states the conditions are unrelated or when another guideline exists that specifically requires a documented linkage between two conditions (e.g., sepsis guideline for 'acute organ dysfunction that is not clearly associated with the sepsis')."[2]

ADVICE/ALERT NOTE

Per ICD-10-CM Guideline Section I(A.15), the "word 'with' or 'in' should be interpreted to mean 'associated with' or 'due to' when it appears in a code title, the Alphabetic Index, or an instructional note in the Tabular List. The classification presumes a causal relationship between the two conditions linked by these terms in the Alphabetic Index or Tabular List. These conditions should be coded as related even in the absence of provider documentation explicitly linking them, unless the documentation clearly states the conditions are unrelated or when another guideline exists that specifically requires a documented linkage between two conditions (e.g., sepsis guideline for 'acute organ dysfunction that is not clearly associated with the sepsis')."[2]

Coding

ICD-10-CM category L89 classifies pressure ulcers, and categories L97 and L98 classify chronic ulcers. Pressure ulcers are coded according to site and stage; chronic ulcers are coded according to site, depth, and presence/absence of necrosis. Pressure ulcers are always going to be caused by pressure exerted on the skin in a patient who is somewhat or entirely immobile. Chronic skin ulcers most commonly occur in the lower extremities, and can have a variety of etiologies, including ischemic ulcers from atherosclerosis, venous stasis ulcers with varicosities, and diabetic foot ulcers.

CODING TIP Do not confuse diabetic foot ulcer classification grades or stages with pressure ulcer stages in ICD-10-CM. The grading systems for diabetic ulcers do not correlate to ICD-10-CM levels of chronic skin ulcer. However, these grades or stages when found in documentation may alert the coder that the physician should be queried about any gangrene, osteomyelitis, or abscess:

Wagner Grade Classification

Grade 0 = Intact skin

Grade 1 = Superficial ulcer of skin or subcutaneous tissue

Grade 2 = Ulcer extends into tendon, bone, or capsule without infection

Grade 3 = Deep ulcer with osteomyelitis, joint infection, or abscess

Grade 4 = Localized gangrene

Grade 5 = Extensive gangrene

University of Texas (Grade and Stage) Diabetic Foot Ulcer Classification

Pick one grade and one stage:

Grade 0 = Pre- or post-ulcerative site that has healed

Grade 1 = Superficial wound not involving tendon, capsule, or bone

Grade 2 = Wound penetrating to tendon or capsule

Grade 3 = Wound penetrating to bone or joint

Stage A = Clean wounds

Stage B = Non-ischemic infected wounds

Stage C = Ischemic non-infected wounds

Stage D = Ischemic infected wounds

For ICD-10-CM 2018, more than 60 new codes were added for chronic ulcers in which each site received new codes to identify chronic ulcers to the level of bone without necrosis, to the level of muscle without necrosis, and "with other specified severity." Before 2018, any chronic ulcer to the level or muscle or bone was by default reported as "with necrosis," which caused some confusion among coders for cases in which the level of bone or muscle was reached but no necrosis was documented. Visual inspection is the basis of staging or assigning levels for both pressure ulcer and chronic ulcer staging. It is acceptable to abstract the stage or level of an ulcer from documentation that is from someone other than a qualified healthcare provider, but only when a physician also documents the presence of the ulcer.

ADVICE/ALERT NOTE

Per ICD-10-CM Guideline Section I(B.14), for the "Body Mass Index (BMI), depth of non-pressure chronic ulcers, pressure ulcer stage, coma scale, and NIH stroke scale (NIHSS) codes, code assignment may be based on medical record documentation from clinicians who are not the patient's provider (i.e., physician or other qualified healthcare practitioner legally accountable for establishing the patient's diagnosis), as this information is typically documented by other clinicians involved in the care of the patient (e.g., a dietitian often documents the BMI, a nurse often documents the pressure ulcer stages, and an emergency medical technician often documents the coma scale). However, the associated diagnosis (such as overweight, obesity, acute stroke, or pressure ulcer) must be documented by the patient's provider. If there is conflicting medical record documentation, either from the same clinician or different clinicians, the patient's attending provider should be queried for clarification."[2]

According to ICD-10-CM Guideline Section I(C.12.a), the "[a]ssignment of the code for unstageable pressure ulcer (L89.--0) should be based on the clinical documentation. These codes are used for pressure ulcers whose stage cannot be clinically determined (e.g., the ulcer is covered by eschar or has been treated with a skin or muscle graft) and pressure ulcers that are documented as deep tissue injury but not documented as due to trauma. This code should not be confused with the codes for unspecified stage (L89.--9). When there is no documentation regarding the stage of the pressure ulcer, assign the appropriate code for unspecified stage (L89.--9). Assignment of the pressure ulcer stage code should be guided by clinical documentation of the stage or documentation of the terms found in the Alphabetic Index. For clinical terms describing the stage that are not found in the Alphabetic Index, and there is no documentation of the stage, the physician should be queried. No code is assigned if the documentation states that the pressure ulcer is completely healed."[2]

Code the level of ulcer documented by the physician, even if the ulcer is documented as "healing." A healing stage 4 pressure ulcer will continue to be a stage 4 pressure ulcer until it is totally healed, at which point it is no longer reported. Sometimes pressure ulcers are identified as "deep tissue injury" in documentation. These pressure ulcers have subcutaneous tissue damage that is visible on the surface of the skin as a bruise-like spot, or by a change in the texture of the site during a physical exam. Because the skin is intact, it is not possible to identify the stage of the pressure ulcer. Injury/deep tissue classifies either to a contusion or an unstageable pressure ulcer in ICD-10-CM. If there is not enough information (eg, documented unstageable) in the documentation to abstract the condition as apressure ulcer, query the physician. ICD-10-CM does not differentiate between skin ulcers with infection and those without infections. If the pressure ulcer or chronic ulcer is infected, a second code should be reported to identify the infective agent. Report separately any cellulitis, abscess, or other complicating condition.

CODING TIP A code from L89.4, *Pressure ulcer of contiguous site of back, buttock and hip,* is used for an extensive ulcer that covers more than one of the listed anatomical sites. The ICD-10-CM guidelines inform us that "and" in code descriptions should actually be interpreted to mean "and/or." Report code L89.4 when a pressure ulcer spans two sites (eg, back and hip, back and buttock, or hip and buttock).

ABSTRACT & CODE IT!

Abstract and code the clinical coding example below. Check your answers against the answers in Appendix C.

Patient: Micah Streeham **DOB:** 04/05/47 **DOS:** 10/19/2017

Chief Complaint: Rx refill

Vitals: 10/19/2017 11:15 a.m.

Ht: 5'9" Wt: 147 lbs BMI: 21.7 BP: 124/92 Pulse: 96 O2 Sat: 96%

Allergies: Gabapentin: rash

Medications: Reviewed 10/19/2017

Aspirin 81 mg tablet, delayed release	Take one by mouth in the evening	07/08/14 entered
BD INSULIN SYRINGE ULTRA-FINE 1 ML 30 GAUGE X 1/2"	Use 2 daily	02/15/16
Clopidogrel 75 mg tablet	Take one by mouth daily	10/19/16 prescribed
Furosemide 40 mg tablet	1 tab daily prn	10/19/16 prescribed
Humulin N 100 unit/mL subcutaneous suspension	Inject 52 units subcu twice daily	07/19/16 filled
Humulin R 100 unit/mL injection solution	Use as directed	02/10/16 filled
Losartan 50 mg-hydrochlorothiazide 12.5 mg tablet	Take 1 by mouth daily	10/19/16 prescribed
Metoprolol succinate ER 25 mg tablet, extended release 24 hr	Take one by mouth twice daily	10/19/16 prescribed
OneTouch Delica Lancets	33 gauge	04/24/14 filled
OneTouch Ultra Test strips	Test three times a day for 90 days	04/24/14 filled
Simvastatin 20 mg tablet	Take one by mouth in the evening	10/19/16 prescribed

Problem List:

Amputated foot

Blood chemistry abnormal

Essential hypertension

Peripheral arterial occlusive disease

Diabetic skin ulcer

Chronic kidney disease stage 4

Type 1 diabetes mellitus

Diabetic retinopathy, proliferative, with some vision loss

Alkaline phosphatase raised

Diabetic renal disease

Atherosclerosis of native arteries of the extremities

Diabetic neuropathy

Edema

Pure hypercholesterolemia

Vitamin D deficiency

Depressive disorder

Family History: Adopted; history unknown

Social History: Retired former smoker, married. Drinks two drinks daily. Lives with wife. Does not engage in regular exercise.

Surgical History:

Amputation 5 toes left foot 5/2017

Angioplasty LLE

Colonoscopy – negative

Retinal surgery 2012 and 2014

PMH [past medical history]

Coronary artery disease

Type 1 diabetes mellitus

Elevated cholesterol

Prostate cancer

Hypertension

AAA

Peripheral arterial disease

Diabetic neuropathy

Foot and ankle ulcers

Vitamin D deficiency

HPI [history of present illness]: Patient is here for a six-month check. He is feeling depressed about his amputation and his inability to get out and do things he used to do. His blood glucose levels are higher than what is healthy because he fears hypoglycemic episodes that he experiences when in tight control, and as a result of the Lupron Depot injections. He currently has a diabetic foot ulcer on his left heel, for which he sees his podiatrist twice monthly.

ROS [review of systems]:

Constitutional: Healthy appearing and well-nourished.

Psychiatric: Good judgment; normal mood and affect. Oriented x3.

Neck: No cervical or supraclavicular NAD. No enlargement of thyroid.

Lungs: No dyspnea. No wheezing, rales, or crackles. Good air movement.

Cardiovascular: Normal S1 and S2, no murmurs, rubs, or gallops. RRR.

Musculoskeletal: No cyanosis, edema or clubbing; he is followed by a podiatrist for his diabetic angiopathy and foot ulcers. Recent amputation of all 5 L toes is healing well. Ulcer noted on L heel.

Assessment/Plan:

1. Type 1 diabetes mellitus. He is in need of tighter control. Hemoglobin A1C. Comprehensive metabolic panel.
2. Major depressive disorder. Patient has a recurrent major depressive disorder that dates back to his teens and has required several hospitalizations. He has weaned himself from all antidepressants two years ago, and I discussed with him his new health status and its impact on his depressive disorder, but he refuses to go back on meds.
3. Essential hypertension. Well controlled with medications. His pressure was a bit elevated today, but his podiatrist's records show very stable numbers.
4. Diabetic foot ulcer and amputation. Amputation site is healing well. Ulcer being managed by Dr. Hue.
5. Hypercholesterolemia. Order lipid panel with LDL/HDL ratio.
6. Vitamin D deficiency. Continue taking vitamin supplements daily.

Skin Burns and Severe Conditions

Severe skin burn or condition
HCC 162 0.321

Burns are classified by type, by anatomical site, and by degree. Most burns are thermal burns, but ICD-10-CM also classifies corrosions related to chemicals as burns. Burns can also come from electricity and radiation. A first-degree burn involves the epidermis and causes some mild edema and redness, and is painful to the touch. Second-degree burns involve the epidermis and dermis, and include leaky blisters and the possible loss of some skin. It, too, is painful. A third-degree burn penetrates full-thickness skin and coagulates tissue, creating irreversible skin loss. It is often initially painless and the skin is dry, dark, and leathery.

Burns are also classified by how much body area the burn covers. ICD-10-CM classifies the total body surface area (TBSA) with third-degree burns. The body has a systemic response to large burn areas that may result in respiratory distress, metabolic changes, and a reduced immune response.

Of more than 2 million burn injuries in the US each year, 50,000 people require hospitalization, and nearly half of these have at least 25% of their TBSA affected, according to the CDC.[15] About 4,500 people die each year from their burns, twice that number die from burn-related infections.[15] Severe skin conditions are also captured in HCC 162, *Severe Burns and Skin Conditions.* See Table 4-4.3 for skin conditions that risk-adjust.

TABLE 4-4.3 Risk-Adjusting Severe Skin Conditions

CODE	DESCRIPTION
L12.30	Acquired epidermolysis bullosa, unspecified
L12.31	Epidermolysis bullosa due to drug
L12.35	Other acquired epidermolysis bullosa
L51.1	Stevens-Johnson syndrome
L51.2	Toxic epidermal necrolysis [Lyell]

Physician Documentation

Multiple elements must be included in the documentation to sufficiently capture a burn diagnosis, and each site of a burn should be separately identified and described. (See Figure 4-4.1.)

- **Site:** Identify the specific body part (eg, thumb, single finger, multiple fingers, palm, back of hand, wrist, forearm, elbow, upper arm, axilla, shoulder, or scapular region).
- **Laterality:** Identify right or left.
- **Type of injury:** Specify "burn" for thermal burn and "corrosion" for chemical burns.
- **Source of the burn or corrosion:** Identify the source, place, and intent of the injury (eg, scald burn from accidental coffee spill or corrosion from accidental hydrochloric acid spill).
- **Degree of burn:.** There may be multiple degrees from one injury or for one site of injury. Burns of the eye and internal organs are not reported by degree.
- **TBSA:** Defined as third-degree burn. ICD-10-CM Guideline Section I(C.19.d.6) states, "Assign codes from category T31, Burns classified according to extent of body surface involved, or T32, Corrosions classified according to extent of body surface involved, when the site of the burn is not specified or when there is a need for additional data. It is advisable to use category T31 as additional coding when needed to provide data for evaluating burn mortality, such as that needed by burn units. It is also advisable to use category T31 as an additional code for reporting purposes when there is mention of a third-degree burn involving 20 percent or more of the body surface."[2]
- **Episode of care:** Burns are reported as in initial treatment, subsequent care, or as sequelae.

Also report any shock, systemic inflammatory response syndrome (SIRS), respiratory distress, or other complication resulting from the acute burn.

CLINICAL EXAMPLES

NONSPECIFIC DOCUMENTATION	SPECIFIC DOCUMENTATION
Example 1 Escharotomy of right upper arm burned in a propane explosion.[a]	**Example 1** Escharotomy of right upper arm and axilla, 11% TBSA third-degree burn, from propane explosion and fire. Torso received second-degree burns totaling 12% TBSA.[b]
Example 2 Patient is here for follow-up to respiratory burns experienced when she was exposed to potassium hydroxide.[c]	**Example 2** She is here two months post-accident to assess her pulmonary function following the accident. The patient has experienced second-degree corrosive burns of her larynx, trachea, and lungs due to potassium hydroxide exposure at her place of work.[d] She experienced acute respiratory failure with hypoxemia, and was weaned from the ventilator 10 days ago.

[a] Identify TBSA and degree of burn, and document the circumstances (eg, at home or work). Clearly identify burn from gas fire vs corrosion.

[b] TBSA and degree have been added, as well as the circumstance of the fire.

[c] Clarify that the burn is corrosive when appropriate, so others do not have to consider whether the agent of the burn is flammable. Identify the specific site.

[d] The burns were identified as corrosive burns and the specific anatomy was noted. Noting the timeline of the accident and ventilator weaning is pertinent. This accident occurred at the workplace.

Coding

According to ICD-10-CM Guideline Section I(C.19.d), "ICD-10-CM makes a distinction between burns and corrosions. The burn codes are for thermal burns, except sunburns, that come from a heat source, such as a fire or hot appliance. The burn codes are also for burns resulting from electricity and radiation. Corrosions are burns due to chemicals. The guidelines are the same for burns and corrosions.

FIGURE 4-4.1 Lund-Browder Diagram and Classification Method Table for Burn Estimations

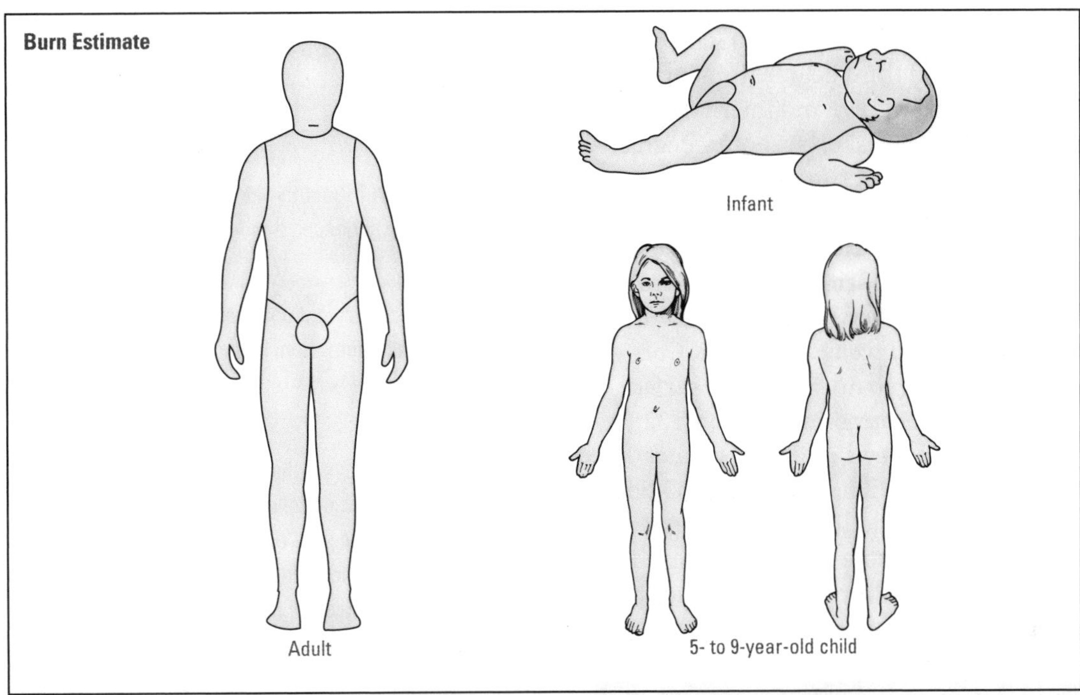

Area	Birth-1 year	1-4 years	5-9 years	10-14 years	15 years	Adult	2 degrees	3 degrees	Total	Donor areas
Head	19	17	13	11	9	7				
Neck	2	2	2	2	2	2				
Ant. trunk	13	13	13	13	13	13				
Post. trunk	13	13	13	13	13	13				
R. buttock	2 1/2	2 1/2	2 1/2	2 1/2	2 1/2	2 1/2				
L. buttock	2 1/2	2 1/2	2 1/2	2 1/2	2 1/2	2 1/2				
Genitalia	1	1	1	1	1	1				
R. U. arm	4	4	4	4	4	4				
L. U. arm	4	4	4	4	4	4				
R. L. arm	3	3	3	3	3	3				
L. L. arm	3	3	3	3	3	3				
R. hand	2 1/2	2 1/2	2 1/2	2 1/2	2 1/2	2 1/2				
L. hand	2 1/2	2 1/2	2 1/2	2 1/2	2 1/2	2 1/2				
R. thigh	5 1/2	6 1/2	8	8 1/2	9	9 1/2				
L. thigh	5 1/2	6 1/2	8	8 1/2	9	9 1/2				
R. leg	5	5	5 1/2	6	6 1/2	7				
L. leg	5	5	5 1/2	6	6 1/2	7				
R. foot	3 1/2	3 1/2	3 1/2	3 1/2	3 1/2	3 1/2				
L. foot	3 1/2	3 1/2	3 1/2	3 1/2	3 1/2	3 1/2				
Total										

The Lund- Browder Classification Method is used for estimating the extent, depth, and percentage of burns, allowing for the varying proportion of body surface in persons of different ages.

Current burns (T20-T25) are classified by depth, extent and by agent (X code). Burns are classified by depth as first degree (erythema), second degree (blistering), and third degree (full-thickness involvement). Burns of the eye and internal organs (T26-T28) are classified by site, but not by degree."[2] When coding burns, at least two codes are required: a code to identify the degree and site of the burn, and a code to identify the percentage of the burn site that is a third-degree burn. These codes are found in categories T31, *Burns classified according to extent of body surface involved*, and T32, *Corrosions classified according to extent of body surface involved*. Only codes in categories T31 and T32 reporting third-degree burns of 10% or greater TBSA risk-adjust. In addition, ICD-10-CM Guidelines Section I(C.19.d.3) and I(C.19.d.4) state that "[n]on-healing burns are coded as acute burns. For any documented infected burn site, use an additional code for the infection."[2]

ADVICE/ALERT NOTE

Per ICD-10-CM Guideline Section I(C.19.d), "ICD-10-CM makes a distinction between burns and corrosions. The burn codes are for thermal burns, except sunburns, that come from a heat source, such as a fire or hot appliance. The burn codes are also for burns resulting from electricity and radiation. Corrosions are burns due to chemicals. The guidelines are the same for burns and corrosions. Current burns (T20-T25) are classified by depth, extent and by agent (X code). Burns are classified by depth as first degree (erythema), second degree (blistering), and third degree (full-thickness involvement). Burns of the eye and internal organs (T26-T28) are classified by site, but not by degree."[2]

Do not add a 7th character for episode of care to categories T31, *Burns classified according to extent of body surface involved*, or T32, *Corrosions classified according to extent of body surface involved*. These codes should have only five characters.

ABSTRACT & CODE IT!

Abstract and code the clinical coding example below. Check your answers against the answers in Appendix C.

Patient 1

Patient is an 18-month-old boy who bit into an electrical cord and experienced a full-thickness burn of his upper lip.

Patient 2

Escharotomy of right upper arm and axilla, 11% TBSA third-degree burn, from home propane fire. Torso received second-degree burns totaling 12% TBSA.

Patient 3

She is here two months post-accident to assess her pulmonary function following the accident. The patient's experienced second-degree corrosive burns of her larynx, trachea, and lungs due to potassium hydroxide exposure at her place of work. She experienced acute respiratory failure with hypoxemia, and was weaned from the ventilator 10 days ago.

Skull Fracture *see* Trauma: Head

Stoma Status

Artificial openings for feeding or elimination
HCC 188 0.571

Ostomies are artificial openings in the body that bypass normal bodily functions. Ostomies can be performed to allow the bowel or urinary system to recover from injury or inflammation or to bypass a blockage. Stomas are the actual end of the organ that protrudes at the opening created to alter urinary or bowel elimination in patients who have had organs removed, or to simplify defecation hygiene practices in patients with incontinence following spinal cord injury. In some cases, the ostomies are later reversed; in other cases, they are permanent.

In an ostomy, the urine or feces of the patient are diverted from the organ involved, and waste is transported to the skin surface through a stoma. The waste is captured there for elimination.

Ostomies can also be created to provide a route for nutritional intake in patients who are too weak to swallow or who have an esophageal blockage. These ostomies are placed in the esophagus (esophagostomy) or the stomach (gastrostomy, or percutaneous endoscopic gastrostomy [PEG] tube). Gastrostomies may be permanent or temporary.

According to the United Ostomy Associations of America, Inc., 750,000 people in the US have temporary or permanent ostomies, and 130,000 people undergo ostomy surgery every year.[16] All ostomies risk-adjust, as they carry a risk of complication and because of the resources consumed in maintaining and monitoring an ostomy site. Tracheostomies risk-adjust, but are grouped with the HCCs for respiratory arrest and failure.

Physician Documentation

All ostomies risk-adjust. Be sure to visualize the ostomy site and document its condition during the physical examination of the patient. Note any complication or requirement for care as it occurs, but document the stoma's inspection in every case (eg, negative for erythema, rash, ulceration, or separation). Be specific in describing the stoma. There are multiple complication codes for ostomy sites, and codes for "attention to" the sites. The status codes, listed here, identify ICD-10-CM's categories for stoma types, and the same language is carried over to the complication and "attention to" codes (see Table 4-4.4).

TABLE 4-4.4 Artificial Opening (Stoma) Status

CODE	DESCRIPTION
Z93.1	Gastrostomy status
Z93.2	Ileostomy status
Z93.3	Colostomy status
Z93.4	Other artificial openings of gastrointestinal tract status
Z93.50	Unspecified cystostomy status
Z93.51	Cutaneous-vesicostomy status
Z93.52	Appendico-vesicostomy status
Z93.59	Other cystostomy status
Z93.6	Other artificial openings of urinary tract status
Z93.8	Other artificial opening status
Z93.9	Artificial opening status, unspecified

Temporary ostomy sites risk-adjust to the same HCCs as permanent ostomy sites. Avoid the words "stoma" or "ostomy" in the medical record, as it is not specific. Instead, specify cystostomy, ileostomy, tracheostomy, etc. Tracheostoma maps to a different HCC, so specificity in identifying the stoma is important for appropriate RA.

Coding

RA coders should carefully review the physical examination of the patient to glean from the record important data regarding the patient's health status (eg, amputation or stoma status). In many cases, notes about the physical examination are the only documentation of these conditions. According to ICD-10-CM Guideline Section I(C.21.c.3), a "status code should not be used with a diagnosis code from one of the body system chapters, if the diagnosis code includes the information provided by the status code. For example, code Z94.1, Heart transplant status, should not be used with a code from subcategory T86.2, Complications of heart transplant. The status code does not provide additional information. The complication code indicates that the patient is a heart transplant patient."[2]

ADVICE/ALERT NOTE

Per ICD-10-CM Guideline Section I(C.21.c.3), a "status code should not be used with a diagnosis code from one of the body system chapters, if the diagnosis code includes the information provided by the status code. For example, code Z94.1, Heart transplant status, should not be used with a code from subcategory T86.2, Complications of heart transplant. The status code does not provide additional information. The complication code indicates that the patient is a heart transplant patient."[2]

Do not report an ostomy status code with an ostomy complication code. To do so is redundant. Instead, report only the complication code. When a patient is undergoing a takedown of a stoma, report the appropriate "attention to" stoma code (eg, when a gastrostomy is being closed, report Z43.1, *Encounter for attention to gastrostomy*). If a surgical encounter is for the creation of an ostomy, do not report an ostomy "status" or "attention to" code. Instead, report the reason for the ostomy (eg, malignant neoplasm of the sigmoid colon).

Systemic Lupus Erythematosus – *see* Arthritis

Thyroid Disorders

Thyroid disorders
RxHCC 42 0.101

The thyroid gland is found at the base of the larynx. It regulates metabolism and produces calcitonin. The thyroid gland produces triiodothyronine (T3) and thyroxine (T4). The pituitary gland releases thyroid-stimulating hormone (TSH) to regulate the amount of T3 and T4 in circulation. Deficiency of the thyroid hormone is called hypothyroidism and it is a common disorder in the US.

The thyroid hormone is manufactured in the thyroid gland, and a decrease in thyroid production is often first diagnosed when the patient becomes symptomatic, with a slowing of mental or physical activity, fatigue, cold intolerance, weight gain with decreased appetite, hair loss, and sleepiness. Often, TSH will be measured if hypothyroidism is suspected, or to evaluate the efficacy of synthetic thyroid prescription in correcting the patient's hypothyroidism. Hypothyroidism is easily reversed with a prescription for synthetic thyroid hormone, but must be regularly monitored. Hashimoto's thyroiditis is often a cause of hypothyroidism. In Hashimoto's disease, the body's immune system attacks the cells that produce T3 and T4.

Goiter describes an enlargement of the thyroid gland to the point that the swollen gland is evidenced by changes in the topography of the neck. In non-toxic goiter, the enlargement is not associated with hyperthyroidism, or overload of the thyroid hormones. Instead, it is usually caused by a chronic deficit in T3 and T4 output leading to an increase in TSH production, which causes the thyroid to enlarge.

Hyperthyroidism is also called thyrotoxicosis and occurs with the overproduction of T3 and T4. In hyperthyroidism, the patient has insomnia, weight loss, nervousness, rapid heartbeat, and tremors. This may be caused by Grave's disease, a condition in which the body produces antibodies called thyroid-stimulating immunoglobulin (TSI). This disease is more common in women. Other causes of hyperthyroidism include the presence of nodules or inflammation. Treatment of hyperthyroidism may include excision of some thyroid tissue, radioactive iodine therapy, or oral medications that interfere with T3 and T4 production.

In hyperthyroidism, a sudden rise in thyroid hormone may cause fever, weakness, confusion, or coma. This is called a thyroid crisis or storm, and is an acute, life-threatening medical emergency usually involving inpatient admission.The American Thyroid Association estimates that 20 million people in the US have a form of thyroid disease, and more than half are unaware of their condition.[17] All thyroid conditions risk-adjust for RxHCCs.

Physician Documentation

For thyroid disorders, document the patient's condition as hypothyroidism, hyperthyroidism, or non-toxic goiter. For goiter, identify the condition as diffuse, multinodular, or with a single nodule. For hypothyroid, identify the cause as congenital, iodine-deficiency related, postinfectious, or postsurgical. Note any goiter. For hyperthyroidism, identify Grave's disease, single or multinodular, from ectopic tissue or factitia. Document any thyrotoxic storm or crisis. For Grave's disease, document all manifestations (eg, exophthalmos, osteoporosis, or polyglandular autoimmune syndrome). A patient with a neoplasm of the thyroid may experience functional disorders (eg, hyperthyroidism or hypothyroidism), as a result of the neoplasm. The functional disorder should be described in addition to the neoplasm.

Two documentation errors are common to thyroid disorders. Foremost, physicians will commonly see hypothyroid documented in PMH and test for TSH to evaluate the therapeutic levels of levothyroxine in the patient's blood. The error comes in not discussing, on paper or in the electronic medical record, the results of the test and the continued care plan for the patient's hypothyroidism. Ensure the record captures the evaluation performed on the patient's hypothyroidism so that the diagnosis can be abstracted appropriately. "Euthyroid" or "euthyroidism" is also often seen in documentation, likely meaning the hypothyroid patient's thyroid levels are at therapeutic levels with levothyroxine. "Euthyroid" is insufficient to for a coder to abstract hypothyroidism. Euthyroid does not appear in the Alphabetic Index of ICD-10-CM and can also be defined as a normal thyroid.

A cautionary note, too, regarding hypothyroid or hyperthyroid in medical transcription services.

The words sound alike and are sometimes misheard. Physicians should review transcribed records carefully and amend the records when these errors are discovered. Coders are not permitted to refer to other encounters to answer questions in the encounter they are abstracting, and contradictory information may be wrongly abstracted. Never abbreviate hyperthyroidism or hypothyroidism, and ensure that any penmanship is clear and transcribed notes are correct.

Coding

Coding of thyroid conditions is relatively straightforward when compared with other conditions in ICD-10-CM. Capture significant manifestations of the thyroid disorder as documented (eg, G73.7, *Myopathy in diseases classified elsewhere,* with E03.9, *Hypothyroidism, unspecified,* for a patient with generalized muscle weakness due to hypothyroidism). In acute thyroiditis, use a second code to identify the infectious agent. For drug-induced thyroiditis or hypothyroidism, identify the drug with a code from categories T36-T65.

Transplant Status

Major organ transplant replacement status
HCC 186 1.000

Kidney transplant status
RxHCC 260 0.330

Lung transplant status
RxHCC 395 1.201

Major organ transplant status, except lung, kidney, and pancreas
RxHCC 396 1.039

Pancreas transplant status
RxHCC 397 0.330

Organ transplants are healthy organs implanted in people with failing organs. Kidneys are the most commonly transplanted organs, accounting for more than half of all transplants. Other transplants include the heart, liver, pancreas, lung and intestines. Transplanted organs are viewed as foreign objects by the body's immune system. The autoimmune process and potential organ rejection is mitigated by carefully matching organ donors to organ recipients through blood and tissue typing and cross-matching. The recipient also will be prescribed immunosuppressants that suppress the body's natural immune responses.

More than 700,000 organ transplants were performed in the US in the past 30 years, according the United Network for Organ Sharing (UNOS), an organization that manages US organ transplant system for the federal government. More than 116,000 people in the US are currently awaiting organs for transplant.[18] Medicare assigns patients with kidney transplants a separate status in RA reimbursement models, making documentation and coding of transplant status essential to compliance.

Physician Documentation

Much of the thought process and evaluation associated with an immunosuppressed patient post-transplant often does not get documented. Organ transplant status is a chronic condition that is always going to affect the care of the patient. For example, a family practice physician should consider the patient's organ transplant status when selecting the appropriate influenza vaccine, possibly choosing an inactive vaccine rather than a live attenuated vaccine. Do not expect others to infer from the PMH that the choice of inactivated vaccine was due to the organ transplant status. Instead, document it.

Transplant status risk-adjusts when the patient has a complication of the transplant or when the patient is in optimal physical health. Always document the organ transplanted, and note the type of medications the patient is prescribed related to the transplant. Complications of a transplant must be clearly linked to the transplant and identified as complications.

Coding

All organ transplants risk-adjust for RxHCCs, and major organ transplants risk-adjust to HCCs as well. Once the presence of a transplanted organ is seen in documentation, coders must determine whether the patient has a transplant status or a transplant complication. When a patient experiences a transplant complication, report the code for the complication.

There is no need for a second code to report the status of the transplant, as that would be redundant.

According to ICD-10-CM Guideline Section I(C.21.c.3), a "status code should not be used with a diagnosis code from one of the body system chapters, if the diagnosis code includes the information provided by the status code. For example, code Z94.1, Heart transplant status, should not be used with a code from subcategory T86.2, Complications of heart transplant. The status code does not provide additional information. The complication code indicates that the patient is a heart transplant patient."[2]

ADVICE/ALERT NOTE

Per ICD-10-CM Guideline Section I(C.21.c.3), a "status code should not be used with a diagnosis code from one of the body system chapters, if the diagnosis code includes the information provided by the status code. For example, code Z94.1, Heart transplant status, should not be used with a code from subcategory T86.2, Complications of heart transplant. The status code does not provide additional information. The complication code indicates that the patient is a heart transplant patient."[2]

A patient with a transplanted organ may still have disorders of that organ (eg, CKD in a kidney transplant or atherosclerosis in a patient with a heart transplant). These disorders are not complications of the transplant. Pre-existing conditions or new medical conditions that develop following a transplant are not considered complications of the transplant unless they are documented as complications.

According to ICD-10-CM Guideline Section I(C.14.a.2), "[p]atients who have undergone kidney transplant may still have some form of chronic kidney disease (CKD) because the kidney transplant may not fully restore kidney function. Therefore, the presence of CKD alone does not constitute a transplant complication. Assign the appropriate N18 code for the patient's stage of CKD and code Z94.0, Kidney transplant status."[2]

ADVICE/ALERT NOTE

Per ICD-10-CM Guideline Section I(C.14.a.2), "[p]atients who have undergone kidney transplant may still have some form of chronic kidney disease (CKD) because the kidney transplant may not fully restore kidney function. Therefore, the presence of CKD alone does not constitute a transplant complication. Assign the appropriate N18 code for the patient's stage of CKD and code Z94.0, Kidney transplant status."[2]

Patients with transplants are at greater risk for infection and cancer because their immune systems are intentionally suppressed to protect them against organ rejection. Occasionally, the immunosuppression of the patient activates an indolent malignant cell in the transplanted organ and the patient develops a malignant neoplasm of the transplanted organ. This is considered a complication of the transplant. Reporting this requires three codes: a transplant complication code, a malignant neoplasm code, and code C80.2, *Malignant neoplasm associated with transplanted organ.*

According to ICD-10-CM Guideline Section I(C.2.r), a "malignant neoplasm of a transplanted organ should be coded as a transplant complication. Assign first the appropriate code from category T86.-, Complications of transplanted organs and tissue, followed by code C80.2, Malignant neoplasm associated with transplanted organ. Use an additional code for the specific malignancy."[2]

ADVICE/ALERT NOTE

Per ICD-10-CM Guideline Section I(C.2.r), a "malignant neoplasm of a transplanted organ should be coded as a transplant complication. Assign first the appropriate code from category T86.-, Complications of transplanted organs and tissue, followed by code C80.2, Malignant neoplasm associated with transplanted organ. Use an additional code for the specific malignancy."[2]

Trauma: Head

Severe head injury
HCC 166 0.584

Major head injury
HCC 167 0.191

The CDC compared people with traumatic brain injury (TBI) to the general population and found that those with TBI were 50 times more likely to have seizures and 11 times more likely to experience an unintentional drug poisoning.[19] They are nine times more prone to infection and six times more likely to get pneumonia. The rate of TBI within the Medicare population is more than double that of any other age group, and 80% of TBIs in patients older than 75 are the result of falls.[19]

Physician Documentation

With head injury, document any coexisting hypoxia, hypotension, seizure, or loss of consciousness.

For skull fracture, document the following:

- Episode of care as initial encounter, subsequent encounter, or sequela
- Site of fracture according to the bone fractured
- The nature of the fracture as open/closed and with nonunion/delayed healing
- Laterality as appropriate

For intracranial injury, document the following:

- Concussion, traumatic cerebral edema, diffuse TBI, focal TBI, contusion, and laceration, or hemorrhage
- Length of loss of consciousness, as appropriate
- Damage to intracranial portion of internal carotid artery, as appropriate
- Site of the hemorrhage as brainstem, cerebrum, epidural, subdural, or subarachnoid
- Laterality as appropriate

Traumatic brain injury (TBI)
Brain function disruption caused by an external force or penetrating injury (eg, a fall or a bullet). TBI may be mild or severe, and the injury may impair motor or sensory skills, cognitive ability, personality, or any combination of these.

Cerebral edema
Swelling of the brain caused by excessive fluid; a medical emergency as the brain is encased in bone and swelling increases intracranial pressure, which can impede blood flow to the brain and cause ischemia or infarction.

Coding

Carefully follow instructions in the ICD-10-CM code set when coding skull fractures and brain injuries. A brain injury often involves several anatomical parts, and each site and type of injury must be identified and abstracted from the record. Often, there is a code from S02, *Fracture of skull and facial bones*, a code from S06, *Intracranial injury*, a code or multiple codes from subcategory R40.2, *Coma*, and external cause codes to describe the circumstances of the injury. Any associated open wounds are also reported with a code from S01, *Open wound of head*, and injury-related convulsions are reported with code R56.1, *Post traumatic seizures*.

According to AHA's *Coding Clinic* (Fourth Quarter, 2016), concussion with loss of consciousness of greater than 30 minutes should be reported with code S06.0X9-, *Concussion with loss of consciousness of unspecified duration*.[20]

CODING TIP Concussion with loss of consciousness of greater than 30 minutes should be reported with code S06.0X9-, *Concussion with loss of consciousness of unspecified duration*, according to AHA's *Coding Clinic* (Fourth Quarter, 2016).[20] Other concussion codes identify concussion without loss of consciousness, or concussion with loss of consciousness of 30 minutes or less. Append the 7th character for code S06.0X9- to report the episode of care.

Trauma: Hip

Hip fracture/dislocation
HCC 170 0.418

Hip fractures occur in the upper portion of the femur, and may be the result of severe impact (eg, an automobile accident or a fall, generally seen in aging people with osteoporosis). The most common site for fracture is in the neck of the femur, the narrowest segment of the femur that bears significant stress in a fall on the hip or side of the body.

Hip fractures generate a significant increase in morbidity and mortality among adults in the US. This is in part because of the risks associated with breaking the largest bone in the body and the subsequent surgery to repair the hip and restore mobility. It is also due in part to comorbidities that may have contributed to the fall leading to the fracture, and the secondary issues that arise when a patient is bedridden for a long period of time, as is the case with a healing hip fracture.

One-year mortality rates for patients with hip fractures vary from 12% to 50%, depending on the source and the range of years studied; however, all studies show a decline in the mortality rates and in the rates of fracture over time in the US. According to the Dartmouth Atlas of Health Care, the incidence of hospitalization for hip fracture in the Medicare population in 2014 was about 6 per 1,000 enrollees.[21] The rate for women was higher, at almost 8 per 1,000 enrollees.[21]

Hip dislocations are uncommon, and usually occur because of a traumatic injury (eg, automobile accident). They may occur with a fracture of the acetabulum, and sometimes lead to femoral head necrosis or sciatic nerve injury. All hip fractures and dislocations risk-adjust. All fractures of the femur risk-adjust, whether within the hip joint or distal to it. Only initial encounters for these conditions risk-adjust.

Physician Documentation

When documenting fracture of the femur, identify:

- **Circumstances** (eg, trauma, osteoporosis, neoplasm, etc)
- **Site** on the femur
  - Head and neck: intracapsular, head of femur, epiphysis, midcervical, base of neck, articular head
  - Pertrochanteric: greater trochanter, lesser trochanter, apopyhyseal, intertrochanteric
  - Subtrochanteric
  - Shaft, by type: transverse, oblique, spiral, comminuted, segmental
  - Lower end: lateral condyle, medial condyle, lower epiphysis, supracondylar, with or without intracondylar extension
- **Laterality**
- **Open or closed** (if open, identify Gustilo classification as type I, II, IIIA, IIIB, or IIIC)
- **Displaced, nondisplaced**
- **Episode of care** (eg, initial, subsequent, sequela)
- Identify any delay in healing, malunion, or nonunion

For dislocation of the hip, identify:

- Subluxation or dislocation
- Site as posterior, obturator, anterior, or central
- Laterality
- Episode of care (eg, initial, subsequent, sequela)

Intracapsular
In a femur fracture, describing a fracture of the neck, which may be described as head, subcapital, transcervical, or basicervical.

Pertrochanteric
In a femur fracture, an extracapsular hip fracture through the intertrochanteric region or the greater or lesser trochanters.

Subtrochanteric
In a femur fracture, relating to the 5 cm distal to the pertrochateric region.

DOCUMENTATION TIP The Gustilo classification system characterizes open fractures of the femur to provide a framework for risk assessment.

Gustilo Open Fracture Classification

Type I

- Wound less than 1 cm with minimal soft tissue injury
- Wound bed is clean
- Fracture is usually a simple transverse, short oblique fracture, with minimal comminution

Type II

- Wound is greater than 1 cm with moderate soft tissue injury
- Fracture is usually a simple transverse, short oblique fracture, with minimal comminution

Type III

Open fracture with extensive soft-tissue laceration (greater than 10 cm), damage, or loss or an open segmental fracture. This type also includes open fractures caused by farm injuries, fractures requiring vascular repair, or fractures having been open for 8 hours or more prior to treatment.

Subtype IIIA

- Adequate soft tissue coverage despite soft tissue laceration or flaps or high energy trauma irrespective of the size of the wound
- Includes segmental or severely comminuted fractures

Subtype IIIB

- Extensive soft tissue lost with periosteal stripping and bony exposure
- Usually associated with massive contamination

Subtype IIIC

- Fracture in which there is a major arterial injury requiring repair for limb salvage

Coding

If a diagnostic test result inserted in the medical record supports the physician's diagnosis and adds more specificity to it (eg, a radiology report identifying the fracture as one of the lesser trochanter of the femur, while the physician documented a pertrochanteric fracture), the radiology report may be used to abstract a more specific diagnosis. Test results cannot, however, be used to change a physician diagnosis (eg, from hip fracture to hip dislocation). When asked how to report a "diagnosis based on the physician's orders of questionable kidney stone, while the abdominal X ray reveals 'bilateral nephrolithiasis with staghorn calculi' without other available documentation," the AHA's *Coding Clinic* (First Quarter, 2017) advised:

> Code to the highest degree of certainty. The radiologist is a physician, and when the x-ray has been interpreted by the radiologist, code the confirmed or definitive diagnosis. The Official Guidelines for Coding and Reporting, Diagnostic Outpatient Services Section IV.K., state, "For outpatient encounters for diagnostic tests that have been interpreted by a physician, and the final report is available at the time of coding, code any confirmed or definitive diagnosis(es) documented in the interpretation.[22]

According to ICD-10-CM Guideline Section I(C.19.a):

> Most categories in chapter 19 have a 7th character requirement for each applicable code. Most categories in this chapter have three 7th character values (with the exception of fractures): A, initial encounter, D, subsequent encounter and S, sequela. Categories for traumatic fractures have additional 7th character values. While the patient may be seen by a new or different physician over the course of treatment for an injury, assignment of the 7th character is based on whether the patient is undergoing active treatment and not whether the physician is seeing the patient for the first time.
>
> For complication codes, active treatment refers to treatment for the condition described by the code, even though it may be related to an earlier precipitating problem. For example, code T84.50XA, Infection and inflammatory reaction due to unspecified internal joint prosthesis, initial encounter, is used when active treatment is provided for the infection, even though the condition relates to the prosthetic device, implant or graft that was placed at a previous encounter.

7th character "A" initial encounter is used for each encounter where the patient is receiving active treatment for the condition.

7th character "D" subsequent encounter is used for encounters after the patient has completed active treatment of the condition and is receiving routine care for the condition during the healing or recovery phase.

The aftercare Z codes should not be used for aftercare for conditions such as injuries or poisonings, where 7th characters are provided to identify subsequent care. For example, for aftercare of an injury, assign the acute injury code with the 7th character "D" (subsequent encounter).

7th character "S" sequela, is for use for complications or conditions that arise as a direct result of a condition, such as scar formation after a burn. The scars are sequelae of the burn. When using 7th character "S" it is necessary to use both the injury code that precipitated the sequela and the code for the sequela itself. The "S" is added only to the injury code, not the sequela code. The 7th character "S" identifies the injury responsible for the sequela. The specific type of sequela (e.g., scar) is sequenced first, followed by the injury code.[2]

Always start a code search in the Alphabetic Index. Not all femoral fractures are classified to category S72, *Fracture of femur.* Age-related osteoporosis in femur fracture is reported with codes from subcategory M80.05, *Age-related osteoporosis with current pathological fracture, femur,* and physeal fractures of the upper end of the femur and other pathological fracture codes (eg, from neoplastic or other disease, have specific codes) as well. From the Alphabetic Index, confirm the code and read all notes in the ICD-10-CM Tabular List.

Physeal
Of or relating to the growth plate in bone.

Ischemia
Inadequate blood supply to tissue due to a disruption in arterial blood flow.

Aneurysm
Arterial ballooning caused by a weakened arterial wall.

Vascular Disease

Atherosclerosis of the extremities with ulceration or gangrene
HCC 106 1.461

Vascular disease with complications
HCC 107 0.400

Vascular disease
HCC 108 0.298

Venous thromboembolism
RxHCC 215 0.145

Peripheral vascular disease
RxHCC 216 N/A

The vascular system describes the body's network of arteries and veins, which work together to carry oxygenated blood from the heart (arteries) and return deoxygenated blood from the extremities to the heart (veins). Each system has its own unique anatomy and pathologies. The blood within arteries has transport advantages: It is propelled by the contractions of the heart and by gravity. The walls of arteries are thick and muscular to withstand the higher arterial pressure. Arterial blood carries oxygen and nourishment to distal cells. As a result, the blood transports lipids, and these lipids can combine with calcium in the blood to form deposits on the walls of the arteries. This substance can harden into plaque, or atheromas. Arteries can be inflamed and damaged by these deposits, which can significantly narrow the circumference of an artery. This narrowing further increases the pressure of blood moving through the vessel. Issues affecting arteries include high blood pressure, atherosclerosis or arteriosclerosis, and the ischemia and infarction that can happen in distal tissues when blood flow is compromised. Patients with lower-extremity artherosclerosis may feel pain upon walking because the muscle tissue develops reversible ischemia upon exercise. This is called intermittent claudication. If the pain persists once the walking stops, it is called rest pain.

Atherosclerosis, hypertension, hypercholesterolemia, tobacco use, and aging are risk factors for aortic aneurysm. An aneurysm occurs at a full-thickness weakness of an artery wall, when arterial pressure causes the weakness to balloon out. The ballooning segment has a thinner arterial wall and a greater potential of rupturing. Because the aortic artery is the largest in the body, an aneurysm or dissection can be life threatening. Arterial dissections occur when blood slips between weakened layers in the wall of the artery, separating arterial wall layers. This separation further weakens the artery and may lead to a rupture of the artery wall.

In contrast, veins rely on the contraction of distal muscles to push venous blood back toward the heart, usually against the pull of gravity. The pressure within veins is lower than the pressure in arteries. The walls of veins are thin and contain semilunar valves to prevent the backflow of blood. At any given time in the human body, there is roughly twice as much spent venous blood making its way back to the heart as there is freshly oxygenated arterial blood.

Plaque does not develop in veins. Disorders of the veins occur when the valves fail and chronic backflow leads to congestion, usually in the lower extremities. Blood clots may develop due to pooling of blood. Venous disease includes varicose veins, venous stasis, phlebitis, and thrombophlebitis. Ankle edema, varix, and changes in skin color are symptoms of chronic venous insufficiency. Phlebitis and thrombophlebitis occur when venous blood lingers in the vessels. The greatest danger of venous thrombus is that the thrombus will relocate and become lodged in the heart or lung. According to the CDC, as many as 900,000 people are affected by venous thrombosis each year, and one in four is complicated by pulmonary embolism.[23] The clots most commonly form in deep veins. Deep vein thromboses (DVTs) account for 90% of pulmonary embolisms, which cause 25,000 deaths each year.[23]

Physician Documentation

Avoid acronyms like PAD (peripheral arterial disease) and PVD (peripheral venous/vascular disease) when discussing peripheral vascular disease, unless working for an organization that has an approved list that includes these acronyms. A better practice is to identify the specific arterial or venous disorder and site (eg, atherosclerosis of native or varicose veins of lower extremities). Do not document "peripheral vascular alteration," as it does not classify in ICD-10-CM.

When documenting atherosclerosis, identify:

- The type of vessel
  - Native or graft
- If a graft, identify as:
  - Autologous
  - Nonautologous biological
  - Nonautologous nonbiological
- Right, left, or bilateral disease
- Site of any complicating factor:
  - Intermittent claudication (do not simply document claudication)
  - Pain
  - Ulceration (identify specific site and ulcer depth)
  - Gangrene

DOCUMENTATION TIP Do not expect the coder to infer atherosclerosis from documentation of "intermittent claudication." Alone, "intermittent claudication" classifies to code I73.9, *Peripheral vascular disease, unspecified*, but when documented with atherosclerosis, a more specific diagnosis code can be reported (eg, I70.213, *Atherosclerosis of native arteries of extremities with intermittent claudication, bilateral legs*).

Link these conditions to the atherosclerosis using causal language like "due to" or "secondary to." A causal link will automatically be made between atherosclerosis, its complications, and any documented diabetes due to the conventions of ICD-10-CM. Document if another cause is diabetes is not responsible.

Arterial dissection
Separation in the lining of an artery with blood flowing in the space between layers.

Varicose veins
Enlarged and twisted veins that are the result of valve dysfunction and venous reflux.

Phlebitis
Inflammation in the wall of a vein.

Thrombophlebitis
Inflammation of the wall of a vein with formation of a blood clot.

Chronic venous insufficiency
Long-standing inadequacy in the return flow of venous blood to the heart, leading to congestion and venous hypertension.

For thrombophlebitis, identify the vessel, including laterality, and specify whether the condition is acute or chronic, or resolved. In RA documentation and coding, a common source of error is in DVTs, when chronicity is not sufficiently stated. Document a history of DVT only when the thrombosis is completely resolved. Both chronic and acute DVTs risk-adjust; however, a lack of clear direction may result in the wrong diagnosis being reported, will affect productivity when queries are required, and may negatively affect coder quality scores.

AHA's *Coding Clinic for ICD-9-CM* (Fourth Quarter, 2009) issued some advice on the chronicity of embolisms in a discussion of pulmonary embolisms (PEs) that may shed some light on distinguishing between chronic and acute conditions:

> An embolus is a blood clot that most commonly originates in the veins of the legs (deep vein thrombosis). The blood clot can dislodge and travel as an embolus to other organs in the body. A pulmonary embolism is a clot that lodges in the lungs, blocking the pulmonary arteries and reducing blood flow to a region of the lungs.
>
> Pulmonary embolic disease may be acute or chronic (longstanding, having occurred over many weeks, months or years). In the majority of cases acute pulmonary emboli do not cause chronic disease because the body's mechanisms will usually break down the blood clot. An acute embolus is usually treated with anticoagulants (e.g., intravenous heparin and warfarin or oral Coumadin) to dissolve the clot and prevent new ones.
>
> For acute pulmonary embolism, anticoagulant therapy may be carried out for 3 to 6 months. Therapy is discontinued when the embolus dissolves. However, it can persist. In patients with recurrent pulmonary embolic disease while on blood thinners or patients who cannot tolerate blood thinners, a filter can be placed to interrupt the vena cava. The device filters the blood returning to the heart and lungs. In some cases of chronic pulmonary embolism, the clot develops fibrous tissue, and surgery is needed to remove this fibrous tissue.[24]

According to AHA's *Coding Clinic* (Fourth Quarter, 2015), "[i]n general, clinical information and information on documentation best practices published in *Coding Clinic* were not unique to ICD-9-CM, and remain applicable for ICD-10-CM with some caveats."[25]

Aortic aneurysms are often treated medically and monitored closely. The presence of an aortic aneurysm should be documented and its status evaluated at least annually. Document the site of the aortic aneurysm, as in at the valve, root, ascending, descending, abdominal, or thoracic site. Identify severity as ectasia or aneurysm, and describe any dissection or infection.

Coding

The codes in category I70, *Atherosclerosis,* are classified by type of vessel, by site, and by severity. Report the highest level of severity when a patient has multiple symptoms of lower extremity atherosclerosis. There is no need to report lesser diagnoses for the same extremity. The hierarchy, from most severe to least severe is:

- **Gangrene,** with tissue necrosis (highest level)
- **Ulceration,** with non-healing wound
- **Rest pain,** with chronic ischemia
- **Intermittent claudication,** with ischemia upon exertion (lowest specified level)

A diagnosis of atherosclerosis with ulceration and intermittent claudication, for example, would be reported as an ulceration; a diagnosis of ulceration and gangrene would be reported as gangrene. Aortic aneurysm and aortic ectasia are similar disorders, with variance in severity. Ectasia is the lesser dilation. Both types of aortic dilations risk-adjust. When an aneurysm bridges two anatomical sites (eg, aortoiliac), report a code for an aneurysm for each site unless a code for the combination site exists (eg, thoracoabdominal aorta).

CODING TIP Do not report code I73.9 *Peripheral vascular disease, unspecified,* when the documentation states the patient has intermittent claudication and atherosclerosis. Atherosclerosis and intermittent claudication has a causal relationship, according to ICD-10-CM Alphabetic Index conventions. Instead, report a code from category I70.21, *Atherosclerosis of native arteries of extremities with intermittent claudication.* The same holds true for causal relationships between atherosclerosis and rest pain, ulceration, or gangrene.

ABSTRACT & CODE IT!

Abstract and code the clinical coding example below. Check your answers against the answers in Appendix C.

Code the following and also identify the missed RA opportunities under-documented for this encounter.

Patient: Randall Oldham **DOB:** 4/28/1945 **DOS**: 11/5/2017

Chief Complaint: Preoperative clearance for vascular stent placement.

Vitals

Ht: 6'0"	Wt: 208 lb	BMI: 28.2	BP: 134/76	Pulse: 92	Temp: 98.7

Allergies: NKDA [no known drug allergies].

Medications:
Aspirin 325 mg tablet, delayed release, 1 tab daily
Losartan 100 mg-hydrochlorothiazide 25 mg tab daily
Metformin 1000 mg tablet BID

PFSH [past family and social history]:
Widowed and retired; former smoker; occasional social drinker; lives alone.

Surgical History
Total colectomy and ileostomy, 2010
Coronary artery stent, 2002, 2008

PMH:
Colon cancer, 2010
Diabetes
Hypertension
Peripheral arterial disease
Polyneuropathy

HPI: Left foot ulcer slowly improving at this time. Hopeful that the stenting will help circulation in his L leg and foot.

Orders:
HbA1c
Microalbumin, urine
Microalbumin: creatinine ratio, urine

ROS: No fatigue, no orthopnea, dyspnea, dysuria. He has some arthralgias, but no muscle weakness or back pain.

PE
Constitutional: Healthy appearing, well nourished, well developed, NAD [no appreciable disease].

Head: Normocelphalic and atraumatic

Neck: Supple, no masses.

Lymph nodes: no cervical LAD or supraclavicular LAD.

Thyroid: nontender, no enlargement.

Lungs: No dyspnea. No dullness or hyper-resonance upon percussion.

Cardiovascular: Apical impulse not displaced. Normal S1 and S2 and RRR. No JVD or carotid bruits.

Abdomen: No tenderness or guarding; soft, nondistended.

continued

Musculoskeletal: Extremities: 2 cm × 3 cm ulcer, with muscle involvement, L heel with decreased pulses. No necrosis present.

Neurological: Gait normal.

Assessment/Plan:

1. Preoperative clearance. Stent surgery on atherosclerotic LLE. Has already been cleared by his cardiologist.

   Orders:
   CBC w/Diff
   PT/PTT, Plasma
   Urinalysis, complete
   CMP, serum or plasma

2. Peripheral vascular disease. Surgical stenting planned.
3. Diabetes mellitus. Continue metformin but hold the morning of surgery.
4. Coronary arteriosclerosis. Continue losartan. Refuses statin.

Encounter reviewed and approved by Howard Monson, MD 4:45 p.m. 11/5/2017

Ventilator Status *see* Arrest, Shock, Ventilator Status

Vertebral Fracture *see* Osteoporosis and Fragility Fractures

References

1. National Institute of Diabetes and Digestive and Kidney Diseases. Kidney Disease Statistics for the United States. https://www.niddk.nih.gov/health-information/health-statistics/kidney-disease. Accessed Nov 22, 2017.
2. Centers for Disease Control and Prevention. *ICD-10-CM Official Guidelines for Coding and Reporting* (FY 2018). https://www.cdc.gov/nchs/data/icd/10cmguidelines_fy2018_final.pdf. Accessed Oct 30, 2017.
3. American Hospital Association. *Coding Clinic® for ICD-10-CM and ICD-10-PCS Q3.* 2016;3(3):22-23.
4. Centers for Medicare & Medicaid Services. *2008 Risk Adjustment Data Technical Assistance for Medicare Advantage Organizations Participant Guide.* https://www.csscoperations.com/mwg-internal/de5fs23hu73ds/progress?id=04WTUGzH8NVu7krDOTYPeYjddO9VvdH6yE8I9-B9MLA. Accessed Nov 1, 2017.
5. Centers for Disease Control and Prevention. Epilepsy Fast Facts. https://www.cdc.gov/epilepsy/basics/fast-facts.htm. Accessed Nov 1, 2017.
6. Centers for Disease Control and Prevention. Sepsis: Data & Reports. https://www.cdc.gov/sepsis/datareports/index.html. Accessed Nov 1, 2017.
7. American Hospital Association. *Coding Clinic® for ICD-10-CM and ICD-10-PCS Q4.* 2016;3(4):149.
8. American Hospital Association. *Coding Clinic® for ICD-10-CM and ICD-10-PCS Q4.* 2017;4(4):99-100.
9. American Hospital Association. *Coding Clinic® for ICD-10-CM and ICD-10-PCS Q3.* 2016;3(3):8.
10. American Hospital Association. *Coding Clinic® for ICD-10-CM and ICD-10-PCS Q2.* 2017;4(2):8.
11. Maklebust J. Policy implications of using reverse staging to monitor pressure ulcer status. *Adv Wound Care.* 1997; 10(5)32-35. Cited by: National Pressure Ulcer Advisory Panel. The Facts about Reverse Staging in 2000: The NPUAP Position Statement. http://www.npuap.org/wp-content/uploads/2012/01/Reverse-Staging-Position-Statement%E2%80%A8.pdf. Accessed Nov 1, 2017.
12. Maklebust J. Perplexing questions about pressure ulcers. *Decubitus* 1992; 5(4)15. Cited by: National Pressure Ulcer Advisory Panel. The Facts about Reverse Staging in 2000: The NPUAP Position Statement. http://www.npuap.org/wp-content/uploads/2012/01/Reverse-Staging-Position-Statement%E2%80%A8.pdf. Accessed Nov 1, 2017.
13. National Pressure Ulcer Advisory Panel. The Facts about Reverse Staging in 2000: The NPUAP Position Statement. http://www.npuap.org/wp-content/uploads/2012/01/Reverse-Staging-Position-Statement%E2%80%A8.pdf. Accessed Nov 1, 2017.
14. Xakellis G, Frantz RA. Pressure ulcer healing: What is it? What influences it? How is it measured? *Adv Wound Care.* 1997; 10(5)20-26. Cited by: National Pressure Ulcer Advisory Panel. The Facts about Reverse Staging in 2000: The NPUAP Position Statement. http://www.npuap.org/wp-content/uploads/2012/01/Reverse-Staging-Position-Statement%E2%80%A8.pdf. Accessed Nov 1, 2017.
15. Centers for Disease Control and Prevention. Burns. https://www.cdc.gov/masstrauma/factsheets/public/burns.pdf. Accessed Nov 1, 2017.
16. United Ostomy Associations of America, Inc. About Us. http://www.ostomy.org/About_the_UOAA.html. Accessed Dec 7, 2017.
17. American Thyroid Association. General Information/Press Room. https://www.thyroid.org/media-main/about-hypothyroidism/. Accessed Nov 1, 2017.
18. UNOS. Data. https://unos.org/data/. Accessed Nov 1, 2017.
19. Centers for Disease Control and Prevention. Traumatic Brain Injury & Concussion. https://www.cdc.gov/traumaticbraininjury/data/rates_deaths_byage.html. Accessed Nov 1, 2017.
20. American Hospital Association. *Coding Clinic® for ICD-10-CM and ICD-10-PCS Q4.* 2016;3(4):67-68.
21. Dartmouth Atlas of Health. Hospitalization For Hip Fracture Per 1,000 Medicare Enrollees, By Gender. http://www.dartmouthatlas.org/data/table.aspx?ind=67. Accessed Dec 6, 2017.
22. American Hospital Association. *Coding Clinic® for ICD-10-CM and ICD-10-PCS Q1.* 2017;4(1):5.
23. Centers for Disease Control and Prevention. Venous Thromboembolism (Blood Clots): Data & Statistics. https://www.cdc.gov/ncbddd/dvt/data.html. Accessed Dec 6, 2017.
24. American Hospital Association. *Coding Clinic® for ICD-9-CM Q4.* 2009;26(4).
25. American Hospital Association. *Coding Clinic® for ICD-10-CM and ICD-10-PCS Q4.* 2015;2(4):20.

Evaluate Your Understanding

The following questions are critical checkpoints that are meant to let you apply your critical thinking and evaluate your understanding of the content covered in this chapter. The answers for the end-of-chapter exercises are available in Appendix C. In addition, the Internet-based Exercises are additional learning and research opportunities to learn more about the topics related to this chapter.

A Answer Questions

Provide the answer(s) to each of the following questions.

1. Documentation of evaluation or treatment of a chronic condition must occur at which of the following intervals to be captured for risk adjustment?
   A. Quarterly
   B. Twice yearly
   C. Annually
   D. Every other year
2. According to the American Heart Association and the American College of Cardiology, cachexia is defined as a BMI of:
   A. Less than 16.0
   B. 16.00-16.99
   C. 17.00-18.49
   D. None of the above
3. The correct code for acute respiratory distress is:
   A. R06.00
   B. R06.02
   C. R06.03
   D. R06.09
4. A patient documented with a previous diagnosis of an HIV-related illness is seen today for a general health exam. The patient is taking anti-virals, and is in good health. How is this coded?
   A. Personal history of other infectious and parasitic diseases, code Z86.19
   B. HIV disease, code B20
   C. HIV positive, code Z21
   D. As a general health exam, without mention of the patient's HIV status
5. Which of the following is classified to K21.9?
   A. Cardiochalasia
   B. Gastroesophageal reflux
   C. Acid reflux
   D. All of the above

B True/False Questions

Answer true or false for the following statements.

1. A diagnosis of "Alzheimer's disease" requires two codes to capture accurately.
2. Documentation that a patient is in chronic respiratory failure with a pulse oxygen level at 82% is sufficient for the coder to abstract J96.11, *Chronic respiratory failure with hypoxia.*
3. One code is needed to report bilateral rheumatoid arthritis of the wrists.
4. A licensed clinical social worker is an acceptable provider in documentation for a condition of autism spectrum disorder.
5. Report codes from category I69 with codes I60-I67 to identify the type of stroke and its manifestations.
6. A note that the patient uses cannabis recreationally should be reported with F12.90, *Cannabis use, unspecified, uncomplicated.*
7. ICD-10-CM assumes a causal link between Crohn's disease and rectal bleeding.
8. "Acute kidney injury" refers to a traumatic injury.
9. Report I73.9, *Peripheral vascular disease, unspecified*, and I25.10, *Atherosclerotic heart disease of native coronary artery without angina pectoris*, when documentation states the patient has intermittent claudication and atherosclerosis.
10. Documenting a code in an electronic health record is sufficient for documenting a diagnosis.

C Internet-based Exercises

1. Explore the Chronic Disease Indicators data at the Centers for Disease Control and Prevention to learn what the health issues are in your locale at https://www.cdc.gov/cdi/index.html.

2. There were more than 8 million Medicare enrollees with diabetes in 2014, compared to 8,000 Medicare enrollees with cystic fibrosis. Read a report on the Centers for Medicare & Medicaid Services (CMS) website about the illness incidence and complexity of Medicare patients, as well as an analysis of costs and risk adjustment at https://www.cms.gov/Research-Statistics-Data-and-Systems/Statistics-Trends-and-Reports/NationalHealthExpendData/Downloads/HighCostComplexPatients.pdf.

3. CMS has compiled data on the top 10 HCCs by relative prevalence for the years 2004-2012. Take a look here: https://www.ncbi.nlm.nih.gov/pmc/articles/PMC4109819/table/t1-mmrr2014-004-02-a06.

4. American Health Information Management Association (AHIMA) has published some tips on clinical documentation improvement from a physician's perspective. Read about it at http://library.ahima.org/doc?oid=106669#.WaXKS9gzXmQ.

5. For a deeper understanding of pathophysiology and disease processes, search Medscape by topic at http://www.medscape.org/multispecialty.

6. Check out health statistics based on diagnostic code reporting within the Medicare population at http://www.dartmouthatlas.org/data/topic/.

CHAPTER 5

Developing Risk-Adjustment Policies

Most career medical coders share these attributes: They are methodical, they are lifetime learners, and they enjoy a good puzzle. These attributes are essential to successful chart abstraction. A coder gathers the information, researches any unfamiliar terminology, and applies official rules for coding to complete the task.

Professional risk-adjustment (RA) coders know that to use the ICD-10-CM code set, they first review the Alphabetic Index, then the Tabular List section, then the *ICD-10-CM Official Guidelines for Coding and Reporting* (*ICD-10-CM Guidelines*), and then the American Hospital Association's (AHA's) *Coding Clinic for ICD-10-CM and ICD-10-PCS* (*Coding Clinic*) to ensure compliant diagnostic coding. Sometimes, the ICD-10-CM Alphabetic Index or the *ICD-10-CM Guidelines* function to complete the data or establish defaults for coding when documentation is incomplete or imprecise (eg, when diabetes is documented but not the type of diabetes mellitus). The *ICD-10-CM Guidelines* provides the coder with the answer—the default for documented "diabetes" is type 2 diabetes mellitus Section I(C.4.a.2). The ICD-10-CM Alphabetic Index identifies which code to report for "anemia due to blood loss," when the blood loss is not documented as acute or chronic, ie, the default is chronic. The AHA's *Coding Clinic* also covers topics that are not addressed in the ICD-10-CM's Alphabetic Index, Tabular List, or the *ICD-10-CM Guidelines*. For example, per the AHA's *Coding Clinic* (Fourth Quarter, 2012), documentation of open dislocation of the elbow is reported with the dislocation code in addition to the code for unspecified open wound of the elbow.[1]

Occasionally, no coding resource is available to provide direction. For example, there is no specific code in the ICD-10-CM Alphabetic Index for type 1.5 diabetes. As the name suggests, type 1.5 diabetes is a form of diabetes that has elements of both types 1 and 2. How should this be reported? The ICD-10-CM Alphabetic Index or coding guidelines has no answer. The AHA's *Coding Clinic for ICD-9-CM* (Third Quarter, 2013) advised the coder to query the physician in order to assign the most appropriate code; however, that advice was applicable to ICD-9-CM, and it is not always possible to query the physician.[2]

As a result, type 1.5 diabetes has been routinely reported as E10, *Type 1 diabetes mellitus*; E11, *Type 2 diabetes mellitus*, and E13, *Other specified diabetes mellitus*. Which is the correct answer?

In the RA coding community, these areas of uncertainty chew up significant time and resources, as coders, quality assurance (QA) auditors, and managers struggle to code compliantly. Nevertheless, there are ways in which a medical practice, hospital, RA auditing company, or payer can address these gray areas of coding. The development of well-researched and methodically documented internal coding policies can provide a standard for organizations to follow. These policies ensure that all coders within an organization are coding using the same rules. The benefits of an internal coding policy are many, some of which are outlined below:

- Promotes more consistency in reporting and eliminates considerable "noise" during internal coding audits. For RA organizations, these policies can improve quality scores, or inter-rater reliability (IRR), of RA auditors.
- Leads to less research performed by individual coders, increasing productivity.
- Improves the accuracy of data being submitted to the Centers for Medicare & Medicaid Services (CMS) and other payers, which has long-range impact on national policy, payment, and rule making.
- May have direct impact on the hierarchical condition category (HCC) assigned to a code, affecting compliance and payment for the insurer.
- Improves the morale of production coding staff, who now see their concerns addressed by management.

The goal of this chapter is to guide coders and organizations through the policy development and execution process. It will review which sources likely carry the highest credibility, and how to build a policy from multiple sources. Selection of topics for policy, researching, writing, and approval of policy, and dissemination of internal policies to coders will be addressed. Maintenance of the policies will also be discussed.

The best way to present policy development information is through example, so this chapter will walk readers through the development of three policies for coding. Keep in mind that these are examples illustrating how to research and write a policy. Each organization must shoulder the responsibility of researching and writing its own policies, based on its own priorities.

In coding, the first line of defense, when possible, is to query the physician to clarify any questions or issues regarding how the physician would want the diagnosis classified and reported, being certain that the physician's wishes are documented in the encounter being

FYI Per 45 CFR153.630(8), "the initial validation auditor must measure and report to the issuer and the US Department of Health & Human Services (HHS), in a manner and timeframe specified by the HHS, its inter-rater reliability rates among its reviewers. The initial validation auditor must achieve a consistency measure of at least 95 percent for his or her review outcomes. However, for validation of risk adjustment data for the 2014 and 2015 benefit years, the initial validation auditor may meet an inter-rater reliability standard of 85 percent for review outcomes."[3]

Inter-rater reliability
A quality measurement for RA coding identifying consistency of code abstraction. In RA, the accepted standard for IRR is 95%, meaning coders abstracting the same chart should achieve the same results 95% of the time.

coded. In many RA coding organizations, querying the physician is not possible. In these cases, each organization must provide the coder during training its expectations for next steps in the coding process.

Each organization must weigh the risks and benefits of each coding policy it develops, knowing that it may ultimately be disputed. The benefit of a well-developed and referenced policy is that, if disputed, it may protect its author from abuse and fraud fines, and, at best, may lead to a reversal of a denial. The policies written in this chapter provide insight into how to approach the problem, build the case, and write a policy that is short, clear, and well-referenced.

Policies and Procedures

According to the Office of Inspector General (OIG) in its publication, *Compliance Program for Individual and Small Group Physician Practices*, "[w]ritten standards and procedures are a central component of any compliance program. Those standards and procedures help to reduce the prospect of erroneous claims and fraudulent activity by identifying risk areas for the practice and establishing tighter internal controls to counter those risks, while also helping to identify any aberrant billing practices. Many physician practices already have something similar to this called 'practice standards' that include practice policy statements regarding patient care, personnel matters and practice standards and procedures on complying with Federal and State law."[4]

> **! ADVICE/ALERT NOTE**
>
> Per the OIG in its publication, *Compliance Program for Individual and Small Group Physician Practices*, "[w]ritten standards and procedures are a central component of any compliance program. Those standards and procedures help to reduce the prospect of erroneous claims and fraudulent activity by identifying risk areas for the practice and establishing tighter internal controls to counter those risks, while also helping to identify any aberrant billing practices. Many physician practices already have something similar to this called 'practice standards' that include practice policy statements regarding patient care, personnel matters and practice standards and procedures on complying with Federal and State law."[4]

When developing an RA coding policy, the first question is the most important one: Where to begin? Professional RA coders are usually aware of at least some diagnoses requiring frequent clarification, but in some cases, they simply have not researched sufficiently. Coders must be meticulous and thorough in code look-up, which can be tricky at times. Rethinking the main term in look-up is often necessary. For example, "afferent loop syndrome" can be found in the ICD-10-CM Alphabetic Index only under the alphabetical order in S entries, under **Syndrome/afferent loop**, while "Aarskog's syndrome" can be found in the Alphabetic Index only under A entries, under **Aarskog's syndrome**. For a coder to assume all syndrome entries are classified in the same manner would be a mistake. Multiple approaches for code look-up are often necessary. Most conditions and diseases appear multiple times in the Alphabetic Index, but some have only one entry. Stepping back and taking a different approach may solve the mystery, or may validate an answer.

Coders who keep a copy of the electronic file of the ICD-10-CM Alphabetic Index and Tabular List of Diseases and Injuries can streamline index look-ups. For example, performing a search of the electronic files for both "Aarskog's" and "afferent loop" yields immediate results. Therefore, it is a good practice to have a copy of the electronic files of the ICD-10-CM Alphabetic Index, Tabular List, and the *ICD-10-CM Guidelines* on hand. The official ICD-10-CM files are available for download at https://www.cdc.gov/nchs/icd/icd10cm.htm.

> **Main term**
>
> In the ICD-10-CM Alphabetic Index, the main category during lookup, appearing as left-aligned, bolded type and describing the type of disorder or reason for an encounter (eg, Foreign body, Fracture, Status or Syndrome.)

A search of the Tabular List section in the official electronic version of the ICD-10-CM code set may be helpful when the Alphabetic Index yields no results. The goal is to thoroughly investigate whether an answer exists in the code set before beginning the research of a new coding policy.

Targeting Policy Topics

Many coding ambiguities will never be addressed in researched policy because developing coding policies and disseminating and maintaining them is costly and time-consuming. Key to targeting policy development is identifying which gray areas are potential liabilities for the organization. Appropriate targets fall into one of two categories: time and money.

Time is wasted when chronic dissent exists regarding codes that do not risk-adjust. When this occurs, it may be time to consider a coding policy simply to reduce distraction. Dissent accomplishes very little, except to drive down the quality scores of the coders and the productivity of the QA team. An example of a chronic topic of dissent is the nuanced determination of when a family history code is appropriate for abstraction. Although no family-history codes risk-adjust, nearly every medical record has a family-history section. ICD-10-CM Guideline Section IV(J) states that "history codes (categories Z80-Z87) may be used as secondary codes if the historical condition or family history has an impact on current care or influences treatment,"[5] and Section I(C.21.c.4) states that "family history codes are for use when a patient has a family member(s) who has had a particular disease that causes the patient to be at higher risk of also contracting the disease."[5] Some coders abstract all documented family histories, because their sense is the guidelines indicate the patient may be at a higher risk and they want to err on the side of inclusion. Some coders report only those family histories that they judge as aligning with diagnoses evaluated or treated during a specific encounter (eg, family history of osteoporosis in a person with a suspected pathological fracture). Some coders only report family history when it is discussed in the narrative section of the chart and never from the past family and social history (PFSH) section. Some RA organizations have policies that exclude history codes altogether. Because the electronic billing standard, ASC X12 Version 5010, and the paper billing form, CMS-1500, only allow for 12 diagnoses to be reported on one claim, priorities must be made so that all acute and chronic diagnoses addressed during the visit are reported. Determining how an organization wants family histories and personal histories reported, and communicating that policy to coders, can ensure all RA coders are producing similar results.

CLINICAL CODING EXAMPLE

HPI [history of present illness]: The patient is being seen for a follow-up on an abnormal mammogram. The patient reports she is doing well off alcohol, but refuses to attend AA meetings. She has had insomnia for six weeks—insomnia began when she stopped drinking.

Family History (last reviewed 01/12/2018)

Mother—Well adult (alive)
- Alcoholism

Father (alive)
- Aortic valve stenosis, s/p valve replacement
- Diabetes
- Malignant melanoma

Brother (alive)
- Bicupsid aortic valve, s/p bicuspid aortic valve replacement
- Factor V Leiden deficiency
- Pulmonary embolism

Maternal grandmother (deceased)
- Congestive heart failure
- Breast cancer
- Varicose veins of lower extremity
- Tremor in hands

Maternal grandfather (deceased)
- COPD
- Smoker

Paternal grandmother (deceased)
- Ovarian cancer

Paternal grandfather (deceased)
- Malignant tumor of lung
- Smoker
- COPD
- Gallstone

COMMENTS: If a wide net is cast, family history codes for this record could include histories for breast cancer, ovarian cancer, respiratory cancer, other cancer, diabetes mellitus, alcohol dependence, tobacco dependence, blood disorders, heart disease, chronic lung disease, and digestive disorders. All told, at least 11 family history codes would be required to capture all family history diagnoses. It is hard to imagine coders abstracting all these histories. As the physician in this encounter addresses the patient's alcoholism in remission, the family history of alcoholism may be pertinent; however, the physician did not mention it in the HPI. Family histories for breast and ovarian cancers may be pertinent, as both of these cancers can be tied to genetic mutations and the patient has an abnormal mammogram. Perhaps they were mentioned in the assessment/plan. The family histories for breast and ovarian cancer would certainly become clinically important if the patient is diagnosed with breast cancer at a later encounter. At that time, genetic tests may be ordered to guide the patient and her clinical team regarding her treatment and recovery decisions, and the family history codes are reported by the provide medical necessity for the tests.

Sometimes, it is the significance of the diagnosis rather than its frequency that prompts the development of a policy. Disputes surrounding any risk-adjusting diagnosis with a high HCC value must be addressed because there is so much at stake. A wrong step can result in high repayments and fines if a diagnosis is upcoded from a non-HCC code to an HCC code, or from one HCC to a higher-paying HCC. Similarly, revenues are lost if a diagnosis is downcoded to a code that does not risk-adjust or risk-adjusts to a lower-paying HCC.

CLINICAL CODING EXAMPLE

Assessment and Plan

1. Temporal arteritis, responding very well to prednisone. His visual disturbances and headaches have resolved and his sedimentation rate is now 29 mm/hr.

   M31.6 Other giant cell arteritis

2. Insomnia due to prednisone therapy. We will begin to slowly taper the prednisone beginning next week.

   F19.982 Other psychoactive substance use, unspecified with psychoactive substance-induced sleep disorder

   T38.0X5A Adverse effect of glucocorticoids and synthetic analogues, initial encounter

COMMENTS: The issue with this coded scenario is reporting code F19.982, *Other psychoactive substance use, unspecified with psychoactive substance-induced sleep disorder*, which is used to report an adverse effect from a psychoactive drug. A psychoactive drug is a substance, whose primary purpose is temporary changes in perception, mood, or behavior. Prednisone is a corticosteroid, whose primary purpose is to relieve inflammation. Code F19.982 was coded based on the index entry, **Insomnia/due to/drug NEC**. There are no other entries in either the Alphabetic Index or the External Cause Index that address insomnia as an adverse effect of a drug.

What should be done when the Alphabetic Index suggests a term in the Tabular List of Diseases that does not fit the patient's clinical circumstances? According to the AHA's *Coding Clinic* (First Quarter, 2013), "a basic rule of coding is that further research is done if the title of the code suggested by the Index does not identify the condition correctly."[6] As such, another code must be found in the Tabular List of Diseases that does not imply that the patient is taking a psychoactive substance. Code G47.09, *Other insomnia*, fits, recognizing that the adverse effect code that follows, T38.0X5A, supports this as an adverse effect of steroids.

Code F19.982 risk-adjusts to HCC 55, *Drug and Alcohol Dependence*, which carries a weight of 0.420; however, coding this when the patient is not taking a psychoactive medication would raise a compliance

continued

concern. A better choice might be code G47.01, *Insomnia due to medical condition*, or code G47.09, *Other insomnia*, which do not risk-adjust.

This scenario represents an uncommon occurrence, but it may be worthy of a policy because a substantial HCC is involved.

The importance of the QA team in identifying potential policy issues cannot be overstated. The QA team, which generally is charged with sampling charts from all production coders to ensure the coders are maintaining an IRR of 95% or greater, can identify patterns of miscoding and determine whether the mistakes are the result of a training deficit or the absence of official guidance. A QA proposal for policy research usually undergoes approval from management before research begins. Once a policy has been researched and written, management must review the policy and evaluate the ramifications the policy will have on HCCs, if any. Most payers will want to review an RA consulting company's internal policies and procedures before an audit because the policies affect HCC capture. Internal coding policies affect RA scores significantly, as seen in the Example below, which shows two versions of coding for the same chart and their HCCs. RxHCCs would also differ with different coding.

EXAMPLE

HPI: Patient has had type 1 diabetes for 45 years and is being seen today to discuss her A1C, which is 7.8.

PMH [past medical history]: DM type 1, right BKA in 2012 for PAD, lumpectomy in 2017

Medications: Lisinopril, insulin glargine, insulin lispro, trastuzumab, atorvastatin, quetiapine fumarate XR

HPI: Type 1 diabetes, in fair control. Patient says her sugars have been better since completing chemo and radiation for her history of breast cancer. She is still on trastuzumab, but doesn't feel this is affecting her sugars like the chemo did. Checked L foot: free of ulcer or inflammation.

Issue addressed in policies:
Under what circumstances can past medical history be abstracted?

Do all conditions require support?

Can evidence of trastuzumab treatment turn a "history of breast cancer" into "breast cancer"?

CODER A	HCC VALUE
Demographics (weight for age and sex)	0.312
E10.9, *Type 1 diabetes mellitus without complications*	HCC 19: 0.104
Z85.3, *Personal history of malignant neoplasm of breast*	<none>
Risk score	0.416

CODER B	HCC VALUE
Demographics (weight for age and sex)	0.312
E10.51, *Type 1 diabetes mellitus with diabetic peripheral angiopathy without gangrene*	HCC 18: 0.318
C50.919, *Malignant neoplasm of unspecified site of unspecified female breast*	HCC 12: 0.146
Z89.511, *Acquired absence of right leg below knee*	HCC 189: 0.588
Risk score	1.364

Some conditions listed in the past medical history are chronic, incurable conditions. Note also that a diagnosis in the HPI, "history of breast cancer," is still being actively treated. Every organization must determine its own tolerance for risk associated with coding diagnoses with less than perfect documentation, when queries to the physician are not possible.

Sources for Developing RA Policies and Procedures

In coding today, most research is performed online. To be effective in online research, the ability to finely hone an Internet search is crucial. Some researchers find Internet-search results unhelpful or unreliable. Others easily find information on the Internet, although they do not know how to assess its merit or accuracy, or find that there are too many results to sort through in order to find usable information. There are simple methods for making Internet searches more productive and efficient. The first rule in developing coding policy is to define your sources as facts or inferences:

- **Fact:** The information is undisputed, and many sources will tell you the same thing. For example, the names of the ligaments in the foot, or the meaning in medical documentation of the acronym "IDDM" is universal among most medical journals. Anything that comes from CMS addressing HCCs can be viewed as fact. In addition, the ICD-10-CM coding conventions, guidelines, and *Coding Clinic* advice also represent facts. The Documentation Guidelines for Evaluation and Management applicable to Current Procedural Terminology (CPT®) coding contain facts. The most recent consensus statements from professional organizations, such as the definition of diabetes from the American Diabetes Association, the definition of acute myocardial infarction from the American Heart Association, the definition of malnutrition from the Academy of Nutrition and Dietetics, and the staging of chronic kidney disease from *Kidney Disease: Improving Global Outcomes* may be deemed as fact, subject to debate by recovery auditors or other accountability agents. See, for example, the discussion of Sepsis-3 in Part 4 of Chapter 4.
- **Inference:** Opinion that is the result of facts cobbled together in a logical fashion, which can lead to an answer that is both valid and acceptable. In developing coding policy, the writer will collect facts and draw inferences from those facts. For example, a patient's assessment/plan states "SZ, stable. Continue Clozaril." The acronym SZ, which could stand for schizophrenia or for seizure, is ambiguous and normally would not be accepted. But the US Food and Drug Administration (FDA), in its information on clozapine states:

  > Clozapine (marketed as Clozaril, Fazaclo ODT, Versacloz and generics) is an antipsychotic medicine used to treat schizophrenia in patients whose symptoms are not controlled with standard antipsychotic drugs. Clozapine is also used in patients with recurrent suicidal behavior associated with schizophrenia or schizoaffective disorder.

  Because Clozaril is prescribed only as a treatment for schizophrenia, the coder may infer that "SZ" is an abbreviation for "schizophrenia" and abstract the condition. Those same sorts of A-to-B-to-C logic trails, built on facts, are how coding policies are developed.

The Internet provides no expiration date for data. A large amount of online information, especially if it is linked to compliance or coding, is outdated. Old information turns up during searches. Reputable websites carry a note at the bottom of the page identifying when the website was last updated (see Figure 5.1).

Adding the current year to the search terms can be helpful in bringing the most current information to the top of the list, too. For example, a search for "ICD-10-CM CHF coding documentation" generates generic information dating back to the implementation of ICD-10-CM. Add "2017" as the first word of the search string, and the 2017 guideline changes regarding the causal relationship between heart failure and hypertension rise to the top of the search results. Adding "2018" as the first word results in information about the new codes for right-sided heart failure. Omit articles (eg, a, the) and conjunctions (eg, and, or) from the search terms, and be as specific as possible. Although this is no guarantee, it is a place to start. Keep in mind that even government websites can fall behind in updates (eg, much of the Internet Only Manuals [IOMs] at CMS still contain ICD-9-CM codes).

Be a cautious Internet reader. Just because an assertion is written by a person with impressive credentials does not mean that the information is accurate, or the credentials are real. Data posted on the Internet can include everything from hoax to mistake to opinion to fact. The best coding resources are going to be sites that are accessed equally by payers and physicians, and present information objectively. These sites are going to be nationally recognized resources whose ownership

FIGURE 5.1 Example of Website Update Info

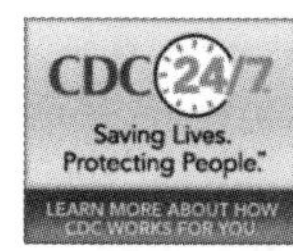

Persistent disparities in cigarette smoking

Despite this progress, disparities in smoking persist across population groups. Cigarette smoking was especially high among males, those aged 25-64 years, people who had less education, American Indians/Alaska Natives, Americans of multiple races, those who had serious psychological distress, those who were uninsured or insured through Medicaid, those living below the poverty level, those who had a disability, those who were lesbian, gay, or bisexual, and those who lived in the Midwest or South.

"The bad news is that cigarette smoking is not declining at the same rate among all population groups," said Brian King Ph.D., deputy director for research translation in CDC's Office on Smoking and Health. "Addressing these disparities with evidence-based interventions is critical to continue the progress we've made in reducing the overall smoking rate."

Reducing smoking-related disease: What more can be done?

Proven population-based interventions – including tobacco price increases, comprehensive smoke-free laws, anti-tobacco mass media campaigns, and barrier-free access to tobacco cessation counseling and medications – are critical to reduce cigarette smoking and smoking-related disease and death among U.S. adults, particularly among populations with the highest rates of use.

Cigarette smoking among U.S. adults has been reduced by more than half since 1964, yet remains the leading preventable cause of disease and death in the United States. It kills more than 480,000 Americans each year. For every person who dies this year from smoking, there are over 30 Americans who continue to live with a smoking-related disease. For more information or for free help quitting, call 1-800-QUIT-NOW or go to www.smokefree.gov.

###

U.S. DEPARTMENT OF HEALTH AND HUMAN SERVICES

Page last reviewed: January 18, 2018
Page last updated: January 18, 2018
Content source: Centers for Disease Control and Prevention

Source: CDC. https://www.cdc.gov/media/releases/2018/p0118-smoking-rates-declining.html. Accessed January 25, 2018.

and authorship is undisputed. The best sites, for the purposes of RA coding policy research, are federal websites, which are sites that coders bookmark and return to regularly. Use these questions as a litmus test for credibility of an Internet site:

- **Why is this source credible?** Do the author's education, credentials, or experience lead a researcher to trust the author's word? What are the motivations behind the article? Is the author selling something? An organization, such as a government entity, specialty society, or medical support organization has more credibility than a Facebook group. Avoid amateurish sites or sites with spelling or grammatical errors. For information on disease, https://www.cdc.gov/diseasesconditions/az/e.html is a top resource site that provides an alphabetized listing of disease and other medical topics, which is operated by the Centers for Disease Control and Prevention (CDC). The CDC site is a good source of information, which will not only describe the disease and its manifestations, but will also address the frequency with which it is seen in the United States (US)—including data on specific geographic locations within the country. National Institutes of Health (NIH) sites have solid information on pathophysiology. The CMS website has significant searchable data, but may not be as useful for claims that are not Medicare- or Medicaid-based (see Figure 5.2). Most physicians have access to a great medical library; consult them on how to gain access.
- **One voice or many?** A writer's work presented on an organization's website, webinar, or live event may not have been peer-reviewed by the organization before posting. There is no implied endorsement from a professional organization when it posts something from an outside author. There is a significant difference between a statement issued by an individual and a statement issued by a credible organization. In addition, the organization may agree to host the information, but that does not necessarily mean the organization endorses it. Therefore, an article by a clinician would carry much less weight than an article authored by a specialty society, even if both are posted on the society's website. That clinician's article, posted on the clinician's website, would carry even less authority. In addition, without the credentials, less still.

FIGURE 5.2 Snapshot of CDC Website

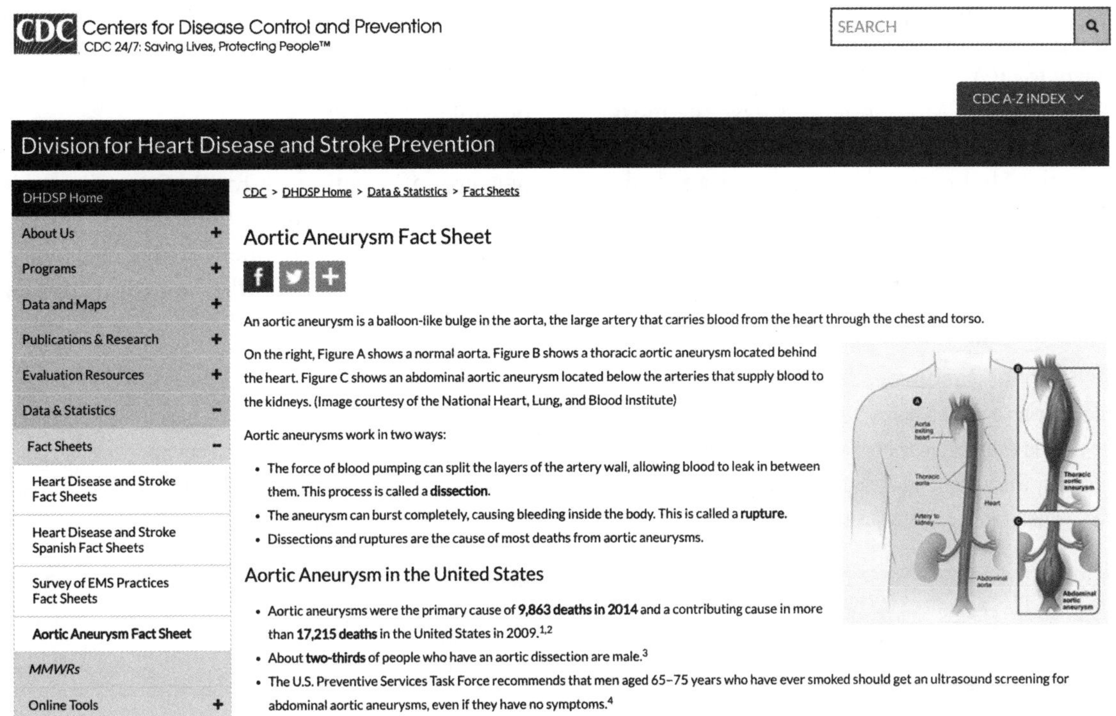

Source: CDC. https://www.cdc.gov/dhdsp/data_statistics/fact_sheets/fs_aortic_aneurysm.htm. Accessed November 3, 2017.

Facebook groups, blogs, magazine columns, and forums are not acceptable sources for coding policy, with one exception: Experienced coders may post links or citations for government documents during online discussions on their professional organization's forums (eg, American Academy of Professional Coders or American Health Information Management Association). The citations are given in response to other coders' questions (eg, "Where did you hear that?"). Follow their links and use the government information as appropriate, but do not follow their advice, bloggers, or groups. Informed people deal in citations, not opinions.

- **Balanced and fair?** An objective website will be cited by physicians, hospitals, and insurance companies because it is factual and does not slant the information in favor of one business segment over another. There are highly charged issues in RA related to what are acceptable documentation and coding practices. Be sure the author is objective. A common trend in the Internet, as well as in print information, is to use a pretext of objectivity to advance an undisclosed agenda, or to support an opinion. This is a slippery slope for coders. Citing a source that is known to disparage insurance companies in a coding policy will not enhance your credibility with the payer reviewing that policy.

The determination of a source's reliability is somewhat dependent upon the audience and the applicable code set. For example, with CPT, the American Medical Association (AMA) and CMS would seem to be two very reliable sources, but there are some issues upon which their policies diverge. In the practical use of codes, any conflict resolution between the AMA and a payer would depend on the topic in the question. The AMA's stance on what a CPT code represents is always going to be the right answer, because the AMA is the owner and creator of the CPT codes. However, the coverage and conventions surrounding the use of modifiers and bundling are going to vary among payers, and each payer's rule will be the final word for claims submitted to that payer (although in some cases, a review of other payer policies can result in a positive outcomes during appeal).

Similarly for RA, official ICD-10-CM guidelines or advice and CMS regulations have the most impact, because the CDC manages ICD-10-CM, CMS owns the Medicare Advantage program and oversees the private-risk pools, and both the CDC and CMS contribute to the *ICD-10-CM Guidelines* and the AHA's *Coding Clinic*. Policies for RA should strive to be based on resources from official sources or compliance documents written by the CMS, HHS, OIG, or other federal agencies, whenever possible.

When researching coding policy, keep a record of every information source that contributed to the final policy, and include citations or links to each source in a source document. These citations are often the clincher in audit reviews and appeals.

Defensibility of Resources Used in Developing Risk-Adjustment Policies

When developing a coding policy, researchers will want to use the most trusted resources that are also the most recent resources. This simple grid example may help in the development of a method for the evaluation of the credibility of a newly developed policy for RA coding. The weighting of sources is based on the accuracy of the source data, and their presumed alignment with federal RA policy. Organizations should use their own experience in audits to alter the categories or authority levels of this grid.

Source → Age of Data ↓	Other Source (Websites, Forums, Coding Blogs)	Specialty Societies (American College of Cardiology, American Urological Association)	Federal Sources (National Institutes of Health; Chronic Conditions Data Warehouse)	CMS Documents (Medicare Learning Network, Medicare Internet-Only Manuals)	RA-Specific Documents From CMS, ICD-10-CM Guidelines, AHA's *Coding Clinic*
Undated	Not recommended	Limited value	N/A	N/A	N/A
Before ICD-10-CM implementation	Not recommended	Limited value for coding; Better value for clinical indicators	Somewhat authoritative	Moderately authoritative	Guidelines, *Coding Clinic* for ICD-9-CM: authoritative when not superseded by new information in ICD-10-CM; CMS RA guidance moderately authoritative
Since ICD-10-CM implementation	Limited value	Authoritative for clinical indicators	Moderately authoritative	Authoritative	Authoritative
In the past 12 months	Limited value	Authoritative for clinical indicators; Limited value for coding advice without government citation	Moderately authoritative	Authoritative	Authoritative

Writing the Policy

Once an issue has been identified and researched, the coding policy can be created. In some cases, two or more policies may be crafted for discussion in a larger audience before the final policy is selected. A policy should have a title that clearly states the issue. Well-written coding policies are concise and well organized, using simple language. They contain no ambiguities. They quickly direct the coder on how to resolve the issue. All policies should be maintained in a searchable document so that a coder can open the document and immediately access all internal policies.

Every coding policy must be supported by a source document that contains the coding policy and all citations used in development of the policy. This source document is much more detailed than the coding policy published internally for coders. The source document should also contain a history of the development and alteration of the policy, and any notes from the author(s). Some organizations will want a record of who in management approved the policy. The source document should be maintained in a location accessible only to staff responsible for its maintenance. Should the need for a policy be eliminated (eg, a new AHA *Coding Clinic* addresses a topic for which a policy was created, the policy may be removed from the coder's resource, but it must be retained in the source document file so that it is available in the event of an audit of past work). A final note on the dispensation of the issue should be appended (eg, did the AHA's *Coding Clinic* advice support the organization's policy or reverse it?). The policy development team may want to develop a procedure for what should be done if official guidance is released that is counter to a long-standing internal policy.

Issues As Examples

What follows are three examples of how coding policies and procedures can be developed. They each identify an issue, its impact, source documentation, and the final policy. These are sample policies for the purpose of illustration; any policies adopted by individual organizations should be researched, carry citations, and be vetted and approved by organization management.

Diabetes Type 1.5

The ICD-10-CM guidelines, instructional notes, and Alphabetical Index have not addressed which diabetes mellitus code to assign to document "type 1.5 diabetes." Type 1.5 diabetes is also known as latent autoimmune diabetes in adults (LADA). As the name suggests, type 1.5 diabetes has elements of type 1 and elements of type 2. While the AHA's *Coding Clinic* advice for ICD-9-CM offers no advice on type 1.5, ICD-10-CM does have the capacity to report specified diabetes that are not type 1, type 2, due to a drug, or due to a disease. Policy could stipulate that an E13.- code be reported for diabetes type 1.5.

Issue and Impact

HCCs associated with diabetes are based on whether the diabetes is associated with complications. The category of diabetes chosen for diabetes type 1.5 does not affect HCC assignment or have financial implications for Medicare Advantage organizations (MAOs) or participants in a health insurance marketplace risk pool. However, coding consistency, individual IRR scores, and productivity are affected when coders cannot easily identify the ICD-10-CM category of diabetes, which are as follows:

E08 Diabetes mellitus due to underlying condition
E09 Drug or chemical induced diabetes mellitus
E10 Type 1 diabetes mellitus
E11 Type 2 diabetes mellitus
E13 Other specified diabetes mellitus

Many practices also want to be sure patients with type 1.5 diabetes are appropriately represented in their claims and in the patient population, and will want all type 1.5 diabetes patients to be represented with the same codes.

Research

An Internet search using key terms "type 1.5 diabetes" nets an article from the American Diabetes Association (ADA), a professional organization of physicians and other professionals invested in diabetes care (http://www.diabetesforecast.org/2010/may/the-other-diabetes-lada-or-type-1-5.html). This article states that type 1.5 diabetes has a progression to insulin dependence that can take months or years. The patient will have autoantibodies, a hallmark of type 1 diabetes, but also an adult onset with some insulin resistance, both common to type 2 diabetes.

The ADA suggests as many as 10% of patients diagnosed with type 2 diabetes actually have type 1.5 diabetes. The ADA states there are 30 million diabetics in the US. This translates into a potential of millions of type 1.5 diabetics in the US.

The AHA's *Coding Clinic for ICD-9-CM* (Third Quarter, 2013) has an entry regarding type 1.5, which states:

> ICD-9-CM does not currently recognize diabetes mellitus type 1.5. Query the provider so the most appropriate code can be assigned. If the physician does not indicate type I, assign code 250.00, Diabetes mellitus type II or unspecified type, not stated as uncontrolled, for diabetes type 1.5. Code 250.00 is the default.[2]

While we can use certain aspects of the AHA's *Coding Clinic for ICD-9-CM* when it does not conflict with ICD-10-CM conventions or supersede guidelines or advice, we must benchmark this advice as to what we experience in the ICD-10-CM environment. Refer to the AHA's *Coding Clinic for ICD-9-CM* (Third Quarter, 2013),[7] which suggests reporting an unspecified type of diabetes when type 1.5 is documented and the physician is not available for query. ICD-10-CM Guideline Section I(C.4.a.2) states that, "[i]f the type of diabetes mellitus is not documented in the medical record, the default is E11.-, *Type 2 diabetes mellitus*."[5] Besides the guidelines, the code set also provides the following pertinent information and notes:

E10 Type 1 diabetes mellitus
  Includes: diabetes (mellitus) due to autoimmune process
E11 Type 2 diabetes mellitus
  Includes: diabetes NOS
  Use additional code to identify control using:
    insulin (Z79.4)
    oral antidiabetic drugs (Z79.84)
E13 Other specified diabetes mellitus
  Includes: diabetes mellitus due to genetic defects of beta-cell function
    diabetes mellitus due to genetic defects to insulin action
  Use additional code to identify control using:
    insulin (Z79.4)
    oral hypoglycemic drugs (Z79.84)
  Excludes1: diabetes (mellitus) due to autoimmune process (E10.-)
    diabetes (mellitus) due to immune mediated pancreatic islet beta-cell destruction (E10.-).

In this case, it seems that type 1.5 diabetes mellitus is not captured accurately with code E10, E11, or E13. How should a coder determine which category is the best fit when the physician is not available for query? First, organize the conflicting data so that the choices can be compared more easily. In this case, the information sorts as outlined in Table 5.1.

TABLE 5-1 Components Weighed for Choosing a Code for Type 1.5 Diabetes Mellitus

CODE CATEGORY	PROS	CONS
E10	E10 reports autoimmune process; *Type 1.5 has autoimmune components.*	*Type 1.5 also has insulin resistance/insulin secretory defects like type 2.*
E11	AHA's *Coding Clinic for ICD-9* citation on Type 1.5 supports 250.00, *which crosswalks to E11.9.*	Reports NOS. Meaning of NOS from guidelines is "unspecified"; *type 1.5 is a specific type of diabetes.*
E13	E13 reports other "specified." Type 1.5 is a specified form of diabetes, and *no Alphabetic Index or Tabular List entries apply to type 1.5; therefore, using "other specified" makes sense.* Excludes autoimmune process (E10); type 1.5 is autoimmune, but *perhaps the exclusion is for E10 specifically.* E13 includes genetic defects of beta cell function; genetic defects to insulin action. *Type 1.5 has these defects.* Excludes immune mediated pancreatic islet beta-cell destruction (E10); type 1.5 is autoimmune, but perhaps the exclusion is for E10 specifically.	

In assembling the evidence, a case could be made for any of the three categories, but the strongest case seems to be for E13, *Other specified diabetes mellitus*. Because there is no HCC component for the decision, the QA department or managers in charge of coding policy could decide how to report type 1.5 diabetes when the physician does not specify a diabetes category for type 1.5 diabetes, and communicate the policy to the staff with a sourced rationale. Monitor the AHA's *Coding Clinic* publication and the *ICD-10-CM Guidelines* and code changes, as these resources could publish guidance on type 1.5 diabetes mellitus coding.

Coder policy should be sparse and concise. While the source rationale should be made available to staff in the initial training related to the policy, it should be omitted from a searchable reference available for daily use by coders. Brevity is the goal in writing a coding policy.

Coding Policy Sample

Type 1.5 diabetes mellitus

Report the appropriate code from category E13, *Other specified diabetes mellitus*, for documented type 1.5 diabetes or latent autoimmune diabetes of adults (LADA), if the physician does not assign a code category in documentation. Long-term use of oral antihyperglycemic drugs or insulin should be reported secondarily.

Sourced Rationale (on file; not in coding policy resource)

- **Coding:** ICD-10-CM Alphabetic Index: Diabetes/specified type NEC E13.9; Tabular rubrics E10, E11, E13
- NEC in guidelines is defined as: "Not elsewhere classifiable." This abbreviation in the Alphabetic Index represents "other specified."
- When a specific code is not available for a condition, the Alphabetic Index directs the coder to the "other specified" code in the Tabular List.
- **Pathophysiology:** Type 1.5 contains elements of types 1 and 2, and is genetic in origin. (http://www.diabetesforecast.org/2010/may/the-other-diabetes-lada-or-type-1-5.html)
- E13 include diabetes due to genetic defects, as is the case for type 1.5.

HCC Risk: None

Resource Defensibility: Authoritative

CLINICAL CODING EXAMPLE

DOS: 12/26/2017

Patient: Dory Martinez **DOB:** 9/23/1973

Surgeon: Alfred Monmichael, MD

CC [chief complaint]: This is a 44-year-old woman being admitted today with a herniated disc at L2-L3 with a large disc fragment pressing the spinal cord.

HPI: The patient states she was exercising a week ago and developed immediate, severe pain radiating down her right leg. The patient was prescribed oxycodone for pain control. The patient is being admitted for surgery.

PMI

Diabetes mellitus type 1.5	Hypertension
Neuropathy in both feet	Hyperlipidemia
Multiple sclerosis	Multiparity

Past Surgical History: Hemorrhoidectomy

Medications

Lantis, Humulin insulin, sliding scale	Ezetimibe 10 mg
Lisinopril one tab per day	Gabapentin 300 mg

continued

PE

Cardiovascular: No chest pain or arm pain, no shortness of breath, no rubs. Regular rate and rhythm; no murmurs.

Respiratory: No rales or rhonchi. Normal respiratory effort; no dyspnea.

Extremities: Patient in obvious discomfort with left-sided sciatica and lumbar pain. Negative for muscle loss; negative for edema.

HEENT [head, ears, eyes, nose, and throat]: Normocephalic. Pupils equal bilaterally. ENT unremarkable. Neck supple and carotid pulses equal bilaterally.

Assessment

1. Herniated disc at L2-L3 with large disc fragment. Surgery in the morning.
2. Hypertension controlled.
3. Type 1.5 diabetes mellitus, controlled. BG [blood glucose] 122 during visit.
4. Neuropathy, managed with gabapentin.

Electronically signed by Alfred Monmichael, MD at 2:45 p.m. 12/26/2017

COMMENTS: Using the new policy for type 1.5 diabetes, report code E13.40. The neuropathy and diabetes have a causal relationship based on ICD-10-CM guidelines regarding Alphabetic Index–entries that contain the word, "with." Multiple sclerosis is in past medical history and has no support in the current note. Therefore, it cannot be abstracted. Radiculopathy refers to pain along a nerve, in this case documented as sciatica. To capture the loose body fragment, see "Loose/body/vertebral," in the Alphabetic Index.

Final Abstraction

E13.40	Other specified diabetes mellitus with diabetic neuropathy, unspecified
I10	Essential (primary) hypertension
M24.08	Loose body, other site
M51.16	Intervertebral disc disorders with radiculopathy, lumbar region

Past Medical History

Past medical history (PMH) is a critical element within the patient record and a component of the past family and/or social history calculation that contributes to different levels of physician evaluation and management (E/M) services. In the 1997 Documentation Guidelines for E/M, PMH is defined as "the patient's past experiences with illnesses, operations, injuries and treatments."[8] The *ICD-10-CM Guidelines* define PMH as a "medical condition that no longer exists and is not receiving any treatment but that has the potential for recurrence, and therefore may require continued monitoring."[5]

The "history of" noted in the history of present illness (HPI) does not contribute to the different levels of physician E/M services. Because HPI represents "present illness," coders may assume the HPI is a current condition, unless the documentation states otherwise (eg, "history of colon cancer, NED," which means "no evidence of disease").

According to the ICD-10-CM Guidelines Section I(C.21.c.4), "[p]ersonal history codes explain a patient's past medical condition that no longer exists and is not receiving any treatment, but that has the potential for recurrence, and therefore may require continued monitoring.

Family history codes are for use when a patient has a family member(s) who has had a particular disease that causes the patient to be at higher risk of also contracting the disease.

Personal history codes may be used in conjunction with follow-up codes and family history codes may be used in conjunction with screening codes to explain the need for a test or procedure. History codes are also acceptable on any medical record regardless of the reason for visit. A history of an illness, even if no longer present, is important information that may alter the type of treatment ordered."[5]

ADVICE/ALERT NOTE

Per ICD-10-CM Guideline Section I(C.21.c.4), "[p]ersonal history codes explain a patient's past medical condition that no longer exists and is not receiving any treatment, but that has the potential for recurrence, and therefore may require continued monitoring.

Family history codes are for use when a patient has a family member(s) who has had a particular disease that causes the patient to be at higher risk of also contracting the disease.

Personal history codes may be used in conjunction with follow-up codes and family history codes may be used in conjunction with screening codes to explain the need for a test or procedure. History codes are also acceptable on any medical record regardless of the reason for visit. A history of an illness, even if no longer present, is important information that may alter the type of treatment ordered."[5]

Issues and Impact of "History of"

From an RA perspective, there are two big obstacles to accurate code abstraction related to "history of":

- **Physician Nomenclature:** Because physicians look at the patient's health continuum in addition to the current encounter, physicians often describe the patient's past and present health as the patient's health "history." A patient may be documented as having a history of prostate cancer in the pre-surgery note before undergoing transurethral resection of prostate for the malignancy. In this case, it is obvious that the patient's prostate cancer is an active condition being treated with prostatectomy. Documentation of a patient with a history of breast cancer being seen for a coin lesion on her lung is less clear: Is the breast cancer active, or is it resolved? If unable to query the physician and without finding further clarification in the record for the encounter, the coder should, according to the guidelines, code as if the breast cancer is resolved.
- **Chart Nomenclature:** PMH is a common category in electronic health records (EHRs), which contains a list of diagnoses the patient has been assigned during previous encounters. Many of the diagnosed conditions will obviously represent resolved conditions, such as tonsillitis, pneumonia, or nasal fracture. Some of the conditions may be recurring or persistent conditions that have been resolved, such as sarcoidosis, hepatitis, and anemia. And some conditions represent chronic, incurable conditions that, by definition, will continue to be active in the patient throughout the patient's life (eg, vascular dementia, multiple sclerosis, rheumatoid arthritis, or chronic obstructive pulmonary disease [COPD]).

Chronic, incurable diseases are sometimes relegated to "history of" conditions by the physician in the HPI or assessment, or by the chart nomenclature as "PMH." In either case, these chronic, incurable diseases are a source of frustration in RA coding. Most chronic, incurable diseases require considerable healthcare resources and therefore, risk-adjust; however, if they are listed as PMH or documented by the physician as "history of," they may not be codeable.

Physicians may, however, document support for the "history of" diagnoses (see Table 5.2).

TABLE 5.2 Physician Supporting Documentation for "History of" Diagnoses

"HISTORY OF" OR "PAST MEDICAL HISTORY"	CHIEF COMPLAINT	SUPPORTING LANGUAGE
Vascular dementia	Follow-up on her osteoporosis and wrist fracture.	"Husband reports further decline in her cognition."
Rheumatoid arthritis	Six month check-up for diabetes.	"ALT is high at 52 U/L. Another liver panel will be done in two weeks to evaluate her for MTX hepatotoxicity."
COPD	Admission for alcohol withdrawal.	"No wheezing, rales, or rhonchi noted. Good results from Mometasone/ formoterolsupple-mented by albuterol sulfate emergency inhaler."

Abbreviations: ALT indicates alanine aminotransferease test and MTX indicates methotrexate.

Note: In these cases, the physician obviously evaluated the condition that was documented as a "history."

Coders can, of course, use their own judgment to pull a "history of" condition into the present when there is documented support, but doing so requires subjectivity, and subjectivity always negatively affects IRR and productivity. Organizations that can provide detailed policies that limit subjectivity are going to have happier coders, better consistency in coding results, and better IRR scores.

Research

The *2008 Risk Adjustment Data Technical Assistance for Medicare Advantage Organizations Participant Guide* (*2008 RA Participant Guide*) recognizes the errors in physician documentation that can occur regarding the use of "history of" for active conditions:

> The physician may actually intend to communicate that a condition is ongoing, but note the "history of" a condition. An example of this is "history of Hepatitis C" (V12.09 personal history of other infectious disease). Hepatitis C generally presents as a chronic condition (070.54, HCC 27) that is rarely fully eradicated. While assigning V12.09 is not necessarily an example of incorrect coding, it may indicate that the physician office is not coding correctly. Again, communication and clear documentation are essential to make the appropriate determination.[9]

When a chronic condition is documented as a "history of," it automatically raises a red flag that this could be an error. In such instances, the coder should query to ensure the physician intended to document the chronic condition as a "history."

Because of the subjectivity of "history of" coding, some organizations rely on the language of the *2008 RA Participant Guide's* "chronic eight" diagnosis list to write policy. Although the ICD-9-CM codes and HCCs in the 2008 guide are outdated, the information within does provide a glimpse into the mindset of CMS concerning chronic conditions:

> Co-existing conditions include chronic, ongoing conditions such as diabetes (250.XX, HCCs 15-19), congestive heart failure (428.0, HCC 80), atrial fibrillation (427.31, HCC 92), chronic obstructive and pulmonary disease (496, HCC 108). These diseases are generally managed by ongoing medication and have the potential for acute exacerbations if not treated properly, particularly if the patient is experiencing other acute conditions. It is likely that these diagnoses would be part of a general overview of the patient's health when treating co-existing conditions for all but the most minor of medical encounters.
>
> Co-existing conditions also include ongoing conditions such as multiple sclerosis (340, HCC 72), hemiplegia (342.9X, HCC 100), rheumatoid arthritis (714.0, HCC 38) and Parkinson's disease (332.0, HCC 73). Although they may not impact every minor healthcare episode, it is likely that patients having these conditions would have their general health status evaluated within a data reporting period, and these diagnoses would be documented and reportable at that time.[9]

Some organizations have developed policies that allow coders to abstract the "chronic eight" diagnoses if they are listed anywhere in the chart, without documentation that shows that the diagnoses were monitored, evaluated, assessed/addressed, and/or treated (MEAT) or affecting care, treatment or management of the patient, including as part of medical decision making (MDM). This may be risky, as CMS and the *ICD-10-CM Guidelines* are explicit in the requirement that documentation support is necessary for diagnoses to be abstracted, which was discussed in Chapter 3. This could take the form of meeting MEAT criteria or documentation by the physician of the diagnosis in the assessment portion of the encounter record or similar field indicating that the diagnoses were considered during the encounter, and were relevant to the care, treatment or management provided at that encounter as well as MDM. Note, for example, this excerpt from the *Risk Adjustment Data Validation of Payments Made to PacifiCare of Texas for Calendar Year 2007*, which is in an audit rebuttal by PacifiCare published by the OIG in 2010, that explains an error OIG found in its submission:

> The OIG found that the documentation submitted for the encounter on 4/26/2006 does not support ICD-9 codes 440.20 (atherosclerosis of the extremities, unspecified) or 443.9 (Peripheral vascular disease, unspecified). The physician documented "PVD" as one of five listed diagnosis [sic] however, this diagnosis did not affect the care, treatment, or management of patient at this encounter.[10]

While this particular issue was only identified by one auditor for one record in this audit (and it was publically reported by OIG that there were 43 invalid records out of 100 records audited), and the issue did not rise to the level of being mentioned in the actual OIG report, this does raise the question of whether in rare circumstances in which the relationship of a particular diagnosis to overall care, treatment, and management is not easily inferred, that it may be prudent for the physician to provide additional documentation to explain relevance as part of his or her assessment/diagnostic statement.

However, that certainly is not a general requirement. In addition, one might conclude that the list of chronic conditions from the *2008 RA Participant Guide* is merely for illustration purposes. The "chronic eight" list was presumably generated without consideration to the possibilities of curing atrial fibrillation through ablation or type 1 diabetes with pancreas transplant.

Nevertheless, regarding the "chronic eight," the *2008 RA Participant Guide* notes that "[i]t is likely that these diagnoses would be part of a general overview of the patient's health when treating co-existing conditions for all but the most minor of medical encounters."[9] Could this guidance be applied to a broader list of chronic, incurable conditions?

ADVICE/ALERT NOTE

Use of "history of." Per the *2008 RA Participant Guide,* "In ICD-9-CM, 'history of' means the patient no longer has the condition and the diagnosis often indexes to a V code not in the HCC models. A physician can make errors in one of two ways with respect to these codes. One error is to code a past condition as active. The opposite error is code a condition as 'history of' when that condition is still active. Both of these errors can impact risk adjustment."[9]

The CDC publishes information on diseases and identifies many of these diseases as chronic, incurable, or lifelong, or discusses how long a patient may survive after diagnosis. A search of the CDC website (https://www.cdc.gov/az/c.html) will reveal dozens of incurable diseases, some stated as such, and some estimating life expectancy for patients with the disease. See the following two examples for amyotrophic lateral sclerosis (ALS) and sickle cell disease (SCD) in Figures 5.3 and 5.4.

FIGURE 5.3 Amyotrophic Lateral Sclerosis (ALS)

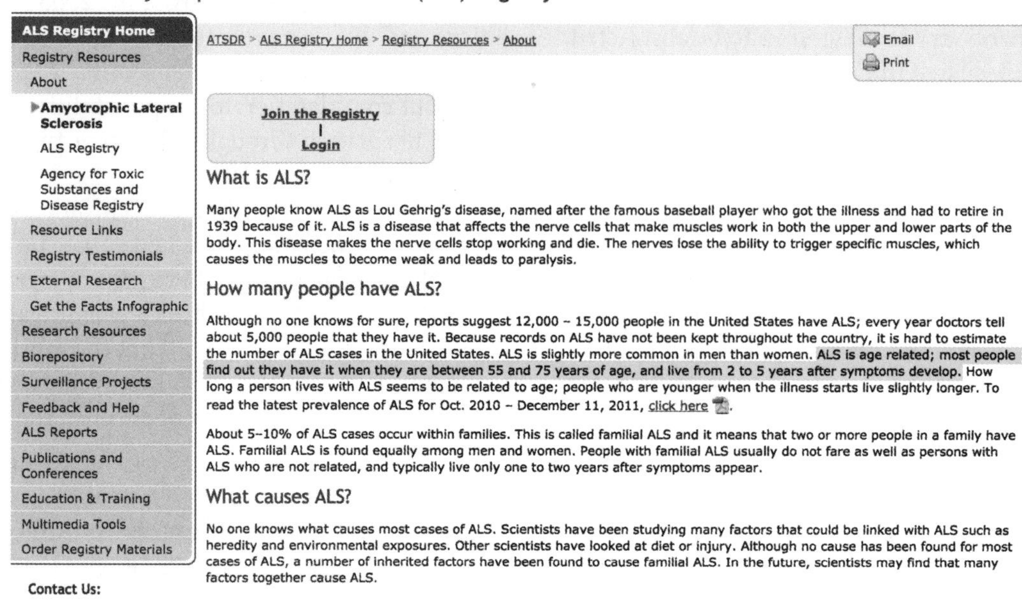

National Amyotrophic Lateral Sclerosis (ALS) Registry

- ALS Registry Home
- Registry Resources
  - About
    - Amyotrophic Lateral Sclerosis
    - ALS Registry
    - Agency for Toxic Substances and Disease Registry
  - Resource Links
  - Registry Testimonials
  - External Research
  - Get the Facts Infographic
- Research Resources
- Biorepository
- Surveillance Projects
- Feedback and Help
- ALS Reports
- Publications and Conferences
- Education & Training
- Multimedia Tools
- Order Registry Materials

Contact Us:

ATSDR > ALS Registry Home > Registry Resources > About

Email
Print

Join the Registry | Login

What is ALS?

Many people know ALS as Lou Gehrig's disease, named after the famous baseball player who got the illness and had to retire in 1939 because of it. ALS is a disease that affects the nerve cells that make muscles work in both the upper and lower parts of the body. This disease makes the nerve cells stop working and die. The nerves lose the ability to trigger specific muscles, which causes the muscles to become weak and leads to paralysis.

How many people have ALS?

Although no one knows for sure, reports suggest 12,000 – 15,000 people in the United States have ALS; every year doctors tell about 5,000 people that they have it. Because records on ALS have not been kept throughout the country, it is hard to estimate the number of ALS cases in the United States. ALS is slightly more common in men than women. ALS is age related; most people find out they have it when they are between 55 and 75 years of age, and live from 2 to 5 years after symptoms develop. How long a person lives with ALS seems to be related to age; people who are younger when the illness starts live slightly longer. To read the latest prevalence of ALS for Oct. 2010 – December 11, 2011, click here.

About 5–10% of ALS cases occur within families. This is called familial ALS and it means that two or more people in a family have ALS. Familial ALS is found equally among men and women. People with familial ALS usually do not fare as well as persons with ALS who are not related, and typically live only one to two years after symptoms appear.

What causes ALS?

No one knows what causes most cases of ALS. Scientists have been studying many factors that could be linked with ALS such as heredity and environmental exposures. Other scientists have looked at diet or injury. Although no cause has been found for most cases of ALS, a number of inherited factors have been found to cause familial ALS. In the future, scientists may find that many factors together cause ALS.

Source: CDC. https://wwwn.cdc.gov/als/WhatisALS.aspx. Accessed November 3, 2017.

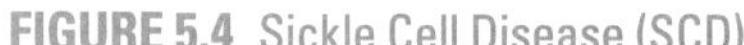

FIGURE 5.4 Sickle Cell Disease (SCD)

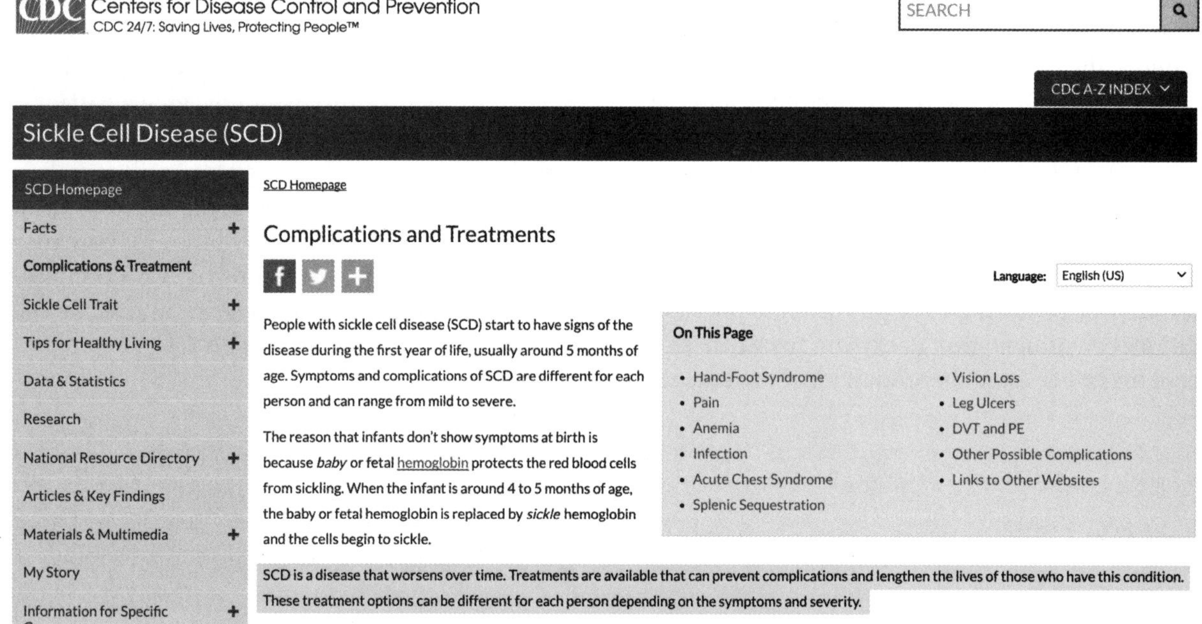

CDC Centers for Disease Control and Prevention
CDC 24/7: Saving Lives, Protecting People™

SEARCH

CDC A-Z INDEX

Sickle Cell Disease (SCD)

- SCD Homepage
- Facts +
- Complications & Treatment
- Sickle Cell Trait +
- Tips for Healthy Living +
- Data & Statistics
- Research
- National Resource Directory +
- Articles & Key Findings
- Materials & Multimedia +
- My Story
- Information for Specific Groups +

SCD Homepage

Complications and Treatments

Language: English (US)

People with sickle cell disease (SCD) start to have signs of the disease during the first year of life, usually around 5 months of age. Symptoms and complications of SCD are different for each person and can range from mild to severe.

The reason that infants don't show symptoms at birth is because *baby* or fetal hemoglobin protects the red blood cells from sickling. When the infant is around 4 to 5 months of age, the baby or fetal hemoglobin is replaced by *sickle* hemoglobin and the cells begin to sickle.

On This Page

- Hand-Foot Syndrome
- Pain
- Anemia
- Infection
- Acute Chest Syndrome
- Splenic Sequestration
- Vision Loss
- Leg Ulcers
- DVT and PE
- Other Possible Complications
- Links to Other Websites

SCD is a disease that worsens over time. Treatments are available that can prevent complications and lengthen the lives of those who have this condition. These treatment options can be different for each person depending on the symptoms and severity.

Source: CDC. https://www.cdc.gov/ncbddd/sicklecell/treatments.html. Accessed November 3, 2017.

The CDC is the umbrella organization of the National Center for Health Statistics, which is responsible for the clinical modification and maintenance of ICD-10-CM. As such, the CDC's statement that a disease is lifelong, chronic, or incurable should substantiate the disease as an active condition for the patient. Nonetheless, support in documentation would still be required. The NIH is another resource for disease information, as is the Chronic Conditions Data Warehouse.

A disease that is incurable or that will last the patient's lifetime is not a "history (of)" disease by clinical definition; however, in ICD-10-CM, the term "history (of)" means that the condition has resolved or is not being treated. Many EHRs treat PMH lists as problem lists for all acute and chronic diagnoses ever assigned to a patient with an automated function that pulls any diagnosis from the assessments in past encounters into the problem list. The *2008 RA Participant Guide* notes that "[f]or CMS' risk adjustment data validation purposes, an acceptable problem list must be comprehensive and show evaluation and treatment of each condition that relates to an ICD-9 code on the date of service."[9]

Based on this statement, it may be acceptable to code a diagnosis when it is listed in PMH or documented as "history of" by the physician if:

1. The diagnosis can be validated as chronic and incurable, and
2. The diagnosis supported in the encounter with MEAT or can be easily inferred to have affected the care, treatment, or management of the patient at the encounter.

The ICD-10-CM Guideline Section IV(G.) states that coders should "list additional codes that describe any coexisting conditions."[5] If the coexisting condition is chronic and incurable, and if the physician documentation has MEAT for the coexisting condition, a coder should query the physician to determine if a diagnosis is active. If the physician is also coding the chart, it is the physician's responsibility to ensure documentation for an active condition is not limited to PMH. In addition, Guideline Section IV(J) states to "[c]ode all documented conditions that coexist at the time of the encounter/visit, and require or affect patient care treatment or management."[5] Furthermore, Guideline Section IV(I) notes that "chronic diseases treated on an ongoing basis may be coded and reported as many times as the patient receives treatment and care for the condition(s)."[5]

Each organization must determine for itself how to address the documentation of chronic, incurable diseases as "past history" in the medical record. Clearly, clinical documentation improvement is the best response, and physician query can achieve results as well. Some organizations may determine that the risk associated with coding from PMH or a "history of" is acceptable under certain conditions for chronic, incurable disorders. Per the *2008 RA Participant Guide*, "MA organizations must submit each required diagnosis at least once during a risk-adjustment reporting period. Therefore, these co-existing conditions should be documented by one of the allowable provider types at least once within the data reporting period."[9] Additional codes that describe any coexisting conditions should be listed, too.[9]

ADVICE/ALERT NOTE

Per the *2008 RA Participant Guide*, "MA organizations must submit each required diagnosis at least once during a risk-adjustment reporting period. Therefore, these co-existing conditions should be documented by one of the allowable provider types at least once within the data reporting period."[9]

FYI

The AHA's *Coding Clinic for ICD-9-CM* (Third Quarter, 2013) states that documentation for the previous encounter may not be clinically pertinent to the current encounter. Documentation for the current encounter should clearly reflect those diagnoses that are current and relevant for that encounter, and that "[i]t is the physician's responsibility to determine the diagnoses applicable to the current encounter and document in the patient's record."[11] In addition, the *Coding Clinic* advises that physicians may need education on the need to document chronic conditions at each encounter, as applicable.

Coding Policy Sample

Past Medical History

The following chronic, incurable conditions, if supported by MEAT or easily inferred to have affected the care, treatment, or management of the patient at the encounter, may be abstracted from documentation stating "history of" or from a Past Medical History list (Note: List is intentionally left incomplete):

- Symptomatic HIV infection, current or in the past
- ALS
- Alzheimer's disease
- Cerebral palsy
- COPD
- Hemiplegia
- Huntington's disease
- Hyperlipidemia
- Multiple sclerosis
- Parkinson's disease
- Rheumatoid arthritis
- Vascular dementia

Examples

- "Patient's nodules of the spine and forearm have not increased in size" in a patient with "history of RA."
- "Patient's blood sugar has remained controlled despite infection" for a patient with "past medical history" of diabetes.

Sourced Rationale

- **Coding:** 2018 ICD-10-CM Guideline Section I(C.21.c.4) defines "history" as a condition that no longer exists. "History" would not apply to chronic, incurable diseases.
- *2008 Risk Adjustment Technical Assistance for MAOs Participant Guide* (6.4), discussion of:
  - chronic disease affecting all but the most minor of complaints, and
  - mistake of coding a chronic condition as a history (Example 9, page 6.9).
- ICD-10-CM Guidelines Sections IV(J) and IV(I) instruct coders to code all coexisting conditions; code chronic diseases as often as they are treated or evaluated.
- **Pathophysiology:** Diseases cited by CDC as chronic/incurable:
  - [List each chronic, incurable disease and the corresponding Internet link that identifies the disease as chronic/incurable/lifelong/etc.]

HCC Risk: Significant. The immediate impact is higher risk-adjustment factor (RAF) scores, and therefore higher risk if the coding of "past medical history" or "history of" is overturned in an audit.

Resource Defensibility: Authoritative

NOTE: This policy is intentionally incomplete. The intent of this chapter is to show how organizations can develop policy, not to provide ready-made policies. Every organization must create policies that address its unique needs. The policies presented here are for illustration only. Each organization must assume the risk associated with policy development.

CLINICAL CODING EXAMPLE

DOS: 3/3/18 **Patient:** Joseph Mendenhall **DOB:** 5/19/1942

CC: Epistaxis and hematemesis

PMI

- Hypertension
- Hyperlipidemia
- Paroxysmal atrial fibrillation
- GERD [gastroesophageal reflux disease]
- Vascular dementia

Medications (updated 3/3/18)

- Lisinopril 40 mg daily
- Metoprolol 12.5 mg BID
- Triamterene-Hydrochlorothiazide 37.5/25
- Ezetimibe10 mg daily
- L-thyroxine .125 mcg
- Rivaroxaban 20 mg daily – *discontinued 3/3/18*
- Omeprazole 20 mg daily

HPI: Mr. Mendenhall presents today with right-sided nasal epistaxis and complaint of hematemesis. Mr. Mendenhall believes the hematemesis is directly related to the epistaxis. He has no other digestive symptoms, except some nausea following a nosebleed. The epistaxis is likely in the setting of rivaroxaban, which I discontinued today. The epistaxis was controlled with posterior packing.

Mr. Mendenhall stated that the nosebleeds have been a chronic problem worsening for several weeks, beginning following an "extraordinary" sneeze. He stated his BP [blood pressure] has been running higher in the past two months, but he did not bring his BP records. He has new-onset anemia.

Laboratory Results: 3/3/18, discussed with patient

- INR 2.9
- Hemoglobin 11.2 (Low)
- Glucose 137 (High)
- BUN 16
- Creatinine 0.94
- Sodium 139
- Potassium 4.2
- Chloride 110

PE

BP: 148/96 Pulse ox: 96 Pulse: 122 Resp: 24 Wt: 182.5 Ht: 72 inches BMI: 24.8

General: W/D, A+O in NAD; tissues packed in nose

Skin: Unremarkable

Head: NC/AT

Eyes: PERRLA, EOMI, non-icteric

Nose: Bright red seepage from nose upon removal of packing

Mouth/Throat: Oropharynx clear, uvula midline

Neck: Good ROM [range of motion], supple, no carotid bruits, no thyromegaly

Lymph: No supraclavicular, cervical, submandibular, submental lymphadenopathy

Chest: CTAB

Heart: RRR, normal S1, S2, no MRG

Abdomen: NT/ND, positive bowel sounds. No HSM. No bruits.

Extremities: No CCE. Good capillary refill. Radial pulses 2+ DP pulses +1

Neuro: Non-focal, 2+ patellar reflexes, nl strength

Assessment/Plan

1. Acute and chronic anterior epistaxis, causing hematemesis. Treated with silver nitrate and nasal packing. Discontinue rivaroxaban. Reminded him of importance of hypertension medications and to come in if his BP is consistently above 130/90. RTC [return to clinic] in two days for re-check of packing.

2. Chronic blood loss anemia, related to chronic epistaxis. This is not his first nosebleed, just the first he has not been able to control at home. Will check HGB when he returns to ensure there is no further drop.

3. Atrial fibrillation, paroxysmal. Discussed with patient the risk of emboli from A-fib vs the short-term benefits of discontinuing rivaroxaban to resolve epistaxis. He agreed to discontinue until epistaxis episode is completely resolved.

Electronically approved by Charles Buchanan, MD, 10:57AM 03/03/2018

continued

COMMENTS: The patient is treated in this encounter for epistaxis and is diagnosed with chronic blood loss anemia. The HPI also discusses the patient's hypertension and atrial fibrillation. Medication reconciliation is documented as having occurred during this encounter. An explanation of the abstraction of diagnoses from the PMH is as follows:

Past Medical History

Hypertension	Also addressed in HPI and supported (Lisinopril)	CODE
Hyperlipidemia	On the chronic list; ezetimibe as support	CODE
Atrial fibrillation	Also addressed in the HPI and supported	CODE
GERD	Not on chronic list; Supported by omeprazole	*OMIT*
Vascular dementia	On the chronic list; no support	*OMIT*

Final Abstraction

D50.0	Iron deficiency anemia secondary to blood loss (chronic)
E78.5	Hyperlipidemia, unspecified
K92.0	Hematemesis
I10	Essential (primary) hypertension
I48.0	Paroxysmal atrial fibrillation
R04.0	Epistaxis

Tamoxifen

Patients who have had surgery, chemotherapy, and/or radiation therapy for breast cancer are often prescribed selective estrogen receptor modulators (SERMs), drugs that block the effects of estrogen on breast cancer. For patients who have had breast cancer, SERMs can fight an existing cancer or act as a prophylaxis against cancer's return. Tamoxifen is a commonly prescribed SERM.

Issues and Consequences

Except for skin cancer, breast cancer is the most common cancer diagnosis among women in the US with more than 250,000 new diagnoses of invasive breast cancer and more than 63,000 cases of *in situ* breast cancer annually, according to the American Cancer Society.[12] Because their survival rate of five years or more is 90%, in 2014, there were more than 3.3 million US women living with breast cancer.[12]

Breast cancer is a very common diagnosis in the Medicare population. It risk-adjusts for HCCs (HCC 12, 0.154) and RxHCCs (RxHCC 19, 0.096). Obviously, if a patient is documented as having "breast cancer" and has a prescription for tamoxifen, the coder will abstract the cancer. The question arises when the physician documents "history of breast cancer" and the patient is prescribed tamoxifen. Does the ongoing prescription of tamoxifen provide evidence of treatment, and therefore evidence of an active cancer? Rejecting active cancer as an option leaves a sizeable HCC behind in RA

Selective estrogen receptor modulators (SERMs)
Drugs that interfere with uptake of estrogen by cells by binding with cellular estrogen receptors; a hormonal treatment for some cancers.

Prophylaxis
A preventive measure against a disease executed in the absence of the disease.

due to the frequency of the disease. Conversely, coding "history of breast cancer" as active cancer because the patient is prescribed tamoxifen could lead to HCC revenue that is wrongly acquired if the tamoxifen is for prophylaxis. As always, a physician query is the best way to resolve this issue. When the physician is not available for query, a policy should be in place.

While no guidance from CMS on tamoxifen as it relates to RA has been issued, the AHA's *Coding Clinic for ICD-9-CM* (Third Quarter, 2009) states that trastuzumab (Herceptin), a monoclonal antibody, is an adjuvant treatment for breast cancer, allowing for the active breast cancer code to be reported, not a "history of breast cancer" code.[13] Many organizations use this citation as the basis for accepting tamoxifen as active treatment in every case.

Research

Patients, physicians, and the ICD-10-CM all have their own definitions of what is "history of cancer." Regardless of those definitions, coders are bound by the definition from the ICD-10-CM Guideline Section I(C.2.d), which states:

> When a primary malignancy has been previously excised or eradicated from its site and there is no further treatment directed to that site and there is no evidence of any existing primary malignancy, a code from category Z85, Personal history of malignant neoplasm, should be used to indicate the former site of the malignancy. Any mention of extension, invasion, or metastasis to another site is coded as a secondary malignant neoplasm to that site. The secondary site may be the principal or first-listed with the Z85 code used as a secondary code.[5]

Patients who have completed surgery, chemotherapy, and radiation therapy for breast cancer may be prescribed medications for up to 10 years following the initial diagnosis. Do all medications constitute "treatment"? If so, could a documented "history of breast cancer" correctly be coded as an active breast cancer? It may depend on the type of drug prescribed.

Each specific SERM medication has its own FDA-approved uses. Raloxifene is a SERM that is used to prevent breast cancer in postmenopausal women at high risk. "High risk" includes women with a personal or family history of breast cancer, or women with a personal history of ductal carcinoma in situ (DCIS). Toremifene, another SERM, is approved by the FDA only for treatment of metastatic breast cancer. Tamoxifen's approved use is more dual in nature. Tamoxifen can be used to treat an active breast cancer or to prevent breast cancer in women at high risk (chemoprevention). Thus, a woman with a "personal history of breast cancer" may be on tamoxifen to treat the cancer, if the history is not a true history, or may be on tamoxifen to prevent the eradicated cancer from returning. To code the underlying reason for tamoxifen use, the documentation must be clear.

Ductal carcinoma in situ
An early form of breast cancer that has not invaded the walls of the milk duct; a common diagnosis among women and not classified as "cancer," but as "carcinoma in situ," because it is still encapsulated.

Chemoprevention
In the case of cancer, the use of a substance as prophylaxis to stop cancer from occurring or from recurring.

ICD-10-CM includes codes for long-term use of drug therapy that address the use of SERMs, and the inclusion notes regarding these codes reveal the duality of SERM therapy:

Z79 Long term (current) drug therapy

Includes: long term (current) drug use for prophylactic purposes
Z79.8 Other long term (current) drug therapy

Z79.81 Long term (current) use of agents affecting estrogen receptors and estrogen levels

Code first, if applicable:
malignant neoplasm of breast (C50.-)
malignant neoplasm of prostate (C61)
Use additional code, if applicable, to identify:
estrogen receptor positive status (Z17.0)
family history of breast cancer (Z80.3)
genetic susceptibility to malignant neoplasm (cancer) (Z15.0-)
personal history of breast cancer (Z85.3)
personal history of prostate cancer (Z85.46)
postmenopausal status (Z78.0)
Excludes1: hormone replacement therapy (Z79.890)

Z79.810 Long term (current) use of selective estrogen receptor modulators (SERMs)
Long term (current) use of raloxifene (Evista)
Long term (current) use of tamoxifen (Nolvadex)
Long term (current) use of toremifene (Fareston)

Z79.811 Long term (current) use of aromatase inhibitors
Long term (current) use of anastrozole (Arimidex)
Long term (current) use of exemestane (Aromasin)
Long term (current) use of letrozole (Femara)

Z79.818 Long term (current) use of other agents affecting estrogen receptors and estrogen levels
Long term (current) use of estrogen receptor downregulators
Long term (current) use of fulvestrant (Faslodex)
Long term (current) use of gonadotropin-releasing hormone (GnRH) agonist
Long term (current) use of goserelin acetate (Zoladex)
Long term (current) use of leuprolide acetate (leuprorelin) (Lupron)
Long term (current) use of megestrol (Megace)

The notes accompanying these codes instruct readers to code first any current breast cancer, or to use an additional code to identify any personal history of breast cancer. While this instruction is directed to a broad list of agents affecting estrogen receptors that may be to either eradicate or prevent cancers, for tamoxifen, it could be used for either purpose. The FDA approves the use of tamoxifen for the following purposes:

- Adjuvant treatment of breast cancer
- Treatment of metastatic breast cancer
- Reduction in breast cancer incidence in high-risk women

Women at high risk for development of the disease are described in an abstract published on the NIH's website (https://www.ncbi.nlm.nih.gov/pmc/articles/PMC3933348/). Women included as "at high risk" are those with a personal history of breast cancer.[14]

In addition, the National Cancer Institute's research on tamoxifen reports that "[f]or some women with breast cancer, taking adjuvant tamoxifen for 10 years after primary treatment leads to a greater reduction in breast cancer recurrences and deaths than taking the drug for only 5 years, according to the results of a large international clinical trial."[15]

Some RA coding organizations reference the AHA's *Coding Clinic ICD-9-CM* (Third Quarter, 2009) advice about Herceptin to defend reporting an active cancer code for documentation of "history of breast cancer" in a patient who is on tamoxifen. According to the advice:

> **Question:** A patient had a malignant breast neoplasm excised three years ago and has completed radiation and chemotherapy. Currently there is no evidence of residual disease on exam, on radiographic images or histologically. However, the patient is receiving consolidative treatment for breast cancer with Herceptin indicated for five years. How is maintenance on Herceptin coded?
>
> **Answer:** Assign code 174.9, *Malignant neoplasm of female breast, unspecified*, as the first-listed diagnosis, since Herceptin is considered cancer treatment. Assign code V58.69, *Long-term (current) use of other medications*, for the Herceptin maintenance. Herceptin therapy is not antineoplastic chemotherapy, but is a biological adjuvant treatment for women with breast cancers that are HER2 positive (with cancer cells overexpressing Human Epidermal Growth Factor Receptor 2).[13]

Trastuzumab (Herceptin) is used to treat cancer. It is not prescribed as prophylaxis. Trastuzumab is an immune targeted therapy, binding to certain antigens within cancer cells. Tamoxifen is a SERM and as such, resides in breast cells, denying the cells access to estrogens. Without the estrogens, any potential cancers cannot take root. Trastuzumab is treatment; tamoxifen can be adjuvant treatment of breast cancer, but also may be prophylaxis or chemoprevention. If a patient is documented with a "history of cancer" and is undergoing trastuzumab therapy, the patient has an active cancer, by virtue of the treatment being performed. But if a patient is documented with "history of cancer" and is undergoing tamoxifen therapy, we can only assume the patient has a history of cancer, as documented, unless there is other evidence of active cancer in the note.

A policy on tamoxifen could argue that a patient on tamoxifen carries additional risk, and therefore, her condition should risk-adjust. This may be a valid argument, but if so, the correct response is for CMS to add code Z79.810, *Long term (current) use of selective estrogen receptor modulators (SERMs)*, to HCC 12 and RxHCC 19 or to provide guidance. Coders must, in the meantime, abstract according to documentation, guidelines, and extrapolated guidance from federal websites. Organizations may choose to draft an RA coding policy stating that "history of cancer" with tamoxifen should be reported as active cancer, and provide citations that support their decision. Other organizations may determine that a policy against coding "history of" cancers as active cancers under any circumstance is appropriate. Again, the policies developed in this chapter are for illustrative purposes only. Each organization must review published regulations and data and understand the risks and rewards when developing its own unique RA coding policies.

Metastatic
In cancer, the extension of the malignancy beyond the initial site where it started.

Adjuvant
In cancer therapy, describing a substance administered after the initial excision or obliteration of the cancer.

Coding Policy Sample

History of breast cancer

- A patient documented with a "history of breast cancer" undergoing trastuzumab therapy has active breast cancer.
- A patient documented with a "history of breast cancer" undergoing tamoxifen therapy has a history of breast cancer.

Sourced Rationale

- **Coding:**
  - ICD-10-CM Tabular List: Z79.81.-, *Long term (current) use of agents affecting estrogen receptors and estrogen levels;* ICD-10-CM Guideline Section I(C.2.d).
  - AHA's *Coding Clinic for ICD-9-CM* (Third Quarter, 2009)
- **Pathophysiology:** FDA labeling for tamoxifen citrate and trastuzumab, accessed through the FDA.gov website
  - https://www.cancer.gov/types/breast/breast-hormone-therapy-fact-sheet for discussion on types of cancer therapies
  - https://www.ncbi.nlm.nih.gov/pmc/articles/PMC3933348/ for information on "high-risk" breast cancer patients
  - https://www.cancer.gov/types/breast/research/10-years-tamoxifen for information on long-term use of tamoxifen

HCC Risk: Critical. Tamoxifen and trastuzumab therapies are common following breast cancer diagnosis; the financial impact is very significant due to the 10-year continuation of tamoxifen prophylaxis. Involve management in formulation of a tamoxifen policy.

Resource Defensibility: Moderately authoritative

CLINICAL CODING EXAMPLE

DOS: 11/21/2017 **Patient:** Laurie Josephsen **DOB:** 6/21/1945

CC: Medicare annual wellness visit

Laurie is being seen today for her annual Medicare exam. She reports she exercises every day, either with a class, weights, aerobics, or bicycle. She reports no issues with activities of daily living.

Problem List (reviewed 11/21/2017)
Midline cystocele
Dyspareunia
Osteoporosis
Malignant neoplasm of right breast

PMI
Cesarean section x2
Tubal libation
Cholecystectomy 3/2/2013
S/P excision and radiation for invasive ductal carcinoma 8/18/2014
DDD [degenerative disc disease] lumbar, CT 6/5/2017
Osteoporosis DEXA 6/15/2017

Medication List (reviewed 11/21/2017)
1000 units vitamin D daily – *new on 11/21/2017*
20 mg tamoxifen daily
Multi-vitamin daily

ROS [review of systems]: Patient reports incontinence and no hematuria. She reports lower back pain. She reports no fever, no night sweats, no significant weight change, and no vision change. She reports no chest pain, no shortness of breath when walking, no shortness of breath when lying down, and no palpitations. She reports no loss of consciousness, no weakness, no numbness, no seizures, no dizziness, no headaches, no tremors, and no memory disturbance. She reports no depression and no insomnia.

Vitals: Ht: 5 ft 2.5 inches Wt: 144 lbs (down 1 lb from last year) BMI: 25.9 BP: 121/72 Pulse: 73 bpm

PE

Constitutional: General appearance is healthy, well developed, and overweight. NAD.

Psychiatric: Good judgment. Normal mood and affect. O&A x3, memory intact.

Head: Normocephalic

Eyes: PERRLA. EOMI. Sclerae: nonicteric. Conjunctiva non-injected.

ENMT: EACs clear, TMs clear. No hearing loss. Nares patent. No nasal discharge. No mouth or lip ulcers; normal dentition. No erythema or exudates in oropharynx.

Neck: Supple, trachea midline. No cervical LAD. Thyroid nontender.

Lungs: No dyspnea, wheezing, rales, rhonchi. Good air movement.

Cardiovascular: Normal S1 and S2 and RRR. No JVD or carotid bruits. Pulses normal.

Breast: Lumpectomy scar, R upper quadrant R breast. Otherwise negative.

Abdomen: Normal bowel sounds. No tenderness or guarding. No distension.

Genitourinary: Defer to OB/Gyn

Musculoskeletal: Normal muscle tone and motor strength.

Neurological: Normal gait and station. No tremor.

Skin: No lesions or rashes. Nail and hair normal.

Assessment/Plan

1. Adult health exam: Well person exam. Immunization schedule reviewed.
2. Osteoporosis: Discussed bisphosphonates again, but she is still unwilling to start them. She has agreed to take 1000 units of Vitamin D daily. She knows the risks of fracture, especially considering her DDD.
3. History of breast cancer: Continue tamoxifen. She is due for her next mammogram in January.

Electronically validated by Bella Morrow, MD, 7:25PM 11/21/2017

COMMENTS: The PMI shows that the breast cancer was surgically excised and therapy completed three years prior to this encounter. The physical exam of the breast was normal, except for the lumpectomy scar. The policy on tamoxifen states that a diagnosis of history of breast cancer is appropriate with tamoxifen, which can be prescribed as chemoprevention. The DDD was discussed in the assessment as an active condition. The AHA's *Coding Clinic* (First Quarter, 2017)[16] defines abnormal findings as new findings.

Final Abstraction

M51.36	Other intervertebral disc degeneration, lumbar region
M81.0	Age-related osteoporosis without current pathological fracture
Z00.00	Encounter for general adult medical examination without abnormal findings
Z79.810	Long term (current) use of selective estrogen receptor modulators (SERMs)
Z85.3	Personal history of malignant neoplasm of breast

Development and Execution of Coding Policies

Every QA team has insight into the areas of ambiguity within its organization's coding, but when beginning the process for coding policy development, it is best to start with the coders. Hold a meeting with all coding staff for input on the biggest issues affecting productivity or quality. If possible, run reports that reveal common errors uncovered by QA. Use HCC and RxHCC factors to weight the errors. Armed with subjective input from QA and coding staff and objective input from coding reports and HCC values, prioritize candidates for policy development. Include management in the meetings and the final prioritization. Some organizations may want to query their clients and include client input into the priorities and final policy decisions if their clients are the MAOs that will be responsible for the codes submitted.

Other topics that may be worth developing internal coding policies include:

- Correct cancer coding when documentation regarding primary vs secondary is ambiguous;
- Obvious cut-and-pasted documentation within an electronic health record (EHR);
- Equivocating language in medical documentation (eg, "I believe," "it is likely due to," or "is consistent with"); and
- Proper coding of acronyms in documentation.

The development, maintenance, and communication of policies consumes resources. Ensure the topics selected for policy development target a significant improvement in coder productivity, better IRR scores, or a reduced risk in an audit.

Work does not end when the policy is written. Communication of new policies must occur in a timely and non-disruptive manner, and management can expect work to be affected as coders begin to apply a new rule to their day-to-day work. QA will want to direct special attention to monitoring codes affected by a new policy to determine whether the training successfully communicated how to code. As recommended by the OIG in its *Compliance Program for Individual and Small Group Physician Practices*, "[i]f updates to the standards and procedures are necessary, those updates should be communicated to employees to keep them informed regarding the practice's operations. New employees can be made aware of the standards and procedures when hired and can be trained on their contents as part of their orientation to the practice. The OIG recommends that the communication of updates and training of new employees occur as soon as possible after either the issuance of a new update or the hiring of a new employee."[4]

Organizations may want to consider a calendar of quarterly updates to coding policies that aligns somewhat with the AHA's *Coding Clinic* publications. In this way, training can capture the *Coding Clinic* changes, annual ICD-10-CM coding updates, and any policy changes as well. Old policies will, at times, need to be changed and/or updated based on the new *Coding Clinic* advice and/or ICD-10-CM codes; however, confining policy changes to a quarterly schedule will reduce disruptions. Similarly, organizations must be flexible as well, should an issue arise that requires staff to create and deploy an immediate coding policy.

ADVICE/ALERT NOTE

Per the OIG in its *Compliance Program for Individual and Small Group Physician Practices*, "[i]f updates to the standards and procedures are necessary, those updates should be communicated to employees to keep them informed regarding the practice's operations. New employees can be made aware of the standards and procedures when hired and can be trained on their contents as part of their orientation to the practice. The OIG recommends that the communication of updates and training of new employees occur as soon as possible after either the issuance of a new update or the hiring of a new employee."[4]

Order Out of Chaos

What is the value of an interesting puzzle if key pieces are missing? Coders love rules, because rules are the key pieces that allow coders to align codes perfectly to documentation. Providing logical and well-constructed coding policies for the gray areas in diagnostic coding has the benefits already mentioned:

- More consistent coding results;
- Reduced risk during an audit;
- Increased productivity; and
- Higher quality scores.

Other benefits are less visible, but equal in value—coding policies communicate that leadership understands the complexity of coding and values coders' focus and expertise. Coding policies let coders know that their emphasis on accurate abstraction is a goal shared by the entire organization. These policies can actually improve recruitment because prospective employees are looking at company philosophies related to quality versus quantity. Well-written coding policies communicate a message that quality counts, and quality is important to most coders.

Coding policies also show CMS auditors that RA organizations have a quality directive. Whether those auditors ultimately agree with the policy or not, evidence of an investment in coding research can demonstrate a desire to code correctly and may carry weight in an auditor's findings.

Processes for New Code Proposal

After research, should your coding team determine that the best answer to a coding problem would be the creation of a new code, the federal government has a process for submission of proposals, which is available at https://www.cdc.gov/nchs/icd/icd10_maintenance.htm.

Proposals for a new code should include:

- Description of the code(s)/change(s) being requested
- Rationale for why the new code/change is needed (including clinical relevancy)
- Supporting clinical references and literature

Proposals should be consistent with the structure and conventions of the classification. For proposal samples, see proposal documents from previous meetings at https://www.cdc.gov/nchs/icd/icd10cm_maintenance.htm.

For proposal submission, email nchsicd10CM@cdc.gov, and for deadlines, visit https://www.cdc.gov/nchs/icd/icd9cm_maintenance.htm.

Once proposals are reviewed, all requestors will be contacted as to whether the proposal has been approved for presentation at the ICD-10-CM Coordination and Maintenance Committee meeting.

References

1. American Hospital Association. *Coding Clinic® for ICD-10-CM and ICD-10-PCS Q4.* 2012;29(4):108.
2. American Hospital Association. *Coding Clinic® for ICD-9-CM Q3.* 2013;30(3):14.
3. Cornell University Legal Information Institute. 45 CFR 153.630—Data validation requirements when HHS operates risk adjustment. https://www.law.cornell.edu/cfr/text/45/153.630. Accessed Nov 3, 2017.
4. Office of Inspector General. OIG Compliance Program for Individual and Small Group Physician Practices." *Fed Regist.* 2000;65(194):59438.
5. Centers for Disease Control and Prevention. *ICD-10-CM Official Guidelines for Coding and Reporting* (FY 2018). https://www.cdc.gov/nchs/data/icd/10cmguidelines_fy2018_final.pdf. Accessed Oct 30, 2017.
6. American Hospital Association. *Coding Clinic® for ICD-9-CM Q1.* 2013;30(1):14.
7. American Hospital Association. *Coding Clinic® for ICD-9-CM Q3.* 2013;30(3):13.
8. Medicare Learning Network. 1997 Documentation Guidelines for Evaluation and Management Services. In: *Evaluation and Management Services.* https://www.cms.gov/Outreach-and-Education/Medicare-Learning-Network-MLN/MLNProducts/Downloads/eval-mgmt-serv-guide-ICN006764.pdf. Accessed Oct 20, 2017.
9. Centers for Medicare and Medicaid Services. *2008 Risk Adjustment Data Technical Assistance for Medicare Advantage Organizations Participant Guide.* https://www.csscoperations.com/Internet/Cssc3.Nsf/files/participant-guide-publish_052909.pdf/$File/participant-guide-publish_052909.pdf. Accessed Nov 1, 2017.
10. Office of Inspector General. Appendix C. In: *Risk Adjustment Data Validation of Payments Made to PacifiCare of Texas for Calendar Year 2007* (Contract Number H4590). https://oig.hhs.gov/oas/reports/region6/60900012.pdf. Accessed Nov 1, 2017.
11. American Hospital Association. *Coding Clinic® for ICD-9-CM Q3.* 2013;30(3):27.
12. American Cancer Society. How Common Is Breast Cancer? https://www.cancer.org/cancer/breast-cancer/about/how-common-is-breast-cancer.html. Accessed Nov 1, 2017.
13. American Hospital Association. *Coding Clinic® for ICD-9-CM Q3.* 2009;26(3):3-4.
14. Nazarali SA, Narod SA. Tamoxifen for women at high risk of breast cancer. *Breast Cancer: Targets and Therapy.* 2014;6:29-36. https://www.ncbi.nlm.nih.gov/pubmed/24648767. Accessed Nov 1, 2017.
15. National Cancer Institute. Ten Years of Tamoxifen Reduces Breast Cancer Recurrences, Improves Survival. https://www.cancer.gov/types/breast/research/10-years-tamoxifen. Accessed Nov 30, 2017.
16. American Hospital Association. *Coding Clinic for ICD-10-CM Q1.* 2017;4(1):17.

Evaluate Your Understanding

The following questions are critical checkpoints that are meant to let you apply your critical thinking and evaluate your understanding of the content covered in this chapter. The answers for the end-of-chapter exercises are available in Appendix C. In addition, the Internet-based Exercises are additional learning and research opportunities to learn more about the topics related to this chapter.

A Answer Questions

Provide the answer(s) to each of the following questions:

1. For most RA organizations, coders must maintain a quality standard of:
   A. 85%
   B. 90%
   C. 95%
   D. 100%
2. Which of the following choices is going to be the most authoritative source of coding advice?
   A. Internet-only manual from CMS
   B. Guidance from a physician posted on a specialty society website
   C. An article from a specialty society
   D. Blog discussion on a coding website
3. Before drafting a coding policy, an organization should:
   A. Assess the frequency of the diagnosis being considered for a policy
   B. Assess the RA impact of a diagnosis being considered for a policy
   C. Thoroughly review ICD-10-CM conventions, guidelines, and *Coding Clinic* to ensure the answer isn't already available in ICD-10-CM resources
   D. All of the above
4. The first line of defense when a coder encounters ambiguous documentation is to:
   A. Petition for a new coding policy
   B. Query the physician
   C. Query the coding manager
   D. Use best judgment to code correctly
5. The patient is diagnosed with a second-degree atrioventricular heart block. The main term to look up in the ICD-10-CM Alphabetic Index is:
   A. Degree
   B. Atrioventricular
   C. Heart
   D. Block
6. The following terms appear in the Past Medical History list on the patient's record for today's date of service. Which one(s) might be considered for coding if supported?
   A. COPD
   B. Histoplasmosis pneumonia
   C. Gestational diabetes
   D. Appendicitis
7. The most important motivation for documenting all resources used in developing a coding policy is:
   A. Citations will help defend coding during an audit.
   B. Coders want to understand the policy development process.
   C. Citations guarantee the policy will be accepted in an audit.
   D. Coders want to check the resources before using the policy to code.
8. Who should have access to RA coding policies?
   A. Coders
   B. Payer clients
   C. RA management team
   D. All of the above
9. In the sample policy developed in this chapter for type 1.5 diabetes mellitus, which of the following statements is true?
   A. The policy has a profound impact on RA payments.
   B. The policy has a moderate impact on RA payments.
   C. The policy has a low impact on RA payments.
   D. The policy has no impact on RA payments.
10. In ICD-10-CM, "history of" indicates:
    A. A condition that continues in the patient's continuum of care
    B. A condition that no longer exists and is not receiving treatment
    C. A condition that is in remission
    D. Any condition documented in a DOS prior to the current DOS

B Internet-based Exercises 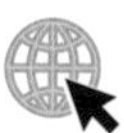

1. See how the Coordination and Maintenance Committee responsible for new code development approaches a coding question by looking at its past and current code proposals here at https://www.cdc.gov/nchs/icd/icd10cm_maintenance.htm.
2. Interested in how diagnostic coding developed in the world? Read the history of the ICD beginning with the *Nosologia methodica*, and *Genera morborum* in the 1700s, through the ICD-10 classification of today at http://www.who.int/classifications/icd/en/HistoryOfICD.pdf.
3. To read the *2008 RA Data Technical Assistance for MAOs*, go to https://www.csscoperations.com/internet/Cssc.nsf/files/2008-resource-guide_060109.pdf/$FIle/2008-resource-guide_060109.pdf.
4. Choose a research topic and head to the NIH website to see what it has to offer at https://www.nih.gov/health-information.
5. The World Health Organization (WHO) has released an early version of ICD-11. To learn how to use the ICD-11 browser, watch WHO videos at http://apps.who.int/classifications/icd11/trainingvideos/. The videos also explain where to find the browser.

C Audit Exercises

1. Review the following clinical scenarios and identify any errors in clinical documentation and a potential coding policy title related to it.

Medical Record:

DOS: 7/16/2017 **Patient:** Kirsten Margula **DOB:** 7/1/1942

CC: Recurrent depression in partial remission

HPI: Kirsten, 66, is being seen today as a follow-up to her depression and a refill for citalopram.

PMI
Depression Hypothyroidism Hyperlipidemia

ROS
Constitutional: No restlessness
Gastrointestinal: Change in appetite
Genitourinary: Patient is post-menopausal
Neuro/Psychiatric: No difficulty concentrating or suicidal ideation

Vital Signs—Taken by RD at 10:12 a.m. 7/16/2017
Ht: 5'0" Wt: 175 lbs BMI: 34.18 BP: 124/82 Temp: 98.4 Pulse: 74 Resp: 18

Medications—Reviewed by Sharon Dearborne at 10:33 a.m. 7/16/2017
Simvastatin: 20 mg daily
Bupropion: 100 mg twice daily
Citalopram: 20 mg daily

PE
Constitutional: Normal, well developed
Psychiatric: Normal, appropriate mood and affect

Assessment/Plan
Kirsten's major depressive disorder and her outlook have improved since adding citalopram. She is now in partial remission, and she is hopeful this is her last recurrence. She stated her primary care physician also adjusted her hyperthyroidism meds, and that has helped.

Electronically signed by Sharon Dearborne at 11:43 a.m. 7/16/2017

2. The note for an 83-year-old man includes the following statement: "Patient diagnosed last year with indolent prostate cancer and is not receiving treatment."

3. Excerpted from an encounter: "The patient has rheumatoid arthritis, COPD, and diabetes mellitus." The medication list was reviewed and dated by the physician. Medications included metformin and prednisone. There were no other mentions of rheumatoid arthritis, COPD, or diabetes mellitus in the encounter.

4. Past surgical history includes a Chopart disarticulation. There is no other mention of lower-extremity amputation in the note.

5 A patient is noted to have a weight of 265 lb, a height of 6'4", and a BMI of 32.3. In the assessment, the physician states:

   1. Carpal tunnel syndrome, right hand. Recommended cock-up brace, NSAIDs, and rest for at least two weeks to see if symptoms improve. I gave him Dr. George's name so he can set up an appointment with the neurology clinic if the problem persists.

   2. Morbid obesity. Patient intends to increase gym attendance from 3x a week to 5x a week to see if it stems his weight gain. He has gained 12 lb over two years.

Appendix A

HCCs and RxHCCs Tables

The HCC tables in Appendix A have been reproduced from Attachment VI of the Center of Medicare & Medicaid Services' (CMS') Announcement of Calendar Year (CY) 2017 Medicare Advantage Capitation Rates and Medicare Advantage and Part D Payment Policies and Final Call Letter. The RxHCC tables have been reproduced from the Announcement of Calendar Year (CY) 2018 Medicare Advantage Capitation Rates and Medicate Advantage and Part D Payment Policies.

Attachment VI is the CMS-HCC and RxHCC risk-adjustment factors section and there are nine tables in Attachment VI. However, only four of the tables have been reproduced in Appendix A: Tables VI-1, VI-2, VI-3, and VI-4.

To download the complete PDFs from CMS, visit https://www.cms.gov/Medicare/Health-Plans/MedicareAdvtgSpecRateStats/Downloads/Announcement2017.pdf and https://www.cms.gov/Medicare/Health-Plans/MedicareAdvtgSpecRateStats/Downloads/Announcement2018.pdf. Note that CMS made no changes to HCCs for 2018, and has instructed that the 2017 tables should be referenced for 2018 HCC information. In this document, the files retain their original 2017 designation, but are, indeed, appropriate for 2018 HCCs.

TABLE VI-1 2017 CMS-HCC Model Relative Factors for Community and Institutional Beneficiaries

Variable	Description Label	Community, NonDual, Aged	Community, NonDual, Disabled	Community, FBDual, Aged	Community, FBDual, Disabled	Community, PBDual, Aged	Community, PBDual, Disabled	Institutional
Female								
0-34 Years		-	0.244	-	0.318	-	0.344	1.031
35-44 Years		-	0.303	-	0.306	-	0.383	0.999
45-54 Years		-	0.322	-	0.338	-	0.374	1.007
55-59 Years		-	0.350	-	0.388	-	0.371	0.986
60-64 Years		-	0.411	-	0.449	-	0.395	1.028
65-69 Years		0.312	-	0.425	-	0.341	-	1.200
70-74 Years		0.374	-	0.511	-	0.406	-	1.092
75-79 Years		0.448	-	0.611	-	0.484	-	0.995
80-84 Years		0.537	-	0.739	-	0.552	-	0.860
85-89 Years		0.664	-	0.917	-	0.678	-	0.749
90-94 Years		0.797	-	1.037	-	0.817	-	0.626
95 Years or Over		0.816	-	1.094	-	0.913	-	0.456
Male								
0-34 Years		-	0.155	-	0.225	-	0.330	1.049
35-44 Years		-	0.190	-	0.204	-	0.267	1.074
45-54 Years		-	0.221	-	0.281	-	0.300	1.008
55-59 Years		-	0.271	-	0.372	-	0.307	1.055
60-64 Years		-	0.303	-	0.486	-	0.343	1.039
65-69 Years		0.300	-	0.492	-	0.334	-	1.269
70-74 Years		0.379	-	0.582	-	0.409	-	1.323
75-79 Years		0.466	-	0.692	-	0.491	-	1.331
80-84 Years		0.561	-	0.816	-	0.546	-	1.189
85-89 Years		0.694	-	1.009	-	0.679	-	1.129
90-94 Years		0.857	-	1.186	-	0.822	-	0.964
95 Years or Over		0.976	-	1.268	-	1.038	-	0.781
Medicaid and Originally Disabled								
Medicaid		-	-	-	-	-	-	0.062
Originally Disabled, Female		0.244	-	0.172	-	0.126	-	-
Originally Disabled, Male		0.152	-	0.192	-	0.105	-	-
Disease Coefficients								
HCC1	HIV/AIDS	0.312	0.288	0.585	0.500	0.550	0.232	1.747
HCC2	Septicemia, Sepsis, Systemic Inflammatory Response Syndrome/ Shock	0.455	0.532	0.596	0.811	0.409	0.417	0.346
HCC6	Opportunistic Infections	0.435	0.704	0.548	0.919	0.482	0.765	0.580
HCC8	Metastatic Cancer and Acute Leukemia	2.625	2.644	2.542	2.767	2.442	2.582	1.143
HCC9	Lung and Other Severe Cancers	0.970	0.927	0.973	1.025	0.955	0.879	0.727

Variable	Description Label	Community, NonDual, Aged	Community, NonDual, Disabled	Community, FBDual, Aged	Community, FBDual, Disabled	Community, PBDual, Aged	Community, PBDual, Disabled	Institutional
HCC10	Lymphoma and Other Cancers	0.677	0.656	0.713	0.761	0.667	0.577	0.401
HCC11	Colorectal, Bladder, and Other Cancers	0.301	0.352	0.332	0.361	0.325	0.400	0.293
HCC12	Breast, Prostate, and Other Cancers and Tumors	0.146	0.202	0.159	0.190	0.152	0.182	0.199
HCC17	Diabetes with Acute Complications	0.318	0.371	0.346	0.431	0.354	0.423	0.441
HCC18	Diabetes with Chronic Complications	0.318	0.371	0.346	0.431	0.354	0.423	0.441
HCC19	Diabetes without Complication	0.104	0.128	0.097	0.160	0.098	0.136	0.160
HCC21	Protein-Calorie Malnutrition	0.545	0.753	0.752	0.845	0.562	0.709	0.260
HCC22	Morbid Obesity	0.273	0.227	0.410	0.373	0.244	0.242	0.511
HCC23	Other Significant Endocrine and Metabolic Disorders	0.228	0.444	0.228	0.353	0.193	0.351	0.337
HCC27	End-Stage Liver Disease	0.962	1.110	1.242	1.349	0.889	0.963	0.962
HCC28	Cirrhosis of Liver	0.390	0.394	0.342	0.491	0.460	0.324	0.390
HCC29	Chronic Hepatitis	0.165	0.267	0.038	0.400	0.263	0.324	0.390
HCC33	Intestinal Obstruction/ Perforation	0.246	0.524	0.369	0.503	0.324	0.510	0.335
HCC34	Chronic Pancreatitis	0.276	0.678	0.333	0.875	0.412	0.849	0.241
HCC35	Inflammatory Bowel Disease	0.294	0.483	0.334	0.613	0.209	0.496	0.244
HCC39	Bone/Joint/Muscle Infections/Necrosis	0.425	0.474	0.552	0.713	0.418	0.491	0.345
HCC40	Rheumatoid Arthritis and Inflammatory Connective Tissue Disease	0.423	0.377	0.370	0.345	0.390	0.290	0.329
HCC46	Severe Hematological Disorders	1.388	3.188	1.219	4.256	1.226	3.529	0.680
HCC47	Disorders of Immunity	0.625	0.848	0.529	0.589	0.449	0.690	0.529
HCC48	Coagulation Defects and Other Specified Hematological Disorders	0.221	0.339	0.268	0.378	0.225	0.382	0.151
HCC54	Drug/Alcohol Psychosis	0.383	0.569	0.706	0.919	0.388	0.613	0.102
HCC55	Drug/Alcohol Dependence	0.383	0.285	0.522	0.366	0.377	0.286	0.102
HCC57	Schizophrenia	0.608	0.395	0.612	0.432	0.547	0.366	0.271
HCC58	Major Depressive, Bipolar, and Paranoid Disorders	0.395	0.209	0.444	0.178	0.413	0.163	0.271

Variable	Description Label	Community, NonDual, Aged	Community, NonDual, Disabled	Community, FBDual, Aged	Community, FBDual, Disabled	Community, PBDual, Aged	Community, PBDual, Disabled	Institutional
HCC70	Quadriplegia	1.314	1.053	1.098	1.056	1.274	1.328	0.497
HCC71	Paraplegia	1.007	0.704	0.920	1.019	0.958	0.908	0.467
HCC72	Spinal Cord Disorders/ Injuries	0.528	0.456	0.552	0.407	0.556	0.384	0.229
HCC73	Amyotrophic Lateral Sclerosis and Other Motor Neuron Disease	0.970	1.082	1.230	1.219	0.570	0.814	0.224
HCC74	Cerebral Palsy	0.280	0.132	-	-	0.158	0.052	-
HCC75	Myasthenia Gravis/ Myoneural Disorders and Guillain-Barre Syndrome/ Inflammatory and Toxic Neuropathy	0.457	0.528	0.436	0.465	0.364	0.331	0.369
HCC76	Muscular Dystrophy	0.505	0.457	0.553	0.512	0.429	0.168	0.104
HCC77	Multiple Sclerosis	0.441	0.540	0.687	0.794	0.407	0.459	-
HCC78	Parkinson's and Huntington's Diseases	0.674	0.585	0.751	0.516	0.629	0.394	0.145
HCC79	Seizure Disorders and Convulsions	0.309	0.227	0.357	0.195	0.349	0.245	0.088
HCC80	Coma, Brain Compression/Anoxic Damage	0.584	0.302	0.946	0.324	0.508	0.155	0.042
HCC82	Respirator Dependence/ Tracheostomy Status	1.055	1.024	2.304	1.575	0.914	0.676	1.631
HCC83	Respiratory Arrest	0.658	0.781	1.033	0.484	0.704	0.429	0.727
HCC84	Cardio-Respiratory Failure and Shock	0.302	0.578	0.471	0.484	0.301	0.429	0.297
HCC85	Congestive Heart Failure	0.323	0.412	0.355	0.415	0.320	0.367	0.191
HCC86	Acute Myocardial Infarction	0.233	0.306	0.473	0.618	0.280	0.438	0.497
HCC87	Unstable Angina and Other Acute Ischemic Heart Disease	0.218	0.306	0.336	0.618	0.280	0.438	0.497
HCC88	Angina Pectoris	0.140	0.121	0.068	0.205	0.175	0.220	0.497
HCC96	Specified Heart Arrhythmias	0.268	0.284	0.369	0.377	0.283	0.258	0.224
HCC99	Cerebral Hemorrhage	0.263	0.282	0.474	0.690	0.278	0.280	0.114
HCC100	Ischemic or Unspecified Stroke	0.263	0.195	0.474	0.357	0.270	0.232	0.114
HCC103	Hemiplegia/ Hemiparesis	0.538	0.324	0.548	0.435	0.603	0.401	0.031
HCC104	Monoplegia, Other Paralytic Syndromes	0.395	0.258	0.374	0.381	0.559	0.401	0.031
HCC106	Atherosclerosis of the Extremities with Ulceration or Gangrene	1.461	1.506	1.744	1.740	1.452	1.601	0.884

Variable	Description Label	Community, NonDual, Aged	Community, NonDual, Disabled	Community, FBDual, Aged	Community, FBDual, Disabled	Community, PBDual, Aged	Community, PBDual, Disabled	Institutional
HCC107	Vascular Disease with Complications	0.400	0.486	0.540	0.756	0.443	0.549	0.321
HCC108	Vascular Disease	0.298	0.333	0.324	0.319	0.316	0.326	0.094
HCC110	Cystic Fibrosis	0.620	2.538	0.985	3.365	0.358	2.861	0.305
HCC111	Chronic Obstructive Pulmonary Disease	0.328	0.262	0.422	0.354	0.358	0.293	0.305
HCC112	Fibrosis of Lung and Other Chronic Lung Disorders	0.209	0.262	0.134	0.322	0.172	0.174	0.057
HCC114	Aspiration and Specified Bacterial Pneumonias	0.599	0.530	0.707	0.490	0.666	0.373	0.067
HCC115	Pneumococcal Pneumonia, Empyema, Lung Abscess	0.221	0.128	0.162	0.049	0.302	0.220	0.067
HCC122	Proliferative Diabetic Retinopathy and Vitreous Hemorrhage	0.217	0.171	0.223	0.284	0.276	0.195	0.460
HCC124	Exudative Macular Degeneration	0.499	0.385	0.278	0.090	0.336	0.115	0.228
HCC134	Dialysis Status	0.422	0.500	0.672	0.637	0.435	0.512	0.462
HCC135	Acute Renal Failure	0.422	0.500	0.672	0.637	0.435	0.512	0.462
HCC136	Chronic Kidney Disease, Stage 5	0.237	0.141	0.244	0.167	0.184	0.147	0.436
HCC137	Chronic Kidney Disease, Severe (Stage 4)	0.237	0.141	0.244	0.079	0.184	0.035	0.202
HCC157	Pressure Ulcer of Skin with Necrosis Through to Muscle, Tendon, or Bone	2.163	2.203	2.879	2.626	2.274	2.655	0.924
HCC158	Pressure Ulcer of Skin with Full Thickness Skin Loss	1.204	1.393	1.576	1.559	1.074	1.237	0.295
HCC161	Chronic Ulcer of Skin, Except Pressure	0.535	0.636	0.757	0.631	0.586	0.620	0.294
HCC162	Severe Skin Burn or Condition	0.321	0.348	0.003	0.537	0.525	0.119	0.076
HCC166	Severe Head Injury	0.584	0.302	0.946	0.324	1.065	0.155	0.042
HCC167	Major Head Injury	0.191	0.044	0.274	0.171	0.133	0.049	-
HCC169	Vertebral Fractures without Spinal Cord Injury	0.495	0.456	0.552	0.407	0.516	0.384	0.209
HCC170	Hip Fracture/ Dislocation	0.418	0.513	0.520	0.668	0.383	0.484	-
HCC173	Traumatic Amputations and Complications	0.266	0.340	0.412	0.383	0.233	0.232	0.267
HCC176	Complications of Specified Implanted Device or Graft	0.597	0.871	0.721	1.156	0.584	0.876	0.502

Variable	Description Label	Community, NonDual, Aged	Community, NonDual, Disabled	Community, FBDual, Aged	Community, FBDual, Disabled	Community, PBDual, Aged	Community, PBDual, Disabled	Institutional
HCC186	Major Organ Transplant or Replacement Status	1.000	0.618	0.816	1.075	0.795	0.655	0.962
HCC188	Artificial Openings for Feeding or Elimination	0.571	0.785	0.775	0.870	0.579	0.867	0.500
HCC189	Amputation Status, Lower Limb/Amputation Complications	0.588	0.455	0.787	1.065	0.737	0.696	0.407
Disease Interactions								
HCC47_gCancer	Immune Disorders*Cancer Group	0.893	0.675	0.815	0.652	0.776	0.808	-
HCC85_gDiabetesMellit	Congestive Heart Failure*Diabetes Group	0.154	0.096	0.205	0.160	0.178	0.139	0.154
HCC85_gCopdCF	Congestive Heart Failure*Chronic Obstructive Pulmonary Disease Group	0.190	0.174	0.240	0.217	0.186	0.181	0.164
HCC85_gRenal	Congestive Heart Failure*Renal Group	0.270	0.493	0.271	0.711	0.299	0.609	-
gRespDepandArre_gCopdCF	Cardiorespiratory Failure Group*Chronic Obstructive Pulmonary Disease Group	0.336	0.256	0.564	0.524	0.460	0.449	0.423
HCC85_HCC96	Congestive Heart Failure*Specified Heart Arrhythmias	0.105	0.285	0.200	0.405	0.116	0.318	-
gSubstanceAbuse_gPsychiatric	Substance Abuse Group*Psychiatric Group	-	0.191	-	0.233	-	0.230	-
SEPSIS_PRESSURE_ULCER	Sepsis*Pressure Ulcer	-	-	-	-	-	-	0.252
SEPSIS_ARTIF_OPENINGS	Sepsis*Artificial Openings for Feeding or Elimination	-	-	-	-	-	-	0.568
ART_OPENINGS_PRESSURE_ULCER	Artificial Openings for Feeding or Elimination*Pressure Ulcer	-	-	-	-	-	-	0.331
gCopdCF_ASP_SPEC_BACT_PNEUM	Chronic Obstructive Pulmonary Disease*Aspiration and Specified Bacterial Pneumonias	-	-	-	-	-	-	0.254
ASP_SPEC_BACT_PNEUM_PRES_ULC	Aspiration and Specified Bacterial Pneumonias*Pressure Ulcer	-	-	-	-	-	-	0.366
SEPSIS_ASP_SPEC_BACT_PNEUM	Sepsis*Aspiration and Specified Bacterial Pneumonias	-	-	-	-	-	-	0.321

Variable	Description Label	Community, NonDual, Aged	Community, NonDual, Disabled	Community, FBDual, Aged	Community, FBDual, Disabled	Community, PBDual, Aged	Community, PBDual, Disabled	Institutional
SCHIZOPHRENIA_ gCopdCF	Schizophrenia*Chronic Obstructive Pulmonary Disease	-	-	-	-	-	-	0.363
SCHIZOPHRENIA_ CHF	Schizophrenia* Congestive Heart Failure	-	-	-	-	-	-	0.173
SCHIZOPHRENIA_ SEIZURES	Schizophrenia*Seizure Disorders and Convulsions	-	-	-	-	-	-	0.483
Disabled/Disease Interactions								
DISABLED_HCC85	Disabled, Congestive Heart Failure	-	-	-	-	-	-	0.321
DISABLED_ PRESSURE_ULCER	Disabled, Pressure Ulcer	-	-	-	-	-	-	0.608
DISABLED_HCC161	Disabled, Chronic Ulcer of the Skin, Except Pressure Ulcer	-	-	-	-	-	-	0.369
DISABLED_HCC39	Disabled, Bone/Joint Muscle Infections/ Necrosis	-	-	-	-	-	-	0.567
DISABLED_HCC77	Disabled, Multiple Sclerosis	-	-	-	-	-	-	0.425
DISABLED_HCC6	Disabled, Opportunistic Infections	-	-	-	-	-	-	0.277

Notes:

1. The denominator is $9,185.29.
2. In the "disease interactions" and "disabled interactions," the variables are defined as follows:
   Immune Disorders = HCC47
   Cancer = HCCs 8-12
   Congestive Heart Failure = HCC 85
   Diabetes = HCCs 17-19
   Chronic Obstructive Pulmonary Disease = HCCs 110-112
   Renal = HCCs 134-137
   Cardiorespiratory Failure = HCCs 82-84
   Specified Heart Arrhythmias = HCC 96
   Substance Abuse = HCCs 54-55
   Psychiatric = HCCs 57-58
   Sepsis = HCC 2
   Pressure Ulcer = HCCs 157-158
   Artificial Openings for Feeding or Elimination = HCC 188
   Aspiration and Specified Bacterial Pneumonias = HCC 114
   Schizophrenia = HCC 57
   Seizure Disorders and Convulsions = HCC 79
   Chronic Ulcer of Skin, except Pressure = HCC 161
   Bone/Joint/Muscle Infections/Necrosis = HCC 39
   Multiple Sclerosis = HCC 77
   Opportunistic Infections = HCC 6

Source: RTI International analysis of 2013-2014 Medicare 100% data and RTI International analysis of 2013-2014 Medicare 100% institutional sample.

TABLE VI-2 2017 CMS-HCC Model Relative Factors for Aged and Disabled New Enrollees

	Non-Medicaid & Non-Originally Disabled	Medicaid & Non-Originally Disabled	Non-Medicaid & Originally Disabled	Medicaid & Originally Disabled
Female				
0-34 Years	0.664	0.985	-	-
35-44 Years	0.936	1.221	-	-
45-54 Years	1.035	1.337	-	-
55-59 Years	1.004	1.342	-	-
60-64 Years	1.122	1.438	-	-
65 Years	0.522	1.059	1.130	1.566
66 Years	0.516	0.946	1.167	1.619
67 Years	0.544	0.946	1.167	1.619
68 Years	0.581	0.946	1.167	1.619
69 Years	0.605	0.946	1.167	1.619
70-74 Years	0.674	0.975	1.167	1.619
75-79 Years	0.892	1.092	1.167	1.619
80-84 Years	1.066	1.395	1.167	1.619
85-89 Years	1.324	1.458	1.167	1.619
90-94 Years	1.324	1.678	1.167	1.619
95 Years or Over	1.324	1.678	1.167	1.619
Male				
0-34 Years	0.456	0.766	-	-
35-44 Years	0.665	1.095	-	-
45-54 Years	0.834	1.357	-	-
55-59 Years	0.889	1.422	-	-
60-64 Years	0.923	1.582	-	-
65 Years	0.514	1.201	0.790	1.613
66 Years	0.533	1.208	0.957	1.613
67 Years	0.575	1.208	1.005	2.202
68 Years	0.641	1.208	1.074	2.202
69 Years	0.671	1.311	1.398	2.202
70-74 Years	0.776	1.311	1.398	2.202
75-79 Years	1.040	1.361	1.398	2.202
80-84 Years	1.270	1.603	1.398	2.202
85-89 Years	1.511	1.850	1.398	2.202
90-94 Years	1.511	1.850	1.398	2.202
95 Years or Over	1.511	1.850	1.398	2.202

Notes:

1. The denominator is $9,185.29.
2. For payment purposes, a new enrollee is a beneficiary who did not have 12 months of Part B eligibility in the data collection year. CMS-HCC new enrollee models are not based on diagnoses, but include factors for different age and gender combinations by Medicaid and the original reason for Medicare entitlement.

Source: RTI International analysis of 2013-2014 100% Medicare data.

TABLE VI-3 2017 CMS-HCC Model Relative Factors for New Enrollees in Chronic Condition Special Needs Plans (C-SNPs)

	Non-Medicaid & Non-Originally Disabled	Medicaid & Non-Originally Disabled	Non-Medicaid & Originally Disabled	Medicaid & Originally Disabled
Female				
0-34 Years	1.136	1.633	-	-
35-44 Years	1.409	1.868	-	-
45-54 Years	1.507	2.068	-	-
55-59 Years	1.618	2.123	-	-
60-64 Years	1.689	2.177	-	-
65 Years	1.003	1.546	1.747	2.161
66 Years	0.997	1.546	1.785	2.214
67 Years	1.063	1.569	1.805	2.272
68 Years	1.100	1.569	1.805	2.272
69 Years	1.123	1.569	1.805	2.272
70-74 Years	1.269	1.776	1.932	2.415
75-79 Years	1.480	1.973	2.096	2.576
80-84 Years	1.687	2.162	2.252	2.844
85-89 Years	1.920	2.381	2.252	2.844
90-94 Years	1.920	2.602	2.252	2.844
95 Years or Over	1.920	2.602	2.252	2.844
Male				
0-34 Years	1.045	1.329	-	-
35-44 Years	1.254	1.658	-	-
45-54 Years	1.503	1.954	-	-
55-59 Years	1.630	2.091	-	-
60-64 Years	1.670	2.187	-	-
65 Years	0.971	1.478	1.655	2.224
66 Years	0.989	1.485	1.691	2.224
67 Years	1.015	1.600	1.705	2.360
68 Years	1.082	1.600	1.734	2.360
69 Years	1.111	1.703	1.780	2.360
70-74 Years	1.302	1.898	1.874	2.356
75-79 Years	1.522	2.080	2.000	2.582
80-84 Years	1.758	2.229	2.254	2.582
85-89 Years	2.047	2.544	2.254	2.582
90-94 Years	2.047	2.544	2.254	2.582
95 Years or Over	2.047	2.544	2.254	2.582

Notes:
1. The denominator is $9,185.29.
2. For payment purposes, a new enrollee is a beneficiary who did not have 12 months of Part B eligibility in the data collection year. CMS-HCC new enrollee models are not based on diagnoses, but include factors for different age and gender combinations by Medicaid and the original reason for Medicare entitlement.
3. The relative factors in this table were calculated by estimating the incremental amount to the standard new enrollee risk model needed to predict the risk scores of continuing enrollees inC-SNPs.

Source: RTI International analysis of 2013-2014 100% Medicare data.

TABLE VI-4 Disease Hierarchies for the 2017 CMS-HCC Model

Hierarchical Condition Category (HCC)	If the Disease Group is Listed in this column . . .	. . . Then drop the Disease Group(s) listed in this column
	Hierarchical Condition Category (HCC) LABEL	
8	Metastatic Cancer and Acute Leukemia	9, 10, 11, 12
9	Lung and Other Severe Cancers	10, 11, 12
10	Lymphoma and Other Cancers	11, 12
11	Colorectal, Bladder, and Other Cancers	12
17	Diabetes with Acute Complications	18, 19
18	Diabetes with Chronic Complications	19
27	End-Stage Liver Disease	28, 29, 80
28	Cirrhosis of Liver	29
46	Severe Hematological Disorders	48
54	Drug/Alcohol Psychosis	55
57	Schizophrenia	58
70	Quadriplegia	71, 72, 103, 104, 169
71	Paraplegia	72, 104, 169
72	Spinal Cord Disorders/Injuries	169
82	Respirator Dependence/Tracheostomy Status	83, 84
83	Respiratory Arrest	84
86	Acute Myocardial Infarction	87, 88
87	Unstable Angina and Other Acute Ischemic Heart Disease	88
99	Cerebral Hemorrhage	100
103	Hemiplegia/Hemiparesis	104
106	Atherosclerosis of the Extremities with Ulceration or Gangrene	107, 108, 161, 189
107	Vascular Disease with Complications	108
110	Cystic Fibrosis	111, 112
111	Chronic Obstructive Pulmonary Disease	112
114	Aspiration and Specified Bacterial Pneumonias	115
134	Dialysis Status	135, 136, 137
135	Acute Renal Failure	136, 137
136	Chronic Kidney Disease, Stage 5	137
157	Pressure Ulcer of Skin with Necrosis Through to Muscle, Tendon, or Bone	158, 161
158	Pressure Ulcer of Skin with Full Thickness Skin Loss	161
166	Severe Head Injury	80, 167

How Payments Are Made With a Disease Hierarchy: If a beneficiary triggers Disease Groups 135 (Acute Renal Failure) and 136 (Chronic Kidney Disease, Stage 5), then DG 136 will be dropped. In other words, payment will always be associated with the DG in column 1, if a DG in column 3 also occurs during the same collection period. Therefore, the organization's payment will be based on DG 135 rather than DG 136.

TABLE VII-1 2018 RxHCC Model Relative Factors for Continuing Enrollees Continuing Enrollees (CE) RxHCC Model Segments

Variable	Disease Group	Community, Non-Low Income, Age≥65	Community, Non-Low Income, Age<65	Community, Low Income, Age≥65	Community, Low Income, Age<65	Institutional
Female						
0-34 Years		-	0.306	-	0.435	1.791
35-44 Years		-	0.450	-	0.625	2.035
45-54 Years		-	0.553	-	0.725	1.716
55-59 Years		-	0.524	-	0.704	1.565
60-64 Years		-	0.485	-	0.638	1.424
65-69 Years		0.239	-	0.389	-	1.488
70-74 Years		0.239	-	0.365	-	1.362
75-79 Years		0.225	-	0.355	-	1.254
80-84 Years		0.205	-	0.316	-	1.159
85-89 Years		0.182	-	0.282	-	1.068
90-94 Years		0.135	-	0.228	-	0.950
95 Years or Over		0.072	-	0.141	-	0.759
Male						
0-34 Years		-	0.271	-	0.474	1.827
35-44 Years		-	0.389	-	0.600	1.818
45-54 Years		-	0.489	-	0.667	1.679
55-59 Years		-	0.524	-	0.674	1.493
60-64 Years		-	0.502	-	0.621	1.366
65-69 Years		0.263	-	0.367	-	1.319
70-74 Years		0.270	-	0.342	-	1.271
75-79 Years		0.245	-	0.342	-	1.199
80-84 Years		0.185	-	0.304	-	1.148
85-89 Years		0.140	-	0.287	-	1.077
90-94 Years		0.083	-	0.240	-	0.986
95 Years or Over		0.047	-	0.224	-	0.867
Originally Disabled Interactions with Sex						
Originally Disabled_Female		0.102	-	0.198	-	0.072
Originally Disabled_Male		-	-	0.135	-	0.072
Disease Coefficients						
RXHCC1	HIV/AIDS	3.192	3.871	3.783	4.127	2.577
RXHCC5	Opportunistic Infections	0.261	0.097	0.175	0.162	0.177
RXHCC15	Chronic Myeloid Leukemia	7.383	7.519	8.142	9.906	4.907
RXHCC16	Multiple Myeloma and Other Neoplastic Disorders	3.946	4.179	3.227	3.663	1.094
RXHCC17	Secondary Cancers of Bone, Lung, Brain, and Other Specified Sites; Liver Cancer	1.771	1.708	1.601	1.588	0.579
RXHCC18	Lung, Kidney, and Other Cancers	0.294	0.260	0.324	0.316	0.069
RXHCC19	Breast and Other Cancers and Tumors	0.096	0.085	0.079	0.115	0.069
RXHCC30	Diabetes with Complications	0.425	0.461	0.501	0.695	0.475
RXHCC31	Diabetes without Complication	0.280	0.262	0.316	0.389	0.321

Variable	Disease Group	Community, Non-Low Income, Age≥65	Community, Non-Low Income, Age<65	Community, Low Income, Age≥65	Community, Low Income, Age<65	Institutional
RXHCC40	Specified Hereditary Metabolic/Immune Disorders	2.990	10.494	3.113	10.451	0.468
RXHCC41	Pituitary, Adrenal Gland, and Other Endocrine and Metabolic Disorders	0.100	0.201	0.060	0.228	0.087
RXHCC42	Thyroid Disorders	0.101	0.178	0.099	0.166	0.076
RXHCC43	Morbid Obesity	0.056	-	0.074	0.068	0.171
RXHCC45	Disorders of Lipoid Metabolism	0.038	-	0.068	0.088	0.052
RXHCC54	Chronic Viral Hepatitis C	3.202	3.685	2.922	2.947	0.945
RXHCC55	Chronic Viral Hepatitis, Except Hepatitis C	0.521	0.335	0.859	0.533	0.371
RXHCC65	Chronic Pancreatitis	0.265	0.188	0.159	0.203	0.173
RXHCC66	Pancreatic Disorders and Intestinal Malabsorption, Except Pancreatitis	0.105	0.188	0.116	0.203	0.117
RXHCC67	Inflammatory Bowel Disease	0.527	0.461	0.458	0.830	0.211
RXHCC68	Esophageal Reflux and Other Disorders of Esophagus	0.076	0.061	0.142	0.169	0.077
RXHCC80	Aseptic Necrosis of Bone	0.177	0.248	0.109	0.144	0.112
RXHCC82	Psoriatic Arthropathy and Systemic Sclerosis	0.769	0.738	1.295	2.065	0.655
RXHCC83	Rheumatoid Arthritis and Other Inflammatory Polyarthropathy	0.377	0.409	0.483	0.805	0.185
RXHCC84	Systemic Lupus Erythematosus, Other Connective Tissue Disorders, and Inflammatory Spondylopathies	0.212	0.333	0.239	0.354	0.168
RXHCC87	Osteoporosis, Vertebral and Pathological Fractures	0.052	0.153	0.121	0.204	-
RXHCC95	Sickle Cell Anemia	0.086	0.288	0.048	0.789	0.343
RXHCC96	Myelodysplastic Syndromes and Myelofibrosis	0.959	1.135	0.772	0.710	0.546
RXHCC97	Immune Disorders	0.553	0.509	0.488	0.454	0.342
RXHCC98	Aplastic Anemia and Other Significant Blood Disorders	0.086	0.155	0.048	0.220	0.044
RXHCC111	Alzheimer's Disease	0.476	0.243	0.177	0.034	-
RXHCC112	Dementia, Except Alzheimer's Disease	0.196	0.104	0.041	-	-
RXHCC130	Schizophrenia	0.261	0.291	0.404	0.700	0.199
RXHCC131	Bipolar Disorders	0.255	0.278	0.284	0.444	0.199
RXHCC132	Major Depression	0.127	0.207	0.143	0.311	0.166
RXHCC133	Specified Anxiety, Personality, and Behavior Disorders	0.127	0.172	0.143	0.311	0.108
RXHCC134	Depression	0.127	0.172	0.137	0.206	0.108
RXHCC135	Anxiety Disorders	0.051	0.113	0.085	0.171	0.108
RXHCC145	Autism	0.127	0.172	0.368	0.374	0.108
RXHCC146	Profound or Severe Intellectual Disability/ Developmental Disorder	-	0.172	0.368	0.334	-
RXHCC147	Moderate Intellectual Disability/Developmental Disorder	-	-	0.240	0.158	-
RXHCC148	Mild or Unspecified Intellectual Disability/ Developmental Disorder	-	-	0.096	0.033	-

Variable	Disease Group	Community, Non-Low Income, Age≥65	Community, Non-Low Income, Age<65	Community, Low Income, Age≥65	Community, Low Income, Age<65	Institutional
RXHCC156	Myasthenia Gravis, Amyotrophic Lateral Sclerosis and Other Motor Neuron Disease	0.361	0.565	0.388	0.574	0.179
RXHCC157	Spinal Cord Disorders	0.114	0.088	0.094	0.057	0.054
RXHCC159	Inflammatory and Toxic Neuropathy	0.171	0.385	0.169	0.331	0.079
RXHCC160	Multiple Sclerosis	2.350	3.951	2.012	4.067	0.970
RXHCC161	Parkinson's and Huntington's Diseases	0.505	0.699	0.316	0.436	0.224
RXHCC163	Intractable Epilepsy	0.298	0.550	0.311	1.031	0.093
RXHCC164	Epilepsy and Other Seizure Disorders, Except Intractable Epilepsy	0.121	0.075	0.048	0.148	-
RXHCC165	Convulsions	0.053	0.024	0.029	0.068	-
RXHCC166	Migraine Headaches	0.138	0.207	0.127	0.141	0.110
RXHCC168	Trigeminal and Postherpetic Neuralgia	0.134	0.294	0.157	0.212	0.193
RXHCC185	Primary Pulmonary Hypertension	0.740	2.201	0.633	1.800	0.255
RXHCC186	Congestive Heart Failure	0.166	0.146	0.225	0.143	0.138
RXHCC187	Hypertension	0.123	0.072	0.189	0.108	0.059
RXHCC188	Coronary Artery Disease	0.125	0.012	0.141	-	0.011
RXHCC193	Atrial Arrhythmias	0.288	0.100	0.140	0.010	0.087
RXHCC206	Cerebrovascular Disease, Except Hemorrhage or Aneurysm	0.044	-	0.040	-	-
RXHCC207	Spastic Hemiplegia	0.191	0.148	0.032	0.160	-
RXHCC215	Venous Thromboembolism	0.145	0.189	0.094	0.107	0.049
RXHCC216	Peripheral Vascular Disease	-	-	0.021	-	-
RXHCC225	Cystic Fibrosis	0.745	5.449	0.364	5.262	1.159
RXHCC226	Chronic Obstructive Pulmonary Disease and Asthma	0.334	0.139	0.364	0.257	0.201
RXHCC227	Pulmonary Fibrosis and Other Chronic Lung Disorders	0.334	0.139	0.174	0.257	0.039
RXHCC241	Diabetic Retinopathy	0.307	0.231	0.226	0.150	0.160
RXHCC243	Open-Angle Glaucoma	0.280	0.235	0.335	0.271	0.228
RXHCC260	Kidney Transplant Status	0.330	0.163	0.380	0.419	0.187
RXHCC261	Dialysis Status	0.246	0.508	0.484	0.928	0.409
RXHCC262	Chronic Kidney Disease Stage 5	0.093	0.119	0.084	0.043	0.057
RXHCC263	Chronic Kidney Disease Stage 4	0.093	0.119	0.084	0.043	0.057
RXHCC311	Chronic Ulcer of Skin, Except Pressure	0.162	0.166	0.102	0.099	0.055
RXHCC314	Pemphigus	0.356	0.650	0.195	0.123	0.041
RXHCC316	Psoriasis, Except with Arthropathy	0.205	0.249	0.408	0.720	0.277
RXHCC355	Narcolepsy and Cataplexy	0.806	1.332	0.649	1.351	0.251
RXHCC395	Lung Transplant Status	1.201	0.781	0.985	0.861	0.871
RXHCC396	Major Organ Transplant Status, Except Lung, Kidney, and Pancreas	1.039	0.781	0.985	0.861	0.187
RXHCC397	Pancreas Transplant Status	0.330	0.163	0.380	0.233	0.187
Non-Aged Disease Interactions						
NonAged_RXHCC1	NonAged * HIV/AIDS	-	-	-	-	0.907

Variable	Disease Group	Community, Non-Low Income, Age≥65	Community, Non-Low Income, Age<65	Community, Low Income, Age≥65	Community, Low Income, Age<65	Institutional
NonAged_ RXHCC130	NonAged * Schizophrenia	-	-	-	-	0.276
NonAged_ RXHCC131	NonAged * Bipolar Disorders	-	-	-	-	0.275
NonAged_ RXHCC132	NonAged * Major Depression	-	-	-	-	0.184
NonAged_ RXHCC133	NonAged * Specified Anxiety, Personality, and Behavior Disorders	-	-	-	-	0.224
NonAged_ RXHCC134	NonAged * Depression	-	-	-	-	0.113
NonAged_ RXHCC135	NonAged * Anxiety Disorders	-	-	-	-	0.189
NonAged_ RXHCC160	NonAged * Multiple Sclerosis	-	-	-	-	1.327
NonAged_ RXHCC163	NonAged * Intractable Epilepsy	-	-	-	-	0.246

Note: The Part D denominator used to calculate relative factors is $1,047.96. This Part D denominator is based on the combined PDP and MA-PD populations.

Source: RTI Analysis of 100% 2015 PDE, 2014 Carrier NCH, 2014 Inpatient SAF, 2014 Outpatient SAF, 2015 HPMS, 2015 CME, 2014-2015 Denominator, Part D Intermediate File, and 2014 Medicare Advantage Diagnoses File.

TABLE VII-2 2018 RxHCC Model Relative Factors for New Enrollees, Non-Low Income

Variable	Not Concurrently ESRD, Not Originally Disabled	Concurrently ESRD, Not Originally Disabled	Originally Disabled, Not Concurrently ESRD	Originally Disabled, Concurrently ESRD
Female				
0-34 Years	0.697	0.946	-	-
35-44 Years	1.208	1.208	-	-
45-54 Years	1.312	1.583	-	-
55-59 Years	1.255	1.744	-	-
60-64 Years	1.245	1.930	-	-
65 Years	0.531	1.930	1.142	1.930
66 Years	0.581	1.930	1.168	1.930
67 Years	0.595	1.930	1.168	1.930
68 Years	0.612	1.930	1.168	1.930
69 Years	0.637	1.930	1.168	1.930
70-74 Years	0.666	1.930	1.057	1.930
75-79 Years	0.685	1.930	0.803	1.930
80-84 Years	0.620	1.930	0.620	1.930
85-89 Years	0.614	1.930	0.614	1.930
90-94 Years	0.351	1.930	0.351	1.930
95 Years or Over	0.351	1.930	0.351	1.930
Male				
0-34 Years	0.462	0.840	-	-
35-44 Years	0.853	1.251	-	-
45-54 Years	1.149	1.584	-	-
55-59 Years	1.223	1.793	-	-
60-64 Years	1.194	2.101	-	-
65 Years	0.594	1.948	1.029	1.948
66 Years	0.639	1.948	1.024	1.948
67 Years	0.656	1.948	1.024	1.948
68 Years	0.686	1.948	1.024	1.948
69 Years	0.706	1.948	1.024	1.948
70-74 Years	0.751	1.948	0.951	1.948
75-79 Years	0.778	1.948	0.778	1.948
80-84 Years	0.705	1.948	0.705	1.948
85-89 Years	0.659	1.948	0.659	1.948
90-94 Years	0.314	1.948	0.314	1.948
95 Years or Over	0.314	1.948	0.314	1.948

Notes:
1. The Part D denominator used to calculate relative factors is $1,047.96. This Part D denominator is based on the combined PDP and MA-PD populations.
2. Originally Disabled is defined as originally entitled to Medicare by disability only (OREC =1).
3. For new enrollees, the concurrent ESRD marker is defined as at least one month in the payment year of ESRD status—dialysis, transplant, or post-graft.

Source: RTI Analysis of 100% 2015 PDE, 2014 Carrier NCH, 2014 Inpatient SAF, 2014 Outpatient SAF, 2015 HPMS, 2015 CME, 2014-2015 Denominator, Part D Intermediate File, and 2014 Medicare Advantage Diagnoses File.

TABLE VII-3 RxHCC Model Relative Factors for New Enrollees, Low Income

Variable	Not Concurrently ESRD, Not Originally Disabled	Concurrently ESRD, Not Originally Disabled	Originally Disabled, Not Concurrently ESRD	Originally Disabled, Concurrently ESRD
Female				
0-34 Years	1.024	2.151	-	-
35-44 Years	1.531	2.198	-	-
45-54 Years	1.583	2.285	-	-
55-59 Years	1.466	2.401	-	-
60-64 Years	1.376	2.234	-	-
65 Years	0.901	2.185	1.249	2.185
66 Years	0.601	2.185	0.836	2.185
67 Years	0.601	2.185	0.836	2.185
68 Years	0.601	2.185	0.836	2.185
69 Years	0.601	2.185	0.836	2.185
70-74 Years	0.606	2.185	0.787	2.185
75-79 Years	0.664	2.185	0.664	2.185
80-84 Years	0.664	2.185	0.664	2.185
85-89 Years	0.664	2.185	0.664	2.185
90-94 Years	0.564	2.185	0.564	2.185
95 Years or Over	0.564	2.185	0.564	2.185
Male				
0-34 Years	0.883	2.248	-	-
35-44 Years	1.264	2.252	-	-
45-54 Years	1.462	2.331	-	-
55-59 Years	1.376	2.189	-	-
60-64 Years	1.289	2.141	-	-
65 Years	0.896	2.033	1.145	2.033
66 Years	0.579	2.033	0.742	2.033
67 Years	0.554	2.033	0.742	2.033
68 Years	0.509	2.033	0.742	2.033
69 Years	0.509	2.033	0.742	2.033
70-74 Years	0.527	2.033	0.591	2.033
75-79 Years	0.545	2.033	0.545	2.033
80-84 Years	0.555	2.033	0.555	2.033
85-89 Years	0.528	2.033	0.528	2.033
90-94 Years	0.412	2.033	0.412	2.033
95 Years or Over	0.412	2.033	0.412	2.033

Notes:

1. The Part D denominator used to calculate relative factors is $1,047.96. This Part D denominator is based on the combined PDP and MA-PD populations.
2. Originally Disabled is defined as originally entitled to Medicare by disability only (OREC =1).
3. For new enrollees, the concurrent ESRD marker is defined as at least one month in the payment year of ESRD status—dialysis, transplant, or post-graft.

Source: RTI Analysis of 100% 2015 PDE, 2014 Carrier NCH, 2014 Inpatient SAF, 2014 Outpatient SAF, 2015 HPMS, 2015 CME, 2014-2015 Denominator, Part D Intermediate File, and 2014 Medicare Advantage Diagnoses File.

TABLE VII-4 RxHCC Model Relative Factors for New Enrollees, Institutional

Variable	Not Concurrently ESRD	Concurrently ESRD
Female		
0-34 Years	2.783	2.796
35-44 Years	2.783	2.796
45-54 Years	2.431	2.796
55-59 Years	2.512	2.796
60-64 Years	2.116	2.796
65 Years	2.204	2.796
66 Years	1.929	2.796
67 Years	1.929	2.796
68 Years	1.929	2.796
69 Years	1.929	2.796
70-74 Years	1.802	2.796
75-79 Years	1.570	2.796
80-84 Years	1.430	2.796
85-89 Years	1.367	2.796
90-94 Years	1.090	2.796
95 Years or Over	1.090	2.796
Male		
0-34 Years	2.419	2.812
35-44 Years	2.603	2.812
45-54 Years	2.374	2.812
55-59 Years	2.166	2.812
60-64 Years	2.109	2.812
65 Years	2.063	2.812
66 Years	1.794	2.812
67 Years	1.794	2.812
68 Years	1.794	2.812
69 Years	1.794	2.812
70-74 Years	1.699	2.812
75-79 Years	1.699	2.812
80-84 Years	1.508	2.812
85-89 Years	1.343	2.812
90-94 Years	1.343	2.812
95 Years or Over	1.343	2.812

Notes:
1. The Part D denominator used to calculate relative factors is $1,047.96. This Part D denominator is based on the combined PDP and MA-PD populations.
2. For new enrollees, the concurrent ESRD marker is defined as at least one month in the payment year of ESRD status—dialysis, transplant, or post-graft.

Source: RTI Analysis of 100% 2015 PDE, 2014 Carrier NCH, 2014 Inpatient SAF, 2014 Outpatient SAF, 2015 HPMS, 2015 CME, 2014-2015 Denominator, Part D Intermediate File, and 2014 Medicare Advantage Diagnoses File.

TABLE VII-5 2018 List of Disease Hierarchies for RxHCC Model

Rx Hierarchical Condition Category (RxHCC)	If the Disease Group is listed in this column . . .	. . . Then drop the RxHCC(s) listed in this column
	Rx Hierarchical Condition Category (RxHCC) LABEL	
15	Chronic Myeloid Leukemia	16, 17, 18, 19, 96, 98
16	Multiple Myeloma and Other Neoplastic Disorders	17, 18, 19, 96, 98
17	Secondary Cancers of Bone, Lung, Brain, and Other Specified Sites; Liver Cancer	18, 19
18	Lung, Kidney, and Other Cancers	19
30	Diabetes with Complications	31
54	Chronic Viral Hepatitis C	55
65	Chronic Pancreatitis	66
82	Psoriatic Arthropathy and Systemic Sclerosis	83, 84, 316
83	Rheumatoid Arthritis and Other Inflammatory Polyarthropathy	84
95	Sickle Cell Anemia	98
96	Myelodysplastic Syndromes and Myelofibrosis	98
111	Alzheimer's Disease	112
130	Schizophrenia	131, 132, 133, 134, 135, 145, 146, 147, 148
131	Bipolar Disorders	132, 133, 134, 135
132	Major Depression	133, 134, 135
133	Specified Anxiety, Personality, and Behavior Disorders	134, 135
134	Depression	135
145	Autism	133, 134, 135, 146, 147, 148
146	Profound or Severe Intellectual Disability/Developmental Disorder	147, 148
147	Moderate Intellectual Disability/Developmental Disorder	148
163	Intractable Epilepsy	164, 165
164	Epilepsy and Other Seizure Disorders, Except Intractable Epilepsy	165
185	Primary Pulmonary Hypertension	186, 187
186	Congestive Heart Failure	187
225	Cystic Fibrosis	226, 227
226	Chronic Obstructive Pulmonary Disease and Asthma	227
260	Kidney Transplant Status	261, 262, 263, 397
261	Dialysis Status	262, 263
262	Chronic Kidney Disease Stage 5	263
395	Lung Transplant Status	396, 397
396	Major Organ Transplant Status, Except Lung, Kidney, and Pancreas	397

How Payments are Made with a Disease Hierarchy: For example, if a beneficiary triggers Disease Groups 163 (Intractable Epilepsy) and 164 (Epilepsy and Other Seizure Disorders, Except Intractable Epilepsy), then DG 164 will be dropped. In other words, payment will always be associated with the DG in column 1 if a DG in column 3 also occurs during the same collection period. Therefore, the organization's payment will be based on DG 163 rather than DG 164.

Source: RTI International.

Appendix B

ICD-10-CM Codes Mapped to HCCs and RxHCCs

Table AB identifies risk-adjusting ICD-10-CM codes with their associated 2018 CMS-HCCs and CMS-RxHCCs. In addition, Table AB consists of only those codes represented in the CMS-HCC Model Category V22 for HCCs and the RxHCC Model Category V05 for the 2018 payment year. Therefore, it is important to reference the complete ICD-10-CM code set when abstracting in order to reference the instructions and guidance from the code set. As with the original Centers for Medicare & Medicaid Services (CMS) files, the decimal points are not included in the codes in Table AB.

If an ICD-10-CM code combines two or more clinical concepts, it may map to more than one payment HCC or RxHCC. When this occurs, both are listed together in Table AB. When the ICD-10-CM code does not map to an HCC or RxHCC, it is indicated by N/A. Code descriptions have been edited due to space constraints, and in some cases, the final digit of the code is represented by a dash (-), and the final digit is provided in a separate key. For example, for codes S32000A through S329XXB, only the following 7th characters risk-adjust: A (initial encounter for closed fracture) and B (initial encounter for open fracture). (See Example.)

Example

Code	Code Descriptors	HCC	RxHCC
For codes S32000- through S329XX-, only the following 7th characters risk-adjust: A intial encounter for closed fracture B intial encounter for open fracture			
S32000-	Wedge compression FX of NOS lumbar vertebra	168	N/A

In this example, valid codes must be "completed," ie, coded to the highest level of specificity, by adding the appropriate digit to the code number, replacing the dash. For example:

S32000A Wedge compression FX of NOS lumbar vertebra, initial encounter for closed fracture

S32000B Wedge compression FX of NOS lumbar vertebra, initial encounter for open fracture

Either code will risk-adjust to HCC 169, but not to an RxHCC.

Acronyms and abbreviations used in the ICD-10-CM descriptors in Table AB are as follows:

& = and
2ndary = secondary
AMI = acute myocardial infarction
ARMD = age-related macular degeneration
BKA = below-knee amputation
BMI = body mass index
CKD = chronic kidney disease
CNS = central nervous system
COPD = chronic obstructive pulmonary disease
D/T = due to
DZ = disease
DKA = diabetic ketoacidosis
DMAC = disseminated mycobacterium avium-intracellulare complex
E. coli = Escherichia coli
ED = emergency room
ESRD = end-stage renal disease
FX = fracture
GCS = Glasgow coma scale
GERD = gastroesophageal reflux disease
HF = heart failure
HIV = human immunodeficiency virus
HR = hour(s)
IgA = immunoglobulin A
IgG = immunoglobulin G
IgM = immunoglobulin M
L = left
LG = large
LOC = loss of consciousness
MAL = NEO malignant neoplasm
N/A = not applicable
NEC = not elsewhere classified (other specified)
NKHHC = nonketotic hyperglycemic hyperosmolar coma
NOS = not otherwise specified (unspecified)
NSTEMI = non-ST elevation myocardial infarction
OAG = open-angle glaucoma
R = right
RF = rheumatoid factor
SIRS = systemic inflammatory response syndrome
SLE = systemic lupus erythematosus
SM = small
STEMI = ST elevation myocardial infarction
TBI = traumatic brain injury
TBSA = total body surface area
W/ = with
W/O = without

TABLE AB CMS-HCC Model Categories V21 and V22 for HCCs and RxHCC Model Category V05 for the 2018 Payment Rate

Code	Code Descriptors	HCC	RxHCC
A0103	Typhoid pneumonia	115	N/A
A0104	Typhoid arthritis	39	N/A
A0105	Typhoid osteomyelitis	39	N/A
A021	Salmonella sepsis	2	N/A
A0222	Salmonella pneumonia	115	N/A
A0223	Salmonella arthritis	39	N/A
A0224	Salmonella osteomyelitis	39	N/A
A065	Amebic lung abscess	115	N/A
A072	Cryptosporidiosis	6	5
A202	Pneumonic plague	115	N/A
A207	Septicemic plague	2	N/A
A212	Pulmonary tularemia	115	N/A
A221	Pulmonary anthrax	115	N/A
A227	Anthrax sepsis	2	N/A
A267	Erysipelothrix sepsis	2	N/A
A310	Pulmonary mycobacterial infection	6	5
A312	DMAC	6	5
A327	Listerial sepsis	2	N/A
A3681	Diphtheritic cardiomyopathy	85	186
A3684	Diphtheritic tubulo-interstitial nephropathy	141	N/A
A391	Waterhouse-Friderichsen syndrome	23	41
A392	Acute meningococcemia	2	N/A
A393	Chronic meningococcemia	2	N/A
A394	Meningococcemia, NOS	2	N/A
A3983	Meningococcal arthritis	39	N/A
A3984	Postmeningococcal arthritis	39	N/A
A400	Sepsis D/T streptococcus, group A	2	N/A
A401	Sepsis D/T streptococcus, group B	2	N/A
A403	Sepsis D/T Streptococcus pneumoniae	2	N/A
A408	Streptococcal sepsis, NEC	2	N/A
A409	Streptococcal sepsis, NOS	2	N/A
A4101	Sepsis D/T MSSA	2	N/A
A4102	Sepsis D/T MRSA	2	N/A
A411	Sepsis D/T staphylococcus, NEC	2	N/A
A412	Sepsis D/T staphylococcus, NOS	2	N/A
A413	Sepsis D/T Hemophilus influenzae	2	N/A
A414	Sepsis D/T anaerobes	2	N/A
A4150	Gram-negative sepsis, NOS	2	N/A
A4151	Sepsis D/T E. coli	2	N/A
A4152	Sepsis D/T Pseudomonas	2	N/A
A4153	Sepsis D/T Serratia	2	N/A
A4159	Gram-negative sepsis, NEC	2	N/A
A4181	Sepsis D/T Enterococcus	2	N/A
A4189	Sepsis, organism NEC	2	N/A
A419	Sepsis, organism NOS	2	N/A
A420	Pulmonary actinomycosis	115	N/A
A427	Actinomycotic sepsis	2	N/A
A430	Pulmonary nocardiosis	115	N/A
A480	Gas gangrene	106	N/A
A481	Legionnaires' DZ	114	N/A
A483	Toxic shock syndrome	2	N/A
A5055	Late congenital syphilitic arthropathy	39	N/A
A5204	Syphilitic cerebral arteritis	N/A	206
A5440	Gonococcal infection of musculoskeletal system, NOS	39	N/A
A5441	Gonococcal spondylopathy	39	N/A
A5442	Gonococcal arthritis	39	N/A
A5443	Gonococcal osteomyelitis	39	N/A
A5449	Gonococcal infection of musculoskeletal tissue, NEC	39	N/A
A5484	Gonococcal pneumonia	115	N/A
A5485	Gonococcal peritonitis	33	N/A
A5486	Gonococcal sepsis	2	N/A
A666	Bone & joint lesions of yaws	39	N/A
A6923	Arthritis D/T Lyme DZ	39	N/A
A8100	Creutzfeldt-Jakob DZ, NOS	52	112
A8101	Variant Creutzfeldt-Jakob DZ	52	112
A8109	Creutzfeldt-Jakob DZ, NEC	52	112
A811	Subacute sclerosing panencephalitis	52	112
A812	Progressive multifocal leukoencephalopathy	52	112
A8181	Kuru	52	112
A8182	Gerstmann-Straussler-Scheinker syndrome	52	112
A8183	Fatal familial insomnia	52	112
A8189	Atypical virus infections of CNS, NEC	52	112
A819	Atypical virus infection of CNS, NOS	52	112
A985	Hemorrhagic fever W/ renal syndrome	141	N/A
B007	Disseminated herpesviral DZ	2	N/A
B0082	Herpes simplex myelitis	72	157
B0112	Varicella myelitis	72	157
B0221	Postherpetic geniculate ganglionitis	N/A	168
B0222	Postherpetic trigeminal neuralgia	N/A	168
B0223	Postherpetic polyneuropathy	N/A	168
B0224	Postherpetic myelitis	72	157
B0229	Postherpetic nervous system involvement, NEC	N/A	168
B0682	Rubella arthritis	39	N/A
B180	Chronic viral hepatitis B W/ delta-agent	29	55
B181	Chronic viral hepatitis B W/O delta-agent	29	55
B182	Chronic viral hepatitis C	29	54
B188	Chronic viral hepatitis, NEC	29	55
B189	Chronic viral hepatitis, NOS	29	55
B20	HIV DZ	1	1

Code	Code Descriptors	HCC	RxHCC
B250	Cytomegaloviral pneumonitis	6	5
B251	Cytomegaloviral hepatitis	6	5
B252	Cytomegaloviral pancreatitis	6	5
B258	Cytomegaloviral DZ, NEC	6	5
B259	Cytomegaloviral DZ, NOS	6	5
B2685	Mumps arthritis	39	N/A
B3324	Viral cardiomyopathy	85	186
B371	Pulmonary candidiasis	6	5
B377	Candidal sepsis	2, 6	5
B3781	Candidal esophagitis	6	5
B380	Acute pulmonary coccidioidomycosis	115	N/A
B381	Chronic pulmonary coccidioidomycosis	115	N/A
B382	Pulmonary coccidioidomycosis, NOS	115	N/A
B390	Acute pulmonary histoplasmosis capsulati	115	N/A
B391	Chronic pulmonary histoplasmosis capsulati	115	N/A
B392	Pulmonary histoplasmosis capsulati, NOS	115	N/A
B400	Acute pulmonary blastomycosis	115	N/A
B401	Chronic pulmonary blastomycosis	115	N/A
B402	Pulmonary blastomycosis, NOS	115	N/A
B410	Pulmonary paracoccidioidomycosis	115	N/A
B4282	Sporotrichosis arthritis	39	N/A
B440	Invasive pulmonary aspergillosis	6	5
B441	Pulmonary aspergillosis, NEC	6	5
B442	Tonsillar aspergillosis	6	5
B447	Disseminated aspergillosis	6	5
B4481	Allergic bronchopulmonary aspergillosis	112	227
B4489	Aspergillosis, NEC	6	5
B449	Aspergillosis, NOS	6	5
B450	Pulmonary cryptococcosis	6	5
B451	Cerebral cryptococcosis	6	5
B452	Cutaneous cryptococcosis	6	5
B453	Osseous cryptococcosis	6	5
B457	Disseminated cryptococcosis	6	5
B458	Cryptococcosis, NEC	6	5
B459	Cryptococcosis, NOS	6	5
B460	Pulmonary mucormycosis	6	5
B461	Rhinocerebral mucormycosis	6	5
B462	Gastrointestinal mucormycosis	6	5
B463	Cutaneous mucormycosis	6	5
B464	Disseminated mucormycosis	6	5
B465	Mucormycosis, NOS	6	5
B468	Aygomycoses, NEC	6	5
B469	Zygomycosis, NOS	6	5
B484	Penicillosis	6	5
B488	Mycoses, NEC	6	5
B520	Plasmodium malariae malaria W/ nephropathy	141	N/A

Code	Code Descriptors	HCC	RxHCC
B582	Toxoplasma meningoencephalitis	6	5
B583	Pulmonary toxoplasmosis	6	5
B59	Pneumocystosis	6	5
B664	Paragonimiasis	115	N/A
B671	Echinococcus granulosus infection of lung	115	N/A
B9735	HIV 2 as cause of DZ classified elsewhere	1	1
C01	MAL NEO of base of tongue	11	N/A
C020	MAL NEO of dorsal surface of tongue	11	N/A
C021	MAL NEO of border of tongue	11	N/A
C022	MAL NEO of ventral surface of tongue	11	N/A
C023	MAL NEO of anterior 2/3 of tongue, NOS	11	N/A
C024	MAL NEO of lingual tonsil	11	N/A
C028	MAL NEO of overlapping sites of tongue	11	N/A
C029	MAL NEO of tongue, NOS	11	N/A
C030	MAL NEO of upper gum	11	N/A
C031	MAL NEO of lower gum	11	N/A
C039	MAL NEO of gum, NOS	11	N/A
C040	MAL NEO of anterior floor of mouth	11	N/A
C041	MAL NEO of lateral floor of mouth	11	N/A
C048	MAL NEO of overlapping sites of floor of mouth	11	N/A
C049	MAL NEO of floor of mouth, NOS	11	N/A
C050	MAL NEO of hard palate	11	N/A
C051	MAL NEO of soft palate	11	N/A
C052	MAL NEO of uvula	11	N/A
C058	MAL NEO of overlapping sites of palate	11	N/A
C059	MAL NEO of palate, NOS	11	N/A
C060	MAL NEO of cheek mucosa	11	N/A
C061	MAL NEO of vestibule of mouth	11	N/A
C062	MAL NEO of retromolar area	11	N/A
C0680	MAL NEO of overlapping sites of mouth, NOS	11	N/A
C0689	MAL NEO of overlapping sites of mouth, NEC	11	N/A
C069	MAL NEO of mouth, NOS	11	N/A
C07	MAL NEO of parotid gland	11	N/A
C080	MAL NEO of submandibular gland	11	N/A
C081	MAL NEO of sublingual gland	11	N/A
C089	MAL NEO of major salivary gland, NOS	11	N/A
C090	MAL NEO of tonsillar fossa	11	N/A
C091	MAL NEO of tonsillar pillar	11	N/A
C098	MAL NEO of overlapping sites of tonsil	11	N/A
C099	MAL NEO of tonsil, NOS	11	N/A
C100	MAL NEO of vallecula	11	N/A
C101	MAL NEO of anterior surface of epiglottis	11	N/A
C102	MAL NEO of lateral wall of oropharynx	11	N/A
C103	MAL NEO of posterior wall of oropharynx	11	N/A

Code	Code Descriptors	HCC	RxHCC
C104	MAL NEO of branchial cleft	11	N/A
C108	MAL NEO of overlapping sites of oropharynx	11	N/A
C109	MAL NEO of oropharynx, NOS	11	N/A
C110	MAL NEO of superior wall of nasopharynx	11	N/A
C111	MAL NEO of posterior wall of nasopharynx	11	N/A
C112	MAL NEO of lateral wall of nasopharynx	11	N/A
C113	MAL NEO of anterior wall of nasopharynx	11	N/A
C118	MAL NEO of overlapping sites of nasopharynx	11	N/A
C119	MAL NEO of nasopharynx, NOS	11	N/A
C12	MAL NEO of pyriform sinus	11	N/A
C130	MAL NEO of postcricoid region	11	N/A
C131	MAL NEO of aryepiglottic fold, hypopharyngeal aspect	11	N/A
C132	MAL NEO of posterior wall of hypopharynx	11	N/A
C138	MAL NEO of overlapping sites of hypopharynx	11	N/A
C139	MAL NEO of hypopharynx, NOS	11	N/A
C140	MAL NEO of pharynx, NOS	11	N/A
C142	MAL NEO of Waldeyer's ring	11	N/A
C148	MAL NEO of overlapping sites of lip, oral cavity & pharynx	11	N/A
C153	MAL NEO of upper 1/3 of esophagus	9	N/A
C154	MAL NEO of middle 1/3 of esophagus	9	N/A
C155	MAL NEO of lower 1/3 of esophagus	9	N/A
C158	MAL NEO of overlapping sites of esophagus	9	N/A
C159	MAL NEO of esophagus, NOS	9	N/A
C160	MAL NEO of cardia	9	18
C161	MAL NEO of fundus of stomach	9	18
C162	MAL NEO of body of stomach	9	18
C163	MAL NEO of pyloric antrum	9	18
C164	MAL NEO of pylorus	9	18
C165	MAL NEO of lesser curvature of stomach, NOS	9	18
C166	MAL NEO of greater curvature of stomach, NOS	9	18
C168	MAL NEO of overlapping sites of stomach	9	18
C169	MAL NEO of stomach, NOS	9	18
C170	MAL NEO of duodenum	9	19
C171	MAL NEO of jejunum	9	19
C172	MAL NEO of ileum	9	19
C173	Meckel's diverticulum, malignant	9	19
C178	MAL NEO of overlapping sites of SM intestine	9	19
C179	MAL NEO of SM intestine, NOS	9	19
C180	MAL NEO of cecum	11	N/A
C181	MAL NEO of appendix	11	N/A
C182	MAL NEO of ascending colon	11	N/A
C183	MAL NEO of hepatic flexure	11	N/A
C184	MAL NEO of transverse colon	11	N/A
C185	MAL NEO of splenic flexure	11	N/A
C186	MAL NEO of descending colon	11	N/A
C187	MAL NEO of sigmoid colon	11	N/A
C188	MAL NEO of overlapping sites of colon	11	N/A
C189	MAL NEO of colon, NOS	11	N/A
C19	MAL NEO of rectosigmoid junction	11	N/A
C20	MAL NEO of rectum	11	N/A
C210	MAL NEO of anus, NOS	11	N/A
C211	MAL NEO of anal canal	11	N/A
C212	MAL NEO of cloacogenic zone	11	N/A
C218	MAL NEO of overlapping sites of rectum, anus & anal canal	11	N/A
C220	Liver cell carcinoma	9	17
C221	Intrahepatic bile duct carcinoma	9	17
C222	Hepatoblastoma	9	17
C223	Angiosarcoma of liver	9	17
C224	Sarcoma of liver, NEC	9	17
C227	Carcinoma of liver, NEC	9	17
C228	MAL NEO of liver, primary, NOS type	9	17
C229	MAL NEO of liver, not specified as primary or 2ndary	9	17
C23	MAL NEO of gallbladder	9	19
C240	MAL NEO of extrahepatic bile duct	9	19
C241	MAL NEO of ampulla of Vater	9	19
C248	MAL NEO of overlapping sites of biliary tract	9	19
C249	MAL NEO of biliary tract, NOS	9	19
C250	MAL NEO of head of pancreas	9	18
C251	MAL NEO of body of pancreas	9	18
C252	MAL NEO of tail of pancreas	9	18
C253	MAL NEO of pancreatic duct	9	18
C254	MAL NEO of endocrine pancreas	9	18
C257	MAL NEO of pancreas, NEC	9	18
C258	MAL NEO of overlapping sites of pancreas	9	18
C259	MAL NEO of pancreas, NOS	9	18
C260	MAL NEO of intestinal tract, part NOS	11	N/A
C261	MAL NEO of spleen	11	N/A
C269	MAL NEO of ill-defined sites in digestive system	11	N/A
C300	MAL NEO of nasal cavity	11	N/A
C301	MAL NEO of middle ear	11	N/A
C310	MAL NEO of maxillary sinus	11	N/A
C311	MAL NEO of ethmoidal sinus	11	N/A
C312	MAL NEO of frontal sinus	11	N/A
C313	MAL NEO of sphenoid sinus	11	N/A

Code	Code Descriptors	HCC	RxHCC
C318	MAL NEO of overlapping sites of accessory sinuses	11	N/A
C319	MAL NEO of accessory sinus, NOS	11	N/A
C320	MAL NEO of glottis	11	N/A
C321	MAL NEO of supraglottis	11	N/A
C322	MAL NEO of subglottis	11	N/A
C323	MAL NEO of laryngeal cartilage	11	N/A
C328	MAL NEO of overlapping sites of larynx	11	N/A
C329	MAL NEO of larynx, NOS	11	N/A
C33	MAL NEO of trachea	9	18
C3400	MAL NEO of NOS main bronchus	9	18
C3401	MAL NEO of R main bronchus	9	18
C3402	MAL NEO of L main bronchus	9	18
C3410	MAL NEO of upper lobe, NOS bronchus or lung	9	18
C3411	MAL NEO of upper lobe, R bronchus or lung	9	18
C3412	MAL NEO of upper lobe, L bronchus or lung	9	18
C342	MAL NEO of middle lobe, bronchus or lung	9	18
C3430	MAL NEO of lower lobe, NOS bronchus or lung	9	18
C3431	MAL NEO of lower lobe, R bronchus or lung	9	18
C3432	MAL NEO of lower lobe, L bronchus or lung	9	18
C3480	MAL NEO of overlapping sites of NOS bronchus & lung	9	18
C3481	MAL NEO of overlapping sites of R bronchus & lung	9	18
C3482	MAL NEO of overlapping sites of L bronchus & lung	9	18
C3490	MAL NEO of NOS part of NOS bronchus or lung	9	18
C3491	MAL NEO of NOS part of R bronchus or lung	9	18
C3492	MAL NEO of NOS part of L bronchus or lung	9	18
C37	MAL NEO of thymus	11	N/A
C380	MAL NEO of heart	11	N/A
C381	MAL NEO of anterior mediastinum	11	N/A
C382	MAL NEO of posterior mediastinum	11	N/A
C383	MAL NEO of mediastinum, part NOS	11	N/A
C384	MAL NEO of pleura	9	18
C388	MAL NEO of overlapping sites of heart, mediastinum & pleura	11	N/A
C390	MAL NEO of upper respiratory tract, part NOS	11	N/A
C399	MAL NEO of lower respiratory tract, part NOS	11	N/A
C4000	MAL NEO of scapula & long bones of NOS upper limb	10	19
C4001	MAL NEO of scapula & long bones of R upper limb	10	19
C4002	MAL NEO of scapula & long bones of L upper limb	10	19
C4010	MAL NEO of short bones of upper limb, NOS	10	19
C4011	MAL NEO of short bones of R upper limb	10	19
C4012	MAL NEO of short bones of L upper limb	10	19
C4020	MAL NEO of long bones of lower limb, NOS	10	19
C4021	MAL NEO of long bones of R lower limb	10	19
C4022	MAL NEO of long bones of L lower limb	10	19
C4030	MAL NEO of short bones of lower limb, NOS	10	19
C4031	MAL NEO of short bones of R lower limb	10	19
C4032	MAL NEO of short bones of L lower limb	10	19
C4080	MAL NEO of overlapping sites of bone & articular cartilage of limb, NOS	10	19
C4081	MAL NEO of overlapping sites of bone & articular cartilage of R limb	10	19
C4082	MAL NEO of overlapping sites of bone & articular cartilage of L limb	10	19
C4090	MAL NEO of NOS bones & articular cartilage of limb, NOS	10	19
C4091	MAL NEO of NOS bones & articular cartilage of R limb	10	19
C4092	MAL NEO of NOS bones & articular cartilage of L limb	10	19
C410	MAL NEO of bones of skull & face	10	19
C411	MAL NEO of mandible	10	19
C412	MAL NEO of vertebral column	10	19
C413	MAL NEO of ribs, sternum & clavicle	10	19
C414	MAL NEO of pelvic bones, sacrum & coccyx	10	19
C419	MAL NEO of bone & articular cartilage, NOS	10	19
C430	Malignant melanoma of lip	12	N/A
C4310	Malignant melanoma of eyelid, NOS, including canthus	12	N/A
C4311	Malignant melanoma of R eyelid, including canthus	12	N/A
C4312	Malignant melanoma of L eyelid, including canthus	12	N/A
C4320	Malignant melanoma of ear & external auricular canal, NOS	12	N/A
C4321	Malignant melanoma of R ear & external auricular canal	12	N/A
C4322	Malignant melanoma of L ear & external auricular canal	12	N/A
C4330	Malignant melanoma of part of face, NOS	12	N/A
C4331	Malignant melanoma of nose	12	N/A
C4339	Malignant melanoma of parts of face, NEC	12	N/A
C434	Malignant melanoma of scalp & neck	12	N/A
C4351	Malignant melanoma of anal skin	12	N/A
C4352	Malignant melanoma of skin of breast	12	N/A
C4359	Malignant melanoma of trunk, NEC	12	N/A
C4360	Malignant melanoma of upper limb, NOS, including shoulder	12	N/A

Code	Code Descriptors	HCC	RXHCC
C4361	Malignant melanoma of R upper limb, including shoulder	12	N/A
C4362	Malignant melanoma of L upper limb, including shoulder	12	N/A
C4370	Malignant melanoma of lower limb, NOS, including hip	12	N/A
C4371	Malignant melanoma of R lower limb, including hip	12	N/A
C4372	Malignant melanoma of L lower limb, including hip	12	N/A
C438	Malignant melanoma of overlapping sites of skin	12	N/A
C439	Malignant melanoma of skin, NOS	12	N/A
C450	Mesothelioma of pleura	9	18
C451	Mesothelioma of peritoneum	9	18
C452	Mesothelioma of pericardium	9	18
C457	Mesothelioma, NEC	9	18
C459	Mesothelioma, NOS	9	18
C460	Kaposi's sarcoma of skin	10	18
C461	Kaposi's sarcoma of soft tissue	10	18
C462	Kaposi's sarcoma of palate	10	18
C463	Kaposi's sarcoma of lymph nodes	10	18
C464	Kaposi's sarcoma of gastrointestinal sites	10	18
C4650	Kaposi's sarcoma of lung, NOS	10	18
C4651	Kaposi's sarcoma of R lung	10	18
C4652	Kaposi's sarcoma of L lung	10	18
C467	Kaposi's sarcoma, NEC	10	18
C469	Kaposi's sarcoma, NOS	10	18
C470	MAL NEO of peripheral nerves of head, face & neck	10	19
C4710	MAL NEO of peripheral nerves of upper limb, NOS, including shoulder	10	19
C4711	MAL NEO of peripheral nerves of R upper limb, including shoulder	10	19
C4712	MAL NEO of peripheral nerves of L upper limb, including shoulder	10	19
C4720	MAL NEO of peripheral nerves of lower limb, NOS, including hip	10	19
C4721	MAL NEO of peripheral nerves of R lower limb, including hip	10	19
C4722	MAL NEO of peripheral nerves of L lower limb, including hip	10	19
C473	MAL NEO of peripheral nerves of thorax	10	19
C474	MAL NEO of peripheral nerves of abdomen	10	16
C475	MAL NEO of peripheral nerves of pelvis	10	19
C476	MAL NEO of peripheral nerves of trunk, NOS	10	19
C478	MAL NEO of overlapping sites of peripheral nerves & autonomic nervous system	10	19
C479	MAL NEO of peripheral nerves & autonomic nervous system, NOS	10	19
C480	MAL NEO of retroperitoneum	9	19

Code	Code Descriptors	HCC	RXHCC
C481	MAL NEO of specified parts of peritoneum	9	19
C482	MAL NEO of peritoneum, NOS	9	19
C488	MAL NEO of overlapping sites of retroperitoneum & peritoneum	9	19
C490	MAL NEO of connective & soft tissue of head, face & neck	10	19
C4910	MAL NEO of connective & soft tissue of upper limb, NOS, including shoulder	10	19
C4911	MAL NEO of connective & soft tissue of R upper limb, including shoulder	10	19
C4912	MAL NEO of connective & soft tissue of L upper limb, including shoulder	10	19
C4920	MAL NEO of connective & soft tissue of NOS lower limb, including hip	10	19
C4921	MAL NEO of connective & soft tissue of R lower limb, including hip	10	19
C4922	MAL NEO of connective & soft tissue of L lower limb, including hip	10	19
C493	MAL NEO of connective & soft tissue of thorax	10	19
C494	MAL NEO of connective & soft tissue of abdomen	10	16
C495	MAL NEO of connective & soft tissue of pelvis	10	19
C496	MAL NEO of connective & soft tissue of trunk, NOS	10	19
C498	MAL NEO of overlapping sites of connective & soft tissue	10	19
C499	MAL NEO of connective & soft tissue, NOS	10	19
C49A0	Gastrointestinal stromal tumor, NOS site	10	16
C49A1	Gastrointestinal stromal tumor of esophagus	10	16
C49A2	Gastrointestinal stromal tumor of stomach	10	16
C49A3	Gastrointestinal stromal tumor of SM intestine	10	16
C49A4	Gastrointestinal stromal tumor of LG intestine	10	16
C49A5	Gastrointestinal stromal tumor of rectum	10	16
C49A9	Gastrointestinal stromal tumor of sites, NEC	10	16
C4A0	Merkel cell carcinoma of lip	12	19
C4A10	Merkel cell carcinoma of NOS eyelid, including canthus	12	19
C4A11	Merkel cell carcinoma of R eyelid, including canthus	12	19
C4A12	Merkel cell carcinoma of L eyelid, including canthus	12	19
C4A20	Merkel cell carcinoma of NOS ear & external auricular canal	12	19
C4A21	Merkel cell carcinoma of R ear & external auricular canal	12	19
C4A22	Merkel cell carcinoma of L ear & external auricular canal	12	19
C4A30	Merkel cell carcinoma of NOS part of face	12	19

Code	Code Descriptors	HCC	RXHCC
C4A31	Merkel cell carcinoma of nose	12	19
C4A39	Merkel cell carcinoma of parts of face, NEC	12	19
C4A4	Merkel cell carcinoma of scalp & neck	12	19
C4A51	Merkel cell carcinoma of anal skin	12	19
C4A52	Merkel cell carcinoma of skin of breast	12	19
C4A59	Merkel cell carcinoma of trunk, NEC	12	19
C4A60	Merkel cell carcinoma of NOS upper limb, including shoulder	12	19
C4A61	Merkel cell carcinoma of R upper limb, including shoulder	12	19
C4A62	Merkel cell carcinoma of L upper limb, including shoulder	12	19
C4A70	Merkel cell carcinoma of NOS lower limb, including hip	12	19
C4A71	Merkel cell carcinoma of R lower limb, including hip	12	19
C4A72	Merkel cell carcinoma of L lower limb, including hip	12	19
C4A8	Merkel cell carcinoma of overlapping sites	12	19
C4A9	Merkel cell carcinoma, NOS	12	19
C50011	MAL NEO of nipple & areola, R female breast	12	19
C50012	MAL NEO of nipple & areola, L female breast	12	19
C50019	MAL NEO of nipple & areola, NOS female breast	12	19
C50021	MAL NEO of nipple & areola, R male breast	12	19
C50022	MAL NEO of nipple & areola, L male breast	12	19
C50029	MAL NEO of nipple & areola, NOS male breast	12	19
C50111	MAL NEO of central portion of R female breast	12	19
C50112	MAL NEO of central portion of L female breast	12	19
C50119	MAL NEO of central portion of NOS female breast	12	19
C50121	MAL NEO of central portion of R male breast	12	19
C50122	MAL NEO of central portion of L male breast	12	19
C50129	MAL NEO of central portion of NOS male breast	12	19
C50211	MAL NEO of upper-inner quadrant of R female breast	12	19
C50212	MAL NEO of upper-inner quadrant of L female breast	12	19
C50219	MAL NEO of upper-inner quadrant of NOS female breast	12	19
C50221	MAL NEO of upper-inner quadrant of R male breast	12	19
C50222	MAL NEO of upper-inner quadrant of L male breast	12	19
C50229	MAL NEO of upper-inner quadrant of NOS male breast	12	19
C50311	MAL NEO of lower-inner quadrant of R female breast	12	19
C50312	MAL NEO of lower-inner quadrant of L female breast	12	19
C50319	MAL NEO of lower-inner quadrant of NOS female breast	12	19
C50321	MAL NEO of lower-inner quadrant of R male breast	12	19
C50322	MAL NEO of lower-inner quadrant of L male breast	12	19
C50329	MAL NEO of lower-inner quadrant of NOS male breast	12	19
C50411	MAL NEO of upper-outer quadrant of R female breast	12	19
C50412	MAL NEO of upper-outer quadrant of L female breast	12	19
C50419	MAL NEO of upper-outer quadrant of NOS female breast	12	19
C50421	MAL NEO of upper-outer quadrant of R male breast	12	19
C50422	MAL NEO of upper-outer quadrant of L male breast	12	19
C50429	MAL NEO of upper-outer quadrant of NOS male breast	12	19
C50511	MAL NEO of lower-outer quadrant of R female breast	12	19
C50512	MAL NEO of lower-outer quadrant of L female breast	12	19
C50519	MAL NEO of lower-outer quadrant of NOS female breast	12	19
C50521	MAL NEO of lower-outer quadrant of R male breast	12	19
C50522	MAL NEO of lower-outer quadrant of L male breast	12	19
C50529	MAL NEO of lower-outer quadrant of NOS male breast	12	19
C50611	MAL NEO of axillary tail of R female breast	12	19
C50612	MAL NEO of axillary tail of L female breast	12	19
C50619	MAL NEO of axillary tail of NOS female breast	12	19
C50621	MAL NEO of axillary tail of R male breast	12	19
C50622	MAL NEO of axillary tail of L male breast	12	19
C50629	MAL NEO of axillary tail of NOS male breast	12	19
C50811	MAL NEO of overlapping sites of R female breast	12	19
C50812	MAL NEO of overlapping sites of L female breast	12	19
C50819	MAL NEO of overlapping sites of NOS female breast	12	19
C50821	MAL NEO of overlapping sites of R male breast	12	19
C50822	MAL NEO of overlapping sites of L male breast	12	19

Code	Code Descriptors	HCC	RXHCC
C50829	MAL NEO of overlapping sites of NOS male breast	12	19
C50911	MAL NEO of NOS site of R female breast	12	19
C50912	MAL NEO of NOS site of L female breast	12	19
C50919	MAL NEO of NOS site of NOS female breast	12	19
C50921	MAL NEO of NOS site of R male breast	12	19
C50922	MAL NEO of NOS site of L male breast	12	19
C50929	MAL NEO of NOS site of NOS male breast	12	19
C510	MAL NEO of labium majus	11	N/A
C511	MAL NEO of labium minus	11	N/A
C512	MAL NEO of clitoris	11	N/A
C518	MAL NEO of overlapping sites of vulva	11	N/A
C519	MAL NEO of vulva, NOS	11	N/A
C52	MAL NEO of vagina	11	N/A
C530	MAL NEO of endocervix	11	N/A
C531	MAL NEO of exocervix	11	N/A
C538	MAL NEO of overlapping sites of cervix uteri	11	N/A
C539	MAL NEO of cervix uteri, NOS	11	N/A
C540	MAL NEO of isthmus uteri	12	N/A
C541	MAL NEO of endometrium	12	N/A
C542	MAL NEO of myometrium	12	N/A
C543	MAL NEO of fundus uteri	12	N/A
C548	MAL NEO of overlapping sites of corpus uteri	12	N/A
C549	MAL NEO of corpus uteri, NOS	12	N/A
C55	MAL NEO of uterus, part NOS	12	N/A
C561	MAL NEO of R ovary	10	N/A
C562	MAL NEO of L ovary	10	N/A
C569	MAL NEO of NOS ovary	10	N/A
C5700	MAL NEO of NOS fallopian tube	10	N/A
C5701	MAL NEO of R fallopian tube	10	N/A
C5702	MAL NEO of L fallopian tube	10	N/A
C5710	MAL NEO of NOS broad ligament	10	N/A
C5711	MAL NEO of R broad ligament	10	N/A
C5712	MAL NEO of L broad ligament	10	N/A
C5720	MAL NEO of NOS round ligament	10	N/A
C5721	MAL NEO of R round ligament	10	N/A
C5722	MAL NEO of L round ligament	10	N/A
C573	MAL NEO of parametrium	10	N/A
C574	MAL NEO of uterine adnexa, NOS	10	N/A
C577	MAL NEO of NEC female genital organs	11	N/A
C578	MAL NEO of overlapping sites of female genital organs	11	N/A
C579	MAL NEO of female genital organ, NOS	11	N/A
C58	MAL NEO of placenta	10	N/A
C600	MAL NEO of prepuce	12	N/A
C601	MAL NEO of glans penis	12	N/A

Code	Code Descriptors	HCC	RXHCC
C602	MAL NEO of body of penis	12	N/A
C608	MAL NEO of overlapping sites of penis	12	N/A
C609	MAL NEO of penis, NOS	12	N/A
C61	MAL NEO of prostate	12	N/A
C6200	MAL NEO of NOS undescended testis	12	N/A
C6201	MAL NEO of undescended R testis	12	N/A
C6202	MAL NEO of undescended L testis	12	N/A
C6210	MAL NEO of NOS descended testis	12	N/A
C6211	MAL NEO of descended R testis	12	N/A
C6212	MAL NEO of descended L testis	12	N/A
C6290	MAL NEO of NOS testis, NOS whether descended or undescended	12	N/A
C6291	MAL NEO of R testis, NOS whether descended or undescended	12	N/A
C6292	MAL NEO of L testis, NOS whether descended or undescended	12	N/A
C6300	MAL NEO of NOS epididymis	12	N/A
C6301	MAL NEO of R epididymis	12	N/A
C6302	MAL NEO of L epididymis	12	N/A
C6310	MAL NEO of NOS spermatic cord	12	N/A
C6311	MAL NEO of R spermatic cord	12	N/A
C6312	MAL NEO of L spermatic cord	12	N/A
C632	MAL NEO of scrotum	12	N/A
C637	MAL NEO of NEC male genital organs	12	N/A
C638	MAL NEO of overlapping sites of male genital organs	12	N/A
C639	MAL NEO of male genital organ, NOS	12	N/A
C641	MAL NEO of R kidney, except renal pelvis	11	18
C642	MAL NEO of L kidney, except renal pelvis	11	18
C649	MAL NEO of NOS kidney, except renal pelvis	11	18
C651	MAL NEO of R renal pelvis	11	18
C652	MAL NEO of L renal pelvis	11	18
C659	MAL NEO of NOS renal pelvis	11	18
C661	MAL NEO of R ureter	11	N/A
C662	MAL NEO of L ureter	11	N/A
C669	MAL NEO of NOS ureter	11	N/A
C670	MAL NEO of trigone of bladder	11	N/A
C671	MAL NEO of dome of bladder	11	N/A
C672	MAL NEO of lateral wall of bladder	11	N/A
C673	MAL NEO of anterior wall of bladder	11	N/A
C674	MAL NEO of posterior wall of bladder	11	N/A
C675	MAL NEO of bladder neck	11	N/A
C676	MAL NEO of ureteric orifice	11	N/A
C677	MAL NEO of urachus	11	N/A
C678	MAL NEO of overlapping sites of bladder	11	N/A
C679	MAL NEO of bladder, NOS	11	N/A
C680	MAL NEO of urethra	11	N/A
C681	MAL NEO of paraurethral glands	11	N/A

Code	Code Descriptors	HCC	RXHCC
C688	MAL NEO of overlapping sites of urinary organs	11	N/A
C689	MAL NEO of urinary organ, NOS	11	N/A
C6900	MAL NEO of NOS conjunctiva	12	N/A
C6901	MAL NEO of R conjunctiva	12	N/A
C6902	MAL NEO of L conjunctiva	12	N/A
C6910	MAL NEO of NOS cornea	12	N/A
C6911	MAL NEO of R cornea	12	N/A
C6912	MAL NEO of L cornea	12	N/A
C6920	MAL NEO of NOS retina	12	N/A
C6921	MAL NEO of R retina	12	N/A
C6922	MAL NEO of L retina	12	N/A
C6930	MAL NEO of NOS choroid	12	N/A
C6931	MAL NEO of R choroid	12	N/A
C6932	MAL NEO of L choroid	12	N/A
C6940	MAL NEO of NOS ciliary body	12	N/A
C6941	MAL NEO of R ciliary body	12	N/A
C6942	MAL NEO of L ciliary body	12	N/A
C6950	MAL NEO of NOS lacrimal gland & duct	12	N/A
C6951	MAL NEO of R lacrimal gland & duct	12	N/A
C6952	MAL NEO of L lacrimal gland & duct	12	N/A
C6960	MAL NEO of NOS orbit	12	N/A
C6961	MAL NEO of R orbit	12	N/A
C6962	MAL NEO of L orbit	12	N/A
C6980	MAL NEO of overlapping sites of NOS eye & adnexa	12	N/A
C6981	MAL NEO of overlapping sites of R eye & adnexa	12	N/A
C6982	MAL NEO of overlapping sites of L eye & adnexa	12	N/A
C6990	MAL NEO of NOS site of NOS eye	12	N/A
C6991	MAL NEO of NOS site of R eye	12	N/A
C6992	MAL NEO of NOS site of L eye	12	N/A
C700	MAL NEO of cerebral meninges	10	N/A
C701	MAL NEO of spinal meninges	10	N/A
C709	MAL NEO of meninges, NOS	10	N/A
C710	MAL NEO of cerebrum, except lobes & ventricles	10	N/A
C711	MAL NEO of frontal lobe	10	N/A
C712	MAL NEO of temporal lobe	10	N/A
C713	MAL NEO of parietal lobe	10	N/A
C714	MAL NEO of occipital lobe	10	N/A
C715	MAL NEO of cerebral ventricle	10	N/A
C716	MAL NEO of cerebellum	10	N/A
C717	MAL NEO of brain stem	10	N/A
C718	MAL NEO of overlapping sites of brain	10	N/A
C719	MAL NEO of brain, NOS	10	N/A
C720	MAL NEO of spinal cord	10	N/A

Code	Code Descriptors	HCC	RXHCC
C721	MAL NEO of cauda equina	10	N/A
C7220	MAL NEO of NOS olfactory nerve	10	N/A
C7221	MAL NEO of R olfactory nerve	10	N/A
C7222	MAL NEO of L olfactory nerve	10	N/A
C7230	MAL NEO of NOS optic nerve	10	N/A
C7231	MAL NEO of R optic nerve	10	N/A
C7232	MAL NEO of L optic nerve	10	N/A
C7240	MAL NEO of NOS acoustic nerve	10	N/A
C7241	MAL NEO of R acoustic nerve	10	N/A
C7242	MAL NEO of L acoustic nerve	10	N/A
C7250	MAL NEO of NOS cranial nerve	10	N/A
C7259	MAL NEO of NEC cranial nerves	10	N/A
C729	MAL NEO of CNS, NOS	10	N/A
C73	MAL NEO of thyroid gland	12	19
C7400	MAL NEO of cortex of NOS adrenal gland	10	19
C7401	MAL NEO of cortex of R adrenal gland	10	19
C7402	MAL NEO of cortex of L adrenal gland	10	19
C7410	MAL NEO of medulla of NOS adrenal gland	10	19
C7411	MAL NEO of medulla of R adrenal gland	10	19
C7412	MAL NEO of medulla of L adrenal gland	10	19
C7490	MAL NEO of NOS part of NOS adrenal gland	10	19
C7491	MAL NEO of NOS part of R adrenal gland	10	19
C7492	MAL NEO of NOS part of L adrenal gland	10	19
C750	MAL NEO of parathyroid gland	12	19
C751	MAL NEO of pituitary gland	10	N/A
C752	MAL NEO of craniopharyngeal duct	10	N/A
C753	MAL NEO of pineal gland	10	N/A
C754	MAL NEO of carotid body	12	19
C755	MAL NEO of aortic body & other paraganglia	12	19
C758	MAL NEO W/ pluriglandular involvement, NOS	12	19
C759	MAL NEO of endocrine gland, NOS	12	19
C760	MAL NEO of head, face & neck	12	N/A
C761	MAL NEO of thorax	12	N/A
C762	MAL NEO of abdomen	12	N/A
C763	MAL NEO of pelvis	12	N/A
C7640	MAL NEO of NOS upper limb	12	N/A
C7641	MAL NEO of R upper limb	12	N/A
C7642	MAL NEO of L upper limb	12	N/A
C7650	MAL NEO of NOS lower limb	12	N/A
C7651	MAL NEO of R lower limb	12	N/A
C7652	MAL NEO of L lower limb	12	N/A
C768	MAL NEO of NEC ill-defined sites	12	N/A
C770	2ndary & NOS MAL NEO of lymph nodes of head, face & neck	8	19
C771	2ndary & NOS MAL NEO of intrathoracic lymph nodes	8	19

Code	Code Descriptors	HCC	RXHCC
C772	2ndary & NOS MAL NEO of intra-abdominal lymph nodes	8	19
C773	2ndary & NOS MAL NEO of axilla & upper limb lymph nodes	10	19
C774	2ndary & NOS MAL NEO of inguinal & lower limb lymph nodes	8	19
C775	2ndary & NOS MAL NEO of intrapelvic lymph nodes	8	19
C778	2ndary & NOS MAL NEO of lymph nodes of multiple regions	8	19
C779	2ndary & NOS MAL NEO of lymph node, NOS	10	19
C7800	2ndary MAL NEO of lung, NOS	8	17
C7801	2ndary MAL NEO of R lung	8	17
C7802	2ndary MAL NEO of L lung	8	17
C781	2ndary MAL NEO of mediastinum	8	17
C782	2ndary MAL NEO of pleura	8	17
C7830	2ndary MAL NEO of respiratory organ, NOS	8	17
C7839	2ndary MAL NEO of respiratory organs, NEC	8	17
C784	2ndary MAL NEO of SM intestine	8	18
C785	2ndary MAL NEO of LG intestine & rectum	8	18
C786	2ndary MAL NEO of retroperitoneum & peritoneum	8	18
C787	2ndary MAL NEO of liver & intrahepatic bile duct	8	17
C7880	2ndary MAL NEO of NOS digestive organ	8	18
C7889	2ndary MAL NEO of NEC digestive organs	8	18
C7900	2ndary MAL NEO of NOS kidney & renal pelvis	8	17
C7901	2ndary MAL NEO of R kidney & renal pelvis	8	17
C7902	2ndary MAL NEO of L kidney & renal pelvis	8	17
C7910	2ndary MAL NEO of urinary organs, NOS	8	18
C7911	2ndary MAL NEO of bladder	8	18
C7919	2ndary MAL NEO of urinary organs, NEC	8	18
C792	2ndary MAL NEO of skin	10	18
C7931	2ndary MAL NEO of brain	8	17
C7932	2ndary MAL NEO of cerebral meninges	8	17
C7940	2ndary MAL NEO of part of nervous system, NOS	8	17
C7949	2ndary MAL NEO of NEC parts of nervous system, NEC	8	17
C7951	2ndary MAL NEO of bone	8	17
C7952	2ndary MAL NEO of bone marrow	8	17
C7960	2ndary MAL NEO of ovary, NOS	8	18
C7961	2ndary MAL NEO of R ovary	8	18
C7962	2ndary MAL NEO of L ovary	8	18
C7970	2ndary MAL NEO of adrenal gland, NOS	8	17
C7971	2ndary MAL NEO of R adrenal gland	8	17
C7972	2ndary MAL NEO of L adrenal gland	8	17
C7981	2ndary MAL NEO of breast	10	18

Code	Code Descriptors	HCC	RXHCC
C7982	2ndary MAL NEO of genital organs	10	18
C7989	2ndary MAL NEO of NEC sites	8	18
C799	2ndary MAL NEO of NOS site	8	18
C7A00	Malignant carcinoid tumor of NOS site	12	19
C7A010	Malignant carcinoid tumor of duodenum	12	19
C7A011	Malignant carcinoid tumor of jejunum	12	19
C7A012	Malignant carcinoid tumor of ileum	12	19
C7A019	Malignant carcinoid tumor of SM intestine, NOS portion	12	19
C7A020	Malignant carcinoid tumor of appendix	12	19
C7A021	Malignant carcinoid tumor of cecum	12	19
C7A022	Malignant carcinoid tumor of ascending colon	12	19
C7A023	Malignant carcinoid tumor of transverse colon	12	19
C7A024	Malignant carcinoid tumor of descending colon	12	19
C7A025	Malignant carcinoid tumor of sigmoid colon	12	19
C7A026	Malignant carcinoid tumor of rectum	12	19
C7A029	Malignant carcinoid tumor of LG intestine, NOS portion	12	19
C7A090	Malignant carcinoid tumor of bronchus & lung	12	19
C7A091	Malignant carcinoid tumor of thymus	12	19
C7A092	Malignant carcinoid tumor of stomach	12	19
C7A093	Malignant carcinoid tumor of kidney	12	19
C7A094	Malignant carcinoid tumor of foregut, NOS	12	19
C7A095	Malignant carcinoid tumor of midgut, NOS	12	19
C7A096	Malignant carcinoid tumor of hindgut, NOS	12	19
C7A098	Malignant carcinoid tumor, NEC	12	19
C7A1	Malignant poorly differentiated neuroendocrine tumors	12	19
C7A8	Malignant neuroendocrine tumor, NEC	12	19
C7B00	2ndary carcinoid tumors, NOS	8	18
C7B01	2ndary carcinoid tumors of distant lymph nodes	8	19
C7B02	2ndary carcinoid tumors of liver	8	17
C7B03	2ndary carcinoid tumors of bone	8	17
C7B04	2ndary carcinoid tumors of peritoneum	8	18
C7B09	2ndary carcinoid tumors of sites, NEC	8	18
C7B1	2ndary Merkel cell carcinoma	8	18
C7B8	2ndary neuroendocrine tumors, NEC	8	18
C800	Disseminated MAL NEO, NOS	8	18
C801	Malignant (primary) neoplasm, NOS	12	N/A
C802	MAL NEO associated W/ transplanted organ	12	N/A
C8100	Nodular lymphocyte predominant Hodgkin lymphoma, NOS site	10	N/A
C8101	Nodular lymphocyte predominant Hodgkin lymphoma, lymph nodes of head, face, & neck	10	N/A

Code	Code Descriptors	HCC	RXHCC
C8102	Nodular lymphocyte predominant Hodgkin lymphoma, intrathoracic lymph nodes	10	N/A
C8103	Nodular lymphocyte predominant Hodgkin lymphoma, intra-abdominal lymph nodes	10	N/A
C8104	Nodular lymphocyte predominant Hodgkin lymphoma, lymph nodes of axilla & upper limb	10	N/A
C8105	Nodular lymphocyte predominant Hodgkin lymphoma, lymph nodes of inguinal region & lower limb	10	N/A
C8106	Nodular lymphocyte predominant Hodgkin lymphoma, intrapelvic lymph nodes	10	N/A
C8107	Nodular lymphocyte predominant Hodgkin lymphoma, spleen	10	N/A
C8108	Nodular lymphocyte predominant Hodgkin lymphoma, lymph nodes of multiple sites	10	N/A
C8109	Nodular lymphocyte predominant Hodgkin lymphoma, extranodal & solid organ sites	10	N/A
C8110	Nodular sclerosis Hodgkin lymphoma, NOS site	10	N/A
C8111	Nodular sclerosis Hodgkin lymphoma, lymph nodes of head, face, & neck	10	N/A
C8112	Nodular sclerosis Hodgkin lymphoma, intrathoracic lymph nodes	10	N/A
C8113	Nodular sclerosis Hodgkin lymphoma, intra-abdominal lymph nodes	10	N/A
C8114	Nodular sclerosis Hodgkin lymphoma, lymph nodes of axilla & upper limb	10	N/A
C8115	Nodular sclerosis Hodgkin lymphoma, lymph nodes of inguinal region & lower limb	10	N/A
C8116	Nodular sclerosis Hodgkin lymphoma, intrapelvic lymph nodes	10	N/A
C8117	Nodular sclerosis Hodgkin lymphoma, spleen	10	N/A
C8118	Nodular sclerosis Hodgkin lymphoma, lymph nodes of multiple sites	10	N/A
C8119	Nodular sclerosis Hodgkin lymphoma, extranodal & solid organ sites	10	N/A
C8120	Mixed cellularity Hodgkin lymphoma, NOS site	10	N/A
C8121	Mixed cellularity Hodgkin lymphoma, lymph nodes of head, face, & neck	10	N/A
C8122	Mixed cellularity Hodgkin lymphoma, intrathoracic lymph nodes	10	N/A
C8123	Mixed cellularity Hodgkin lymphoma, intra-abdominal lymph nodes	10	N/A
C8124	Mixed cellularity Hodgkin lymphoma, lymph nodes of axilla & upper limb	10	N/A
C8125	Mixed cellularity Hodgkin lymphoma, lymph nodes of inguinal region & lower limb	10	N/A
C8126	Mixed cellularity Hodgkin lymphoma, intrapelvic lymph nodes	10	N/A
C8127	Mixed cellularity Hodgkin lymphoma, spleen	10	N/A
C8128	Mixed cellularity Hodgkin lymphoma, lymph nodes of multiple sites	10	N/A
C8129	Mixed cellularity Hodgkin lymphoma, extranodal & solid organ sites	10	N/A
C8130	Lymphocyte depleted Hodgkin lymphoma, NOS site	10	N/A
C8131	Lymphocyte depleted Hodgkin lymphoma, lymph nodes of head, face, & neck	10	N/A
C8132	Lymphocyte depleted Hodgkin lymphoma, intrathoracic lymph nodes	10	N/A
C8133	Lymphocyte depleted Hodgkin lymphoma, intra- abdominal lymph nodes	10	N/A
C8134	Lymphocyte depleted Hodgkin lymphoma, lymph nodes of axilla & upper limb	10	N/A
C8135	Lymphocyte depleted Hodgkin lymphoma, lymph nodes of inguinal region & lower limb	10	N/A
C8136	Lymphocyte depleted Hodgkin lymphoma, intrapelvic lymph nodes	10	N/A
C8137	Lymphocyte depleted Hodgkin lymphoma, spleen	10	N/A
C8138	Lymphocyte depleted Hodgkin lymphoma, lymph nodes of multiple sites	10	N/A
C8139	Lymphocyte depleted Hodgkin lymphoma, extranodal & solid organ sites	10	N/A
C8140	Lymphocyte-rich Hodgkin lymphoma, NOS site	10	N/A
C8141	Lymphocyte-rich Hodgkin lymphoma, lymph nodes of head, face, & neck	10	N/A
C8142	Lymphocyte-rich Hodgkin lymphoma, intrathoracic lymph nodes	10	N/A
C8143	Lymphocyte-rich Hodgkin lymphoma, intra-abdominal lymph nodes	10	N/A
C8144	Lymphocyte-rich Hodgkin lymphoma, lymph nodes of axilla & upper limb	10	N/A
C8145	Lymphocyte-rich Hodgkin lymphoma, lymph nodes of inguinal region & lower limb	10	N/A
C8146	Lymphocyte-rich Hodgkin lymphoma, intrapelvic lymph nodes	10	N/A
C8147	Lymphocyte-rich Hodgkin lymphoma, spleen	10	N/A
C8148	Lymphocyte-rich Hodgkin lymphoma, lymph nodes of multiple sites	10	N/A
C8149	Lymphocyte-rich Hodgkin lymphoma, extranodal & solid organ sites	10	N/A
C8170	Other Hodgkin lymphoma, NOS site	10	N/A
C8171	Other Hodgkin lymphoma, lymph nodes of head, face, & neck	10	N/A
C8172	Other Hodgkin lymphoma, intrathoracic lymph nodes	10	N/A
C8173	Other Hodgkin lymphoma, intra-abdominal lymph nodes	10	N/A
C8174	Other Hodgkin lymphoma, lymph nodes of axilla & upper limb	10	N/A
C8175	Other Hodgkin lymphoma, lymph nodes of inguinal region & lower limb	10	N/A

Code	Code Descriptors	HCC	RXHCC
C8176	Other Hodgkin lymphoma, intrapelvic lymph nodes	10	N/A
C8177	Other Hodgkin lymphoma, spleen	10	N/A
C8178	Other Hodgkin lymphoma, lymph nodes of multiple sites	10	N/A
C8179	Other Hodgkin lymphoma, extranodal & solid organ sites	10	N/A
C8190	Hodgkin lymphoma, NOS, NOS site	10	N/A
C8191	Hodgkin lymphoma, NOS, lymph nodes of head, face, & neck	10	N/A
C8192	Hodgkin lymphoma, NOS, intrathoracic lymph nodes	10	N/A
C8193	Hodgkin lymphoma, NOS, intra-abdominal lymph nodes	10	N/A
C8194	Hodgkin lymphoma, NOS, lymph nodes of axilla & upper limb	10	N/A
C8195	Hodgkin lymphoma, NOS, lymph nodes of inguinal region & lower limb	10	N/A
C8196	Hodgkin lymphoma, NOS, intrapelvic lymph nodes	10	N/A
C8197	Hodgkin lymphoma, NOS, spleen	10	N/A
C8198	Hodgkin lymphoma, NOS, lymph nodes of multiple sites	10	N/A
C8199	Hodgkin lymphoma, NOS, extranodal & solid organ sites	10	N/A
C8200	Follicular lymphoma grade I, NOS	10	N/A
C8201	Follicular lymphoma grade I, lymph nodes of head, face, & neck	10	N/A
C8202	Follicular lymphoma grade I, intrathoracic lymph nodes	10	N/A
C8203	Follicular lymphoma grade I, intra-abdominal lymph nodes	10	N/A
C8204	Follicular lymphoma grade I, lymph nodes of axilla & upper limb	10	N/A
C8205	Follicular lymphoma grade I, lymph nodes of inguinal region & lower limb	10	N/A
C8206	Follicular lymphoma grade I, intrapelvic lymph nodes	10	N/A
C8207	Follicular lymphoma grade I, spleen	10	N/A
C8208	Follicular lymphoma grade I, lymph nodes of multiple sites	10	N/A
C8209	Follicular lymphoma grade I, extranodal & solid organ sites	10	N/A
C8210	Follicular lymphoma grade II, NOS site	10	N/A
C8211	Follicular lymphoma grade II, lymph nodes of head, face, & neck	10	N/A
C8212	Follicular lymphoma grade II, intrathoracic lymph nodes	10	N/A
C8213	Follicular lymphoma grade II, intra-abdominal lymph nodes	10	N/A
C8214	Follicular lymphoma grade II, lymph nodes of axilla & upper limb	10	N/A

Code	Code Descriptors	HCC	RXHCC
C8215	Follicular lymphoma grade II, lymph nodes of inguinal region & lower limb	10	N/A
C8216	Follicular lymphoma grade II, intrapelvic lymph nodes	10	N/A
C8217	Follicular lymphoma grade II, spleen	10	N/A
C8218	Follicular lymphoma grade II, lymph nodes of multiple sites	10	N/A
C8219	Follicular lymphoma grade II, extranodal & solid organ sites	10	N/A
C8220	Follicular lymphoma grade III, NOS, NOS site	10	N/A
C8221	Follicular lymphoma grade III, NOS, lymph nodes of head, face, & neck	10	N/A
C8222	Follicular lymphoma grade III, NOS, intrathoracic lymph nodes	10	N/A
C8223	Follicular lymphoma grade III, NOS, intra-abdominal lymph nodes	10	N/A
C8224	Follicular lymphoma grade III, NOS, lymph nodes of axilla & upper limb	10	N/A
C8225	Follicular lymphoma grade III, NOS, lymph nodes of inguinal region & lower limb	10	N/A
C8226	Follicular lymphoma grade III, NOS, intrapelvic lymph nodes	10	N/A
C8227	Follicular lymphoma grade III, NOS, spleen	10	N/A
C8228	Follicular lymphoma grade III, NOS, lymph nodes of multiple sites	10	N/A
C8229	Follicular lymphoma grade III, NOS, extranodal & solid organ sites	10	N/A
C8230	Follicular lymphoma grade IIIa, NOS site	10	N/A
C8231	Follicular lymphoma grade IIIa, lymph nodes of head, face, & neck	10	N/A
C8232	Follicular lymphoma grade IIIa, intrathoracic lymph nodes	10	N/A
C8233	Follicular lymphoma grade IIIa, intra-abdominal lymph nodes	10	N/A
C8234	Follicular lymphoma grade IIIa, lymph nodes of axilla & upper limb	10	N/A
C8235	Follicular lymphoma grade IIIa, lymph nodes of inguinal region & lower limb	10	N/A
C8236	Follicular lymphoma grade IIIa, intrapelvic lymph nodes	10	N/A
C8237	Follicular lymphoma grade IIIa, spleen	10	N/A
C8238	Follicular lymphoma grade IIIa, lymph nodes of multiple sites	10	N/A
C8239	Follicular lymphoma grade IIIa, extranodal & solid organ sites	10	N/A
C8240	Follicular lymphoma grade IIIb, NOS site	10	N/A
C8241	Follicular lymphoma grade IIIb, lymph nodes of head, face, & neck	10	N/A
C8242	Follicular lymphoma grade IIIb, intrathoracic lymph nodes	10	N/A
C8243	Follicular lymphoma grade IIIb, intra-abdominal lymph nodes	10	N/A

Code	Code Descriptors	HCC	RXHCC
C8244	Follicular lymphoma grade IIIb, lymph nodes of axilla & upper limb	10	N/A
C8245	Follicular lymphoma grade IIIb, lymph nodes of inguinal region & lower limb	10	N/A
C8246	Follicular lymphoma grade IIIb, intrapelvic lymph nodes	10	N/A
C8247	Follicular lymphoma grade IIIb, spleen	10	N/A
C8248	Follicular lymphoma grade IIIb, lymph nodes of multiple sites	10	N/A
C8249	Follicular lymphoma grade IIIb, extranodal & solid organ sites	10	N/A
C8250	Diffuse follicle center lymphoma, NOS site	10	N/A
C8251	Diffuse follicle center lymphoma, lymph nodes of head, face, & neck	10	N/A
C8252	Diffuse follicle center lymphoma, intrathoracic lymph nodes	10	N/A
C8253	Diffuse follicle center lymphoma, intra-abdominal lymph nodes	10	N/A
C8254	Diffuse follicle center lymphoma, lymph nodes of axilla & upper limb	10	N/A
C8255	Diffuse follicle center lymphoma, lymph nodes of inguinal region & lower limb	10	N/A
C8256	Diffuse follicle center lymphoma, intrapelvic lymph nodes	10	N/A
C8257	Diffuse follicle center lymphoma, spleen	10	N/A
C8258	Diffuse follicle center lymphoma, lymph nodes of multiple sites	10	N/A
C8259	Diffuse follicle center lymphoma, extranodal & solid organ sites	10	N/A
C8260	Cutaneous follicle center lymphoma, NOS site	10	N/A
C8261	Cutaneous follicle center lymphoma, lymph nodes of head, face, & neck	10	N/A
C8262	Cutaneous follicle center lymphoma, intrathoracic lymph nodes	10	N/A
C8263	Cutaneous follicle center lymphoma, intra-abdominal lymph nodes	10	N/A
C8264	Cutaneous follicle center lymphoma, lymph nodes of axilla & upper limb	10	N/A
C8265	Cutaneous follicle center lymphoma, lymph nodes of inguinal region & lower limb	10	N/A
C8266	Cutaneous follicle center lymphoma, intrapelvic lymph nodes	10	N/A
C8267	Cutaneous follicle center lymphoma, spleen	10	N/A
C8268	Cutaneous follicle center lymphoma, lymph nodes of multiple sites	10	N/A
C8269	Cutaneous follicle center lymphoma, extranodal & solid organ sites	10	N/A
C8280	Other types of follicular lymphoma, NOS site	10	N/A
C8281	Other types of follicular lymphoma, lymph nodes of head, face, & neck	10	N/A
C8282	Other types of follicular lymphoma, intrathoracic lymph nodes	10	N/A

Code	Code Descriptors	HCC	RXHCC
C8283	Other types of follicular lymphoma, intra-abdominal lymph nodes	10	N/A
C8284	Other types of follicular lymphoma, lymph nodes of axilla & upper limb	10	N/A
C8285	Other types of follicular lymphoma, lymph nodes of inguinal region & lower limb	10	N/A
C8286	Other types of follicular lymphoma, intrapelvic lymph nodes	10	N/A
C8287	Other types of follicular lymphoma, spleen	10	N/A
C8288	Other types of follicular lymphoma, lymph nodes of multiple sites	10	N/A
C8289	Other types of follicular lymphoma, extranodal & solid organ sites	10	N/A
C8290	Follicular lymphoma, NOS, NOS site	10	N/A
C8291	Follicular lymphoma, NOS, lymph nodes of head, face, & neck	10	N/A
C8292	Follicular lymphoma, NOS, intrathoracic lymph nodes	10	N/A
C8293	Follicular lymphoma, NOS, intra-abdominal lymph nodes	10	N/A
C8294	Follicular lymphoma, NOS, lymph nodes of axilla & upper limb	10	N/A
C8295	Follicular lymphoma, NOS, lymph nodes of inguinal region & lower limb	10	N/A
C8296	Follicular lymphoma, NOS, intrapelvic lymph nodes	10	N/A
C8297	Follicular lymphoma, NOS, spleen	10	N/A
C8298	Follicular lymphoma, NOS, lymph nodes of multiple sites	10	N/A
C8299	Follicular lymphoma, NOS, extranodal & solid organ sites	10	N/A
C8300	SM cell B-cell lymphoma, NOS site	10	N/A
C8301	SM cell B-cell lymphoma, lymph nodes of head, face, & neck	10	N/A
C8302	SM cell B-cell lymphoma, intrathoracic lymph nodes	10	N/A
C8303	SM cell B-cell lymphoma, intra-abdominal lymph nodes	10	N/A
C8304	SM cell B-cell lymphoma, lymph nodes of axilla & upper limb	10	N/A
C8305	SM cell B-cell lymphoma, lymph nodes of inguinal region & lower limb	10	N/A
C8306	SM cell B-cell lymphoma, intrapelvic lymph nodes	10	N/A
C8307	SM cell B-cell lymphoma, spleen	10	N/A
C8308	SM cell B-cell lymphoma, lymph nodes of multiple sites	10	N/A
C8309	SM cell B-cell lymphoma, extranodal & solid organ sites	10	N/A
C8310	Mantle cell lymphoma, NOS site	10	N/A
C8311	Mantle cell lymphoma, lymph nodes of head, face, & neck	10	N/A

Code	Code Descriptors	HCC	RXHCC
C8312	Mantle cell lymphoma, intrathoracic lymph nodes	10	N/A
C8313	Mantle cell lymphoma, intra-abdominal lymph nodes	10	N/A
C8314	Mantle cell lymphoma, lymph nodes of axilla & upper limb	10	N/A
C8315	Mantle cell lymphoma, lymph nodes of inguinal region & lower limb	10	N/A
C8316	Mantle cell lymphoma, intrapelvic lymph nodes	10	N/A
C8317	Mantle cell lymphoma, spleen	10	N/A
C8318	Mantle cell lymphoma, lymph nodes of multiple sites	10	N/A
C8319	Mantle cell lymphoma, extranodal & solid organ sites	10	N/A
C8330	Diffuse LG B-cell lymphoma, NOS site	10	N/A
C8331	Diffuse LG B-cell lymphoma, lymph nodes of head, face, & neck	10	N/A
C8332	Diffuse LG B-cell lymphoma, intrathoracic lymph nodes	10	N/A
C8333	Diffuse LG B-cell lymphoma, intra-abdominal lymph nodes	10	N/A
C8334	Diffuse LG B-cell lymphoma, lymph nodes of axilla & upper limb	10	N/A
C8335	Diffuse LG B-cell lymphoma, lymph nodes of inguinal region & lower limb	10	N/A
C8336	Diffuse LG B-cell lymphoma, intrapelvic lymph nodes	10	N/A
C8337	Diffuse LG B-cell lymphoma, spleen	10	N/A
C8338	Diffuse LG B-cell lymphoma, lymph nodes of multiple sites	10	N/A
C8339	Diffuse LG B-cell lymphoma, extranodal & solid organ sites	10	N/A
C8350	Lymphoblastic lymphoma, NOS site	10	N/A
C8351	Lymphoblastic lymphoma, lymph nodes of head, face, & neck	10	N/A
C8352	Lymphoblastic lymphoma, intrathoracic lymph nodes	10	N/A
C8353	Lymphoblastic lymphoma, intra-abdominal lymph nodes	10	N/A
C8354	Lymphoblastic lymphoma, lymph nodes of axilla & upper limb	10	N/A
C8355	Lymphoblastic lymphoma, lymph nodes of inguinal region & lower limb	10	N/A
C8356	Lymphoblastic lymphoma, intrapelvic lymph nodes	10	N/A
C8357	Lymphoblastic lymphoma, spleen	10	N/A
C8358	Lymphoblastic lymphoma, lymph nodes of multiple sites	10	N/A
C8359	Lymphoblastic lymphoma, extranodal & solid organ sites	10	N/A
C8370	Burkitt lymphoma, NOS site	10	N/A

Code	Code Descriptors	HCC	RXHCC
C8371	Burkitt lymphoma, lymph nodes of head, face, & neck	10	N/A
C8372	Burkitt lymphoma, intrathoracic lymph nodes	10	N/A
C8373	Burkitt lymphoma, intra-abdominal lymph nodes	10	N/A
C8374	Burkitt lymphoma, lymph nodes of axilla & upper limb	10	N/A
C8375	Burkitt lymphoma, lymph nodes of inguinal region & lower limb	10	N/A
C8376	Burkitt lymphoma, intrapelvic lymph nodes	10	N/A
C8377	Burkitt lymphoma, spleen	10	N/A
C8378	Burkitt lymphoma, lymph nodes of multiple sites	10	N/A
C8379	Burkitt lymphoma, extranodal & solid organ sites	10	N/A
C8380	Other non-follicular lymphoma, NOS site	10	N/A
C8381	Other non-follicular lymphoma, lymph nodes of head, face, & neck	10	N/A
C8382	Other non-follicular lymphoma, intrathoracic lymph nodes	10	N/A
C8383	Other non-follicular lymphoma, intra-abdominal lymph nodes	10	N/A
C8384	Other non-follicular lymphoma, lymph nodes of axilla & upper limb	10	N/A
C8385	Other non-follicular lymphoma, lymph nodes of inguinal region & lower limb	10	N/A
C8386	Other non-follicular lymphoma, intrapelvic lymph nodes	10	N/A
C8387	Other non-follicular lymphoma, spleen	10	N/A
C8388	Other non-follicular lymphoma, lymph nodes of multiple sites	10	N/A
C8389	Other non-follicular lymphoma, extranodal & solid organ sites	10	N/A
C8390	Non-follicular lymphoma, NOS, NOS site	10	N/A
C8391	Non-follicular lymphoma, NOS, lymph nodes of head, face, & neck	10	N/A
C8392	Non-follicular lymphoma, NOS, intrathoracic lymph nodes	10	N/A
C8393	Non-follicular lymphoma, NOS, intra-abdominal lymph nodes	10	N/A
C8394	Non-follicular lymphoma, NOS, lymph nodes of axilla & upper limb	10	N/A
C8395	Non-follicular lymphoma, NOS, lymph nodes of inguinal region & lower limb	10	N/A
C8396	Non-follicular lymphoma, NOS, intrapelvic lymph nodes	10	N/A
C8397	Non-follicular lymphoma, NOS, spleen	10	N/A
C8398	Non-follicular lymphoma, NOS, lymph nodes of multiple sites	10	N/A
C8399	Non-follicular lymphoma, NOS, extranodal & solid organ sites	10	N/A
C8400	Mycosis fungoides, NOS site	10	18

Code	Code Descriptors	HCC	RXHCC
C8401	Mycosis fungoides, lymph nodes of head, face, & neck	10	18
C8402	Mycosis fungoides, intrathoracic lymph nodes	10	18
C8403	Mycosis fungoides, intra-abdominal lymph nodes	10	18
C8404	Mycosis fungoides, lymph nodes of axilla & upper limb	10	18
C8405	Mycosis fungoides, lymph nodes of inguinal region & lower limb	10	18
C8406	Mycosis fungoides, intrapelvic lymph nodes	10	18
C8407	Mycosis fungoides, spleen	10	18
C8408	Mycosis fungoides, lymph nodes of multiple sites	10	18
C8409	Mycosis fungoides, extranodal & solid organ sites	10	18
C8410	Sezary DZ, NOS site	10	18
C8411	Sezary DZ, lymph nodes of head, face, & neck	10	18
C8412	Sezary DZ, intrathoracic lymph nodes	10	18
C8413	Sezary DZ, intra-abdominal lymph nodes	10	18
C8414	Sezary DZ, lymph nodes of axilla & upper limb	10	18
C8415	Sezary DZ, lymph nodes of inguinal region & lower limb	10	18
C8416	Sezary DZ, intrapelvic lymph nodes	10	18
C8417	Sezary DZ, spleen	10	18
C8418	Sezary DZ, lymph nodes of multiple sites	10	18
C8419	Sezary DZ, extranodal & solid organ sites	10	18
C8440	Peripheral T-cell lymphoma, not classified, NOS site	10	N/A
C8441	Peripheral T-cell lymphoma, not classified, lymph nodes of head, face, & neck	10	N/A
C8442	Peripheral T-cell lymphoma, not classified, intrathoracic lymph nodes	10	N/A
C8443	Peripheral T-cell lymphoma, not classified, intra- abdominal lymph nodes	10	N/A
C8444	Peripheral T-cell lymphoma, not classified, lymph nodes of axilla & upper limb	10	N/A
C8445	Peripheral T-cell lymphoma, not classified, lymph nodes of inguinal region & lower limb	10	N/A
C8446	Peripheral T-cell lymphoma, not classified, intrapelvic lymph nodes	10	N/A
C8447	Peripheral T-cell lymphoma, not classified, spleen	10	N/A
C8448	Peripheral T-cell lymphoma, not classified, lymph nodes of multiple sites	10	N/A
C8449	Peripheral T-cell lymphoma, not classified, extranodal & solid organ sites	10	N/A
C8460	Anaplastic LG cell lymphoma, ALK-positive, NOS site	10	N/A
C8461	Anaplastic LG cell lymphoma, ALK-positive, lymph nodes of head, face, & neck	10	N/A

Code	Code Descriptors	HCC	RXHCC
C8462	Anaplastic LG cell lymphoma, ALK-positive, intrathoracic lymph nodes	10	N/A
C8463	Anaplastic LG cell lymphoma, ALK-positive, intra- abdominal lymph nodes	10	N/A
C8464	Anaplastic LG cell lymphoma, ALK-positive, lymph nodes of axilla & upper limb	10	N/A
C8465	Anaplastic LG cell lymphoma, ALK-positive, lymph nodes of inguinal region & lower limb	10	N/A
C8466	Anaplastic LG cell lymphoma, ALK-positive, intrapelvic lymph nodes	10	N/A
C8467	Anaplastic LG cell lymphoma, ALK-positive, spleen	10	N/A
C8468	Anaplastic LG cell lymphoma, ALK-positive, lymph nodes of multiple sites	10	N/A
C8469	Anaplastic LG cell lymphoma, ALK-positive, extranodal & solid organ sites	10	N/A
C8470	Anaplastic LG cell lymphoma, ALK-negative, NOS site	10	N/A
C8471	Anaplastic LG cell lymphoma, ALK-negative, lymph nodes of head, face, & neck	10	N/A
C8472	Anaplastic LG cell lymphoma, ALK-negative, intrathoracic lymph nodes	10	N/A
C8473	Anaplastic LG cell lymphoma, ALK-negative, intra- abdominal lymph nodes	10	N/A
C8474	Anaplastic LG cell lymphoma, ALK-negative, lymph nodes of axilla & upper limb	10	N/A
C8475	Anaplastic LG cell lymphoma, ALK-negative, lymph nodes of inguinal region & lower limb	10	N/A
C8476	Anaplastic LG cell lymphoma, ALK-negative, intrapelvic lymph nodes	10	N/A
C8477	Anaplastic LG cell lymphoma, ALK-negative, spleen	10	N/A
C8478	Anaplastic LG cell lymphoma, ALK-negative, lymph nodes of multiple sites	10	N/A
C8479	Anaplastic LG cell lymphoma, ALK-negative, extranodal & solid organ sites	10	N/A
C8490	Mature T/NK-cell lymphomas, NOS, NOS site	10	N/A
C8491	Mature T/NK-cell lymphomas, NOS, lymph nodes of head, face, & neck	10	N/A
C8492	Mature T/NK-cell lymphomas, NOS, intrathoracic lymph nodes	10	N/A
C8493	Mature T/NK-cell lymphomas, NOS, intra- abdominal lymph nodes	10	N/A
C8494	Mature T/NK-cell lymphomas, NOS, lymph nodes of axilla & upper limb	10	N/A
C8495	Mature T/NK-cell lymphomas, NOS, lymph nodes of inguinal region & lower limb	10	N/A
C8496	Mature T/NK-cell lymphomas, NOS, intrapelvic lymph nodes	10	N/A
C8497	Mature T/NK-cell lymphomas, NOS, spleen	10	N/A
C8498	Mature T/NK-cell lymphomas, NOS, lymph nodes of multiple sites	10	N/A

Code	Code Descriptors	HCC	RXHCC
C8499	Mature T/NK-cell lymphomas, NOS, extranodal & solid organ sites	10	N/A
C84A0	Cutaneous T-cell lymphoma, NOS, NOS site	10	N/A
C84A1	Cutaneous T-cell lymphoma, NOS lymph nodes of head, face, & neck	10	N/A
C84A2	Cutaneous T-cell lymphoma, NOS, intrathoracic lymph nodes	10	N/A
C84A3	Cutaneous T-cell lymphoma, NOS, intra-abdominal lymph nodes	10	N/A
C84A4	Cutaneous T-cell lymphoma, NOS, lymph nodes of axilla & upper limb	10	N/A
C84A5	Cutaneous T-cell lymphoma, NOS, lymph nodes of inguinal region & lower limb	10	N/A
C84A6	Cutaneous T-cell lymphoma, NOS, intrapelvic lymph nodes	10	N/A
C84A7	Cutaneous T-cell lymphoma, NOS, spleen	10	N/A
C84A8	Cutaneous T-cell lymphoma, NOS, lymph nodes of multiple sites	10	N/A
C84A9	Cutaneous T-cell lymphoma, NOS, extranodal & solid organ sites	10	N/A
C84Z0	Other mature T/NK-cell lymphomas, NOS site	10	N/A
C84Z1	Other mature T/NK-cell lymphomas, lymph nodes of head, face, & neck	10	N/A
C84Z2	Other mature T/NK-cell lymphomas, intrathoracic lymph nodes	10	N/A
C84Z3	Other mature T/NK-cell lymphomas, intra-abdominal lymph nodes	10	N/A
C84Z4	Other mature T/NK-cell lymphomas, lymph nodes of axilla & upper limb	10	N/A
C84Z5	Other mature T/NK-cell lymphomas, lymph nodes of inguinal region & lower limb	10	N/A
C84Z6	Other mature T/NK-cell lymphomas, intrapelvic lymph nodes	10	N/A
C84Z7	Other mature T/NK-cell lymphomas, spleen	10	N/A
C84Z8	Other mature T/NK-cell lymphomas, lymph nodes of multiple sites	10	N/A
C84Z9	Other mature T/NK-cell lymphomas, extranodal & solid organ sites	10	N/A
C8510	NOS B-cell lymphoma, NOS site	10	N/A
C8511	NOS B-cell lymphoma, lymph nodes of head, face, & neck	10	N/A
C8512	NOS B-cell lymphoma, intrathoracic lymph nodes	10	N/A
C8513	NOS B-cell lymphoma, intra-abdominal lymph nodes	10	N/A
C8514	NOS B-cell lymphoma, lymph nodes of axilla & upper limb	10	N/A
C8515	NOS B-cell lymphoma, lymph nodes of inguinal region & lower limb	10	N/A
C8516	NOS B-cell lymphoma, intrapelvic lymph nodes	10	N/A
C8517	NOS B-cell lymphoma, spleen	10	N/A

Code	Code Descriptors	HCC	RXHCC
C8518	NOS B-cell lymphoma, lymph nodes of multiple sites	10	N/A
C8519	NOS B-cell lymphoma, extranodal & solid organ sites	10	N/A
C8520	Mediastinal LG B-cell lymphoma, NOS site	10	N/A
C8521	Mediastinal LG B-cell lymphoma, lymph nodes of head, face, & neck	10	N/A
C8522	Mediastinal LG B-cell lymphoma, intrathoracic lymph nodes	10	N/A
C8523	Mediastinal LG B-cell lymphoma, intra-abdominal lymph nodes	10	N/A
C8524	Mediastinal LG B-cell lymphoma, lymph nodes of axilla & upper limb	10	N/A
C8525	Mediastinal LG B-cell lymphoma, lymph nodes of inguinal region & lower limb	10	N/A
C8526	Mediastinal LG B-cell lymphoma, intrapelvic lymph nodes	10	N/A
C8527	Mediastinal LG B-cell lymphoma, spleen	10	N/A
C8528	Mediastinal LG B-cell lymphoma, lymph nodes of multiple sites	10	N/A
C8529	Mediastinal LG B-cell lymphoma, extranodal & solid organ sites	10	N/A
C8580	NEC types of non-Hodgkin lymphoma, NOS site	10	N/A
C8581	NEC types of non-Hodgkin lymphoma, lymph nodes of head, face, & neck	10	N/A
C8582	NEC types of non-Hodgkin lymphoma, intrathoracic lymph nodes	10	N/A
C8583	NEC types of non-Hodgkin lymphoma, intra-abdominal lymph nodes	10	N/A
C8584	NEC types of non-Hodgkin lymphoma, lymph nodes of axilla & upper limb	10	N/A
C8585	NEC types of non-Hodgkin lymphoma, lymph nodes of inguinal region & lower limb	10	N/A
C8586	NEC types of non-Hodgkin lymphoma, intrapelvic lymph nodes	10	N/A
C8587	NEC types of non-Hodgkin lymphoma, spleen	10	N/A
C8588	NEC types of non-Hodgkin lymphoma, lymph nodes of multiple sites	10	N/A
C8589	NEC types of non-Hodgkin lymphoma, extranodal & solid organ sites	10	N/A
C8590	Non-Hodgkin lymphoma, NOS, NOS site	10	N/A
C8591	Non-Hodgkin lymphoma, NOS, lymph nodes of head, face, & neck	10	N/A
C8592	Non-Hodgkin lymphoma, NOS, intrathoracic lymph nodes	10	N/A
C8593	Non-Hodgkin lymphoma, NOS, intra-abdominal lymph nodes	10	N/A
C8594	Non-Hodgkin lymphoma, NOS, lymph nodes of axilla & upper limb	10	N/A
C8595	Non-Hodgkin lymphoma, NOS, lymph nodes of inguinal region & lower limb	10	N/A

Code	Code Descriptors	HCC	RXHCC
C8596	Non-Hodgkin lymphoma, NOS, intrapelvic lymph nodes	10	N/A
C8597	Non-Hodgkin lymphoma, NOS, spleen	10	N/A
C8598	Non-Hodgkin lymphoma, NOS, lymph nodes of multiple sites	10	N/A
C8599	Non-Hodgkin lymphoma, NOS, extranodal & solid organ sites	10	N/A
C860	Extranodal NK/T-cell lymphoma, nasal type	10	N/A
C861	Hepatosplenic T-cell lymphoma	10	N/A
C862	Enteropathy-type T-cell lymphoma	10	N/A
C863	Subcutaneous panniculitis-like T-cell lymphoma	10	N/A
C864	Blastic NK-cell lymphoma	10	N/A
C865	Angioimmunoblastic T-cell lymphoma	10	N/A
C866	Primary cutaneous CD30-positive T-cell proliferations	10	N/A
C880	Waldenstrom macroglobulinemia	23	N/A
C882	Heavy chain DZ	10	N/A
C883	Immunoproliferative SM intestinal DZ	10	N/A
C884	Extranodal marginal zone B-cell lymphoma of mucosa-associated lymphoid tissue [MALT- lymphoma]	10	N/A
C888	Malignant immunoproliferative DZ, NEC	10	N/A
C889	Malignant immunoproliferative DZ, NOS	10	N/A
For codes C900- through C944-, use the following 5th character: 0 not having achieved remission 1 in remission 2 in relapse			
C900-	Multiple myeloma	9	16
C901-	Plasma cell leukemia	9	16
C902-	Extramedullary plasmacytoma	9	16
C903-	Solitary plasmacytoma	10	16
C910-	Acute lymphoblastic leukemia	8	N/A
C911-	Chronic lymphocytic leukemia of B-cell type	10	N/A
C913-	Prolymphocytic leukemia of B-cell type	10	N/A
C914-	Hairy cell leukemia	10	N/A
C915-	Adult T-cell lymphoma/leukemia (HTLV-1-associated)	10	N/A
C916-	Prolymphocytic leukemia of T-cell type	10	N/A
C919-	Lymphoid leukemia, NOS	10	N/A
C91A-	Mature B-cell leukemia Burkitt-type	10	N/A
C91Z-	Other lymphoid leukemia	10	N/A
C920-	Acute myeloblastic leukemia	8	N/A
C921-	Chronic myeloid leukemia, BCR/ABL-positive	9	15
C922-	Atypical chronic myeloid leukemia, BCR/ ABL- negative	9	18
C923-	Myeloid sarcoma	9	18
C924-	Acute promyelocytic leukemia	8	N/A
C925-	Acute myelomonocytic leukemia	8	N/A

Code	Code Descriptors	HCC	RXHCC
C926-	Acute myeloid leukemia W/ 11q23-abnormality	8	N/A
C929-	Myeloid leukemia, NOS	9	18
C92A-	Acute myeloid leukemia W/ multilineage dysplasia	8	N/A
C92Z-	Other myeloid leukemia	9	18
C930-	Acute monoblastic/monocytic leukemia	8	N/A
C931-	Chronic myelomonocytic leukemia	9	18
C933-	Juvenile myelomonocytic leukemia	9	18
C939-	Monocytic leukemia, NOS	9	18
C93Z-	Other monocytic leukemia	9	18
C940-	Acute erythroid leukemia	8	N/A
C942-	Acute megakaryoblastic leukemia	8	N/A
C943-	Mast cell leukemia	9	18
C944-	Acute panmyelosis W/ myelofibrosis	8	N/A
C946	Myelodysplastic DZ, not classified	48	N/A
For codes C948- through C959-, use the following 5th character: 0 not having achieved remission 1 in remission 2 in relapse			
C948-	Leukemia, NEC	9	18
C950-	Acute leukemia of NOS cell type	8	N/A
C951-	Chronic leukemia of NOS cell type	10	N/A
C959-	Leukemia, NOS	10	N/A
C960	Multifocal & multisystemic (disseminated) Langerhans-cell histiocytosis	10	N/A
C9620	Malignant mast cell neoplasm, unspecified	10	18
C9621	Aggressive systemic mastocytosis	10	18
C9622	Mast cell sarcoma	10	18
C9629	Other malignant mast cell neoplasm	10	18
C964	Sarcoma of dendritic cells (accessory cells)	10	N/A
C965	Multifocal & unisystemic Langerhans-cell histiocytosis	10	N/A
C966	Unifocal Langerhans-cell histiocytosis	10	N/A
C969	MAL NEO of lymphoid, hematopoietic & related tissue, NOS	10	N/A
C96A	Histiocytic sarcoma	10	N/A
C96Z	NEC MAL NEOs of lymphoid, hematopoietic & related tissue	10	N/A
D030	Melanoma in situ of lip	12	N/A
D0310	Melanoma in situ of NOS eyelid, including canthus	12	N/A
D0311	Melanoma in situ of R eyelid, including canthus	12	N/A
D0312	Melanoma in situ of L eyelid, including canthus	12	N/A
D0320	Melanoma in situ of NOS ear & external auricular canal	12	N/A
D0321	Melanoma in situ of R ear & external auricular canal	12	N/A

Code	Code Descriptors	HCC	RXHCC
D0322	Melanoma in situ of L ear & external auricular canal	12	N/A
D0330	Melanoma in situ of NOS part of face	12	N/A
D0339	Melanoma in situ of other parts of face	12	N/A
D034	Melanoma in situ of scalp & neck	12	N/A
D0351	Melanoma in situ of anal skin	12	N/A
D0352	Melanoma in situ of breast (skin) (soft tissue)	12	N/A
D0359	Melanoma in situ of other part of trunk	12	N/A
D0360	Melanoma in situ of NOS upper limb, including shoulder	12	N/A
D0361	Melanoma in situ of R upper limb, including shoulder	12	N/A
D0362	Melanoma in situ of L upper limb, including shoulder	12	N/A
D0370	Melanoma in situ of NOS lower limb, including hip	12	N/A
D0371	Melanoma in situ of R lower limb, including hip	12	N/A
D0372	Melanoma in situ of L lower limb, including hip	12	N/A
D038	Melanoma in situ, NEC	12	N/A
D039	Melanoma in situ, NOS	12	N/A
D1802	Hemangioma of intracranial structures	12	N/A
D320	Benign neoplasm of cerebral meninges	12	N/A
D321	Benign neoplasm of spinal meninges	12	N/A
D329	Benign neoplasm of meninges, NOS	12	N/A
D330	Benign neoplasm of brain, supratentorial	12	N/A
D331	Benign neoplasm of brain, infratentorial	12	N/A
D332	Benign neoplasm of brain, NOS	12	N/A
D333	Benign neoplasm of cranial nerves	12	N/A
D334	Benign neoplasm of spinal cord	12	N/A
D337	Benign neoplasm of NEC parts of CNS	12	N/A
D339	Benign neoplasm of CNS, NOS	12	N/A
D352	Benign neoplasm of pituitary gland	12	N/A
D353	Benign neoplasm of craniopharyngeal duct	12	N/A
D354	Benign neoplasm of pineal gland	12	N/A
D420	Neoplasm of uncertain behavior of cerebral meninges	12	N/A
D421	Neoplasm of uncertain behavior of spinal meninges	12	N/A
D429	Neoplasm of uncertain behavior of meninges, NOS	12	N/A
D430	Neoplasm of uncertain behavior of brain, supratentorial	12	N/A
D431	Neoplasm of uncertain behavior of brain, infratentorial	12	N/A
D432	Neoplasm of uncertain behavior of brain, NOS	12	N/A
D433	Neoplasm of uncertain behavior of cranial nerves	12	N/A

Code	Code Descriptors	HCC	RXHCC
D434	Neoplasm of uncertain behavior of spinal cord	12	N/A
D438	Neoplasm of uncertain behavior of NEC parts of CNS	12	N/A
D439	Neoplasm of uncertain behavior of CNS, NOS	12	N/A
D443	Neoplasm of uncertain behavior of pituitary gland	12	N/A
D444	Neoplasm of uncertain behavior of craniopharyngeal duct	12	N/A
D445	Neoplasm of uncertain behavior of pineal gland	12	N/A
D446	Neoplasm of uncertain behavior of carotid body	12	N/A
D447	Neoplasm of uncertain behavior of aortic body & other paraganglia	12	N/A
D45	Polycythemia vera	48	N/A
D460	Refractory anemia W/O ring sideroblasts, so stated	46	96
D461	Refractory anemia W/ ring sideroblasts	46	96
D4620	Refractory anemia W/ excess of blasts, NOS	46	96
D4621	Refractory anemia W/ excess of blasts 1	46	96
D4622	Refractory anemia W/ excess of blasts 2	46	96
D464	Refractory anemia, NOS	46	96
D469	Myelodysplastic syndrome, NOS	46	96
D46A	Refractory cytopenia W/ multilineage dysplasia	46	96
D46B	Refractory cytopenia W/ multilineage dysplasia & ring sideroblasts	46	96
D46C	Myelodysplastic syndrome W/ isolated del(5q) chromosomal abnormality	46	16
D46Z	Other myelodysplastic syndromes	46	96
D471	Chronic myeloproliferative DZ	48	N/A
D473	Essential (hemorrhagic) thrombocythemia	48	N/A
D474	Osteomyelofibrosis	46	96
D479	Neoplasm of uncertain behavior of lymphoid, hematopoietic & related tissue, NOS	48	N/A
D47Z1	Post-transplant lymphoproliferative disorder (PTLD)	48	N/A
D47Z2	Castleman DZ	48	N/A
D47Z9	NEC neoplasms of uncertain behavior of lymphoid, hematopoietic & related tissue	48	N/A
D496	Neoplasm of NOS behavior of brain	12	N/A
D550	Anemia D/T glucose-6-phosphate dehydrogenase [G6PD] deficiency	48	N/A
D551	Anemia D/T other disorders of glutathione metabolism	48	N/A
D552	Anemia D/T disorders of glycolytic enzymes	48	N/A
D553	Anemia D/T disorders of nucleotide metabolism	48	N/A
D558	Other anemias D/T enzyme disorders	48	N/A

Code	Code Descriptors	HCC	RXHCC
D559	Anemia D/T enzyme disorder, NOS	48	N/A
D560	Alpha thalassemia	48	98
D561	Beta thalassemia	48	98
D562	Delta-beta thalassemia	48	N/A
D564	Hereditary persistence of fetal hemoglobin [HPFH]	48	N/A
D565	Hemoglobin E-beta thalassemia	48	98
D568	Other thalassemias	48	N/A
D5700	Hb-SS DZ W/ crisis, NOS	46	95
D5701	Hb-SS DZ W/ acute chest syndrome	46	95, 98
D5702	Hb-SS DZ W/ splenic sequestration	46	95, 98
D571	Sickle-cell DZ W/O crisis	46	95
D5720	Sickle-cell/Hb-C DZ W/O crisis	46	98
D57211	Sickle-cell/Hb-C DZ W/ acute chest syndrome	46	98
D57212	Sickle-cell/Hb-C DZ W/ splenic sequestration	46	98
D57219	Sickle-cell/Hb-C DZ W/ crisis, NOS	46	98
D573	Sickle-cell trait	48	N/A
D5740	Sickle-cell thalassemia W/O crisis	46	98
D57411	Sickle-cell thalassemia W/ acute chest syndrome	46	98
D57412	Sickle-cell thalassemia W/ splenic sequestration	46	98
D57419	Sickle-cell thalassemia W/ crisis, NOS	46	98
D5780	Other sickle-cell disorders W/O crisis	46	98
D57811	Other sickle-cell disorders W/ acute chest syndrome	46	98
D57812	Other sickle-cell disorders W/ splenic sequestration	46	98
D57819	Other sickle-cell disorders W/ crisis, NOS	46	98
D580	Hereditary spherocytosis	48	N/A
D581	Hereditary elliptocytosis	48	N/A
D582	Hemoglobinopathies, NEC	48	N/A
D588	Hereditary hemolytic anemia, NEC	48	N/A
D589	Hereditary hemolytic anemia, NOS	48	N/A
D590	Drug-induced autoimmune hemolytic anemia	46	98
D591	Other autoimmune hemolytic anemias	46	98
D592	Drug-induced nonautoimmune hemolytic anemia	46	98
D593	Hemolytic-uremic syndrome	46	98
D594	Nonautoimmune hemolytic anemias, NEC	46	98
D595	Paroxysmal nocturnal hemoglobinuria [Marchiafava- Micheli]	46	98
D596	Hemoglobinuria D/T hemolysis from other external causes	46	98
D598	Acquired hemolytic anemias, NEC	46	98
D599	Acquired hemolytic anemia, NOS	46	98

Code	Code Descriptors	HCC	RXHCC
D600	Chronic acquired pure red cell aplasia	46	98
D601	Transient acquired pure red cell aplasia	46	98
D608	Acquired pure red cell aplasia, NEC	46	98
D609	Acquired pure red cell aplasia, NOS	46	98
D6101	Constitutional (pure) red blood cell aplasia	46	98
D6109	Constitutional aplastic anemia, NEC	46	98
D611	Drug-induced aplastic anemia	46	98
D612	Aplastic anemia D/T other external agents	46	98
D613	Idiopathic aplastic anemia	46	98
D61810	Antineoplastic chemotherapy induced pancytopenia	47	N/A
D61811	Drug-induced pancytopenia, NEC	47	N/A
D61818	Pancytopenia, NEC	47	N/A
D6182	Myelophthisis	46	98
D6189	Aplastic anemias & other bone marrow failure syndromes, NEC	46	98
D619	Aplastic anemia, NOS	46	98
D640	Hereditary sideroblastic anemia	48	98
D641	2ndary sideroblastic anemia D/T DZ	48	98
D642	2ndary sideroblastic anemia D/T drugs & toxins	48	98
D643	Sideroblastic anemia, NEC	48	98
D65	Disseminated intravascular coagulation [defibrination syndrome]	48	N/A
D66	Hereditary factor VIII deficiency	46	N/A
D67	Hereditary factor IX deficiency	46	N/A
D680	Von Willebrand's DZ	48	N/A
D681	Hereditary factor XI deficiency	48	N/A
D682	Hereditary deficiency of clotting factor NEC	48	N/A
D68311	Acquired hemophilia	48	N/A
D68312	Antiphospholipid antibody W/ hemorrhagic disorder	48	N/A
D68318	Hemorrhagic disorder D/T intrinsic circulating anticoagulants, antibodies, or inhibitors, NEC	48	N/A
D6832	Hemorrhagic disorder D/T extrinsic circulating anticoagulants	48	N/A
D684	Acquired coagulation factor deficiency	48	N/A
D6851	Activated protein C resistance	48	98
D6852	Prothrombin gene mutation	48	98
D6859	Primary thrombophilia, NEC	48	98
D6861	Antiphospholipid syndrome	48	98
D6862	Lupus anticoagulant syndrome	48	98
D6869	Thrombophilia, NEC	48	98
D688	Coagulation defect, NEC	48	N/A
D689	Coagulation defect, NOS	48	N/A
D690	Allergic purpura	48	N/A
D691	Qualitative platelet defects	48	N/A
D692	Nonthrombocytopenic purpura, NEC	48	N/A

Code	Code Descriptors	HCC	RXHCC
D693	Immune thrombocytopenic purpura	48	N/A
D6941	Evans syndrome	48	N/A
D6942	Congenital & hereditary thrombocytopenia purpura	48	N/A
D6949	Primary thrombocytopenia, NEC	48	N/A
D696	Thrombocytopenia, NOS	48	N/A
D698	Hemorrhagic condition, NEC	48	N/A
D699	Hemorrhagic condition, NOS	48	N/A
D700	Congenital agranulocytosis	47	N/A
D701	Agranulocytosis 2ndary to cancer chemotherapy	47	N/A
D702	Drug-induced agranulocytosis, NEC	47	N/A
D703	Neutropenia D/T infection	47	N/A
D704	Cyclic neutropenia	47	N/A
D708	Neutropenia, NEC	47	N/A
D709	Neutropenia, NOS	47	N/A
D71	Functional disorder of polymorphonuclear neutrophils	47	N/A
D720	Genetic anomalies of leukocytes	47	N/A
D7581	Myelofibrosis	46	96
D7582	Heparin induced thrombocytopenia (HIT)	48	N/A
D761	Hemophagocytic lymphohistiocytosis	47	N/A
D762	Hemophagocytic syndrome, infection-associated	47	N/A
D763	Histiocytosis syndrome, NEC	47	N/A
D800	Hereditary hypogammaglobulinemia	47	97
D801	Nonfamilial hypogammaglobulinemia	47	97
D802	Selective deficiency of IgA	47	97
D803	Selective deficiency of IgG subclasses	47	97
D804	Selective deficiency of IgM	47	97
D805	Immunodeficiency W/ increased IgM	47	97
D806	Antibody deficiency W/ near-normal immunoglobulins or W/ hyperimmunoglobulinemia	47	97
D807	Transient hypogammaglobulinemia of infancy	47	97
D808	Immunodeficiencies W/ predominantly antibody defects, NEC	47	97
D809	Immunodeficiency W/ predominantly antibody defects, NOS	47	97
D810	Severe combined immunodeficiency [SCID] W/ reticular dysgenesis	47	97
D811	Severe combined immunodeficiency [SCID] W/ low T & B-cell numbers	47	97
D812	Severe combined immunodeficiency [SCID] W/ low or normal B-cell numbers	47	97
D813	Adenosine deaminase [ADA] deficiency	47	97
D814	Nezelof's syndrome	47	97
D815	Purine nucleoside phosphorylase [PNP] deficiency	47	97

Code	Code Descriptors	HCC	RXHCC
D816	Major histocompatibility complex class I deficiency	47	97
D817	Major histocompatibility complex class II deficiency	47	97
D8189	Combined immunodeficiency, NEC	47	97
D819	Combined immunodeficiency, NOS	47	97
D820	Wiskott-Aldrich syndrome	47	97
D821	Di George's syndrome	47	97
D822	Immunodeficiency W/ short-limbed stature	47	97
D823	Immunodeficiency following hereditary defective response to Epstein-Barr virus	47	97
D824	Hyperimmunoglobulin E [IgE] syndrome	47	97
D828	Immunodeficiency associated W/ major defect, NEC	47	97
D829	Immunodeficiency associated W/ major defect, NOS	47	97
D830	Common variable immunodeficiency W/ predominant abnormalities of B-cell numbers & function	47	97
D831	Common variable immunodeficiency W/ predominant immunoregulatory T-cell disorders	47	97
D832	Common variable immunodeficiency W/ autoantibodies to B- or T-cells	47	97
D838	Common variable immunodeficiency, NEC	47	97
D839	Common variable immunodeficiency, NOS	47	97
D840	Lymphocyte function antigen-1 [LFA-1] defect	47	97
D841	Defects in complement system	23	40
D848	Immunodeficiency, NEC	47	97
D849	Immunodeficiency, NOS	47	97
D860	Sarcoidosis of lung	112	N/A
D862	Sarcoidosis of lung W/ sarcoidosis of lymph nodes	112	N/A
D8682	Multiple cranial nerve palsies in sarcoidosis	75	159
D8684	Sarcoid pyelonephritis	141	N/A
D891	Cryoglobulinemia	23	N/A
D893	Immune reconstitution syndrome	47	97
D8940	Mast cell activation, NOS	47	97
D8941	Monoclonal mast cell activation syndrome	47	97
D8942	Idiopathic mast cell activation syndrome	47	97
D8943	2ndary mast cell activation	47	97
D8949	Other mast cell activation disorder	47	97
D89810	Acute graft-versus-host DZ	47	396
D89811	Chronic graft-versus-host DZ	47	396
D89812	Acute on chronic graft-versus-host DZ	47	396
D89813	Graft-versus-host DZ, NOS	47	396
D8982	Autoimmune lymphoproliferative syndrome	47	97
D8989	Disorder involving immune mechanism, NEC	47	97
D899	Disorder involving immune mechanism, NOS	47	97

Code	Code Descriptors	HCC	RXHCC
E000	Congenital iodine-deficiency syndrome, neurological type	N/A	42
E001	Congenital iodine-deficiency syndrome, myxedematous type	N/A	42
E002	Congenital iodine-deficiency syndrome, mixed type	N/A	42
E009	Congenital iodine-deficiency syndrome, NOS	N/A	42
E010	Iodine-deficiency related diffuse (endemic) goiter	N/A	42
E011	Iodine-deficiency related multinodular (endemic) goiter	N/A	42
E012	Iodine-deficiency related (endemic) goiter, NOS	N/A	42
E018	Other iodine-deficiency related thyroid disorders & allied conditions	N/A	42
E02	Subclinical iodine-deficiency hypothyroidism	N/A	42
E030	Congenital hypothyroidism W/ diffuse goiter	N/A	42
E031	Congenital hypothyroidism W/O goiter	N/A	42
E032	Hypothyroidism D/T medicaments & other exogenous substances	N/A	42
E033	Postinfectious hypothyroidism	N/A	42
E034	Atrophy of thyroid (acquired)	N/A	42
E035	Myxedema coma	23	42
E038	Hypothyroidism, NEC	N/A	42
E039	Hypothyroidism, NOS	N/A	42
E040	Nontoxic diffuse goiter	N/A	42
E041	Nontoxic single thyroid nodule	N/A	42
E042	Nontoxic multinodular goiter	N/A	42
E048	Nontoxic goiter, NEC	N/A	42
E049	Nontoxic goiter, NOS	N/A	42
E0500	Thyrotoxicosis W/ diffuse goiter W/O thyrotoxic crisis or storm	N/A	42
E0501	Thyrotoxicosis W/ diffuse goiter W/ thyrotoxic crisis or storm	N/A	42
E0510	Thyrotoxicosis W/ toxic single thyroid nodule W/O thyrotoxic crisis or storm	N/A	42
E0511	Thyrotoxicosis W/ toxic single thyroid nodule W/ thyrotoxic crisis or storm	N/A	42
E0520	Thyrotoxicosis W/ toxic multinodular goiter W/O thyrotoxic crisis or storm	N/A	42
E0521	Thyrotoxicosis W/ toxic multinodular goiter W/ thyrotoxic crisis or storm	N/A	42
E0530	Thyrotoxicosis from ectopic thyroid tissue W/O thyrotoxic crisis or storm	N/A	42
E0531	Thyrotoxicosis from ectopic thyroid tissue W/ thyrotoxic crisis or storm	N/A	42
E0540	Thyrotoxicosis factitia W/O thyrotoxic crisis or storm	N/A	42
E0541	Thyrotoxicosis factitia W/ thyrotoxic crisis or storm	N/A	42
E0580	Thyrotoxicosis, NEC, W/O thyrotoxic crisis or storm	N/A	42

Code	Code Descriptors	HCC	RXHCC
E0581	Thyrotoxicosis, NEC, W/ thyrotoxic crisis or storm	N/A	42
E0590	Thyrotoxicosis, NOS, W/O thyrotoxic crisis or storm	N/A	42
E0591	Thyrotoxicosis, NOS, W/ thyrotoxic crisis or storm	N/A	42
E060	Acute thyroiditis	N/A	42
E061	Subacute thyroiditis	N/A	42
E062	Chronic thyroiditis W/ transient thyrotoxicosis	N/A	42
E063	Autoimmune thyroiditis	N/A	42
E064	Drug-induced thyroiditis	N/A	42
E065	Chronic thyroiditis, NEC	N/A	42
E069	Thyroiditis, NOS	N/A	42
E070	Hypersecretion of calcitonin	N/A	42
E071	Dyshormogenetic goiter	N/A	42
E0789	Disorder of thyroid, NEC	N/A	42
E079	Disorder of thyroid, NOS	N/A	42
E0800	DM D/T underlying condition W/ hyperosmolarity W/O NKHHC	17	30
E0801	DM D/T underlying condition W/ hyperosmolarity W/ coma	17	30
E0810	DM D/T underlying condition W/ DKA W/O coma	17	30
E0811	DM D/T underlying condition W/ DKA W/ coma	17	30
E0821	DM D/T underlying condition W/ diabetic nephropathy	18, 141	30
E0822	DM D/T underlying condition W/ diabetic CKD	18, 139	30
E0829	DM D/T underlying condition W/ other diabetic kidney complication	18, 141	30
E08311	DM D/T underlying condition W/ NOS diabetic retinopathy W/ macular edema	18	30, 241
E08319	DM D/T underlying condition W/ NOS diabetic retinopathy W/O macular edema	18	30, 241
For codes E08321- through E08359-, use the following 7th character: 1 Right eye 2 Left eye 3 Bilateral eye 9 Eye, NOS			
E08321-	DM D/T underlying condition W/ mild nonproliferative diabetic retinopathy W/ macular edema	18	30, 241
E08329-	DM D/T underlying condition W/ mild nonproliferative diabetic retinopathy W/O macular edema	18	30, 241
E08331-	DM D/T underlying condition W/ moderate nonproliferative diabetic retinopathy W/ macular edema	18	30, 241
E08339-	DM D/T underlying condition W/ moderate nonproliferative diabetic retinopathy W/O macular edema	18	30, 241

Code	Code Descriptors	HCC	RXHCC
E08341-	DM D/T underlying condition W/ severe nonproliferative diabetic retinopathy W/ macular edema	18	30, 241
E08349-	DM D/T underlying condition W/ severe nonproliferative diabetic retinopathy W/O macular edema	18	30, 241
E08351-	DM D/T underlying condition W/ proliferative diabetic retinopathy W/ macular edema	18, 122	30, 241
E08352-	DM D/T underlying condition W/ proliferative diabetic retinopathy W/ traction retinal detachment involving maculae	18, 122	30, 241
E08353-	DM D/T underlying condition W/ proliferative diabetic retinopathy W/ traction retinal detachment not involving macula	18, 122	30, 241
E08354-	DM D/T underlying condition W/ proliferative diabetic retinopathy W/ combined traction retinal detachment & rhegmatogenous retinal detachment	18, 122	30, 241
E08355-	DM D/T underlying condition W/ stable proliferative diabetic retinopathy	18, 122	30, 241
E08359-	DM D/T underlying condition W/ proliferative diabetic retinopathy W/O macular edema	18, 122	30, 241
E0836	DM D/T underlying condition W/ diabetic cataract	18	30
E0837X1	DM D/T underlying condition W/ diabetic macular edema, resolved following treatment, R eye	18	30
E0837X2	DM D/T underlying condition W/ diabetic macular edema, resolved following treatment, L eye	18	30
E0837X3	DM D/T underlying condition W/ diabetic macular edema, resolved following treatment, bilateral	18	30
E0837X9	DM D/T underlying condition W/ diabetic macular edema, resolved following treatment, NOS eye	18	30
E0839	DM D/T underlying condition W/ other diabetic ophthalmic complication	18	30
E0840	DM D/T underlying condition W/ diabetic neuropathy, NOS	18, 75	30
E0841	DM D/T underlying condition W/ diabetic mononeuropathy	18	30
E0842	DM D/T underlying condition W/ diabetic polyneuropathy	18, 75	30
E0843	DM D/T underlying condition W/ diabetic autonomic (poly)neuropathy	18	30
E0844	DM D/T underlying condition W/ diabetic amyotrophy	18	30
E0849	DM D/T underlying condition W/ diabetic neurological complication, NEC	18	30
E0851	DM D/T underlying condition W/ diabetic peripheral angiopathy W/O gangrene	18, 108	30, 216

Code	Code Descriptors	HCC	RXHCC
E0852	DM D/T underlying condition W/ diabetic peripheral angiopathy W/ gangrene	18, 106, 108	30, 216
E0859	DM D/T underlying condition W/ circulatory complication, NEC	18	30
E08610	DM D/T underlying condition W/ diabetic neuropathic arthropathy	18	30
E08618	DM D/T underlying condition W/ other diabetic arthropathy	18	30
E08620	DM D/T underlying condition W/ diabetic dermatitis	18	30
E08621	DM D/T underlying condition W/ foot ulcer	18, 161	30, 311
E08622	DM D/T underlying condition W/ skin ulcer, NEC	18, 161	30, 311
E08628	DM D/T underlying condition W/ skin complication, NEC	18	30
E08630	DM D/T underlying condition W/ periodontal DZ	18	30
E08638	DM D/T underlying condition W/ oral complication, NEC	18	30
E08641	DM D/T underlying condition W/ hypoglycemia W/ coma	17	30
E08649	DM D/T underlying condition W/ hypoglycemia W/O coma	18	30
E0865	DM D/T underlying condition W/ hyperglycemia	18	30
E0869	DM D/T underlying condition W/ NEC complication	18	30
E088	DM D/T underlying condition W/ NOS complications	18	30
E089	DM D/T underlying condition W/O complications	19	31
E0900	Drug or chemical induced DM W/ NKHHC	17	30
E0901	Drug or chemical induced DM W/ hyperosmolarity W/ coma	17	30
E0910	Drug or chemical induced DM W/ DKA W/O coma	17	30
E0911	Drug or chemical induced DM W/ DKA W/ coma	17	30
E0921	Drug or chemical induced DM W/ diabetic nephropathy	18, 141	30
E0922	Drug or chemical induced DM W/ diabetic CKD	18, 139	30
E0929	Drug or chemical induced DM W/ diabetic kidney complication, NEC	18, 141	30
E09311	Drug or chemical induced DM W/ NOS diabetic retinopathy W/ macular edema	18	30, 241
E09319	Drug or chemical induced DM W/ NOS diabetic retinopathy W/O macular edema	18	30, 241

Code	Code Descriptors	HCC	RXHCC
For codes E09321- through E09359-, use the following 7th character: 1 Right eye 2 Left eye 3 Bilateral eye 9 Eye, NOS			
E09331-	Drug or chemical induced DM W/ moderate nonproliferative diabetic retinopathy W/ macular edema	18	30, 241
E09339-	Drug or chemical induced DM W/ moderate nonproliferative diabetic retinopathy W/O macular edema	18	30, 241
E09341-	Drug or chemical induced DM W/ severe nonproliferative diabetic retinopathy W/ macular edema	18	30, 241
E09349-	Drug or chemical induced DM W/ severe nonproliferative diabetic retinopathy W/O macular edemaye	18	30, 241
E09351-	Drug or chemical induced DM W/ proliferative diabetic retinopathy W/ macular edemaye	18, 122	30, 241
E09352-	Drug or chemical induced DM W/ proliferative diabetic retinopathy W/ traction retinal detachment involving macula	18, 122	30, 241
E09353-	Drug or chemical induced DM W/ proliferative diabetic retinopathy W/ traction retinal detachment not involving maculae	18, 122	30, 241
E09354-	Drug or chemical induced DM W/ proliferative diabetic retinopathy W/ combined traction retinal detachment & rhegmatogenous retinal detachment	18, 122	30, 241
E09355-	Drug or chemical induced DM W/ stable proliferative diabetic retinopathy	18, 122	30, 241
E09359-	Drug or chemical induced DM W/ proliferative diabetic retinopathy W/O macular edema	18, 122	30, 241
E0936	Drug or chemical induced DM W/ diabetic cataract	18	30
E0937X1	Drug or chemical induced DM W/ diabetic macular edema, resolved following treatment, R eye	18	30
E0937X2	Drug or chemical induced DM W/ diabetic macular edema, resolved following treatment, L eye	18	30
E0937X3	Drug or chemical induced DM W/ diabetic macular edema, resolved following treatment, bilateral	18	30
E0937X9	Drug or chemical induced DM W/ diabetic macular edema, resolved following treatment, NOS eye	18	30
E0939	Drug or chemical induced DM W/ diabetic ophthalmic complication, NEC	18	30
E0940	Drug or chemical induced DM W/ neurological complications W/ diabetic neuropathy, NOS	18, 75	30

Code	Code Descriptors	HCC	RXHCC
E0941	Drug or chemical induced DM W/ neurological complications W/ diabetic mononeuropathy	18	30
E0942	Drug or chemical induced DM W/ neurological complications W/ diabetic polyneuropathy	18, 75	30
E0943	Drug or chemical induced DM W/ neurological complications W/ diabetic autonomic (poly)neuropathy	18	30
E0944	Drug or chemical induced DM W/ neurological complications W/ diabetic amyotrophy	18	30
E0949	Drug or chemical induced DM W/ neurological complications W/ diabetic neurological complication, NEC	18	30
E0951	Drug or chemical induced DM W/ diabetic peripheral angiopathy W/O gangrene	18, 108	30, 216
E0952	Drug or chemical induced DM W/ diabetic peripheral angiopathy W/ gangrene	18, 106, 108	30, 216
E0959	Drug or chemical induced DM W/ circulatory complication, NEC	18	30
E09610	Drug or chemical induced DM W/ diabetic neuropathic arthropathy	18	30
E09618	Drug or chemical induced DM W/ diabetic arthropathy, NEC	18	30
E09620	Drug or chemical induced DM W/ diabetic dermatitis	18	30
E09621	Drug or chemical induced DM W/ foot ulcer	18, 161	30, 311
E09622	Drug or chemical induced DM W/ skin ulcer, NEC	18, 161	30, 311
E09628	Drug or chemical induced DM W/ skin complication, NEC	18	30
E09630	Drug or chemical induced DM W/ periodontal DZ	18	30
E09638	Drug or chemical induced DM W/ oral complication, NEC	18	30
E09641	Drug or chemical induced DM W/ hypoglycemia W/ coma	17	30
E09649	Drug or chemical induced DM W/ hypoglycemia W/O coma	18	30
E0965	Drug or chemical induced DM W/ hyperglycemia	18	30
E0969	Drug or chemical induced DM W/ NEC complication	18	30
E098	Drug or chemical induced DM W/ NOS complications	18	30
E099	Drug or chemical induced DM W/O complications	19	31
E1010	Type 1 DM W/ DKA W/O coma	17	30
E1011	Type 1 DM W/ DKA W/ coma	17	30
E1021	Type 1 DM W/ diabetic nephropathy	18, 141	30
E1022	Type 1 DM W/ diabetic CKD	18, 139	30

Code	Code Descriptors	HCC	RXHCC
E1029	Type 1 DM W/ diabetic kidney complication, NEC	18, 141	30
E10311	Type 1 DM W/ NOS diabetic retinopathy W/ macular edema	18	30, 241
E10319	Type 1 DM W/ NOS diabetic retinopathy W/O macular edema	18	30, 241
For codes E10321- through E10359-, use the following 7th character: 1 Right eye 2 Left eye 3 Bilateral eye 9 Eye, NOS			
E10321-	Type 1 DM W/ mild nonproliferative diabetic retinopathy W/ macular edema	18	30, 241
E10329-	Type 1 DM W/ mild nonproliferative diabetic retinopathy W/O macular edema	18	30, 241
E10331-	Type 1 DM W/ moderate nonproliferative diabetic retinopathy W/ macular edema	18	30, 241
E10339-	Type 1 DM W/ moderate nonproliferative diabetic retinopathy W/O macular edema	18	30, 241
E10341-	Type 1 DM W/ severe nonproliferative diabetic retinopathy W/ macular edema,	18	30, 241
E10349-	Type 1 DM W/ severe nonproliferative diabetic retinopathy W/O macular edema	18	30, 241
E10351-	Type 1 DM W/ proliferative diabetic retinopathy W/ macular edema	18, 122	30, 241
E10352-	Type 1 DM W/ proliferative diabetic retinopathy W/ traction retinal detachment involving macula	18, 122	30, 241
E10353-	Type 1 DM W/ proliferative diabetic retinopathy W/ traction retinal detachment not involving the macula	18, 122	30, 241
E10354-	Type 1 DM W/ proliferative diabetic retinopathy W/ combined traction retinal detachment & rhegmatogenous retinal detachment	18, 122	30, 241
E10354-	Type 1 DM W/ proliferative diabetic retinopathy W/ combined traction retinal detachment & rhegmatogenous retinal detachment	18, 122	30, 241
E10359-	Type 1 DM W/ proliferative diabetic retinopathy W/O macular edema	18, 122	30, 241
E1036	Type 1 DM W/ diabetic cataract	18	30
E1037X1	Type 1 DM W/ diabetic macular edema, resolved following treatment, R eye	18	30
E1037X2	Type 1 DM W/ diabetic macular edema, resolved following treatment, L eye	18	30
E1037X3	Type 1 DM W/ diabetic macular edema, resolved following treatment, bilateral	18	30
E1037X9	Type 1 DM W/ diabetic macular edema, resolved following treatment, NOS eye	18	30
E1039	Type 1 DM W/ diabetic ophthalmic complication, NEC	18	30
E1040	Type 1 DM W/ diabetic neuropathy, NOS	18, 75	30
E1041	Type 1 DM W/ diabetic mononeuropathy	18	30
E1042	Type 1 DM W/ diabetic polyneuropathy	18, 75	30

Code	Code Descriptors	HCC	RXHCC
E1043	Type 1 DM W/ diabetic autonomic (poly) neuropathy	18	30
E1044	Type 1 DM W/ diabetic amyotrophy	18	30
E1049	Type 1 DM W/ other diabetic neurological complication	18	30
E1051	Type 1 DM W/ diabetic peripheral angiopathy W/O gangrene	18, 108	30, 216
E1052	Type 1 DM W/ diabetic peripheral angiopathy W/ gangrene	18, 106, 108	30, 216
E1059	Type 1 DM W/ circulatory complication, NEC	18	30
E10610	Type 1 DM W/ diabetic neuropathic arthropathy	18	30
E10618	Type 1 DM W/ diabetic arthropathy, NEC	18	30
E10620	Type 1 DM W/ diabetic dermatitis	18, 161	30, 311
E10621	Type 1 DM W/ foot ulcer	18, 161	30, 311
E10622	Type 1 DM W/ skin ulcer, NEC	18	30
E10628	Type 1 DM W/ skin complication, NEC	18	30
E10630	Type 1 DM W/ periodontal DZ	18	30
E10638	Type 1 DM W/ oral complication, NEC	18	30
E10641	Type 1 DM W/ hypoglycemia W/ coma	17	30
E10649	Type 1 DM W/ hypoglycemia W/O coma	18	30
E1065	Type 1 DM W/ hyperglycemia	18	30
E1069	Type 1 DM W/ NEC complication	18	30
E108	Type 1 DM W/ NOS complications	18	30
E109	Type 1 DM W/O complications	19	31
E1100	Type 2 DM W/ NKHHC	17	30
E1101	Type 2 DM W/ hyperosmolarity W/ coma	17	30
E1110	Type 2 DM W/ DKA W/O coma	17	30
E1111	Type 2 DM W/ DKA W coma	17	30
E1121	Type 2 DM W/ diabetic nephropathy	18, 141	30
E1122	Type 2 DM W/ diabetic CKD	18, 139	30
E1129	Type 2 DM W/ diabetic kidney complication, NEC	18, 141	30
E11311	Type 2 DM W/ NOS diabetic retinopathy W/ macular edema	18	30, 241
E11319	Type 2 DM W/ NOS diabetic retinopathy W/O macular edema	18	30, 241
For codes E11321- through E11359-, use the following 7th character: 1 Right eye 2 Left eye 3 Bilateral eye 9 Eye, NOS			
E11321-	Type 2 DM W/ mild nonproliferative diabetic retinopathy W/ macular edema	18	30, 241
E11329-	Type 2 DM W/ mild nonproliferative diabetic retinopathy W/O macular edema	18	30, 241
E11331-	Type 2 DM W/ moderate nonproliferative diabetic retinopathy W/ macular edema	18	30, 241

Code	Code Descriptors	HCC	RXHCC
E11339-	Type 2 DM W/ moderate nonproliferative diabetic retinopathy W/O macular edema	18	30, 241
E11341-	Type 2 DM W/ severe nonproliferative diabetic retinopathy W/ macular edema, R eye	18	30, 241
E11349-	Type 2 DM W/ severe nonproliferative diabetic retinopathy W/O macular edema	18	30, 241
E11351-	Type 2 DM W/ proliferative diabetic retinopathy W/ macular edema	18, 122	30, 241
E11352-	Type 2 DM W/ proliferative diabetic retinopathy W/ traction retinal detachment involving macula	18, 122	30, 241
E11353-	Type 2 DM W/ proliferative diabetic retinopathy W/ traction retinal detachment not involving the macula	18, 122	30, 241
E11354-	Type 2 DM W/ proliferative diabetic retinopathy W/ combined traction retinal detachment & rhegmatogenous retinal detachment	18, 122	30, 241
E11355-	Type 2 DM W/ stable proliferative diabetic retinopathy	18, 122	30, 241
E11359-	Type 2 DM W/ proliferative diabetic retinopathy W/O macular edema	18, 122	30, 241
E1136	Type 2 DM W/ diabetic cataract	18	30
E1137X1	Type 2 DM W/ diabetic macular edema, resolved following treatment, R eye	18	30
E1137X2	Type 2 DM W/ diabetic macular edema, resolved following treatment, L eye	18	30
E1137X3	Type 2 DM W/ diabetic macular edema, resolved following treatment, bilateral	18	30
E1137X9	Type 2 DM W/ diabetic macular edema, resolved following treatment, NOS eye	18	30
E1139	Type 2 DM W/ diabetic ophthalmic complication, NEC	18	30
E1140	Type 2 DM W/ diabetic neuropathy, NOS	18, 75	30
E1141	Type 2 DM W/ diabetic mononeuropathy	18	30
E1142	Type 2 DM W/ diabetic polyneuropathy	18, 75	30
E1143	Type 2 DM W/ diabetic autonomic (poly) neuropathy	18	30
E1144	Type 2 DM W/ diabetic amyotrophy	18	30
E1149	Type 2 DM W/ diabetic neurological complication, NEC	18	30
E1151	Type 2 DM W/ diabetic peripheral angiopathy W/O gangrene	18, 108	30, 216
E1152	Type 2 DM W/ diabetic peripheral angiopathy W/ gangrene	18, 106, 108	30, 216
E1159	Type 2 DM W/ circulatory complication, NEC	18	30
E11610	Type 2 DM W/ diabetic neuropathic arthropathy	18	30
E11618	Type 2 DM W/ other diabetic arthropathy	18	30
E11620	Type 2 DM W/ diabetic dermatitis	18	30
E11621	Type 2 DM W/ foot ulcer	18, 161	30, 311

Code	Code Descriptors	HCC	RXHCC
E11622	Type 2 DM W/ skin ulcer, NEC	18, 161	30, 311
E11628	Type 2 DM W/ skin complication, NEC	18	30
E11630	Type 2 DM W/ periodontal DZ	18	30
E11638	Type 2 DM W/ oral complication, NEC	18	30
E11641	Type 2 DM W/ hypoglycemia W/ coma	17	30
E11649	Type 2 DM W/ hypoglycemia W/O coma	18	30
E1165	Type 2 DM W/ hyperglycemia	18	30
E1169	Type 2 DM W/ NEC complication	18	30
E118	Type 2 DM W/ NOS complication	18	30
E119	Type 2 DM W/O complications	19	31
E1300	NEC DM W/ hyperosmolarity W/O NKHHC	17	30
E1301	NEC DM W/ hyperosmolarity W/ coma	17	30
E1310	NEC DM W/ DKA W/O coma	17	30
E1311	NEC DM W/ DKA W/ coma	17	30
E1321	NEC DM W/ diabetic nephropathy	18, 141	30
E1322	NEC DM W/ diabetic CKD	18, 139	30
E1329	NEC DM W/ diabetic kidney complication, NEC	18, 141	30
E13311	NEC DM W/ NOS diabetic retinopathy W/ macular edema	18	30, 241
E13319	NEC DM W/ NOS diabetic retinopathy W/O macular edema	18	30, 241
For codes E13321- through E13359-, use the following 7th character: **1 Right eye** **2 Left eye** **3 Bilateral eye** **9 Eye, NOS**			
E13321-	NEC DM W/ mild nonproliferative diabetic retinopathy W/ macular edema	18	30, 241
E13329-	NEC DM W/ mild nonproliferative diabetic retinopathy W/O macular edema	18	30, 241
E13331-	NEC DM W/ moderate nonproliferative diabetic retinopathy W/ macular edema	18	30, 241
E13339-	NEC DM W/ moderate nonproliferative diabetic retinopathy W/O macular edema	18	30, 241
E13341-	NEC DM W/ severe nonproliferative diabetic retinopathy W/ macular edema	18	30, 241
E13349-	NEC DM W/ severe nonproliferative diabetic retinopathy W/O macular edema	18	30, 241
E13351-	NEC DM W/ proliferative diabetic retinopathy W/ macular edema	18, 122	30, 241
E13352-	NEC DM W/ proliferative diabetic retinopathy W/ traction retinal detachment involving macula	18, 122	30, 241
E13353-	NEC DM W/ proliferative diabetic retinopathy W/ traction retinal detachment not involving macula	18, 122	30, 241
E13354-	NEC DM W/ proliferative diabetic retinopathy W/ combined traction retinal detachment & rhegmatogenous retinal detachment	18, 122	30, 241

Code	Code Descriptors	HCC	RXHCC
E13355-	NEC DM W/ stable proliferative diabetic retinopathy	18, 122	30, 241
E13359-	NEC DM W/ proliferative diabetic retinopathy W/O macular edema	18, 122	30, 241
E1336	NEC DM W/ diabetic cataract	18	30
E1337X1	NEC DM W/ diabetic macular edema, resolved following treatment, R eye	18	30
E1337X2	NEC DM W/ diabetic macular edema, resolved following treatment, L eye	18	30
E1337X3	NEC DM W/ diabetic macular edema, resolved following treatment, bilateral	18	30
E1337X9	NEC DM W/ diabetic macular edema, resolved following treatment, NOS eye	18	30
E1339	NEC DM W/ diabetic ophthalmic complication, NEC	18	30
E1340	NEC DM W/ diabetic neuropathy, NOS	18, 75	30
E1341	NEC DM W/ diabetic mononeuropathy	18	30
E1342	NEC DM W/ diabetic polyneuropathy	18, 75	30
E1343	NEC DM W/ diabetic autonomic (poly) neuropathy	18	30
E1344	NEC DM W/ diabetic amyotrophy	18	30
E1349	NEC DM W/ diabetic neurological complication, NEC	18	30
E1351	NEC DM W/ diabetic peripheral angiopathy W/O gangrene	18, 108	30, 216
E1352	NEC DM W/ diabetic peripheral angiopathy W/ gangrene	18, 106, 108	30, 216
E1359	NEC DM W/ circulatory complication, NECs	18	30
E13610	NEC DM W/ diabetic neuropathic arthropathy	18	30
E13618	NEC DM W/ diabetic arthropathy, NEC	18	30
E13620	NEC DM W/ diabetic dermatitis	18, 161	30, 311
E13621	NEC DM W/ foot ulcer	18, 161	30, 311
E13622	NEC DM W/ skin ulcer, NEC	18	30
E13628	NEC DM W/ skin complication, NEC	18	30
E13630	NEC DM W/ periodontal DZ	18	30
E13638	NEC DM W/ oral complication, NEC	18	30
E13641	NEC DM W/ hypoglycemia W/ coma	17	30
E13649	NEC DM W/ hypoglycemia W/O coma	18	30
E1365	NEC DM W/ hyperglycemia	18	30
E1369	NEC DM W/ NEC complication	18	30
E138	NEC DM W/ NOS complication	18	30
E139	NEC DM W/O complications	19	31
E15	Nondiabetic hypoglycemic coma	23	N/A
E163	Increased secretion of glucagon	N/A	66
E164	Increased secretion of gastrin	N/A	66
E168	Disorder of pancreatic internal secretion, NEC	N/A	66

Code	Code Descriptors	HCC	RXHCC
E169	Disorder of pancreatic internal secretion, NOS	N/A	66
E200	Idiopathic hypoparathyroidism	23	41
E208	Hypoparathyroidism, NEC	23	41
E209	Hypoparathyroidism, NOS	23	41
E210	Primary hyperparathyroidism	23	41
E211	2ndary hyperparathyroidism, NEC	23	41
E212	Hyperparathyroidism, NEC	23	41
E213	Hyperparathyroidism, NOS	23	41
E214	Disorder of parathyroid gland, NEC	23	41
E215	Disorder of parathyroid gland, NOS	23	41
E220	Acromegaly & pituitary gigantism	23	41
E221	Hyperprolactinemia	23	41
E222	Syndrome of inappropriate secretion of antidiuretic hormone	23	41
E228	Hyperfunction of pituitary gland, NEC	23	41
E229	Hyperfunction of pituitary gland, NOS	23	41
E230	Hypopituitarism	23	41
E231	Drug-induced hypopituitarism	23	41
E232	Diabetes insipidus	23	41
E233	Hypothalamic dysfunction, NEC	23	41
E236	Disorder of pituitary gland, NEC	23	41
E237	Disorder of pituitary gland, NOS	23	41
E240	Pituitary-dependent Cushing's DZ	23	41
E241	Nelson's syndrome	23	41
E242	Drug-induced Cushing's syndrome	23	41
E243	Ectopic ACTH syndrome	23	41
E244	Alcohol-induced pseudo-Cushing's syndrome	23	41
E248	Cushing's syndrome, NEC	23	41
E249	Cushing's syndrome, NOS	23	41
E250	Congenital adrenogenital disorders associated W/ enzyme deficiency	23	41
E258	Adrenogenital disorder, NEC	23	41
E259	Adrenogenital disorder, NOS	23	41
E2601	Conn's syndrome	23	41
E2602	Glucocorticoid-remediable aldosteronism	23	41
E2609	Primary hyperaldosteronism, NEC	23	41
E261	2ndary hyperaldosteronism	23	41
E2681	Bartter's syndrome	23	41
E2689	Hyperaldosteronism, NEC	23	41
E269	Hyperaldosteronism, NOS	23	41
E270	Adrenocortical overactivity, NEC	23	41
E271	Primary adrenocortical insufficiency	23	41
E272	Addisonian crisis	23	41
E273	Drug-induced adrenocortical insufficiency	23	41
E2740	NOS adrenocortical insufficiency	23	41
E2749	NEC adrenocortical insufficiency	23	41

Code	Code Descriptors	HCC	RXHCC
E275	Adrenomedullary hyperfunction	23	41
E278	Disorder of adrenal gland, NEC	23	41
E279	Disorder of adrenal gland, NOS	23	41
E310	Autoimmune polyglandular failure	23	41
E311	Polyglandular hyperfunction	23	41
E3120	Multiple endocrine neoplasia [MEN] syndrome, NOS	23	41
E3121	Multiple endocrine neoplasia type I	23	41
E3122	Multiple endocrine neoplasia type IIA	23	41
E3123	Multiple endocrine neoplasia type IIB	23	41
E318	Polyglandular dysfunction, NEC	23	41
E319	Polyglandular dysfunction, NOS	23	41
E320	Persistent hyperplasia of thymus	23	41
E321	Abscess of thymus	23	41
E328	DZ of thymus, NEC	23	41
E329	DZ of thymus, NOS	23	41
E340	Carcinoid syndrome	12	19
E344	Constitutional tall stature	23	41
E40	Kwashiorkor	21	N/A
E41	Nutritional marasmus	21	N/A
E42	Marasmic kwashiorkor	21	N/A
E43	NOS severe protein-calorie malnutrition	21	N/A
E440	Moderate protein-calorie malnutrition	21	N/A
E441	Mild protein-calorie malnutrition	21	N/A
E45	Retarded development following protein-calorie malnutrition	21	N/A
E46	NOS protein-calorie malnutrition	21	N/A
E550	Rickets, active	N/A	87
E640	Sequelae of protein-calorie malnutrition	21	N/A
E6601	Morbid (severe) obesity D/T excess calories	22	43
E662	Morbid (severe) obesity W/ alveolar hypoventilation	22	43
E700	Classical phenylketonuria	23	41
E701	Hyperphenylalaninemia, NEC	23	41
E7020	Disorder of tyrosine metabolism, NOS	23	41
E7021	Tyrosinemia	23	41
E7029	Disorder of tyrosine metabolism, NEC	23	41
E7030	Albinism, NOS	23	41
E70310	X-linked ocular albinism	23	41
E70311	Autosomal recessive ocular albinism	23	41
E70318	Ocular albinism, NEC	23	41
E70319	Ocular albinism, NOS	23	41
E70320	Tyrosinase negative oculocutaneous albinism	23	41
E70321	Tyrosinase positive oculocutaneous albinism	23	41
E70328	Oculocutaneous albinism, NEC	23	41
E70329	Oculocutaneous albinism, NOS	23	41
E70330	Chediak-Higashi syndrome	23	41
E70331	Hermansky-Pudlak syndrome	23	41
E70338	Albinism W/ hematologic abnormality, NEC	23	41
E70339	Albinism W/ hematologic abnormality, NOS	23	41
E7039	Albinism, NEC	23	41
E7040	Disorders of histidine metabolism, NOS	23	41
E7041	Histidinemia	23	41
E7049	Disorders of histidine metabolism, NEC	23	41
E705	Disorders of tryptophan metabolism	23	41
E708	Disorder of aromatic amino-acid metabolism, NEC	23	41
E709	Disorder of aromatic amino-acid metabolism, NOS	23	41
E710	Maple-syrup-urine DZ	23	41
E71110	Isovaleric acidemia	23	41
E71111	3-methylglutaconic aciduria	23	41
E71118	Other branched-chain organic acidurias	23	41
E71120	Methylmalonic acidemia	23	41
E71121	Propionic acidemia	23	41
E71128	Disorders of propionate metabolism, NEC	23	41
E7119	Disorder of branched-chain amino-acid metabolism, NEC	23	41
E712	Disorder of branched-chain amino-acid metabolism, NOS	23	41
E7130	Disorder of fatty-acid metabolism, NOS	N/A	45
E71310	Long chain/very long chain acyl CoA dehydrogenase deficiency	23	41
E71311	Medium chain acyl CoA dehydrogenase deficiency	23	41
E71312	Short chain acyl CoA dehydrogenase deficiency	23	41
E71313	Glutaric aciduria type II	23	41
E71314	Muscle carnitine palmitoyltransferase deficiency	23	41
E71318	Disorders of fatty-acid oxidation, NEC	23	41
E7132	Disorders of ketone metabolism	23	41
E7139	Ddisorders of fatty-acid metabolism, NEC	23	41
E7140	Disorder of carnitine metabolism, NOS	23	41
E7141	Primary carnitine deficiency	23	41
E7142	Carnitine deficiency D/T inborn errors of metabolism	23	41
E7143	Iatrogenic carnitine deficiency	23	41
E71440	Ruvalcaba-Myhre-Smith syndrome	23	41
E71448	2ndary carnitine deficiency, NEC	23	41
E7150	Peroxisomal disorder, NOS	23	41
E71510	Zellweger syndrome	23	41
E71511	Neonatal adrenoleukodystrophy	23	41
E71518	Disorder of peroxisome biogenesis, NEC	23	41
E71520	Childhood cerebral X-linked adrenoleukodystrophy	23	41

Code	Code Descriptors	HCC	RXHCC
E71521	Adolescent X-linked adrenoleukodystrophy	23	41
E71522	Adrenomyeloneuropathy	23	41
E71528	X-linked adrenoleukodystrophy, NEC type	23	41
E71529	X-linked adrenoleukodystrophy, NOS type	23	41
E7153	Group 2 peroxisomal disorder, NEC	23	41
E71540	Rhizomelic chondrodysplasia punctata	23	41
E71541	Zellweger-like syndrome	23	41
E71542	Group 3 peroxisomal disorder, NEC	23	41
E71548	Other peroxisomal disorders	23	41
E7200	Disorders of amino-acid transport, NOS	23	41
E7201	Cystinuria	23	41
E7202	Hartnup's DZ	23	41
E7203	Lowe's syndrome	23	41
E7204	Cystinosis	23	41
E7209	Disorders of amino-acid transport, NEC	23	41
E7210	Disorders of sulfur-bearing amino-acid metabolism, NOS	23	41
E7211	Homocystinuria	23	41
E7212	Methylenetetrahydrofolate reductase deficiency	23	41
E7219	Other disorders of sulfur-bearing amino-acid metabolism	23	41
E7220	Disorder of urea cycle metabolism, NOS	23	41
E7221	Argininemia	23	41
E7222	Arginosuccinic aciduria	23	41
E7223	Citrullinemia	23	41
E7229	Disorder of urea cycle metabolism, NEC	23	41
E723	Disorder of lysine & hydroxylysine metabolism	23	41
E724	Disorder of ornithine metabolism	23	41
E7250	Disorder of glycine metabolism, NOS	23	41
E7251	Non-ketotic hyperglycinemia	23	41
E7252	Trimethylaminuria	23	41
E7253	Hyperoxaluria	23	41
E7259	Disorder of glycine metabolism, NEC	23	41
E728	Disorder of amino-acid metabolism, NEC	23	41
E729	Disorder of amino-acid metabolism, NOS	23	41
E7400	Glycogen storage DZ, NOS	23	41
E7401	von Gierke DZ	23	41
E7402	Pompe DZ	23	41
E7403	Cori DZ	23	41
E7404	McArdle DZ	23	41
E7409	Glycogen storage DZ, NEC	23	41
E7420	Disorders of galactose metabolism, NOS	23	41
E7421	Galactosemia	23	41
E7429	Disorders of galactose metabolism, NEC	23	41
E744	Disorders of pyruvate metabolism & gluconeogenesis	23	41

Code	Code Descriptors	HCC	RXHCC
E748	Disorder of carbohydrate metabolism, NEC	23	41
E749	Disorder of carbohydrate metabolism, NOS	23	41
E7500	GM2 gangliosidosis, NOS	52	112
E7501	Sandhoff DZ	52	112
E7502	Tay-Sachs DZ	52	112
E7509	GM2 gangliosidosis, NEC	52	112
E7510	Gangliosidosis, NOS	52	112
E7511	Mucolipidosis IV	52	112
E7519	Gangliosidosis, NEC	52	112
E7521	Fabry (-Anderson) DZ	23	41
E7522	Gaucher DZ	23	41
E7523	Krabbe DZ	52	112
E75240	Niemann-Pick DZ type A	23	41
E75241	Niemann-Pick DZ type B	23	41
E75242	Niemann-Pick DZ type C	23	41
E75243	Niemann-Pick DZ type D	23	41
E75248	Niemann-Pick DZ, NEC	23	41
E75249	Niemann-Pick DZ, NOS	23	41
E7525	Metachromatic leukodystrophy	52	112
E7529	Sphingolipidosis, NEC	52	112
E753	Sphingolipidosis, NOS	23	41
E754	Neuronal ceroid lipofuscinosis	52	112
E755	Lipid storage disorder, NEC	N/A	45
E756	Lipid storage disorder, NOS	N/A	45
E7601	Hurler's syndrome	23	41
E7602	Hurler-Scheie syndrome	23	41
E7603	Scheie's syndrome	23	41
E761	Mucopolysaccharidosis, type II	23	41
E76210	Morquio A mucopolysaccharidoses	23	41
E76211	Morquio B mucopolysaccharidoses	23	41
E76219	Morquio mucopolysaccharidoses, NOS	23	41
E7622	Sanfilippo mucopolysaccharidoses	23	41
E7629	Mucopolysaccharidosis, NEC	23	41
E763	Mucopolysaccharidosis, NOS	23	41
E768	Disorder of glucosaminoglycan metabolism, NEC	23	41
E769	Glucosaminoglycan metabolism disorder, NOS	23	41
E770	Defects in post-translational modification of	23	41
E771	Defects in glycoprotein degradation	23	41
E778	Disorder of glycoprotein metabolism, NEC	23	41
E779	Disorder of glycoprotein metabolism, NOS	23	41
E7800	Pure hypercholesterolemia, NOS	N/A	45
E7801	Familial hypercholesterolemia	N/A	45
E781	Pure hyperglyceridemia	N/A	45
E782	Mixed hyperlipidemia	N/A	45
E783	Hyperchylomicronemia	N/A	45

Code	Code Descriptors	HCC	RXHCC
E784	Hyperlipidemia, NEC	N/A	45
E785	Hyperlipidemia, NOS	N/A	45
E786	Lipoprotein deficiency	N/A	45
E7870	Disorder of bile acid & cholesterol metabolism, NOS	N/A	45
E7879	Disorder of bile acid & cholesterol metabolism, NEC	N/A	45
E7881	Lipoid dermatoarthritis	N/A	45
E7889	Disorder of lipoprotein metabolism, NEC	N/A	45
E789	Disorder of lipoprotein metabolism, NOS	N/A	45
E791	Lesch-Nyhan syndrome	23	41
E792	Myoadenylate deaminase deficiency	23	41
E798	Disorder of purine & pyrimidine metabolism, NEC	23	41
E799	Disorder of purine & pyrimidine metabolism, NOS	23	41
E800	Hereditary erythropoietic porphyria	23	41
E801	Porphyria cutanea tarda	23	41
E8020	Porphyria, NOS	23	41
E8021	Acute intermittent (hepatic) porphyria	23	41
E8029	Porphyria, NEC	23	41
E803	Defects of catalase & peroxidase	23	41
E8300	Disorder of copper metabolism, NOS	N/A	41
E8301	Wilson's DZ	N/A	41
E8309	Disorder of copper metabolism, NEC	N/A	41
E8310	Disorder of iron metabolism, NOS	N/A	41
E83110	Hereditary hemochromatosis	23	41
E83118	Hemochromatosis, NEC	N/A	41
E83119	Hemochromatosis, NOS	N/A	41
E8319	Disorder of iron metabolism, NEC	N/A	41
E8330	Disorder of phosphorus metabolism, NOS	N/A	41
E8331	Familial hypophosphatemia	N/A	41
E8332	Hereditary vitamin D-dependent rickets (type 1) (type 2)	N/A	41
E8339	Disorder of phosphorus metabolism, NEC	N/A	41
E840	Cystic fibrosis W/ pulmonary manifestations	110	225
E8411	Meconium ileus in cystic fibrosis	110	225
E8419	Cystic fibrosis W/ other intestinal manifestations	110	225
E848	Cystic fibrosis W/ other manifestations	110	225
E849	Cystic fibrosis, NOS	110	225
E850	Non-neuropathic heredofamilial amyloidosis	23	N/A
E851	Neuropathic heredofamilial amyloidosis	23	N/A
E852	Heredofamilial amyloidosis, NOS	23	N/A
E853	2ndary systemic amyloidosis	23	N/A
E854	Organ-limited amyloidosis	23	N/A
E8581	Light chain (AL) amyloidosis	23	N/A

Code	Code Descriptors	HCC	RXHCC
E8582	Wild-type transthyretin-related (ATTR) amyloidosis	23	N/A
E8589	Amyloidosis, NEC	23	N/A
E859	Amyloidosis, NOS	23	N/A
E8801	Alpha-1-antitrypsin deficiency	23	40
E882	Lipomatosis, NEC	N/A	45
E8840	Mitochondrial metabolism disorder, NOS	23	41
E8841	MELAS syndrome	23	41
E8842	MERRF syndrome	23	41
E8849	Mitochondrial metabolism disorder, NEC	23	41
E8889	Metabolic disorder, NEC	23	41
E890	Postprocedural hypothyroidism	N/A	42
E892	Postprocedural hypoparathyroidism	23	41
E893	Postprocedural hypopituitarism	23	41
E896	Postprocedural adrenocortical hypofunction	23	41
F0150	Vascular dementia W/O behavioral disturbance	52	112
F0151	Vascular dementia W/ behavioral disturbance	51	112
F0280	Dementia in other DZ classified elsewhere W/O behavioral disturbance	52	112
F0281	Dementia in other DZ classified elsewhere W/ behavioral disturbance	51	112
F0390	NOS dementia W/O behavioral disturbance	52	112
F0391	NOS dementia W/ behavioral disturbance	51	112
F04	Amnestic disorder D/T known physiological condition	52	112
F10120	Alcohol abuse W/ intoxication, uncomplicated	55	N/A
F10121	Alcohol abuse W/ intoxication delirium	55	N/A
F10129	Alcohol abuse W/ intoxication, NOS	55	N/A
F1014	Alcohol abuse W/ alcohol-induced mood disorder	55	N/A
F10150	Alcohol abuse W/ alcohol-induced psychotic disorder W/ delusions	54	N/A
F10151	Alcohol abuse W/ alcohol-induced psychotic disorder W/ hallucinations	54	N/A
F10159	Alcohol abuse W/ alcohol-induced psychotic disorder, NOS	54	N/A
F10180	Alcohol abuse W/ alcohol-induced anxiety disorder	55	N/A
F10181	Alcohol abuse W/ alcohol-induced sexual dysfunction	55	N/A
F10182	Alcohol abuse W/ alcohol-induced sleep disorder	55	N/A
F10188	Alcohol abuse W/ alcohol-induced disorder, NEC	55	N/A
F1019	Alcohol abuse W/ alcohol-induced disorder, NOS	55	N/A
F1020	Alcohol dependence, uncomplicated	55	N/A
F1021	Alcohol dependence, in remission	55	N/A

Code	Code Descriptors	HCC	RXHCC
F10220	Alcohol dependence W/ intoxication, uncomplicated	55	N/A
F10221	Alcohol dependence W/ intoxication delirium	55	N/A
F10229	Alcohol dependence W/ intoxication, NOS	55	N/A
F10230	Alcohol dependence W/ withdrawal, uncomplicated	55	N/A
F10231	Alcohol dependence W/ withdrawal delirium	54	N/A
F10232	Alcohol dependence W/ withdrawal W/ perceptual disturbance	54	N/A
F10239	Alcohol dependence W/ withdrawal, NOS	55	N/A
F1024	Alcohol dependence W/ alcohol-induced mood disorder	55	N/A
F10250	Alcohol dependence W/ alcohol-induced psychotic disorder W/ delusions	54	N/A
F10251	Alcohol dependence W/ alcohol-induced psychotic disorder W/ hallucinations	54	N/A
F10259	Alcohol dependence W/ alcohol-induced psychotic disorder, NOS	54	N/A
F1026	Alcohol dependence W/ alcohol-induced persisting amnestic disorder	54	N/A
F1027	Alcohol dependence W/ alcohol-induced persisting dementia	54	N/A
F10280	Alcohol dependence W/ alcohol-induced anxiety disorder	55	N/A
F10281	Alcohol dependence W/ alcohol-induced sexual dysfunction	55	N/A
F10282	Alcohol dependence W/ alcohol-induced sleep disorder	55	N/A
F10288	Alcohol dependence W/ alcohol-induced disorder, NEC	55	N/A
F1029	Alcohol dependence W/ alcohol-induced disorder, NOS	55	N/A
F10920	Alcohol use, NOS W/ intoxication, uncomplicated	55	N/A
F10921	Alcohol use, NOS W/ intoxication delirium	55	N/A
F10929	Alcohol use, NOS W/ intoxication, NOS	55	N/A
F1094	Alcohol use, NOS W/ alcohol-induced mood disorder	55	N/A
F10950	Alcohol use, NOS W/ alcohol-induced psychotic disorder W/ delusions	54	N/A
F10951	Alcohol use, NOS W/ alcohol-induced psychotic disorder W/ hallucinations	54	N/A
F10959	Alcohol use, NOS W/ alcohol-induced psychotic disorder, NOS	54	N/A
F1096	Alcohol use, NOS W/ alcohol-induced persisting amnestic disorder	54	N/A
F1097	Alcohol use, NOS W/ alcohol-induced persisting dementia	54	N/A
F10980	Alcohol use, NOS W/ alcohol-induced anxiety disorder	55	N/A
F10981	Alcohol use, NOS W/ alcohol-induced sexual dysfunction	55	N/A

Code	Code Descriptors	HCC	RXHCC
F10982	Alcohol use, NOS W/ alcohol-induced sleep disorder	55	N/A
F10988	Alcohol use, NOS W/ alcohol-induced disorder, NEC	55	N/A
F1099	Alcohol use, NOS W/ alcohol-induced disorder, NOS	55	N/A
F11120	Opioid abuse W/ intoxication, uncomplicated	55	N/A
F11121	Opioid abuse W/ intoxication delirium	55	N/A
F11122	Opioid abuse W/ intoxication W/ perceptual disturbance	55	N/A
F11129	Opioid abuse W/ intoxication, NOS	55	N/A
F1114	Opioid abuse W/ opioid-induced mood disorder	55	N/A
F11150	Opioid abuse W/ opioid-induced psychotic disorder W/ delusions	54	N/A
F11151	Opioid abuse W/ opioid-induced psychotic disorder W/ hallucinations	54	N/A
F11159	Opioid abuse W/ opioid-induced psychotic disorder, NOS	54	N/A
F11181	Opioid abuse W/ opioid-induced sexual dysfunction	55	N/A
F11182	Opioid abuse W/ opioid-induced sleep disorder	55	N/A
F11188	Opioid abuse W/ other opioid-induced disorder	55	N/A
F1119	Opioid abuse W/ NOS opioid-induced disorder	55	N/A
F1120	Opioid dependence, uncomplicated	55	N/A
F1121	Opioid dependence, in remission	55	N/A
F11220	Opioid dependence W/ intoxication, uncomplicated	55	N/A
F11221	Opioid dependence W/ intoxication delirium	55	N/A
F11222	Opioid dependence W/ intoxication W/ perceptual disturbance	55	N/A
F11229	Opioid dependence W/ intoxication, NOS	55	N/A
F1123	Opioid dependence W/ withdrawal	55	N/A
F1124	Opioid dependence W/ opioid-induced mood disorder	55	N/A
F11250	Opioid dependence W/ opioid-induced psychotic disorder W/ delusions	54	N/A
F11251	Opioid dependence W/ opioid-induced psychotic disorder W/ hallucinations	54	N/A
F11259	Opioid dependence W/ opioid-induced psychotic disorder, NOS	54	N/A
F11281	Opioid dependence W/ opioid-induced sexual dysfunction	55	N/A
F11282	Opioid dependence W/ opioid-induced sleep disorder	55	N/A
F11288	Opioid dependence W/ opioid-induced disorder, NEC	55	N/A
F1129	Opioid dependence W/ opioid-induced disorder, NOS	55	N/A

Code	Code Descriptors	HCC	RXHCC
F11920	Opioid use, NOS W/ intoxication, uncomplicated	55	N/A
F11921	Opioid use, NOS W/ intoxication delirium	55	N/A
F11922	Opioid use, NOS W/ intoxication W/ perceptual disturbance	55	N/A
F11929	Opioid use, NOS W/ intoxication, NOS	55	N/A
F1193	Opioid use, NOS W/ withdrawal	55	N/A
F1194	Opioid use, NOS W/ opioid-induced mood disorder	55	N/A
F11950	Opioid use, NOS W/ opioid-induced psychotic disorder W/ delusions	54	N/A
F11951	Opioid use, NOS W/ opioid-induced psychotic disorder W/ hallucinations	54	N/A
F11959	Opioid use, NOS W/ opioid-induced psychotic disorder, NOS	54	N/A
F11981	Opioid use, NOS W/ opioid-induced sexual dysfunction	55	N/A
F11982	Opioid use, NOS W/ opioid-induced sleep disorder	55	N/A
F11988	Opioid use, NOS W/ opioid-induced disorder, NEC	55	N/A
F1199	Opioid use, NOS W/ opioid-induced disorder, NOS	55	N/A
F12120	Cannabis abuse W/ intoxication, uncomplicated	55	N/A
F12121	Cannabis abuse W/ intoxication delirium	55	N/A
F12122	Cannabis abuse W/ intoxication W/ perceptual disturbance	55	N/A
F12129	Cannabis abuse W/ intoxication, NOS	55	N/A
F12150	Cannabis abuse W/ psychotic disorder W/ delusions	54	N/A
F12151	Cannabis abuse W/ psychotic disorder W/ hallucinations	54	N/A
F12159	Cannabis abuse W/ psychotic disorder, NOS	54	N/A
F12180	Cannabis abuse W/ cannabis-induced anxiety disorder	55	N/A
F12188	Cannabis abuse W/ cannabis-induced disorder, NEC	55	N/A
F1219	Cannabis abuse W/ cannabis-induced disorder, NOS	55	N/A
F1220	Cannabis dependence, uncomplicated	55	N/A
F1221	Cannabis dependence, in remission	55	N/A
F12220	Cannabis dependence W/ intoxication, uncomplicated	55	N/A
F12221	Cannabis dependence W/ intoxication delirium	55	N/A
F12222	Cannabis dependence W/ intoxication W/ perceptual disturbance	55	N/A
F12229	Cannabis dependence W/ intoxication, NOS	55	N/A
F12250	Cannabis dependence W/ psychotic disorder W/ delusions	54	N/A
F12251	Cannabis dependence W/ psychotic disorder W/ hallucinations	54	N/A

Code	Code Descriptors	HCC	RXHCC
F12259	Cannabis dependence W/ psychotic disorder, NOS	54	N/A
F12280	Cannabis dependence W/ cannabis-induced anxiety disorder	55	N/A
F12288	Cannabis dependence W/ cannabis-induced disorder, NEC	55	N/A
F1229	Cannabis dependence W/ cannabis-induced disorder, NOS	55	N/A
F12920	Cannabis use, NOS W/ intoxication, uncomplicated	55	N/A
F12921	Cannabis use, NOS W/ intoxication delirium	55	N/A
F12922	Cannabis use, NOS W/ intoxication W/ perceptual disturbance	55	N/A
F12929	Cannabis use, NOS W/ intoxication, NOS	55	N/A
F12950	Cannabis use, NOS W/ psychotic disorder W/ delusions	54	N/A
F12951	Cannabis use, NOS W/ psychotic disorder W/ hallucinations	54	N/A
F12959	Cannabis use, NOS W/ psychotic disorder, NOS	54	N/A
F12980	Cannabis use, NOS W/ anxiety disorder	55	N/A
F12988	Cannabis use, NOS W/ other cannabis-induced disorder	55	N/A
F1299	Cannabis use, NOS W/ NOS cannabis-induced disorder	55	N/A
F13120	Sedative, hypnotic or anxiolytic abuse W/ intoxication, uncomplicated	55	N/A
F13121	Sedative, hypnotic or anxiolytic abuse W/ intoxication delirium	55	N/A
F13129	Sedative, hypnotic or anxiolytic abuse W/ intoxication, NOS	55	N/A
F1314	Sedative, hypnotic or anxiolytic abuse W/ sedative, hypnotic or anxiolytic-induced mood disorder	55	N/A
F13150	Sedative, hypnotic or anxiolytic abuse W/ sedative, hypnotic or anxiolytic-induced psychotic disorder W/ delusions	54	N/A
F13151	Sedative, hypnotic or anxiolytic abuse W/ sedative, hypnotic or anxiolytic-induced psychotic disorder W/ hallucinations	54	N/A
F13159	Sedative, hypnotic or anxiolytic abuse W/ sedative, hypnotic or anxiolytic-induced psychotic disorder, NOS	54	N/A
F13180	Sedative, hypnotic or anxiolytic abuse W/ sedative, hypnotic or anxiolytic-induced anxiety disorder	55	N/A
F13181	Sedative, hypnotic or anxiolytic abuse W/ sedative, hypnotic or anxiolytic-induced sexual dysfunction	55	N/A
F13182	Sedative, hypnotic or anxiolytic abuse W/ sedative, hypnotic or anxiolytic-induced sleep disorder	55	N/A
F13188	Sedative, hypnotic or anxiolytic abuse W/ sedative, hypnotic or anxiolytic-induced disorder, NEC	55	N/A

Code	Code Descriptors	HCC	RXHCC
F1319	Sedative, hypnotic or anxiolytic abuse W/ sedative, hypnotic or anxiolytic-induced disorder, NOS	55	N/A
F1320	Sedative, hypnotic or anxiolytic dependence, uncomplicated	55	N/A
F1321	Sedative, hypnotic or anxiolytic dependence, in remission	55	N/A
F13220	Sedative, hypnotic or anxiolytic dependence W/ intoxication, uncomplicated	55	N/A
F13221	Sedative, hypnotic or anxiolytic dependence W/ intoxication delirium	55	N/A
F13229	Sedative, hypnotic or anxiolytic dependence W/ intoxication, NOS	55	N/A
F13230	Sedative, hypnotic or anxiolytic dependence W/ withdrawal, uncomplicated	55	N/A
F13231	Sedative, hypnotic or anxiolytic dependence W/ withdrawal delirium	54	N/A
F13232	Sedative, hypnotic or anxiolytic dependence W/ withdrawal W/ perceptual disturbance	54	N/A
F13239	Sedative, hypnotic or anxiolytic dependence W/ withdrawal, NOS	55	N/A
F1324	Sedative, hypnotic or anxiolytic dependence W/ sedative, hypnotic or anxiolytic-induced mood disorder	55	N/A
F13250	Sedative, hypnotic or anxiolytic dependence W/ sedative, hypnotic or anxiolytic-induced psychotic disorder W/ delusions	54	N/A
F13251	Sedative, hypnotic or anxiolytic dependence W/ sedative, hypnotic or anxiolytic-induced psychotic disorder W/ hallucinations	54	N/A
F13259	Sedative, hypnotic or anxiolytic dependence W/ sedative, hypnotic or anxiolytic-induced psychotic disorder, NOS	54	N/A
F1326	Sedative, hypnotic or anxiolytic dependence W/ sedative, hypnotic or anxiolytic-induced persisting amnestic disorder	54	N/A
F1327	Sedative, hypnotic or anxiolytic dependence W/ sedative, hypnotic or anxiolytic-induced persisting dementia	54	N/A
F13280	Sedative, hypnotic or anxiolytic dependence W/ sedative, hypnotic or anxiolytic-induced anxiety disorder	55	N/A
F13281	Sedative, hypnotic or anxiolytic dependence W/ sedative, hypnotic or anxiolytic-induced sexual dysfunction	55	N/A
F13282	Sedative, hypnotic or anxiolytic dependence W/ sedative, hypnotic or anxiolytic-induced sleep disorder	55	N/A
F13288	Sedative, hypnotic or anxiolytic dependence W/ sedative, hypnotic or anxiolytic-induced disorder, NEC	55	N/A
F1329	Sedative, hypnotic or anxiolytic dependence W/ sedative, hypnotic or anxiolytic-induced disorder, NOS	55	N/A
F13920	Sedative, hypnotic or anxiolytic use, NOS W/ intoxication, uncomplicated	55	N/A

Code	Code Descriptors	HCC	RXHCC
F13921	Sedative, hypnotic or anxiolytic use, NOS W/ intoxication delirium	55	N/A
F13929	Sedative, hypnotic or anxiolytic use, NOS W/ intoxication, NOS	55	N/A
F13930	Sedative, hypnotic or anxiolytic use, NOS W/ withdrawal, uncomplicated	55	N/A
F13931	Sedative, hypnotic or anxiolytic use, NOS W/ withdrawal delirium	54	N/A
F13932	Sedative, hypnotic or anxiolytic use, NOS W/ withdrawal W/ perceptual disturbances	54	N/A
F13939	Sedative, hypnotic or anxiolytic use, NOS W/ withdrawal, NOS	55	N/A
F1394	Sedative, hypnotic or anxiolytic use, NOS W/ sedative, hypnotic or anxiolytic-induced mood disorder	55	N/A
F13950	Sedative, hypnotic or anxiolytic use, NOS W/ sedative, hypnotic or anxiolytic-induced psychotic disorder W/ delusions	54	N/A
F13951	Sedative, hypnotic or anxiolytic use, NOS W/ sedative, hypnotic or anxiolytic-induced psychotic disorder W/ hallucinations	54	N/A
F13959	Sedative, hypnotic or anxiolytic use, NOS W/ sedative, hypnotic or anxiolytic-induced psychotic disorder, NOS	54	N/A
F1396	Sedative, hypnotic or anxiolytic use, NOS W/ sedative, hypnotic or anxiolytic-induced persisting amnestic disorder	54	N/A
F1397	Sedative, hypnotic or anxiolytic use, NOS W/ sedative, hypnotic or anxiolytic-induced persisting dementia	54	N/A
F13980	Sedative, hypnotic or anxiolytic use, NOS W/ sedative, hypnotic or anxiolytic-induced anxiety disorder	55	N/A
F13981	Sedative, hypnotic or anxiolytic use, NOS W/ sedative, hypnotic or anxiolytic-induced sexual dysfunction	55	N/A
F13982	Sedative, hypnotic or anxiolytic use, NOS W/ sedative, hypnotic or anxiolytic-induced sleep disorder	55	N/A
F13988	Sedative, hypnotic or anxiolytic use, NOS W/ sedative, hypnotic or anxiolytic-induced disorder, NEC	55	N/A
F1399	Sedative, hypnotic or anxiolytic use, NOS W/ sedative, hypnotic or anxiolytic-induced disorder, NOS	55	N/A
F14120	Cocaine abuse W/ intoxication, uncomplicated	55	N/A
F14121	Cocaine abuse W/ intoxication W/ delirium	55	N/A
F14122	Cocaine abuse W/ intoxication W/ perceptual disturbance	55	N/A
F14129	Cocaine abuse W/ intoxication, NOS	55	N/A
F1414	Cocaine abuse W/ cocaine-induced mood disorder	55	N/A
F14150	Cocaine abuse W/ cocaine-induced psychotic disorder W/ delusions	54	N/A

Code	Code Descriptors	HCC	RXHCC
F14151	Cocaine abuse W/ cocaine-induced psychotic disorder W/ hallucinations	54	N/A
F14159	Cocaine abuse W/ cocaine-induced psychotic disorder, NOS	54	N/A
F14180	Cocaine abuse W/ cocaine-induced anxiety disorder	55	N/A
F14181	Cocaine abuse W/ cocaine-induced sexual dysfunction	55	N/A
F14182	Cocaine abuse W/ cocaine-induced sleep disorder	55	N/A
F14188	Cocaine abuse W/ cocaine-induced disorder, NEC	55	N/A
F1419	Cocaine abuse W/ cocaine-induced disorder, NOS	55	N/A
F1420	Cocaine dependence, uncomplicated	55	N/A
F1421	Cocaine dependence, in remission	55	N/A
F14220	Cocaine dependence W/ intoxication, uncomplicated	55	N/A
F14221	Cocaine dependence W/ intoxication delirium	55	N/A
F14222	Cocaine dependence W/ intoxication W/ perceptual disturbance	55	N/A
F14229	Cocaine dependence W/ intoxication, NOS	55	N/A
F1423	Cocaine dependence W/ withdrawal	55	N/A
F1424	Cocaine dependence W/ cocaine-induced mood disorder	55	N/A
F14250	Cocaine dependence W/ cocaine-induced psychotic disorder W/ delusions	54	N/A
F14251	Cocaine dependence W/ cocaine-induced psychotic disorder W/ hallucinations	54	N/A
F14259	Cocaine dependence W/ cocaine-induced psychotic disorder, NOS	54	N/A
F14280	Cocaine dependence W/ cocaine-induced anxiety disorder	55	N/A
F14281	Cocaine dependence W/ cocaine-induced sexual dysfunction	55	N/A
F14282	Cocaine dependence W/ cocaine-induced sleep disorder	55	N/A
F14288	Cocaine dependence W/ cocaine-induced disorder, NEC	55	N/A
F1429	Cocaine dependence W/ cocaine-induced disorder, NOS	55	N/A
F14920	Cocaine use, NOS W/ intoxication, uncomplicated	55	N/A
F14921	Cocaine use, NOS W/ intoxication delirium	55	N/A
F14922	Cocaine use, NOS W/ intoxication W/ perceptual disturbance	55	N/A
F14929	Cocaine use, NOS W/ intoxication, NOS	55	N/A
F1494	Cocaine use, NOS W/ cocaine-induced mood disorder	55	N/A
F14950	Cocaine use, NOS W/ cocaine-induced psychotic disorder W/ delusions	54	N/A

Code	Code Descriptors	HCC	RXHCC
F14951	Cocaine use, NOS W/ cocaine-induced psychotic disorder W/ hallucinations	54	N/A
F14959	Cocaine use, NOS W/ cocaine-induced psychotic disorder, NOS	54	N/A
F14980	Cocaine use, NOS W/ cocaine-induced anxiety disorder	55	N/A
F14981	Cocaine use, NOS W/ cocaine-induced sexual dysfunction	55	N/A
F14982	Cocaine use, NOS W/ cocaine-induced sleep disorder	55	N/A
F14988	Cocaine use, NOS W/ cocaine-induced disorder, NEC	55	N/A
F1499	Cocaine use, NOS W/ cocaine-induced disorder, NOS	55	N/A
F15120	Other stimulant abuse W/ intoxication, uncomplicated	55	N/A
F15121	Other stimulant abuse W/ intoxication delirium	55	N/A
F15122	Other stimulant abuse W/ intoxication W/ perceptual disturbance	55	N/A
F15129	Other stimulant abuse W/ intoxication, NOS	55	N/A
F1514	Other stimulant abuse W/ stimulant-induced mood disorder	55	N/A
F15150	Other stimulant abuse W/ stimulant-induced psychotic disorder W/ delusions	54	N/A
F15151	Other stimulant abuse W/ stimulant-induced psychotic disorder W/ hallucinations	54	N/A
F15159	Other stimulant abuse W/ stimulant-induced psychotic disorder, NOS	54	N/A
F15180	Other stimulant abuse W/ stimulant-induced anxiety disorder	55	N/A
F15181	Other stimulant abuse W/ stimulant-induced sexual dysfunction	55	N/A
F15182	Other stimulant abuse W/ stimulant-induced sleep disorder	55	N/A
F15188	Other stimulant abuse W/ stimulant-induced disorder, nEC	55	N/A
F1519	Other stimulant abuse W/ stimulant-induced disorder, NOS	55	N/A
F1520	Other stimulant dependence, uncomplicated	55	N/A
F1521	Other stimulant dependence, in remission	55	N/A
F15220	Other stimulant dependence W/ intoxication, uncomplicated	55	N/A
F15221	Other stimulant dependence W/ intoxication delirium	55	N/A
F15222	Other stimulant dependence W/ intoxication W/ perceptual disturbance	55	N/A
F15229	Other stimulant dependence W/ intoxication, NOS	55	N/A
F1523	Other stimulant dependence W/ withdrawal	55	N/A
F1524	Other stimulant dependence W/ stimulant-induced mood disorder	55	N/A

Code	Code Descriptors	HCC	RXHCC
F15250	Other stimulant dependence W/ stimulant-induced psychotic disorder W/ delusions	54	N/A
F15251	Other stimulant dependence W/ stimulant-induced psychotic disorder W/ hallucinations	54	N/A
F15259	Other stimulant dependence W/ stimulant-induced psychotic disorder, NOS	54	N/A
F15280	Other stimulant dependence W/ stimulant-induced anxiety disorder	55	N/A
F15281	Other stimulant dependence W/ stimulant-induced sexual dysfunction	55	N/A
F15282	Other stimulant dependence W/ stimulant-induced sleep disorder	55	N/A
F15288	Other stimulant dependence W/ stimulant-induced disorder, NEC	55	N/A
F1529	Other stimulant dependence W/ stimulant-induced disorder, NOS	55	N/A
F15920	Other stimulant use, NOS W/ intoxication, uncomplicated	55	N/A
F15921	Other stimulant use, NOS W/ intoxication delirium	55	N/A
F15922	Other stimulant use, NOS W/ intoxication W/ perceptual disturbance	55	N/A
F15929	Other stimulant use, NOS W/ intoxication, NOS	55	N/A
F1593	Other stimulant use, NOS W/ withdrawal	55	N/A
F1594	Other stimulant use, NOS W/ stimulant-induced mood disorder	55	N/A
F15950	Other stimulant use, NOS W/ stimulant-induced psychotic disorder W/ delusions	54	N/A
F15951	Other stimulant use, NOS W/ stimulant-induced psychotic disorder W/ hallucinations	54	N/A
F15959	Other stimulant use, NOS W/ stimulant-induced psychotic disorder, NOS	54	N/A
F15980	Other stimulant use, NOS W/ stimulant-induced anxiety disorder	55	N/A
F15981	Other stimulant use, NOS W/ stimulant-induced sexual dysfunction	55	N/A
F15982	Other stimulant use, NOS W/ stimulant-induced sleep disorder	55	N/A
F15988	Other stimulant use, NOS W/ stimulant-induced disorder, NEC	55	N/A
F1599	Other stimulant use, NOS W/ stimulant-induced disorder, NOS	55	N/A
F16120	Hallucinogen abuse W/ intoxication, uncomplicated	55	N/A
F16121	Hallucinogen abuse W/ intoxication W/ delirium	55	N/A
F16122	Hallucinogen abuse W/ intoxication W/ perceptual disturbance	55	N/A
F16129	Hallucinogen abuse W/ intoxication, NOS	55	N/A
F1614	Hallucinogen abuse W/ hallucinogen-induced mood disorder	55	N/A
F16150	Hallucinogen abuse W/ hallucinogen-induced psychotic disorder W/ delusions	54	N/A
F16151	Hallucinogen abuse W/ hallucinogen-induced psychotic disorder W/ hallucinations	54	N/A
F16159	Hallucinogen abuse W/ hallucinogen-induced psychotic disorder, NOS	54	N/A
F16180	Hallucinogen abuse W/ hallucinogen-induced anxiety disorder	55	N/A
F16183	Hallucinogen abuse W/ hallucinogen persisting perception disorder (flashbacks)	55	N/A
F16188	Hallucinogen abuse W/ other hallucinogen-induced disorder	55	N/A
F1619	Hallucinogen abuse W/ NOS hallucinogen-induced disorder	55	N/A
F1620	Hallucinogen dependence, uncomplicated	55	N/A
F1621	Hallucinogen dependence, in remission	55	N/A
F16220	Hallucinogen dependence W/ intoxication, uncomplicated	55	N/A
F16221	Hallucinogen dependence W/ intoxication W/ delirium	55	N/A
F16229	Hallucinogen dependence W/ intoxication, NOS	55	N/A
F1624	Hallucinogen dependence W/ hallucinogen-induced mood disorder	55	N/A
F16250	Hallucinogen dependence W/ hallucinogen-induced psychotic disorder W/ delusions	54	N/A
F16251	Hallucinogen dependence W/ hallucinogen-induced psychotic disorder W/ hallucinations	54	N/A
F16259	Hallucinogen dependence W/ hallucinogen-induced psychotic disorder, NOS	54	N/A
F16280	Hallucinogen dependence W/ hallucinogen-induced anxiety disorder	55	N/A
F16283	Hallucinogen dependence W/ hallucinogen persisting perception disorder (flashbacks)	55	N/A
F16288	Hallucinogen dependence W/ hallucinogen-induced disorder, NEC	55	N/A
F1629	Hallucinogen dependence W/ hallucinogen-induced disorder, NOS	55	N/A
F16920	Hallucinogen use, NOS W/ intoxication, uncomplicated	55	N/A
F16921	Hallucinogen use, NOS W/ intoxication W/ delirium	55	N/A
F16929	Hallucinogen use, NOS W/ intoxication, NOS	55	N/A
F1694	Hallucinogen use, NOS W/ hallucinogen-induced mood disorder	55	N/A
F16950	Hallucinogen use, NOS W/ hallucinogen-induced psychotic disorder W/ delusions	54	N/A
F16951	Hallucinogen use, NOS W/ hallucinogen-induced psychotic disorder W/ hallucinations	54	N/A
F16959	Hallucinogen use, NOS W/ hallucinogen-induced psychotic disorder, NOS	54	N/A

Code	Code Descriptors	HCC	RXHCC
F16980	Hallucinogen use, NOS W/ hallucinogen-induced anxiety disorder	55	N/A
F16983	Hallucinogen use, NOS W/ hallucinogen persisting perception disorder (flashbacks)	55	N/A
F16988	Hallucinogen use, NOS W/ other hallucinogen- induced disorder	55	N/A
F1699	Hallucinogen use, NOS W/ NOS hallucinogen- induced disorder	55	N/A
F18120	Inhalant abuse W/ intoxication, uncomplicated	55	N/A
F18121	Inhalant abuse W/ intoxication delirium	55	N/A
F18129	Inhalant abuse W/ intoxication, NOS	55	N/A
F1814	Inhalant abuse W/ inhalant-induced mood disorder	55	N/A
F18150	Inhalant abuse W/ inhalant-induced psychotic disorder W/ delusions	54	N/A
F18151	Inhalant abuse W/ inhalant-induced psychotic disorder W/ hallucinations	54	N/A
F18159	Inhalant abuse W/ inhalant-induced psychotic disorder, NOS	54	N/A
F1817	Inhalant abuse W/ inhalant-induced dementia	54	N/A
F18180	Inhalant abuse W/ inhalant-induced anxiety disorder	55	N/A
F18188	Inhalant abuse W/ inhalant-induced disorder, NEC	55	N/A
F1819	Inhalant abuse W/ inhalant-induced disorder, NOS	55	N/A
F1820	Inhalant dependence, uncomplicated	55	N/A
F1821	Inhalant dependence, in remission	55	N/A
F18220	Inhalant dependence W/ intoxication, uncomplicated	55	N/A
F18221	Inhalant dependence W/ intoxication delirium	55	N/A
F18229	Inhalant dependence W/ intoxication, NOS	55	N/A
F1824	Inhalant dependence W/ inhalant-induced mood disorder	55	N/A
F18250	Inhalant dependence W/ inhalant-induced psychotic disorder W/ delusions	54	N/A
F18251	Inhalant dependence W/ inhalant-induced psychotic disorder W/ hallucinations	54	N/A
F18259	Inhalant dependence W/ inhalant-induced psychotic disorder, NOS	54	N/A
F1827	Inhalant dependence W/ inhalant-induced dementia	54	N/A
F18280	Inhalant dependence W/ inhalant-induced anxiety disorder	55	N/A
F18288	Inhalant dependence W/ inhalant-induced disorder, NEC	55	N/A
F1829	Inhalant dependence W/ inhalant-induced disorder, NOS	55	N/A
F18920	Inhalant use, NOS W/ intoxication, uncomplicated	55	N/A

Code	Code Descriptors	HCC	RXHCC
F18921	Inhalant use, NOS W/ intoxication W/ delirium	55	N/A
F18929	Inhalant use, NOS W/ intoxication, NOS	55	N/A
F1894	Inhalant use, NOS W/ inhalant-induced mood disorder	55	N/A
F18950	Inhalant use, NOS W/ inhalant-induced psychotic disorder W/ delusions	54	N/A
F18951	Inhalant use, NOS W/ inhalant-induced psychotic disorder W/ hallucinations	54	N/A
F18959	Inhalant use, NOS W/ inhalant-induced psychotic disorder, NOS	54	N/A
F1897	Inhalant use, NOS W/ inhalant-induced persisting dementia	54	N/A
F18980	Inhalant use, NOS W/ inhalant-induced anxiety disorder	55	N/A
F18988	Inhalant use, NOS W/ inhalant-induced disorder, NEC	55	N/A
F1899	Inhalant use, NOS W/ inhalant-induced disorder, NOS	55	N/A
F19121	Other psychoactive substance abuse W/ intoxication delirium	55	N/A
F19122	Other psychoactive substance abuse W/ intoxication W/ perceptual disturbances	55	N/A
F19129	Other psychoactive substance abuse W/ intoxication, NOS	55	N/A
F1914	Other psychoactive substance abuse W/ psychoactive substance-induced mood disorder	55	N/A
F19150	Other psychoactive substance abuse W/ psychoactive substance-induced psychotic disorder W/ delusions	54	N/A
F19151	Other psychoactive substance abuse W/ psychoactive substance-induced psychotic disorder W/ hallucinations	54	N/A
F19159	Other psychoactive substance abuse W/ psychoactive substance-induced psychotic disorder, NOS	54	N/A
F1916	Other psychoactive substance abuse W/ psychoactive substance-induced persisting amnestic disorder	54	N/A
F1917	Other psychoactive substance abuse W/ psychoactive substance-induced persisting dementia	54	N/A
F19180	Other psychoactive substance abuse W/ psychoactive substance-induced anxiety disorder	55	N/A
F19181	Other psychoactive substance abuse W/ psychoactive substance-induced sexual dysfunction	55	N/A
F19182	Other psychoactive substance abuse W/ psychoactive substance-induced sleep disorder	55	N/A
F19188	Other psychoactive substance abuse W/ psychoactive substance-induced disorder, NEC	55	N/A

Code	Code Descriptors	HCC	RXHCC
F1919	Other psychoactive substance abuse W/ psychoactive substance-induced disorder, NOS	55	N/A
F1920	Other psychoactive substance dependence, uncomplicated	55	N/A
F1921	Other psychoactive substance dependence, in remission	55	N/A
F19220	Other psychoactive substance dependence W/ intoxication, uncomplicated	55	N/A
F19221	Other psychoactive substance dependence W/ intoxication delirium	55	N/A
F19222	Other psychoactive substance dependence W/ intoxication W/ perceptual disturbance	55	N/A
F19229	Other psychoactive substance dependence W/ intoxication, NOS	55	N/A
F19230	Other psychoactive substance dependence W/ withdrawal, uncomplicated	55	N/A
F19231	Other psychoactive substance dependence W/ withdrawal delirium	54	N/A
F19232	Other psychoactive substance dependence W/ withdrawal W/ perceptual disturbance	54	N/A
F19239	Other psychoactive substance dependence W/ withdrawal, NOS	55	N/A
F1924	Other psychoactive substance dependence W/ psychoactive substance-induced mood disorder	55	N/A
F19250	Other psychoactive substance dependence W/ psychoactive substance-induced psychotic disorder W/ delusions	54	N/A
F19251	Other psychoactive substance dependence W/ psychoactive substance-induced psychotic disorder W/ hallucinations	54	N/A
F19259	Other psychoactive substance dependence W/ psychoactive substance-induced psychotic disorder, NOS	54	N/A
F1926	Other psychoactive substance dependence W/ psychoactive substance-induced persisting amnestic disorder	54	N/A
F1927	Other psychoactive substance dependence W/ psychoactive substance-induced persisting dementia	54	N/A
F19280	Other psychoactive substance dependence W/ psychoactive substance-induced anxiety disorder	55	N/A
F19281	Other psychoactive substance dependence W/ psychoactive substance-induced sexual dysfunction	55	N/A
F19282	Other psychoactive substance dependence W/ psychoactive substance-induced sleep disorder	55	N/A
F19288	Other psychoactive substance dependence W/ psychoactive substance-induced disorder, NEC	55	N/A
F1929	Other psychoactive substance dependence W/ psychoactive substance-induced disorder, NOS	55	N/A

Code	Code Descriptors	HCC	RXHCC
F19920	Other psychoactive substance use, NOS W/ intoxication, uncomplicated	55	N/A
F19921	Other psychoactive substance use, NOS W/ intoxication W/ delirium	55	N/A
F19922	Other psychoactive substance use, NOS W/ intoxication W/ perceptual disturbance	55	N/A
F19929	Other psychoactive substance use, NOS W/ intoxication, NOS	55	N/A
F19930	Other psychoactive substance use, NOS W/ withdrawal, uncomplicated	55	N/A
F19931	Other psychoactive substance use, NOS W/ withdrawal delirium	54	N/A
F19932	Other psychoactive substance use, NOS W/ withdrawal W/ perceptual disturbance	54	N/A
F19939	Other psychoactive substance use, NOS W/ withdrawal, NOS	55	N/A
F1994	Other psychoactive substance use, NOS W/ psychoactive substance-induced mood disorder	55	N/A
F19950	Other psychoactive substance use, NOS W/ psychoactive substance-induced psychotic disorder W/ delusions	54	N/A
F19951	Other psychoactive substance use, NOS W/ psychoactive substance-induced psychotic disorder W/ hallucinations	54	N/A
F19959	Other psychoactive substance use, NOS W/ psychoactive substance-induced psychotic disorder, NOS	54	N/A
F1996	Other psychoactive substance use, NOS W/ psychoactive substance-induced persisting amnestic disorder	54	N/A
F1997	Other psychoactive substance use, NOS W/ psychoactive substance-induced persisting dementia	54	N/A
F19980	Other psychoactive substance use, NOS W/ psychoactive substance-induced anxiety disorder	55	N/A
F19981	Other psychoactive substance use, NOS W/ psychoactive substance-induced sexual dysfunction	55	N/A
F19982	Other psychoactive substance use, NOS W/ psychoactive substance-induced sleep disorder	55	N/A
F19988	Other psychoactive substance use, NOS W/ psychoactive substance-induced disorder, NEC	55	N/A
F1999	Other psychoactive substance use, NOS W/ psychoactive substance-induced disorder, NOS	55	N/A
F200	Paranoid schizophrenia	57	130
F201	Disorganized schizophrenia	57	130
F202	Catatonic schizophrenia	57	130
F203	Undifferentiated schizophrenia	57	130
F205	Residual schizophrenia	57	130
F2081	Schizophreniform disorder	57	130

Code	Code Descriptors	HCC	RXHCC
F2089	Schizophrenia, NEC	57	130
F209	Schizophrenia, NOS	57	130
F22	Delusional disorders	58	N/A
F24	Shared psychotic disorder	58	N/A
F250	Schizoaffective disorder, bipolar type	57	130
F251	Schizoaffective disorder, depressive type	57	130
F258	Schizoaffective disorder, NEC	57	130
F259	Schizoaffective disorder, NOS	57	130
F3010	Manic episode W/O psychotic symptoms, NOS	58	131
F3011	Manic episode W/O psychotic symptoms, mild	58	131
F3012	Manic episode W/O psychotic symptoms, moderate	58	131
F3013	Manic episode, severe, W/O psychotic symptoms	58	131
F302	Manic episode, severe W/ psychotic symptoms	58	131
F303	Manic episode in partial remission	58	131
F304	Manic episode in full remission	58	131
F308	Manic episode, NEC	58	131
F309	Manic episode, NOS	58	131
F310	Bipolar disorder, current episode hypomanic	58	131
F3110	Bipolar disorder, current episode manic W/O psychotic features, NOS	58	131
F3111	Bipolar disorder, current episode manic W/O psychotic features, mild	58	131
F3112	Bipolar disorder, current episode manic W/O psychotic features, moderate	58	131
F3113	Bipolar disorder, current episode manic W/O psychotic features, severe	58	131
F312	Bipolar disorder, current episode manic severe W/ psychotic features	58	131
F3130	Bipolar disorder, current episode depressed, mild or moderate severity, NOS	58	131
F3131	Bipolar disorder, current episode depressed, mild	58	131
F3132	Bipolar disorder, current episode depressed, moderate	58	131
F314	Bipolar disorder, current episode depressed, severe, W/O psychotic features	58	131
F315	Bipolar disorder, current episode depressed, severe, W/ psychotic features	58	131
F3160	Bipolar disorder, current episode mixed, NOS	58	131
F3161	Bipolar disorder, current episode mixed, mild	58	131
F3162	Bipolar disorder, current episode mixed, moderate	58	131
F3163	Bipolar disorder, current episode mixed, severe, W/O psychotic features	58	131
F3164	Bipolar disorder, current episode mixed, severe, W/ psychotic features	58	131

Code	Code Descriptors	HCC	RXHCC
F3170	Bipolar disorder, currently in remission, most recent episode NOS	58	131
F3171	Bipolar disorder, in partial remission, most recent episode hypomanic	58	131
F3172	Bipolar disorder, in full remission, most recent episode hypomanic	58	131
F3173	Bipolar disorder, in partial remission, most recent episode manic	58	131
F3174	Bipolar disorder, in full remission, most recent episode manic	58	131
F3175	Bipolar disorder, in partial remission, most recent episode depressed	58	131
F3176	Bipolar disorder, in full remission, most recent episode depressed	58	131
F3177	Bipolar disorder, in partial remission, most recent episode mixed	58	131
F3178	Bipolar disorder, in full remission, most recent episode mixed	58	131
F3181	Bipolar II disorder	58	131
F3189	Bipolar disorder, NEC	58	131
F319	Bipolar disorder, NOS	58	131
F320	Major depressive disorder, single episode, mild	58	132
F321	Major depressive disorder, single episode, moderate	58	132
F322	Major depressive disorder, single episode, severe W/O psychotic features	58	132
F323	Major depressive disorder, single episode, severe W/ psychotic features	58	132
F324	Major depressive disorder, single episode, in partial remission	58	132
F325	Major depressive disorder, single episode, in full remission	58	132
F3281	Premenstrual dysphoric disorder	N/A	134
F3289	Depressive episode, NEC	N/A	134
F329	Major depressive disorder, single episode, NOS	N/A	134
F330	Major depressive disorder, recurrent, mild	58	132
F331	Major depressive disorder, recurrent, moderate	58	132
F332	Major depressive disorder, recurrent severe W/O psychotic features	58	132
F333	Major depressive disorder, recurrent, severe W/ psychotic symptoms	58	132
F3340	Major depressive disorder, recurrent, in remission, NOS	58	132
F3341	Major depressive disorder, recurrent, in partial remission	58	132
F3342	Major depressive disorder, recurrent, in full remission	58	132
F338	Recurrent depressive disorder, NEC	58	132
F339	Major depressive disorder, recurrent, NOS	58	132
F340	Cyclothymic disorder	N/A	134

Code	Code Descriptors	HCC	RXHCC
F341	Dysthymic disorder	N/A	134
F3481	Disruptive mood dysregulation disorder	58	131
F3489	Persistent mood disorder, NEC	58	131
F349	Persistent mood [affective] disorder, NOS	58	131
F39	Mood [affective] disorder, NOS	58	131
F4000	Agoraphobia, NOS	N/A	135
F4001	Agoraphobia W/ panic disorder	N/A	135
F4002	Agoraphobia W/O panic disorder	N/A	135
F4010	Social phobia, NOS	N/A	135
F4011	Social phobia, generalized	N/A	135
F40210	Arachnophobia	N/A	135
F40218	Other animal type phobia	N/A	135
F40220	Fear of thunderstorms	N/A	135
F40228	Other natural environment type phobia	N/A	135
F40230	Fear of blood	N/A	135
F40231	Fear of injections & transfusions	N/A	135
F40232	Fear of other medical care	N/A	135
F40233	Fear of injury	N/A	135
F40240	Claustrophobia	N/A	135
F40241	Acrophobia	N/A	135
F40242	Fear of bridges	N/A	135
F40243	Fear of flying	N/A	135
F40248	Situational type phobia, NEC	N/A	135
F40290	Androphobia	N/A	135
F40291	Gynephobia	N/A	135
F40298	Phobia, NEC	N/A	135
F408	Phobic anxiety disorder, NEC	N/A	135
F409	Phobic anxiety disorder, NOS	N/A	135
F410	Panic disorder [episodic paroxysmal anxiety]	N/A	135
F411	Generalized anxiety disorder	N/A	135
F422	Mixed obsessional thoughts & acts	N/A	133
F423	Hoarding disorder	N/A	133
F424	Excoriation (skin-picking) disorder	N/A	133
F428	Obsessive-compulsive disorder, NEC	N/A	133
F429	Obsessive-compulsive disorder, NOS	N/A	133
F4310	Post-traumatic stress disorder, NOS	N/A	133
F4311	Post-traumatic stress disorder, acute	N/A	133
F4312	Post-traumatic stress disorder, chronic	N/A	133
F440	Dissociative amnesia	N/A	133
F441	Dissociative fugue	N/A	133
F442	Dissociative stupor	N/A	135
F444	Conversion disorder W/ motor symptom or deficit	N/A	135
F445	Conversion disorder W/ seizures or convulsions	N/A	135
F446	Conversion disorder W/ sensory symptom or deficit	N/A	135
F447	Conversion disorder W/ mixed symptom presentation	N/A	135
F4481	Dissociative identity disorder	N/A	133
F4489	Dissociative & conversion disorder, NEC	N/A	135
F449	Dissociative & conversion disorder, NOS	N/A	135
F450	Somatization disorder	N/A	135
F451	Undifferentiated somatoform disorder	N/A	135
F4520	Hypochondriacal disorder, NOS	N/A	135
F4521	Hypochondriasis	N/A	135
F4522	Body dysmorphic disorder	N/A	135
F4529	Hypochondriacal disorder, NEC	N/A	135
F458	Somatoform disorder, NEC	N/A	135
F459	Somatoform disorder, NOS	N/A	135
F481	Depersonalization-derealization syndrome	N/A	133
F5000	Anorexia nervosa, NOS	N/A	133
F5001	Anorexia nervosa, restricting type	N/A	133
F5002	Anorexia nervosa, binge eating/purging type	N/A	133
F502	Bulimia nervosa	N/A	133
F603	Borderline personality disorder	N/A	133
F605	Obsessive-compulsive personality disorder	N/A	133
F630	Pathological gambling	N/A	133
F631	Pyromania	N/A	133
F632	Kleptomania	N/A	133
F633	Trichotillomania	N/A	133
F6381	Intermittent explosive disorder	N/A	133
F6389	Impulse disorder, NEC	N/A	133
F639	Impulse disorder, NOS	N/A	133
F6810	Factitious disorder, NOS	N/A	135
F6811	Factitious disorder W/ predominantly psychological signs & symptoms	N/A	135
F6812	Factitious disorder W/ predominantly physical signs & symptoms	N/A	135
F6813	Factitious disorder W/ combined psychological & physical signs & symptoms	N/A	135
F70	Mild intellectual disabilities	N/A	148
F71	Moderate intellectual disabilities	N/A	147
F72	Severe intellectual disabilities	N/A	146
F73	Profound intellectual disabilities	N/A	146
F78	Intellectual disability, NEC	N/A	148
F79	Intellectual disability, NOS	N/A	148
F840	Autistic disorder	N/A	145
F842	Rett's syndrome	N/A	145
F843	Childhood disintegrative disorder, NEC	N/A	145
F845	Asperger's syndrome	N/A	145
F848	Pervasive developmental disorder, NEC	N/A	145
F849	Pervasive developmental disorder, NOS	N/A	145

Code	Code Descriptors	HCC	RXHCC
F900	Attention-deficit hyperactivity disorder, predominantly inattentive type	N/A	133
F901	Attention-deficit hyperactivity disorder, predominantly hyperactive type	N/A	133
F902	Attention-deficit hyperactivity disorder, combined type	N/A	133
F908	Attention-deficit hyperactivity disorder, NEC type	N/A	133
F909	Attention-deficit hyperactivity disorder, NOS type	N/A	133
F910	Conduct disorder confined to family context	N/A	133
F911	Conduct disorder, childhood-onset type	N/A	133
F912	Conduct disorder, adolescent-onset type	N/A	133
F913	Oppositional defiant disorder	N/A	133
F918	Conduct disorder, NEC	N/A	133
F919	Conduct disorder, NOS	N/A	133
F952	Tourette's disorder	N/A	133
F984	Stereotyped movement disorders	N/A	133
G041	Tropical spastic paraplegia	72	157
G0489	Myelitis, NEC	72	157
G0491	Myelitis, NOS	72	157
G054	Myelitis in DZ classified elsewhere	72	157
G10	Huntington's DZ	78	161
G110	Congenital nonprogressive ataxia	72	N/A
G111	Early-onset cerebellar ataxia	72	N/A
G112	Late-onset cerebellar ataxia	72	N/A
G113	Cerebellar ataxia W/ defective DNA repair	72	N/A
G114	Hereditary spastic paraplegia	72	N/A
G118	Hereditary ataxia, NEC	72	N/A
G119	Hereditary ataxia, NOS	72	N/A
G120	Infantile spinal muscular atrophy, type I [Werdnig- Hoffman]	72	157
G121	Inherited spinal muscular atrophy, NEC	72	157
G1220	Motor neuron DZ, NOS	73	156
G1221	Amyotrophic lateral sclerosis	73	156
G1222	Progressive bulbar palsy	73	156
G1223	Primary lateral sclerosis	73	156
G1224	Familial motor neuron disease	73	156
G1225	Progressive spinal muscle atrophy	73	156
G1229	Motor neuron DZ, NEC	73	156
G128	Spinal muscular atrophies & related syndromes, NEC	72	157
G129	Spinal muscular atrophy, NOS	72	157
G130	Paraneoplastic neuromyopathy & neuropathy	75	159
G131	Systemic atrophy primarily affecting CNS in neoplastic DZ, NEC	75	159
G132	Systemic atrophy primarily affecting CNS in myxedema	52	112
G138	Systemic atrophy primarily affecting CNS in other DZ classified elsewhere	52	112
G20	Parkinson's DZ	78	161
G2111	Neuroleptic induced parkinsonism	78	161
G2119	Other drug induced 2ndary parkinsonism	78	161
G212	2ndary parkinsonism D/T other external agents	78	161
G213	Postencephalitic parkinsonism	78	161
G214	Vascular parkinsonism	78	161
G218	2ndary parkinsonism, NEC	78	161
G219	2ndary parkinsonism, NOS	78	161
G230	Hallervorden-Spatz DZ	78	N/A
G231	Progressive supranuclear ophthalmoplegia [Steele- Richardson-Olszewski]	78	N/A
G232	Striatonigral degeneration	78	N/A
G238	Degenerative DZ of basal ganglia, NEC	78	N/A
G239	Degenerative DZ of basal ganglia, NOS	78	N/A
G300	Alzheimer's DZ W/ early onset	52	111
G301	Alzheimer's DZ W/ late onset	52	111
G308	Alzheimer's DZ, NEC	52	111
G309	Alzheimer's DZ, NOS	52	111
G3101	Pick's DZ	52	112
G3109	Other frontotemporal dementia	52	112
G311	Senile degeneration of brain, NEC	52	112
G312	Degeneration of nervous system D/T alcohol	52	112
G3181	Alpers DZ	52	112
G3182	Leigh's DZ	52	112
G3183	Dementia W/ Lewy bodies	52	112
G3185	Corticobasal degeneration	52	112
G3189	Degenerative DZ of nervous system, NEC	52	112
G319	Degenerative DZ of nervous system, NOS	52	112
G320	Subacute combined degeneration of spinal cord in DZ classified elsewhere	72	157
G3281	Cerebellar ataxia in DZ classified elsewhere	72	N/A
G35	Multiple sclerosis	77	160
G360	Neuromyelitis optica [Devic]	77	160
G361	Acute & subacute hemorrhagic leukoencephalitis [Hurst]	77	N/A
G368	Acute disseminated demyelination, NEC	77	N/A
G369	Acute disseminated demyelination, NOS	77	N/A
G370	Diffuse sclerosis of CNS	77	160
G371	Central demyelination of corpus callosum	77	N/A
G372	Central pontine myelinolysis	77	N/A
G373	Acute transverse myelitis in demyelinating CNS DZ	72	157
G374	Subacute necrotizing myelitis of CNS	72	157
G375	Concentric sclerosis [Balo] of CNS	77	160
G378	Demyelinating DZ of CNS, NEC	77	N/A

Code	Code Descriptors	HCC	RXHCC
G379	Demyelinating DZ of CNS, NOS	77	N/A
G40001	Localization-related idiopathic epilepsy & epileptic syndromes W/ seizures of localized onset, not intractable, W/ status epilepticus	79	164
G40009	Localization-related idiopathic epilepsy & epileptic syndromes W/ seizures of localized onset, not intractable, W/O status epilepticus	79	164
G40011	Localization-related idiopathic epilepsy & epileptic syndromes W/ seizures of localized onset, intractable, W/ status epilepticus	79	163
G40019	Localization-related idiopathic epilepsy & epileptic syndromes W/ seizures of localized onset, intractable, W/O status epilepticus	79	163
G40101	Localization-related symptomatic epilepsy & epileptic syndromes W/ simple partial seizures, not intractable, W/ status epilepticus	79	164
G40109	Localization-related symptomatic epilepsy & epileptic syndromes W/ simple partial seizures, not intractable, W/O status epilepticus	79	164
G40111	Localization-related symptomatic epilepsy & epileptic syndromes W/ simple partial seizures, intractable, W/ status epilepticus	79	163
G40119	Localization-related symptomatic epilepsy & epileptic syndromes W/ simple partial seizures, intractable, W/O status epilepticus	79	163
G40201	Localization-related symptomatic epilepsy & epileptic syndromes W/ complex partial seizures, not intractable, W/ status epilepticus	79	164
G40209	Localization-related symptomatic epilepsy & epileptic syndromes W/ complex partial seizures, not intractable, W/O status epilepticus	79	164
G40211	Localization-related symptomatic epilepsy & epileptic syndromes W/ complex partial seizures, intractable, W/ status epilepticus	79	163
G40219	Localization-related symptomatic epilepsy & epileptic syndromes W/ complex partial seizures, intractable, W/O status epilepticus	79	163
G40301	Generalized idiopathic epilepsy & epileptic syndromes, not intractable, W/ status epilepticus	79	164
G40309	Generalized idiopathic epilepsy & epileptic syndromes, not intractable, W/O status epilepticus	79	164
G40311	Generalized idiopathic epilepsy & epileptic syndromes, intractable, W/ status epilepticus	79	163
G40319	Generalized idiopathic epilepsy & epileptic syndromes, intractable, W/O status epilepticus	79	163
G40401	Other generalized epilepsy & epileptic syndromes, not intractable, W/ status epilepticus	79	164

Code	Code Descriptors	HCC	RXHCC
G40409	Other generalized epilepsy & epileptic syndromes, not intractable, W/O status epilepticus	79	164
G40411	Other generalized epilepsy & epileptic syndromes, intractable, W/ status epilepticus	79	163
G40419	Other generalized epilepsy & epileptic syndromes, intractable, W/O status epilepticus	79	163
G40501	Epileptic seizures related to external causes, not intractable, W/ status epilepticus	79	164
G40509	Epileptic seizures related to external causes, not intractable, W/O status epilepticus	79	164
G40801	Other epilepsy, not intractable, W/ status epilepticus	79	164
G40802	Other epilepsy, not intractable, W/O status epilepticus	79	164
G40803	Other epilepsy, intractable, W/ status epilepticus	79	163
G40804	Other epilepsy, intractable, W/O status epilepticus	79	163
G40811	Lennox-Gastaut syndrome, not intractable, W/ status epilepticus	79	164
G40812	Lennox-Gastaut syndrome, not intractable, W/O status epilepticus	79	164
G40813	Lennox-Gastaut syndrome, intractable, W/ status epilepticus	79	163
G40814	Lennox-Gastaut syndrome, intractable, W/O status epilepticus	79	163
G40821	Epileptic spasms, not intractable, W/ status epilepticus	79	164
G40822	Epileptic spasms, not intractable, W/O status epilepticus	79	164
G40823	Epileptic spasms, intractable, W/ status epilepticus	79	163
G40824	Epileptic spasms, intractable, W/O status epilepticus	79	163
G4089	Seizures, NEC	79	164
G40901	Epilepsy, NOS, not intractable, W/ status epilepticus	79	164
G40909	Epilepsy, NOS, not intractable, W/O status epilepticus	79	164
G40911	Epilepsy, NOS, intractable, W/ status epilepticus	79	163
G40919	Epilepsy, NOS, intractable, W/O status epilepticus	79	163
G40A01	Absence epileptic syndrome, not intractable, W/ status epilepticus	79	164
G40A09	Absence epileptic syndrome, not intractable, W/O status epilepticus	79	164
G40A11	Absence epileptic syndrome, intractable, W/ status epilepticus	79	163
G40A19	Absence epileptic syndrome, intractable, W/O status epilepticus	79	163

Code	Code Descriptors	HCC	RXHCC
G40B01	Juvenile myoclonic epilepsy, not intractable, W/ status epilepticus	79	164
G40B09	Juvenile myoclonic epilepsy, not intractable, W/O status epilepticus	79	164
G40B11	Juvenile myoclonic epilepsy, intractable, W/ status epilepticus	79	163
G40B19	Juvenile myoclonic epilepsy, intractable, W/O status epilepticus	79	163
For codes G4300- through G4391-, use the following 6th character: 1 with status migrainosus 9 without status migrainosus			
G4300-	Migraine W/O aura, not intractable	N/A	166
G4301-	Migraine W/O aura, intractable	N/A	166
G4310-	Migraine W/ aura, not intractable	N/A	166
G4311-	Migraine W/ aura, intractable	N/A	166
G4340-	Hemiplegic migraine, not intractable	N/A	166
G4341-	Hemiplegic migraine, intractable	N/A	166
G4350-	Persistent migraine aura W/O cerebral infarction, not intractable	N/A	166
G4351-	Persistent migraine aura W/O cerebral infarction, intractable	N/A	166
G4360-	Persistent migraine aura W/ cerebral infarction, not intractable	N/A	166
G4361-	Persistent migraine aura W/ cerebral infarction, intractable	N/A	166
G4370-	Chronic migraine W/O aura, not intractable	N/A	166
G4371-	Chronic migraine W/O aura, intractable	N/A	166
G4380-	Migraine NEC, not intractable	N/A	166
G4381-	Migraine NEC, intractable	N/A	166
G4382-	Menstrual migraine, not intractable	N/A	166
G4383-	Menstrual migraine, intractable	N/A	166
G4390-	Migraine, NOS, not intractable	N/A	166
G4391-	Migraine, NOS, intractable	N/A	166
G43A0	Cyclical vomiting, not intractable	N/A	166
G43A1	Cyclical vomiting, intractable	N/A	166
G43B0	Ophthalmoplegic migraine, not intractable	N/A	166
G43B1	Ophthalmoplegic migraine, intractable	N/A	166
G43C0	Periodic headache syndromes in child or adult, not intractable	N/A	166
G43C1	Periodic headache syndromes in child or adult, intractable	N/A	166
G43D0	Abdominal migraine, not intractable	N/A	166
G43D1	Abdominal migraine, intractable	N/A	166
G450	Vertebro-basilar artery syndrome	N/A	206
G451	Carotid artery syndrome (hemispheric)	N/A	206
G452	Multiple & bilateral precerebral artery syndromes	N/A	206
G458	Transient cerebral ischemic attacks & related syndromes, NEC	N/A	206
G459	Transient cerebral ischemic attack, NOS	N/A	206

Code	Code Descriptors	HCC	RXHCC
G460	Middle cerebral artery syndrome	N/A	206
G461	Anterior cerebral artery syndrome	N/A	206
G462	Posterior cerebral artery syndrome	N/A	206
G463	Brain stem stroke syndrome	N/A	206
G464	Cerebellar stroke syndrome	N/A	206
G465	Pure motor lacunar syndrome	N/A	206
G466	Pure sensory lacunar syndrome	N/A	206
G467	Lacunar syndrome, NEC	N/A	206
G468	Vascular syndromes of brain in cerebrovascular DZ, NEC	N/A	206
G47411	Narcolepsy W/ cataplexy	N/A	355
G47419	Narcolepsy W/O cataplexy	N/A	355
G47421	Narcolepsy in conditions classified elsewhere W/ cataplexy	N/A	355
G47429	Narcolepsy in conditions classified elsewhere W/O cataplexy	N/A	355
G500	Trigeminal neuralgia	N/A	168
G501	Atypical facial pain	N/A	168
G508	Disorder of trigeminal nerve, NEC	N/A	168
G509	Disorder of trigeminal nerve, NOS	N/A	168
G546	Phantom limb syndrome W/ pain	189	N/A
G547	Phantom limb syndrome W/O pain	189	N/A
G600	Hereditary motor & sensory neuropathy	75	N/A
G601	Refsum's DZ	75	N/A
G602	Neuropathy in association W/ hereditary ataxia	75	N/A
G603	Idiopathic progressive neuropathy	75	N/A
G608	Hereditary & idiopathic neuropathy, NEC	75	N/A
G609	Hereditary & idiopathic neuropathy, NOS	75	N/A
G610	Guillain-Barre syndrome	75	159
G611	Serum neuropathy	75	159
G6181	Chronic inflammatory demyelinating polyneuritis	75	159
G6182	Multifocal motor neuropathy	75	159
G6189	Inflammatory polyneuropathy, NEC	75	159
G619	Inflammatory polyneuropathy, NOS	75	159
G620	Drug-induced polyneuropathy	75	159
G621	Alcoholic polyneuropathy	75	159
G622	Polyneuropathy D/T toxic agent NEC	75	159
G6281	Critical illness polyneuropathy	75	159
G6282	Radiation-induced polyneuropathy	75	159
G6289	Polyneuropathy, NEC	75	N/A
G629	Polyneuropathy, NOS	75	N/A
G63	Polyneuropathy in DZ classified elsewhere	75	159
G64	Disorders of peripheral nervous system, NEC	75	N/A
G650	Sequelae of Guillain-Barre syndrome	75	159
G651	Sequelae of inflammatory polyneuropathy, NEC	75	159

Code	Code Descriptors	HCC	RXHCC
G652	Sequelae of toxic polyneuropathy	75	159
G7000	Myasthenia gravis W/O exacerbation	75	156
G7001	Myasthenia gravis W/ exacerbation	75	156
G701	Toxic myoneural disorders	75	156
G702	Congenital & developmental myasthenia	75	156
G7080	Lambert-Eaton syndrome, NOS	75	156
G7081	Lambert-Eaton syndrome in DZ classified elsewhere	75	156
G7089	Myoneural disorder, NEC	75	156
G709	Myoneural disorder, NOS	75	156
G710	Muscular dystrophy	76	N/A
G7111	Myotonic muscular dystrophy	76	N/A
G7112	Myotonia congenita	75	N/A
G7113	Myotonic chondrodystrophy	75	N/A
G7114	Drug induced myotonia	75	N/A
G7119	Myotonic disorder, NEC	75	N/A
G712	Congenital myopathies	76	N/A
G713	Mitochondrial myopathy, NEC	75	N/A
G718	Primary disorder of muscle, NEC	75	N/A
G719	Primary disorder of muscle, NOS	75	N/A
G720	Drug-induced myopathy	75	N/A
G721	Alcoholic myopathy	75	N/A
G722	Myopathy D/T toxic agents NEC	75	N/A
G723	Periodic paralysis	75	N/A
G7241	Inclusion body myositis	75	N/A
G7249	Other inflammatory & immune myopathies, NEC	75	N/A
G7281	Critical illness myopathy	75	N/A
G7289	Myopathy, NEC	75	N/A
G729	Myopathy, NOS	75	N/A
G731	Lambert-Eaton syndrome in neoplastic DZ	75	156
G733	Myasthenic syndromes in other DZ classified elsewhere	75	156
G737	Myopathy in DZ classified elsewhere	75	N/A
G800	Spastic quadriplegic cerebral palsy	74	N/A
G801	Spastic diplegic cerebral palsy	74	N/A
G802	Spastic hemiplegic cerebral palsy	74	N/A
G803	Athetoid cerebral palsy	74	N/A
G804	Ataxic cerebral palsy	74	N/A
G808	Cerebral palsy, NEC	74	N/A
G809	Cerebral palsy, NOS	74	N/A
For codes G810- through G819-, use the following 5th character: 0 affecting unspecified side 1 affecting right dominant side 2 affecting left dominant side 3 affecting right non-dominant side 4 affecting left non-dominant side			
G810-	Flaccid hemiplegia	103	N/A
G811-	Spastic hemiplegia	103	207
G819-	Hemiplegia, NOS	103	N/A
G8220	Paraplegia, NOS	71	N/A
G8221	Paraplegia, complete	71	N/A
G8222	Paraplegia, incomplete	71	N/A
G8250	Quadriplegia, NOS	70	N/A
G8251	Quadriplegia, C1-C4 complete	70	N/A
G8252	Quadriplegia, C1-C4 incomplete	70	N/A
G8253	Quadriplegia, C5-C7 complete	70	N/A
G8254	Quadriplegia, C5-C7 incomplete	70	N/A
G830	Diplegia of upper limbs	104	N/A
For codes G831- through G833-, use the following 5th character: 0 affecting unspecified side 1 affecting right dominant side 2 affecting left dominant side 3 affecting right non-dominant side 4 affecting left non-dominant side			
G831-	Monoplegia of lower limb	104	N/A
G832-	Monoplegia of upper limb	104	N/A
G833-	Monoplegia, NOS	104	N/A
G834	Cauda equina syndrome	72	157
G835	Locked-in state	104	N/A
G8381	Brown-Sequard syndrome	104	N/A
G8382	Anterior cord syndrome	104	N/A
G8383	Posterior cord syndrome	104	N/A
G8384	Todd's paralysis (postepileptic)	104	N/A
G8389	Paralytic syndrome, NEC	104	N/A
G839	Paralytic syndrome, NOS	104	N/A
G9001	Carotid sinus syncope	75	N/A
G9009	Idiopathic peripheral autonomic neuropathy, NEC	75	N/A
G901	Familial dysautonomia [Riley-Day]	72	157
G902	Horner's syndrome	75	N/A
G903	Multi-system degeneration of autonomic nervous system	78	N/A
G904	Autonomic dysreflexia	75	N/A
G9050	Complex regional pain syndrome I, NOS	75	N/A
G90511	Complex regional pain syndrome I of R upper limb	75	N/A
G90512	Complex regional pain syndrome I of L upper limb	75	N/A
G90513	Complex regional pain syndrome I of upper limb, bilateral	75	N/A
G90519	Complex regional pain syndrome I of NOS upper limb	75	N/A
G90521	Complex regional pain syndrome I of R lower limb	75	N/A
G90522	Complex regional pain syndrome I of L lower limb	75	N/A
G90523	Complex regional pain syndrome I of lower limb, bilateral	75	N/A

Code	Code Descriptors	HCC	RXHCC
G90529	Complex regional pain syndrome I of NOS lower limb	75	N/A
G9059	Complex regional pain syndrome I of NEC site	75	N/A
G908	Disorder of autonomic nervous system, NEC	75	N/A
G909	Disorder of autonomic nervous system, NOS	75	N/A
G910	Communicating hydrocephalus	51	N/A
G911	Obstructive hydrocephalus	51	N/A
G912	Normal pressure hydrocephalus	51	N/A
G913	Post-traumatic hydrocephalus, NOS	51	N/A
G914	Hydrocephalus in DZ classified elsewhere	51	N/A
G918	Hydrocephalus, NEC	51	N/A
G919	Hydrocephalus, NOS	51	N/A
G931	Anoxic brain damage, NEC	80	N/A
G935	Compression of brain	80	N/A
G936	Cerebral edema	80	N/A
G937	Reye's syndrome	52	112
G950	Syringomyelia & syringobulbia	72	157
G9511	Acute infarction of spinal cord	72	157
G9519	Vascular myelopathy, NEC	72	157
G9520	Cord compression, NOS	72	157
G9529	Cord compression, NEC	72	157
G9581	Conus medullaris syndrome	72	157
G9589	DZ of spinal cord, NEC	72	157
G959	DZ of spinal cord, NOS	72	157
G990	Autonomic neuropathy in DZ classified elsewhere	75	N/A
G992	Myelopathy in DZ classified elsewhere	72	157
For codes H35321- through H35329-, use the following 7th character: 0 stage NOS 1 with active choroidal neovascularization 2 with inactive choroidal neovascularization 3 with inactive scar			
H35321-	Exudative ARMD, R eye	124	N/A
H35322-	Exudative ARMD, L eye	124	N/A
H35323-	Exudative ARMD, bilateralOS	124	N/A
H35329-	Exudative ARMD, NOS eye	124	N/A
For codes H4010X- through H40139-, use the following 7th character: 0 stage unspecified 1 mild stage 2 moderate stage 3 severe stage 4 indeterminate stage			
H4010X-	NOS OAG	N/A	243
H40111-	Primary OAG, R eye	N/A	243
H40112-	Primary OAG, L eye	N/A	243
H40113-	Primary OAG, bilateral	N/A	243
H40119-	Primary OAG, NOS eye	N/A	243

Code	Code Descriptors	HCC	RXHCC
H40121-	Low-tension glaucoma, R eye	N/A	243
H40122-	Low-tension glaucoma, L eye	N/A	243
H40123-	Low-tension glaucoma, bilateral	N/A	243
H40129-	Low-tension glaucoma, NOS eye	N/A	243
H40131-	Pigmentary glaucoma, R eye	N/A	243
H40132-	Pigmentary glaucoma, L eye	N/A	243
H40133-	Pigmentary glaucoma, bilateral	N/A	243
H40139-	Pigmentary glaucoma, NOS eye	N/A	243
H40151	Residual stage of OAG, R eye	N/A	243
H40152	Residual stage of OAG, L eye	N/A	243
H40153	Residual stage of OAG, bilateral	N/A	243
H40159	Residual stage of OAG, NOS eye	N/A	243
H4310	Vitreous hemorrhage, NOS eye	122	N/A
H4311	Vitreous hemorrhage, R eye	122	N/A
H4312	Vitreous hemorrhage, L eye	122	N/A
H4313	Vitreous hemorrhage, bilateral	122	N/A
H49811	Kearns-Sayre syndrome, R eye	23	41
H49812	Kearns-Sayre syndrome, L eye	23	41
H49813	Kearns-Sayre syndrome, bilateral	23	41
H49819	Kearns-Sayre syndrome, NOS eye	23	41
I0981	Rheumatic HF	85	186
I10	Essential (primary) hypertension	N/A	187
I110	Hypertensive heart DZ W/ HF	85	186
I119	Hypertensive heart DZ W/O HF	N/A	187
I120	Hypertensive CKD W/ stage 5 CKD or ESRD	136	187, 262
I129	Hypertensive CKD W/ stage 1 through stage 4 CKD, or NOS CKD	139	187
I130	Hypertensive heart & CKD W/ HF & stage 1-4 CKD, or CKD NOS	85, 139	186
I1310	Hypertensive heart & CKD W/O HF, W/ stage 1-4 CKD, or CKD NOS	139	187
I1311	Hypertensive heart & CKD W/O HF, W/ stage 5 CKD, or ESRD	136	187, 262
I132	Hypertensive heart & CKD W/ HF & W/ stage 5 CKD, or ESRD	85, 136	186, 262
I150	Renovascular hypertension	N/A	187
I151	Hypertension 2ndary to other renal disorder	N/A	187
I152	Hypertension 2ndary to endocrine disorder	N/A	187
I158	2ndary hypertension, NEC	N/A	187
I159	2ndary hypertension, NOS	N/A	187
I160	Hypertensive urgency	N/A	187
I161	Hypertensive emergency	N/A	187
I169	Hypertensive crisis, NOS	N/A	187
I200	Unstable angina	87	188
I201	Angina pectoris W/ documented spasm	88	188
I208	Angina pectoris, NEC	88	188
I209	Angina pectoris, NOS	88	188

Code	Code Descriptors	HCC	RXHCC
I2101	STEMI involving L main coronary artery	86	188
I2102	STEMI involving L anterior descending coronary artery	86	188
I2109	STEMI involving other coronary artery of anterior wall	86	188
I2111	STEMI involving R coronary artery	86	188
I2119	STEMI involving other coronary artery of inferior wall	86	188
I2121	STEMI involving L circumflex coronary artery	86	188
I2129	STEMI of NEC site	86	188
I213	STEMI of NOS site	86	188
I214	NSTEMI	86	188
I220	Subsequent STEMI of anterior wall	86	188
I221	Subsequent STEMI of inferior wall	86	188
I222	Subsequent NSTEMI	86	188
I228	Subsequent STEMI of NEC site	86	188
I229	Subsequent STEMI of NOS site	86	188
I21A1	Myocardial infarction type 2	86	188
I21A9	Myocardial infarction type NEC	86	188
I230	Hemopericardium as current complication following AMI	87	188
I231	Atrial septal defect as current complication following AMI	87	188
I232	Ventricular septal defect as current complication following AMI	87	188
I233	Rupture of cardiac wall W/O hemopericardium as current complication following AMI	87	188
I234	Rupture of chordae tendineae as current complication following AMI	86	188
I235	Rupture of papillary muscle as current complication following AMI	86	188
I236	Thrombosis of atrium, auricular appendage, & ventricle as current complications following AMI	87	188
I237	Postinfarction angina	87	188
I238	Other current complications following AMI	87	188
I240	Acute coronary thrombosis not resulting in myocardial infarction	87	188
I241	Dressler's syndrome	87	188
I248	Acute ischemic heart DZ, NEC	87	188
I249	Acute ischemic heart DZ, NOS	87	188
I2510	Atherosclerotic heart DZ of native coronary artery W/O angina pectoris	N/A	188
I25110	Atherosclerotic heart DZ of native coronary artery W/ unstable angina pectoris	87	188
I25111	Atherosclerotic heart DZ of native coronary artery W/ angina pectoris W/ documented spasm	88	188
I25118	Atherosclerotic heart DZ of native coronary artery W/ other forms of angina pectoris	88	188

Code	Code Descriptors	HCC	RXHCC
I25119	Atherosclerotic heart DZ of native coronary artery W/ NOS angina pectoris	88	188
I252	Old myocardial infarction	N/A	188
I253	Aneurysm of heart	N/A	188
I2541	Coronary artery aneurysm	N/A	188
I2542	Coronary artery dissection	N/A	188
I255	Ischemic cardiomyopathy	N/A	188
I256	Silent myocardial ischemia	N/A	188
I25700	Atherosclerosis of coronary artery bypass graft(s), NOS, W/ unstable angina pectoris	87	188
I25701	Atherosclerosis of coronary artery bypass graft(s), NOS, W/ angina pectoris W/ documented spasm	88	188
I25708	Atherosclerosis of coronary artery bypass graft(s), NOS, W/ other forms of angina pectoris	88	188
I25709	Atherosclerosis of coronary artery bypass graft(s), NOS, W/ NOS angina pectoris	88	188
I25710	Atherosclerosis of autologous vein coronary artery bypass graft(s) W/ unstable angina pectoris	87	188
I25711	Atherosclerosis of autologous vein coronary artery bypass graft(s) W/ angina pectoris W/ documented spasm	88	188
I25718	Atherosclerosis of autologous vein coronary artery bypass graft(s) W/ other forms of angina pectoris	88	188
I25719	Atherosclerosis of autologous vein coronary artery bypass graft(s) W/ NOS angina pectoris	88	188
I25720	Atherosclerosis of autologous artery coronary artery bypass graft(s) W/ unstable angina pectoris	87	188
I25721	Atherosclerosis of autologous artery coronary artery bypass graft(s) W/ angina pectoris W/ documented spasm	88	188
I25728	Atherosclerosis of autologous artery coronary artery bypass graft(s) W/ other forms of angina pectoris	88	188
I25729	Atherosclerosis of autologous artery coronary artery bypass graft(s) W/ NOS angina pectoris	88	188
I25730	Atherosclerosis of nonautologous biological coronary artery bypass graft(s) W/ unstable angina pectoris	87	188
I25731	Atherosclerosis of nonautologous biological coronary artery bypass graft(s) W/ angina pectoris W/ documented spasm	88	188
I25738	Atherosclerosis of nonautologous biological coronary artery bypass graft(s) W/ other forms of angina pectoris	88	188
I25739	Atherosclerosis of nonautologous biological coronary artery bypass graft(s) W/ NOS angina pectoris	88	188

Code	Code Descriptors	HCC	RXHCC
I25750	Atherosclerosis of native coronary artery of transplanted heart W/ unstable angina	87	188
I25751	Atherosclerosis of native coronary artery of transplanted heart W/ angina pectoris W/ documented spasm	88	188
I25758	Atherosclerosis of native coronary artery of transplanted heart W/ other forms of angina pectoris	88	188
I25759	Atherosclerosis of native coronary artery of transplanted heart W/ NOS angina pectoris	88	188
I25760	Atherosclerosis of bypass graft of coronary artery of transplanted heart W/ unstable angina	87	188
I25761	Atherosclerosis of bypass graft of coronary artery of transplanted heart W/ angina pectoris W/ documented spasm	88	188
I25768	Atherosclerosis of bypass graft of coronary artery of transplanted heart W/ other forms of angina pectoris	88	188
I25769	Atherosclerosis of bypass graft of coronary artery of transplanted heart W/ NOS angina pectoris	88	188
I25790	Atherosclerosis of other coronary artery bypass graft(s) W/ unstable angina pectoris	87	188
I25791	Atherosclerosis of other coronary artery bypass graft(s) W/ angina pectoris W/ documented spasm	88	188
I25798	Atherosclerosis of other coronary artery bypass graft(s) W/ other forms of angina pectoris	88	188
I25799	Atherosclerosis of other coronary artery bypass graft(s) W/ NOS angina pectoris	88	188
I25810	Atherosclerosis of coronary artery bypass graft(s) W/O angina pectoris	N/A	188
I25811	Atherosclerosis of native coronary artery of transplanted heart W/O angina pectoris	N/A	188
I25812	Atherosclerosis of bypass graft of coronary artery of transplanted heart W/O angina pectoris	N/A	188
I2582	Chronic total occlusion of coronary artery	N/A	188
I2583	Coronary atherosclerosis D/T lipid rich plaque	N/A	188
I2584	Coronary atherosclerosis D/T calcified coronary lesion	N/A	188
I2589	Chronic ischemic heart DZ, NEC	N/A	188
I259	Chronic ischemic heart DZ, NOS	N/A	188
I2601	Septic pulmonary embolism W/ acute cor pulmonale	85, 107	186, 215
I2602	Saddle embolus of pulmonary artery W/ acute cor pulmonale	85, 107	186, 215
I2609	Other pulmonary embolism W/ acute cor pulmonale	85, 107	186, 215
I2690	Septic pulmonary embolism W/O acute cor pulmonale	107	215

Code	Code Descriptors	HCC	RXHCC
I2692	Saddle embolus of pulmonary artery W/O acute cor pulmonale	107	215
I2699	Other pulmonary embolism W/O acute cor pulmonale	107	215
I270	Primary pulmonary hypertension	85	185
I271	Kyphoscoliotic heart DZ	85	186
I2720	Pulmonary hypertension, NOS	85	186
I2721	2ndary pulmonary arterial hypertension	85	186
I2722	Pulmonary hypertension D/T left heart disease	85	186
I2723	Pulmonary hypertension D/T lung disease & hypoxia	85	186
I2724	Chronic thromboembolic pulmonary hypertension	85	186
I2729	2ndary pulmonary hypertension, NEC	85	186
I2781	Cor pulmonale	85	186
I2782	Chronic pulmonary embolism	107	215
I2783	Eisenmenger's syndrome	85	185
I2789	Pulmonary heart DZ, NEC	85	186
I279	Pulmonary heart DZ, NOS	85	186
I280	Arteriovenous fistula of pulmonary vessels	85	186
I281	Aneurysm of pulmonary artery	85	186
I288	DZ of pulmonary vessels, NEC	85	186
I289	DZ of pulmonary vessels, NOS	85	186
I420	Dilated cardiomyopathy	85	186
I421	Obstructive hypertrophic cardiomyopathy	85	186
I422	Other hypertrophic cardiomyopathy	85	186
I423	Endomyocardial (eosinophilic) DZ	85	186
I424	Endocardial fibroelastosis	85	186
I425	Restrictive cardiomyopathy, NEC	85	186
I426	Alcoholic cardiomyopathy	85	186
I427	Cardiomyopathy D/T drug & external agent	85	186
I428	Cardiomyopathy, NEC	85	186
I429	Cardiomyopathy, NOS	85	186
I43	Cardiomyopathy in DZ classified elsewhere	85	186
I442	Atrioventricular block, complete	96	N/A
I462	Cardiac arrest D/T underlying cardiac condition	84	N/A
I468	Cardiac arrest D/T other underlying condition	84	N/A
I469	Cardiac arrest, cause NOS	84	N/A
I470	Re-entry ventricular arrhythmia	96	N/A
I471	Supraventricular tachycardia	96	193
I472	Ventricular tachycardia	96	N/A
I479	Paroxysmal tachycardia, NOS	96	193
I480	Paroxysmal atrial fibrillation	96	193
I481	Persistent atrial fibrillation	96	193
I482	Chronic atrial fibrillation	96	193

Code	Code Descriptors	HCC	RXHCC
I483	Typical atrial flutter	96	193
I484	Atypical atrial flutter	96	193
I4891	Atrial fibrillation, NOS	96	193
I4892	Atrial flutter, NOS	96	193
I4901	Ventricular fibrillation	84	N/A
I4902	Ventricular flutter	84	N/A
I492	Junctional premature depolarization	96	193
I495	Sick sinus syndrome	96	N/A
I501	L ventricular failure, NOS	85	186
I5020	Systolic HF, NOS	85	186
I5021	Acute systolic HF	85	186
I5022	Chronic systolic HF	85	186
I5023	Acute on chronic systolic HF	85	186
I5030	Diastolic HF, NOS	85	186
I5031	Acute diastolic HF	85	186
I5032	Chronic diastolic HF	85	186
I5033	Acute on chronic diastolic HF	85	186
I5040	Combined systolic & diastolic HF, NOS	85	186
I5041	Acute combined systolic & diastolic HF	85	186
I5042	Chronic combined systolic & diastolic HF	85	186
I5043	Acute on chronic combined systolic & diastolic HF	85	186
I50810	R HF, NOS	85	186
I50811	Acute R HF	85	186
I50812	Chronic R HF	85	186
I50813	Acute on chronic R HF	85	186
I50814	R HF due to L HF	85	186
I5082	Biventricular HF	85	186
I5083	High output HF	85	186
I5084	End stage HF	85	186
I5089	HF, NEC	85	186
I509	HF, NOS	85	186
I511	Rupture of chordae tendineae, NEC	86	188
I512	Rupture of papillary muscle, NEC	86	188
I514	Myocarditis, NOS	85	186
I515	Myocardial degeneration	85	186
I6000	Nontraumatic subarachnoid hemorrhage from NOS carotid siphon & bifurcation	99	N/A
I6001	Nontraumatic subarachnoid hemorrhage from R carotid siphon & bifurcation	99	N/A
I6002	Nontraumatic subarachnoid hemorrhage from L carotid siphon & bifurcation	99	N/A
I6010	Nontraumatic subarachnoid hemorrhage from NOS middle cerebral artery	99	N/A
I6011	Nontraumatic subarachnoid hemorrhage from R middle cerebral artery	99	N/A
I6012	Nontraumatic subarachnoid hemorrhage from L middle cerebral artery	99	N/A
I602	Nontraumatic subarachnoid hemorrhage from anterior communicating artery	99	N/A
I6030	Nontraumatic subarachnoid hemorrhage from NOS posterior communicating artery	99	N/A
I6031	Nontraumatic subarachnoid hemorrhage from R posterior communicating artery	99	N/A
I6032	Nontraumatic subarachnoid hemorrhage from L posterior communicating artery	99	N/A
I604	Nontraumatic subarachnoid hemorrhage from basilar artery	99	N/A
I6050	Nontraumatic subarachnoid hemorrhage from NOS vertebral artery	99	N/A
I6051	Nontraumatic subarachnoid hemorrhage from R vertebral artery	99	N/A
I6052	Nontraumatic subarachnoid hemorrhage from L vertebral artery	99	N/A
I606	Nontraumatic subarachnoid hemorrhage from other intracranial arteries	99	N/A
I607	Nontraumatic subarachnoid hemorrhage from intracranial artery, NOS	99	N/A
I608	Nontraumatic subarachnoid hemorrhage, NEC	99	N/A
I609	Nontraumatic subarachnoid hemorrhage, NOS	99	N/A
I610	Nontraumatic intracerebral hemorrhage in hemisphere, subcortical	99	N/A
I611	Nontraumatic intracerebral hemorrhage in hemisphere, cortical	99	N/A
I612	Nontraumatic intracerebral hemorrhage in hemisphere, NOS	99	N/A
I613	Nontraumatic intracerebral hemorrhage in brain stem	99	N/A
I614	Nontraumatic intracerebral hemorrhage in cerebellum	99	N/A
I615	Nontraumatic intracerebral hemorrhage, intraventricular	99	N/A
I616	Nontraumatic intracerebral hemorrhage, multiple localized	99	N/A
I618	Nontraumatic intracerebral hemorrhage NEC	99	N/A
I619	Nontraumatic intracerebral hemorrhage, NOS	99	N/A
I6200	Nontraumatic subdural hemorrhage, NOS	99	N/A
I6201	Nontraumatic acute subdural hemorrhage	99	N/A
I6202	Nontraumatic subacute subdural hemorrhage	99	N/A
I6203	Nontraumatic chronic subdural hemorrhage	99	N/A
I621	Nontraumatic extradural hemorrhage	99	N/A
I629	Nontraumatic intracranial hemorrhage, NOS	99	N/A
I6300	Cerebral infarction D/T thrombosis of NOS precerebral artery	100	206
I63011	Cerebral infarction D/T thrombosis of R vertebral artery	100	206

Code	Code Descriptors	HCC	RXHCC
I63012	Cerebral infarction D/T thrombosis of L vertebral artery	100	206
I63013	Cerebral infarction D/T thrombosis of bilateral vertebral arteries	100	206
I63019	Cerebral infarction D/T thrombosis of NOS vertebral artery	100	206
I6302	Cerebral infarction D/T thrombosis of basilar artery	100	206
I63031	Cerebral infarction D/T thrombosis of R carotid artery	100	206
I63032	Cerebral infarction D/T thrombosis of L carotid artery	100	206
I63033	Cerebral infarction D/T thrombosis of bilateral carotid arteries	100	206
I63039	Cerebral infarction D/T thrombosis of NOS carotid artery	100	206
I6309	Cerebral infarction D/T thrombosis of other precerebral artery	100	206
I6310	Cerebral infarction D/T embolism of NOS precerebral artery	100	206
I63111	Cerebral infarction D/T embolism of R vertebral artery	100	206
I63112	Cerebral infarction D/T embolism of L vertebral artery	100	206
I63113	Cerebral infarction D/T embolism of bilateral vertebral arteries	100	206
I63119	Cerebral infarction D/T embolism of NOS vertebral artery	100	206
I6312	Cerebral infarction D/T embolism of basilar artery	100	206
I63131	Cerebral infarction D/T embolism of R carotid artery	100	206
I63132	Cerebral infarction D/T embolism of L carotid artery	100	206
I63133	Cerebral infarction D/T embolism of bilateral carotid arteries	100	206
I63139	Cerebral infarction D/T embolism of NOS carotid artery	100	206
I6319	Cerebral infarction D/T embolism of other precerebral artery	100	206
I6320	Cerebral infarction D/T NOS occlusion or stenosis of NOS precerebral arteries	100	206
I63211	Cerebral infarction D/T NOS occlusion or stenosis of R vertebral artery	100	206
I63212	Cerebral infarction D/T NOS occlusion or stenosis of L vertebral artery	100	206
I63213	Cerebral infarction D/T NOS occlusion or stenosis of bilateral vertebral arteries	100	206
I63219	Cerebral infarction D/T NOS occlusion or stenosis of NOS vertebral arteries	100	206
I6322	Cerebral infarction D/T NOS occlusion or stenosis of basilar artery	100	206
I63231	Cerebral infarction D/T NOS occlusion or stenosis of R carotid arteries	100	206

Code	Code Descriptors	HCC	RXHCC
I63232	Cerebral infarction D/T NOS occlusion or stenosis of L carotid arteries	100	206
I63233	Cerebral infarction D/T NOS occlusion or stenosis of bilateral carotid arteries	100	206
I63239	Cerebral infarction D/T NOS occlusion or stenosis of NOS carotid arteries	100	206
I6329	Cerebral infarction D/T NOS occlusion or stenosis of other precerebral arteries	100	206
I6330	Cerebral infarction D/T thrombosis of NOS cerebral artery	100	206
I63311	Cerebral infarction D/T thrombosis of R middle cerebral artery	100	206
I63312	Cerebral infarction D/T thrombosis of L middle cerebral artery	100	206
I63313	Cerebral infarction D/T thrombosis of bilateral middle cerebral arteries	100	206
I63319	Cerebral infarction D/T thrombosis of NOS middle cerebral artery	100	206
I63321	Cerebral infarction D/T thrombosis of R anterior cerebral artery	100	206
I63322	Cerebral infarction D/T thrombosis of L anterior cerebral artery	100	206
I63323	Cerebral infarction D/T thrombosis of bilateral anterior cerebral arteries	100	206
I63329	Cerebral infarction D/T thrombosis of NOS anterior cerebral artery	100	206
I63331	Cerebral infarction D/T thrombosis of R posterior cerebral artery	100	206
I63332	Cerebral infarction D/T thrombosis of L posterior cerebral artery	100	206
I63333	Cerebral infarction to thrombosis of bilateral posterior cerebral arteries	100	206
I63339	Cerebral infarction D/T thrombosis of NOS posterior cerebral artery	100	206
I63341	Cerebral infarction D/T thrombosis of R cerebellar artery	100	206
I63342	Cerebral infarction D/T thrombosis of L cerebellar artery	100	206
I63343	Cerebral infarction to thrombosis of bilateral cerebellar arteries	100	206
I63349	Cerebral infarction D/T thrombosis of NOS cerebellar artery	100	206
I6339	Cerebral infarction D/T thrombosis of other cerebral artery	100	206
I6340	Cerebral infarction D/T embolism of NOS cerebral artery	100	206
I63411	Cerebral infarction D/T embolism of R middle cerebral artery	100	206
I63412	Cerebral infarction D/T embolism of L middle cerebral artery	100	206
I63413	Cerebral infarction D/T embolism of bilateral middle cerebral arteries	100	206
I63419	Cerebral infarction D/T embolism of NOS middle cerebral artery	100	206

Code	Code Descriptors	HCC	RXHCC
I63421	Cerebral infarction D/T embolism of R anterior cerebral artery	100	206
I63422	Cerebral infarction D/T embolism of L anterior cerebral artery	100	206
I63423	Cerebral infarction D/T embolism of bilateral anterior cerebral arteries	100	206
I63429	Cerebral infarction D/T embolism of NOS anterior cerebral artery	100	206
I63431	Cerebral infarction D/T embolism of R posterior cerebral artery	100	206
I63432	Cerebral infarction D/T embolism of L posterior cerebral artery	100	206
I63433	Cerebral infarction D/T embolism of bilateral posterior cerebral arteries	100	206
I63439	Cerebral infarction D/T embolism of NOS posterior cerebral artery	100	206
I63441	Cerebral infarction D/T embolism of R cerebellar artery	100	206
I63442	Cerebral infarction D/T embolism of L cerebellar artery	100	206
I63443	Cerebral infarction D/T embolism of bilateral cerebellar arteries	100	206
I63449	Cerebral infarction D/T embolism of NOS cerebellar artery	100	206
I6349	Cerebral infarction D/T embolism of other cerebral artery	100	206
I6350	Cerebral infarction D/T NOS occlusion or stenosis of NOS cerebral artery	100	206
I63511	Cerebral infarction D/T NOS occlusion or stenosis of R middle cerebral artery	100	206
I63512	Cerebral infarction D/T NOS occlusion or stenosis of L middle cerebral artery	100	206
I63513	Cerebral infarction D/T NOS occlusion or stenosis of bilateral middle cerebral arteries	100	206
I63519	Cerebral infarction D/T NOS occlusion or stenosis of NOS middle cerebral artery	100	206
I63521	Cerebral infarction D/T NOS occlusion or stenosis of R anterior cerebral artery	100	206
I63522	Cerebral infarction D/T NOS occlusion or stenosis of L anterior cerebral artery	100	206
I63523	Cerebral infarction D/T NOS occlusion or stenosis of bilateral anterior cerebral arteries	100	206
I63529	Cerebral infarction D/T NOS occlusion or stenosis of NOS anterior cerebral artery	100	206
I63531	Cerebral infarction D/T NOS occlusion or stenosis of R posterior cerebral artery	100	206
I63532	Cerebral infarction D/T NOS occlusion or stenosis of L posterior cerebral artery	100	206
I63533	Cerebral infarction D/T NOS occlusion or stenosis of bilateral posterior cerebral arteries	100	206
I63539	Cerebral infarction D/T NOS occlusion or stenosis of NOS posterior cerebral artery	100	206

Code	Code Descriptors	HCC	RXHCC
I63541	Cerebral infarction D/T NOS occlusion or stenosis of R cerebellar artery	100	206
I63542	Cerebral infarction D/T NOS occlusion or stenosis of L cerebellar artery	100	206
I63543	Cerebral infarction D/T NOS occlusion or stenosis of bilateral cerebellar arteries	100	206
I63549	Cerebral infarction D/T NOS occlusion or stenosis of NOS cerebellar artery	100	206
I6359	Cerebral infarction D/T NOS occlusion or stenosis of other cerebral artery	100	206
I636	Cerebral infarction D/T cerebral venous thrombosis, nonpyogenic	100	206
I638	Cerebral infarction, NEC	100	206
I639	Cerebral infarction, NOS	100	206
I6501	Occlusion & stenosis of R vertebral artery	N/A	206
I6502	Occlusion & stenosis of L vertebral artery	N/A	206
I6503	Occlusion & stenosis of bilateral vertebral arteries	N/A	206
I6509	Occlusion & stenosis of NOS vertebral artery	N/A	206
I651	Occlusion & stenosis of basilar artery	N/A	206
I6521	Occlusion & stenosis of R carotid artery	N/A	206
I6522	Occlusion & stenosis of L carotid artery	N/A	206
I6523	Occlusion & stenosis of bilateral carotid arteries	N/A	206
I6529	Occlusion & stenosis of NOS carotid artery	N/A	206
I658	Occlusion & stenosis of other precerebral arteries	N/A	206
I659	Occlusion & stenosis of NOS precerebral artery	N/A	206
I6601	Occlusion & stenosis of R middle cerebral artery	N/A	206
I6602	Occlusion & stenosis of L middle cerebral artery	N/A	206
I6603	Occlusion & stenosis of bilateral middle cerebral arteries	N/A	206
I6609	Occlusion & stenosis of NOS middle cerebral artery	N/A	206
I6611	Occlusion & stenosis of R anterior cerebral artery	N/A	206
I6612	Occlusion & stenosis of L anterior cerebral artery	N/A	206
I6613	Occlusion & stenosis of bilateral anterior cerebral arteries	N/A	206
I6619	Occlusion & stenosis of NOS anterior cerebral artery	N/A	206
I6621	Occlusion & stenosis of R posterior cerebral artery	N/A	206
I6622	Occlusion & stenosis of L posterior cerebral artery	N/A	206
I6623	Occlusion & stenosis of bilateral posterior cerebral arteries	N/A	206

Code	Code Descriptors	HCC	RXHCC
I6629	Occlusion & stenosis of NOS posterior cerebral artery	N/A	206
I663	Occlusion & stenosis of cerebellar arteries	N/A	206
I668	Occlusion & stenosis of other cerebral arteries	N/A	206
I669	Occlusion & stenosis of NOS cerebral artery	N/A	206
I670	Dissection of cerebral arteries, nonruptured	107	N/A
I672	Cerebral atherosclerosis	N/A	206
I673	Progressive vascular leukoencephalopathy	52	112
I674	Hypertensive encephalopathy	N/A	187
I675	Moyamoya DZ	N/A	206
I676	Nonpyogenic thrombosis of intracranial venous system	N/A	206
I677	Cerebral arteritis, NEC	N/A	206
I6781	Acute cerebrovascular insufficiency	N/A	206
I6782	Cerebral ischemia	N/A	206
I67841	Reversible cerebrovascular vasoconstriction syndrome	N/A	206
I67848	Other cerebrovascular vasospasm & vasoconstriction	N/A	206
I6789	Cerebrovascular DZ, NEC	N/A	206
I679	Cerebrovascular DZ, NOS	N/A	206
I680	Cerebral amyloid angiopathy	N/A	206
I682	Cerebral arteritis in other DZ classified elsewhere	N/A	206
I688	Cerebrovascular disorders in DZ classified elsewhere, NEC	N/A	206
For codes I6903- through I6905-, use the following 7th character: **1 affecting right dominant side** **2 affecting left dominant side** **3 affecting right non-dominant side** **4 affecting left non-dominant side** **9 affecting unspecified side**			
I6903-	Monoplegia of upper limb following nontraumatic subarachnoid hemorrhage	104	N/A
I6904-	Monoplegia of lower limb following nontraumatic subarachnoid hemorrhage	104	N/A
I6905-	Hemiplegia & hemiparesis following nontraumatic subarachnoid hemorrhage	103	N/A
I69061	Other paralytic syndrome following nontraumatic subarachnoid hemorrhage affecting R dominant side	104	N/A
I69062	Other paralytic syndrome following nontraumatic subarachnoid hemorrhage affecting L dominant side	104	N/A
I69063	Other paralytic syndrome following nontraumatic subarachnoid hemorrhage affecting R non-dominant side	104	N/A
I69064	Other paralytic syndrome following nontraumatic subarachnoid hemorrhage affecting L non-dominant side	104	N/A
I69065	Other paralytic syndrome following nontraumatic subarachnoid hemorrhage, bilateral	104	N/A
I69069	Other paralytic syndrome following nontraumatic subarachnoid hemorrhage affecting NOS side	104	N/A
For codes I6913- through I6915-, use the following 7th character: **1 affecting right dominant side** **2 affecting left dominant side** **3 affecting right non-dominant side** **4 affecting left non-dominant side** **9 affecting unspecified side**			
I6913-	Monoplegia of upper limb following nontraumatic intracerebral hemorrhage e	104	N/A
I6914-	Monoplegia of lower limb following nontraumatic intracerebral hemorrhage	104	N/A
I6915-	Hemiplegia & hemiparesis following nontraumatic intracerebral hemorrhage	103	N/A
I69161	Other paralytic syndrome following nontraumatic intracerebral hemorrhage affecting R dominant side	104	N/A
I69162	Other paralytic syndrome following nontraumatic intracerebral hemorrhage affecting L dominant side	104	N/A
I69163	Other paralytic syndrome following nontraumatic intracerebral hemorrhage affecting R non-dominant side	104	N/A
I69164	Other paralytic syndrome following nontraumatic intracerebral hemorrhage affecting L non-dominant side	104	N/A
I69165	Other paralytic syndrome following nontraumatic intracerebral hemorrhage, bilateral	104	N/A
I69169	Other paralytic syndrome following nontraumatic intracerebral hemorrhage affecting NOS side	104	N/A
For codes I6923- through I6925-, use the following 7th character: **1 affecting right dominant side** **2 affecting left dominant side** **3 affecting right non-dominant side** **4 affecting left non-dominant side** **9 affecting unspecified side**			
I6923-	Monoplegia of upper limb following other nontraumatic intracranial hemorrhage	104	N/A
I6924-	Monoplegia of lower limb following other nontraumatic intracranial hemorrhage	104	N/A
I6925-	Hemiplegia & hemiparesis following other nontraumatic intracranial hemorrhage	103	N/A
I69261	Other paralytic syndrome following other nontraumatic intracranial hemorrhage affecting R dominant side	104	N/A
I69262	Other paralytic syndrome following other nontraumatic intracranial hemorrhage affecting L dominant side	104	N/A
I69263	Other paralytic syndrome following other nontraumatic intracranial hemorrhage affecting R non-dominant side	104	N/A

Code	Code Descriptors	HCC	RXHCC
I69264	Other paralytic syndrome following other nontraumatic intracranial hemorrhage affecting L non-dominant side	104	N/A
I69265	Other paralytic syndrome following other nontraumatic intracranial hemorrhage, bilateral	104	N/A
I69269	Other paralytic syndrome following other nontraumatic intracranial hemorrhage affecting NOS side	104	N/A
For codes I6933- through I6935-, use the following 7th character: **1 affecting right dominant side** **2 affecting left dominant side** **3 affecting right non-dominant side** **4 affecting left non-dominant side** **9 affecting unspecified side**			
I6933-	Monoplegia of upper limb following cerebral infarction	104	N/A
I6934-	Monoplegia of lower limb following cerebral infarction	104	N/A
I6935-	Hemiplegia & hemiparesis following cerebral infarction	103	N/A
I69361	Other paralytic syndrome following cerebral infarction, affecting R dominant side	104	N/A
I69362	Other paralytic syndrome following cerebral infarction affecting L dominant side	104	N/A
I69363	Other paralytic syndrome following cerebral infarction affecting R non-dominant side	104	N/A
I69364	Other paralytic syndrome following cerebral infarction affecting L non-dominant side	104	N/A
I69365	Other paralytic syndrome following cerebral infarction, bilateral	104	N/A
I69369	Other paralytic syndrome following cerebral infarction affecting NOS side	104	N/A
For codes I6983- through I6985-, use the following 7th character: **1 affecting right dominant side** **2 affecting left dominant side** **3 affecting right non-dominant side** **4 affecting left non-dominant side** **9 affecting unspecified side**			
I6983-	Monoplegia of upper limb following other cerebrovascular DZ	104	N/A
I6984-	Monoplegia of lower limb following other cerebrovascular DZ	104	N/A
I6985-	Hemiplegia & hemiparesis following other cerebrovascular DZ	103	N/A
I69861	Other paralytic syndrome following other cerebrovascular DZ affecting R dominant side	104	N/A
I69862	Other paralytic syndrome following other cerebrovascular DZ affecting L dominant side	104	N/A
I69863	Other paralytic syndrome following other cerebrovascular DZ affecting R non-dominant side	104	N/A

Code	Code Descriptors	HCC	RXHCC
I69864	Other paralytic syndrome following other cerebrovascular DZ affecting L non-dominant side	104	N/A
I69865	Other paralytic syndrome following other cerebrovascular DZ, bilateral	104	N/A
I69869	Other paralytic syndrome following other cerebrovascular DZ affecting NOS side	104	N/A
For codes I6993- through I6995-, use the following 7th character: **1 affecting right dominant side** **2 affecting left dominant side** **3 affecting right non-dominant side** **4 affecting left non-dominant side** **9 affecting unspecified side**			
I6993-	Monoplegia of upper limb following NOS cerebrovascular DZ ide	104	N/A
I6994-	Monoplegia of lower limb following NOS cerebrovascular DZ	104	N/A
I6995-	Hemiplegia & hemiparesis following NOS cerebrovascular DZ	103	N/A
I69961	Other paralytic syndrome following NOS cerebrovascular DZ affecting R dominant side	104	N/A
I69962	Other paralytic syndrome following NOS cerebrovascular DZ affecting L dominant side	104	N/A
I69963	Other paralytic syndrome following NOS cerebrovascular DZ affecting R non-dominant side	104	N/A
I69964	Other paralytic syndrome following NOS cerebrovascular DZ affecting L non-dominant side	104	N/A
I69965	Other paralytic syndrome following NOS cerebrovascular DZ, bilateral	104	N/A
I69969	Other paralytic syndrome following NOS cerebrovascular DZ affecting NOS side	104	N/A
I700	Atherosclerosis of aorta	108	216
I701	Atherosclerosis of renal artery	108	216
For codes I7020- through I7022-, use the following 6th character: **1 right leg** **2 left leg** **3 bilateral leg** **8 other extremity** **9 extremity NOS**			
I7020-	NOS atherosclerosis of native arteries of extremities	108	216
I7021-	Atherosclerosis of native arteries of extremities W/ intermittent claudication	108	216
I7022-	Atherosclerosis of native arteries of extremities W/ rest pain	108	216
I70231	Atherosclerosis of native arteries of R leg W/ ulceration of thigh	106, 161	311
I70232	Atherosclerosis of native arteries of R leg W/ ulceration of calf	106, 161	311
I70233	Atherosclerosis of native arteries of R leg W/ ulceration of ankle	106, 161	311

Code	Code Descriptors	HCC	RXHCC
I70234	Atherosclerosis of native arteries of R leg W/ ulceration of heel & midfoot	106, 161	311
I70235	Atherosclerosis of native arteries of R leg W/ ulceration of other part of foot	106, 161	311
I70238	Atherosclerosis of native arteries of R leg W/ ulceration of other part of lower R leg	106, 161	311
I70239	Atherosclerosis of native arteries of R leg W/ ulceration of NOS site	106, 161	311
I70241	Atherosclerosis of native arteries of L leg W/ ulceration of thigh	106, 161	311
I70242	Atherosclerosis of native arteries of L leg W/ ulceration of calf	106, 161	311
I70243	Atherosclerosis of native arteries of L leg W/ ulceration of ankle	106, 161	311
I70244	Atherosclerosis of native arteries of L leg W/ ulceration of heel & midfoot	106, 161	311
I70245	Atherosclerosis of native arteries of L leg W/ ulceration of other part of foot	106, 161	311
I70248	Atherosclerosis of native arteries of L leg W/ ulceration of other part of lower L leg	106, 161	311
I70249	Atherosclerosis of native arteries of L leg W/ ulceration of NOS site	106, 161	311
I7025	Atherosclerosis of native arteries of other extremities W/ ulceration	106, 161	311
I70261	Atherosclerosis of native arteries of extremities W/ gangrene, R leg	106	N/A
I70262	Atherosclerosis of native arteries of extremities W/ gangrene, L leg	106	N/A
I70263	Atherosclerosis of native arteries of extremities W/ gangrene, bilateral legs	106	N/A
I70268	Atherosclerosis of native arteries of extremities W/ gangrene, other extremity	106	N/A
I70269	Atherosclerosis of native arteries of extremities W/ gangrene, NOS extremity	106	N/A
I70291	Other atherosclerosis of native arteries of extremities, R leg	108	216
I70292	Other atherosclerosis of native arteries of extremities, L leg	108	216
I70293	Other atherosclerosis of native arteries of extremities, bilateral legs	108	216
I70298	Other atherosclerosis of native arteries of extremities, other extremity	108	216
I70299	Other atherosclerosis of native arteries of extremities, NOS extremity	108	216
I70301	NOS atherosclerosis of NOS type of bypass graft(s) of extremities, R leg	108	216
I70302	NOS atherosclerosis of NOS type of bypass graft(s) of extremities, L leg	108	216
I70303	NOS atherosclerosis of NOS type of bypass graft(s) of extremities, bilateral legs	108	216
I70308	NOS atherosclerosis of NOS type of bypass graft(s) of extremities, other extremity	108	216
I70309	NOS atherosclerosis of NOS type of bypass graft(s) of extremities, NOS extremity	108	216

Code	Code Descriptors	HCC	RXHCC
For codes I7031- through I7032-, use the following 6th character: **1 right leg** **2 left leg** **3 bilateral leg** **8 other extremity** **9 extremity NOS**			
I7031-	Atherosclerosis of NOS type of bypass graft(s) of extremities W/ intermittent claudication	108	216
I7032-	Atherosclerosis of NOS type of bypass graft(s) of the extremities W/ rest pain	108	216
I70331	Atherosclerosis of NOS type of bypass graft(s) of the R leg W/ ulceration of thigh	106, 161	311
I70332	Atherosclerosis of NOS type of bypass graft(s) of the R leg W/ ulceration of calf	106, 161	311
I70333	Atherosclerosis of NOS type of bypass graft(s) of the R leg W/ ulceration of ankle	106, 161	311
I70334	Atherosclerosis of NOS type of bypass graft(s) of the R leg W/ ulceration of heel & midfoot	106, 161	311
I70335	Atherosclerosis of NOS type of bypass graft(s) of R leg W/ ulceration of other part of foot	106, 161	311
I70338	Atherosclerosis of NOS type of bypass graft(s) of R leg W/ ulceration of other part of lower leg	106, 161	311
I70339	Atherosclerosis of NOS type of bypass graft(s) of the R leg W/ ulceration of NOS site	106, 161	311
I70341	Atherosclerosis of NOS type of bypass graft(s) of the L leg W/ ulceration of thigh	106, 161	311
I70342	Atherosclerosis of NOS type of bypass graft(s) of the L leg W/ ulceration of calf	106, 161	311
I70343	Atherosclerosis of NOS type of bypass graft(s) of the L leg W/ ulceration of ankle	106, 161	311
I70344	Atherosclerosis of NOS type of bypass graft(s) of the L leg W/ ulceration of heel & midfoot	106, 161	311
I70345	Atherosclerosis of NOS type of bypass graft(s) of the L leg W/ ulceration of other part of foot	106, 161	311
I70348	Atherosclerosis of NOS type of bypass graft(s) of L leg W/ ulceration of other part of lower leg	106, 161	311
I70349	Atherosclerosis of NOS type of bypass graft(s) of the L leg W/ ulceration of NOS site	106, 161	311
I7035	Atherosclerosis of NOS type of bypass graft(s) of other extremity W/ ulceration	106, 161	311
For codes I7036- through I7039-, use the following 6th character: **1 right leg** **2 left leg** **3 bilateral leg** **8 other extremity** **9 extremity NOS**			
I7036-	Atherosclerosis of NOS type of bypass graft(s) of the extremities W/ gangrene	106	N/A

Code	Code Descriptors	HCC	RXHCC
I7039-	Other atherosclerosis of NOS type of bypass graft(s) of extremities	108	216
For codes I7040- through I7042-, use the following 6th character: 1 right leg 2 left leg 3 bilateral leg 8 other extremity 9 extremity NOS			
I7040-	NOS atherosclerosis of autologous vein bypass graft(s) of extremities	108	216
I7041-	Atherosclerosis of autologous vein bypass graft(s) of extremities W/ intermittent claudication	108	216
I7042-	Atherosclerosis of autologous vein bypass graft(s) of extremities W/ rest pain	108	216
I70431	Atherosclerosis of autologous vein bypass graft(s) of R leg W/ ulceration of thigh	106, 161	311
I70432	Atherosclerosis of autologous vein bypass graft(s) of R leg W/ ulceration of calf	106, 161	311
I70433	Atherosclerosis of autologous vein bypass graft(s) of R leg W/ ulceration of ankle	106, 161	311
I70434	Atherosclerosis of autologous vein bypass graft(s) of R leg W/ ulceration of heel & midfoot	106, 161	311
I70435	Atherosclerosis of autologous vein bypass graft(s) of R leg W/ ulceration of other part of foot	106, 161	311
I70438	Atherosclerosis of autologous vein bypass graft(s) of R leg W/ ulceration of other part of lower leg	106, 161	311
I70439	Atherosclerosis of autologous vein bypass graft(s) of R leg W/ ulceration of NOS site	106, 161	311
I70441	Atherosclerosis of autologous vein bypass graft(s) of L leg W/ ulceration of thigh	106, 161	311
I70442	Atherosclerosis of autologous vein bypass graft(s) of L leg W/ ulceration of calf	106, 161	311
I70443	Atherosclerosis of autologous vein bypass graft(s) of L leg W/ ulceration of ankle	106, 161	311
I70444	Atherosclerosis of autologous vein bypass graft(s) of L leg W/ ulceration of heel & midfoot	106, 161	311
I70445	Atherosclerosis of autologous vein bypass graft(s) of L leg W/ ulceration of other part of foot	106, 161	311
I70448	Atherosclerosis of autologous vein bypass graft(s) of L leg W/ ulceration of other part of lower leg	106, 161	311
I70449	Atherosclerosis of autologous vein bypass graft(s) of L leg W/ ulceration of NOS site	106, 161	311
I7045	Atherosclerosis of autologous vein bypass graft(s) of other extremity W/ ulceration	106, 161	311

Code	Code Descriptors	HCC	RXHCC
For codes I7046- through I7052-, use the following 6th character: 1 right leg 2 left leg 3 bilateral leg 8 other extremity 9 extremity NOS			
I7046-	Atherosclerosis of autologous vein bypass graft(s) of extremities W/ gangrene	106	N/A
I7049-	Other atherosclerosis of autologous vein bypass graft(s) of extremities	108	216
I7050-	Atherosclerosis of nonautologous biological bypass graft(s) of extremities, NOS	108	216
I7051-	Atherosclerosis of nonautologous biological bypass graft(s) of extremities W/ intermittent claudication	108	216
I7052-	Atherosclerosis of nonautologous biological bypass graft(s) of extremities W/ rest pain	108	216
I70531	Atherosclerosis of nonautologous biological bypass graft(s) of R leg W/ ulceration of thigh	106, 161	311
I70532	Atherosclerosis of nonautologous biological bypass graft(s) of R leg W/ ulceration of calf	106, 161	311
I70533	Atherosclerosis of nonautologous biological bypass graft(s) of R leg W/ ulceration of ankle	106, 161	311
I70534	Atherosclerosis of nonautologous biological bypass graft(s) of R leg W/ ulceration of heel & midfoot	106, 161	311
I70535	Atherosclerosis of nonautologous biological bypass graft(s) of R leg W/ ulceration of other part of foot	106, 161	311
I70538	Atherosclerosis of nonautologous biological bypass graft(s) of R leg W/ ulceration of other part of lower leg	106, 161	311
I70539	Atherosclerosis of nonautologous biological bypass graft(s) of R leg W/ ulceration of NOS site	106, 161	311
I70541	Atherosclerosis of nonautologous biological bypass graft(s) of L leg W/ ulceration of thigh	106, 161	311
I70542	Atherosclerosis of nonautologous biological bypass graft(s) of L leg W/ ulceration of calf	106, 161	311
I70543	Atherosclerosis of nonautologous biological bypass graft(s) of L leg W/ ulceration of ankle	106, 161	311
I70544	Atherosclerosis of nonautologous biological bypass graft(s) of L leg W/ ulceration of heel & midfoot	106, 161	311
I70545	Atherosclerosis of nonautologous biological bypass graft(s) of L leg W/ ulceration of other part of foot	106, 161	311
I70548	Atherosclerosis of nonautologous biological bypass graft(s) of L leg W/ ulceration of other part of lower leg	106, 161	311
I70549	Atherosclerosis of nonautologous biological bypass graft(s) of L leg W/ ulceration of NOS site	106, 161	311

Code	Code Descriptors	HCC	RXHCC
I7055	Atherosclerosis of nonautologous biological bypass graft(s) of other extremity W/ ulceration	106, 161	311
For codes I7056- through I7062-, use the following 6th character: **1 right leg** **2 left leg** **3 bilateral leg** **8 other extremity** **9 extremity NOS**			
I7056-	Atherosclerosis of nonautologous biological bypass graft(s) of extremities W/ gangrene	106	N/A
I7059-	Other atherosclerosis of nonautologous biological bypass graft(s) of extremities	108	216
I7060-	NOS atherosclerosis of nonbiological bypass graft(s) of extremities	108	216
I7061-	Atherosclerosis of nonbiological bypass graft(s) of extremities W/ intermittent claudication	108	216
I7062-	Atherosclerosis of nonbiological bypass graft(s) of extremities W/ rest pain	108	216
I70631	Atherosclerosis of nonbiological bypass graft(s) of R leg W/ ulceration of thigh	106, 161	311
I70632	Atherosclerosis of nonbiological bypass graft(s) of R leg W/ ulceration of calf	106, 161	311
I70633	Atherosclerosis of nonbiological bypass graft(s) of R leg W/ ulceration of ankle	106, 161	311
I70634	Atherosclerosis of nonbiological bypass graft(s) of R leg W/ ulceration of heel & midfoot	106, 161	311
I70635	Atherosclerosis of nonbiological bypass graft(s) of R leg W/ ulceration of other part of foot	106, 161	311
I70638	Atherosclerosis of nonbiological bypass graft(s) of R leg W/ ulceration of other part of lower leg	106, 161	311
I70639	Atherosclerosis of nonbiological bypass graft(s) of R leg W/ ulceration of NOS site	106, 161	311
I70641	Atherosclerosis of nonbiological bypass graft(s) of L leg W/ ulceration of thigh	106, 161	311
I70642	Atherosclerosis of nonbiological bypass graft(s) of L leg W/ ulceration of calf	106, 161	311
I70643	Atherosclerosis of nonbiological bypass graft(s) of L leg W/ ulceration of ankle	106, 161	311
I70644	Atherosclerosis of nonbiological bypass graft(s) of L leg W/ ulceration of heel & midfoot	106, 161	311
I70645	Atherosclerosis of nonbiological bypass graft(s) of L leg W/ ulceration of other part of foot	106, 161	311
I70648	Atherosclerosis of nonbiological bypass graft(s) of L leg W/ ulceration of other part of lower leg	106, 161	311
I70649	Atherosclerosis of nonbiological bypass graft(s) of L leg W/ ulceration of NOS site	106, 161	311
I7065	Atherosclerosis of nonbiological bypass graft(s) of other extremity W/ ulceration	106, 161	311

Code	Code Descriptors	HCC	RXHCC
For codes I7066- through I7072-, use the following 6th character: **1 right leg** **2 left leg** **3 bilateral leg** **8 other extremity** **9 extremity NOS**			
I7066-	Atherosclerosis of nonbiological bypass graft(s) of extremities W/ gangrene	106	N/A
I7069-	Other atherosclerosis of nonbiological bypass graft(s) of extremities	108	216
I7070-	NOS atherosclerosis of other type of bypass graft(s) of extremities	108	216
I7071-	Atherosclerosis of other type of bypass graft(s) of extremities W/ intermittent claudication	108	216
I7072-	Atherosclerosis of other type of bypass graft(s) of extremities W/ rest pain	108	216
I70731	Atherosclerosis of other type of bypass graft(s) of R leg W/ ulceration of thigh	106, 161	311
I70732	Atherosclerosis of other type of bypass graft(s) of R leg W/ ulceration of calf	106, 161	311
I70733	Atherosclerosis of other type of bypass graft(s) of R leg W/ ulceration of ankle	106, 161	311
I70734	Atherosclerosis of other type of bypass graft(s) of R leg W/ ulceration of heel & midfoot	106, 161	311
I70735	Atherosclerosis of other type of bypass graft(s) of R leg W/ ulceration of other part of foot	106, 161	311
I70738	Atherosclerosis of other type of bypass graft(s) of R leg W/ ulceration of other part of lower leg	106, 161	311
I70739	Atherosclerosis of other type of bypass graft(s) of R leg W/ ulceration of NOS site	106, 161	311
I70741	Atherosclerosis of other type of bypass graft(s) of L leg W/ ulceration of thigh	106, 161	311
I70742	Atherosclerosis of other type of bypass graft(s) of L leg W/ ulceration of calf	106, 161	311
I70743	Atherosclerosis of other type of bypass graft(s) of L leg W/ ulceration of ankle	106, 161	311
I70744	Atherosclerosis of other type of bypass graft(s) of L leg W/ ulceration of heel & midfoot	106, 161	311
I70745	Atherosclerosis of other type of bypass graft(s) of L leg W/ ulceration of other part of foot	106, 161	311
I70748	Atherosclerosis of other type of bypass graft(s) of L leg W/ ulceration of other part of lower leg	106, 161	311
I70749	Atherosclerosis of other type of bypass graft(s) of L leg W/ ulceration of NOS site	106, 161	311
I7075	Atherosclerosis of other type of bypass graft(s) of other extremity W/ ulceration	106, 161	311

Code	Code Descriptors	HCC	RXHCC
For codes I7076- through I7079-, use the following 6th character: 1 right leg 2 left leg 3 bilateral leg 8 other extremity 9 extremity NOS			
I7076-	Atherosclerosis of other type of bypass graft(s) of extremities W/ gangrene	106	N/A
I7079-	Other atherosclerosis of other type of bypass graft(s) of extremity	108	216
I7092	Chronic total occlusion of artery of extremities	108	216
I7100	Dissection of NOS site of aorta	107	N/A
I7101	Dissection of thoracic aorta	107	N/A
I7102	Dissection of abdominal aorta	107	N/A
I7103	Dissection of thoracoabdominal aorta	107	N/A
I711	Thoracic aortic aneurysm, ruptured	107	N/A
I712	Thoracic aortic aneurysm, W/O rupture	108	N/A
I713	Abdominal aortic aneurysm, ruptured	107	N/A
I714	Abdominal aortic aneurysm, W/O rupture	108	N/A
I715	Thoracoabdominal aortic aneurysm, ruptured	107	N/A
I716	Thoracoabdominal aortic aneurysm, W/O rupture	108	N/A
I718	Aortic aneurysm of NOS site, ruptured	107	N/A
I719	Aortic aneurysm of NOS site, W/O rupture	108	N/A
I720	Aneurysm of carotid artery	108	N/A
I721	Aneurysm of artery of upper extremity	108	N/A
I722	Aneurysm of renal artery	108	N/A
I723	Aneurysm of iliac artery	108	N/A
I724	Aneurysm of artery of lower extremity	108	N/A
I725	Aneurysm of other precerebral arteries	108	N/A
I726	Aneurysm of vertebral artery	108	N/A
I728	Aneurysm of NEC arteries	108	N/A
I729	Aneurysm of NOS site	108	N/A
I7301	Raynaud's syndrome W/ gangrene	106	N/A
I731	Thromboangiitis obliterans	108	216
I7381	Erythromelalgia	108	216
I7389	Peripheral vascular DZ, NEC	108	216
I739	Peripheral vascular DZ, NOS	108	216
I7401	Saddle embolus of abdominal aorta	107	N/A
I7409	Other arterial embolism & thrombosis of abdominal aorta	107	N/A
I7410	Embolism & thrombosis of NOS parts of aorta	107	N/A
I7411	Embolism & thrombosis of thoracic aorta	107	N/A
I7419	Embolism & thrombosis of NEC parts of aorta	107	N/A
I742	Embolism & thrombosis of arteries of upper extremities	107	N/A

Code	Code Descriptors	HCC	RXHCC
I743	Embolism & thrombosis of arteries of lower extremities	107	N/A
I744	Embolism & thrombosis of arteries of extremities, NOS	107	N/A
I745	Embolism & thrombosis of iliac artery	107	N/A
I748	Embolism & thrombosis of NEC artery	107	N/A
I749	Embolism & thrombosis of NOS artery	107	N/A
I75011	Atheroembolism of R upper extremity	107	N/A
I75012	Atheroembolism of L upper extremity	107	N/A
I75013	Atheroembolism of bilateral upper extremities	107	N/A
I75019	Atheroembolism of NOS upper extremity	107	N/A
I75021	Atheroembolism of R lower extremity	107	N/A
I75022	Atheroembolism of L lower extremity	107	N/A
I75023	Atheroembolism of bilateral lower extremities	107	N/A
I75029	Atheroembolism of NOS lower extremity	107	N/A
I7581	Atheroembolism of kidney	107	N/A
I7589	Atheroembolism of other site	107	N/A
I76	Septic arterial embolism	107	N/A
I770	Arteriovenous fistula, acquired	108	N/A
I771	Stricture of artery	108	N/A
I772	Rupture of artery	108	N/A
I773	Arterial fibromuscular dysplasia	108	N/A
I774	Celiac artery compression syndrome	108	N/A
I775	Necrosis of artery	108	N/A
I776	Arteritis, NOS	108	N/A
I7770	Dissection of NOS artery	107	N/A
I7771	Dissection of carotid artery	107	N/A
I7772	Dissection of iliac artery	107	N/A
I7773	Dissection of renal artery	107	N/A
I7774	Dissection of vertebral artery	107	N/A
I7775	Dissection of other precerebral arteries	107	N/A
I7776	Dissection of artery of upper extremity	107	N/A
I7777	Dissection of artery of lower extremity	107	N/A
I7779	Dissection of NEC artery	107	N/A
I77810	Thoracic aortic ectasia	108	N/A
I77811	Abdominal aortic ectasia	108	N/A
I77812	Thoracoabdominal aortic ectasia	108	N/A
I77819	Aortic ectasia, NOS site	108	N/A
I7789	Disorder of arteries & arterioles, NEC	108	N/A
I779	Disorder of arteries & arterioles, NOS	108	N/A
I780	Hereditary hemorrhagic telangiectasia	108	N/A
I790	Aneurysm of aorta in DZ classified elsewhere	108	N/A
I791	Aortitis in DZ classified elsewhere	108	216
I798	Other disorders of arteries, arterioles & capillaries in DZ classified elsewhere	108	216

Code	Code Descriptors	HCC	RXHCC
I8010	Phlebitis & thrombophlebitis of NOS femoral vein	108	215
I8011	Phlebitis & thrombophlebitis of R femoral vein	108	215
I8012	Phlebitis & thrombophlebitis of L femoral vein	108	215
I8013	Phlebitis & thrombophlebitis of femoral vein, bilateral	108	215
For codes I8020- through I8029-, use the following 6th character: **1 right** **2 left** **3 bilateral** **9 NOS**			
I8020-	Phlebitis & thrombophlebitis of NOS deep vessels of lower extremity	108	215
I8021-	Phlebitis & thrombophlebitis of iliac vein	108	215
I8022-	Phlebitis & thrombophlebitis of popliteal vein	108	215
I8023-	Phlebitis & thrombophlebitis of tibial vein	108	215
I8029-	Phlebitis & thrombophlebitis of other deep vessels of lower extremity	108	215
I820	Budd-Chiari syndrome	108	215
I82210	Acute embolism & thrombosis of superior vena cava	108	215
I82211	Chronic embolism & thrombosis of superior vena cava	108	215
I82220	Acute embolism & thrombosis of inferior vena cava	108	215
I82221	Chronic embolism & thrombosis of inferior vena cava	108	215
I82290	Acute embolism & thrombosis of other thoracic veins	108	215
I82291	Chronic embolism & thrombosis of other thoracic veins	108	215
I823	Embolism & thrombosis of renal vein	108	215
For codes I8240- through I82C2-, use the following 6th character: **1 right** **2 left** **3 bilateral** **9 NOS**			
I8240-	Acute embolism & thrombosis of NOS deep veins of lower extremity	108	215
I8241-	Acute embolism & thrombosis of femoral vein	108	215
I8242-	Acute embolism & thrombosis of iliac vein	108	215
I8243-	Acute embolism & thrombosis of popliteal vein	108	215
I8244-	Acute embolism & thrombosis of tibial vein	108	215
I8249-	Acute embolism & thrombosis of NEC deep vein of lower extremity	108	215
I824Y-	Acute embolism & thrombosis of NOS deep veins of proximal lower extremity	108	215
I824Z-	Acute embolism & thrombosis of NOS deep veins of distal lower extremity	108	215

Code	Code Descriptors	HCC	RXHCC
I8250-	Chronic embolism & thrombosis of NOS deep veins of lower extremity	108	215
I8251-	Chronic embolism & thrombosis of femoral vein	108	215
I8252-	Chronic embolism & thrombosis of iliac vein	108	215
I8253-	Chronic embolism & thrombosis of popliteal vein	108	215
I8254-	Chronic embolism & thrombosis of tibial vein	108	215
I8259-	Chronic embolism & thrombosis of NEC deep vein of lower extremity	108	215
I825Y-	Chronic embolism & thrombosis of NOS deep veins of proximal lower extremity	108	215
I825Z-	Chronic embolism & thrombosis of NOS deep veins of distal lower extremity	108	215
I8262-	Acute embolism & thrombosis of deep veins of upper extremity	108	215
I8272-	Chronic embolism & thrombosis of deep veins of upper extremity	108	215
I82A1-	Acute embolism & thrombosis of axillary vein	108	215
I82A2-	Chronic embolism & thrombosis of axillary vein	108	215
I82B1-	Acute embolism & thrombosis of subclavian vein	108	215
I82B2-	Chronic embolism & thrombosis of subclavian vein	108	215
I82C1-	Acute embolism & thrombosis of internal jugular vein	108	215
I82C2-	Chronic embolism & thrombosis of internal jugular vein	108	215
I83001	Varicose veins of NOS lower extremity W/ ulcer of thigh	107	N/A
I83002	Varicose veins of NOS lower extremity W/ ulcer of calf	107	N/A
I83003	Varicose veins of NOS lower extremity W/ ulcer of ankle	107	N/A
I83004	Varicose veins of NOS lower extremity W/ ulcer of heel & midfoot	107	N/A
I83005	Varicose veins of NOS lower extremity W/ ulcer other part of foot	107	N/A
I83008	Varicose veins of NOS lower extremity W/ ulcer other part of lower leg	107	N/A
I83009	Varicose veins of NOS lower extremity W/ ulcer of NOS site	107	N/A
I83011	Varicose veins of R lower extremity W/ ulcer of thigh	107	N/A
I83012	Varicose veins of R lower extremity W/ ulcer of calf	107	N/A
I83013	Varicose veins of R lower extremity W/ ulcer of ankle	107	N/A
I83014	Varicose veins of R lower extremity W/ ulcer of heel & midfoot	107	N/A
I83015	Varicose veins of R lower extremity W/ ulcer other part of foot	107	N/A

Code	Code Descriptors	HCC	RXHCC
I83018	Varicose veins of R lower extremity W/ ulcer other part of lower leg	107	N/A
I83019	Varicose veins of R lower extremity W/ ulcer of NOS site	107	N/A
I83021	Varicose veins of L lower extremity W/ ulcer of thigh	107	N/A
I83022	Varicose veins of L lower extremity W/ ulcer of calf	107	N/A
I83023	Varicose veins of L lower extremity W/ ulcer of ankle	107	N/A
I83024	Varicose veins of L lower extremity W/ ulcer of heel & midfoot	107	N/A
I83025	Varicose veins of L lower extremity W/ ulcer other part of foot	107	N/A
I83028	Varicose veins of L lower extremity W/ ulcer other part of lower leg	107	N/A
I83029	Varicose veins of L lower extremity W/ ulcer of NOS site	107	N/A
I83201	Varicose veins of NOS lower extremity W/ both ulcer of thigh & inflammation	107	N/A
I83202	Varicose veins of NOS lower extremity W/ both ulcer of calf & inflammation	107	N/A
I83203	Varicose veins of NOS lower extremity W/ both ulcer of ankle & inflammation	107	N/A
I83204	Varicose veins of NOS lower extremity W/ both ulcer of heel & midfoot & inflammation	107	N/A
I83205	Varicose veins of NOS lower extremity W/ both ulcer other part of foot & inflammation	107	N/A
I83208	Varicose veins of NOS lower extremity W/ both ulcer of other part of lower extremity & inflammation	107	N/A
I83209	Varicose veins of NOS lower extremity W/ both ulcer of NOS site & inflammation	107	N/A
I83211	Varicose veins of R lower extremity W/ both ulcer of thigh & inflammation	107	N/A
I83212	Varicose veins of R lower extremity W/ both ulcer of calf & inflammation	107	N/A
I83213	Varicose veins of R lower extremity W/ both ulcer of ankle & inflammation	107	N/A
I83214	Varicose veins of R lower extremity W/ both ulcer of heel & midfoot & inflammation	107	N/A
I83215	Varicose veins of R lower extremity W/ both ulcer other part of foot & inflammation	107	N/A
I83218	Varicose veins of R lower extremity W/ both ulcer of other part of lower extremity & inflammation	107	N/A
I83219	Varicose veins of R lower extremity W/ both ulcer of NOS site & inflammation	107	N/A
I83221	Varicose veins of L lower extremity W/ both ulcer of thigh & inflammation	107	N/A
I83222	Varicose veins of L lower extremity W/ both ulcer of calf & inflammation	107	N/A
I83223	Varicose veins of L lower extremity W/ both ulcer of ankle & inflammation	107	N/A

Code	Code Descriptors	HCC	RXHCC
I83224	Varicose veins of L lower extremity W/ both ulcer of heel & midfoot & inflammation	107	N/A
I83225	Varicose veins of L lower extremity W/ both ulcer other part of foot & inflammation	107	N/A
I83228	Varicose veins of L lower extremity W/ both ulcer of other part of lower extremity & inflammation	107	N/A
I83229	Varicose veins of L lower extremity W/ both ulcer of NOS site & inflammation	107	N/A
I8500	Esophageal varices W/O bleeding	27	N/A
I8501	Esophageal varices W/ bleeding	27	N/A
I8510	2ndary esophageal varices W/O bleeding	27	N/A
I8511	2ndary esophageal varices W/ bleeding	27	N/A
For codes I8701- through I8733-, use the following 6th character: 1 right lower extremity 2 left lower extremity 3 bilateral lower extremity 9 NOS lower extremity			
I8701-	Postthrombotic syndrome W/ ulcer	107	N/A
I8703-	Postthrombotic syndrome W/ ulcer & inflammation	107	N/A
I8731-	Chronic venous hypertension (idiopathic) W/ ulcer	107	N/A
I8733-	Chronic venous hypertension (idiopathic) W/ ulcer & inflammation	107	N/A
I96	Gangrene, NEC	106	N/A
I97810	Intraoperative cerebrovascular infarction during cardiac surgery	100	206
I97811	Intraoperative cerebrovascular infarction during other surgery	100	206
I97820	Postprocedural cerebrovascular infarction following cardiac surgery	100	206
I97821	Postprocedural cerebrovascular infarction following other surgery	100	206
J13	Pneumonia D/T Streptococcus pneumoniae	115	N/A
J14	Pneumonia D/T Hemophilus influenzae	115	N/A
J150	Pneumonia D/T Klebsiella pneumoniae	114	N/A
J151	Pneumonia D/T Pseudomonas	114	N/A
J1520	Pneumonia D/T staphylococcus, NOS	114	N/A
J15211	Pneumonia D/T MSSA	114	N/A
J15212	Pneumonia D/T MRSA	114	N/A
J1529	Pneumonia D/T staphylococcus, NEC	114	N/A
J153	Pneumonia D/T streptococcus, group B	115	N/A
J154	Pneumonia D/T other streptococci	115	N/A
J155	Pneumonia D/T E. coli	114	N/A
J156	Pneumonia D/T other Gram-negative bacteria	114	N/A
J158	Pneumonia D/T NEC bacteria	114	N/A
J181	Lobar pneumonia, NOS organism	115	N/A
J410	Simple chronic bronchitis	111	226
J411	Mucopurulent chronic bronchitis	111	226

Code	Code Descriptors	HCC	RXHCC
J418	Mixed simple & mucopurulent chronic bronchitis	111	226
J42	NOS chronic bronchitis	111	226
J430	Unilateral pulmonary emphysema	111	226
J431	Panlobular emphysema	111	226
J432	Centrilobular emphysema	111	226
J438	Emphysema, NEC	111	226
J439	Emphysema, NOS	111	226
J440	COPD W/ acute lower respiratory infection	111	226
J441	COPD W/ exacerbation	111	226
J449	COPD, NOS	111	226
For codes J452- through J455-, use the following 5th character: **0 uncomplicated** **1 with exacerbation** **2 with status asthmaticus**			
J452-	Mild intermittent asthma	N/A	226
J453-	Mild persistent asthma	N/A	226
J454-	Moderate persistent asthma	N/A	226
J455-	Severe persistent asthma	N/A	226
J45901	NOS asthma W/ exacerbation	N/A	226
J45902	NOS asthma W/ status asthmaticus	N/A	226
J45909	NOS asthma, uncomplicated	N/A	226
J45990	Exercise induced bronchospasm	N/A	226
J45991	Cough variant asthma	N/A	226
J45998	Other asthma	N/A	226
J470	Bronchiectasis W/ acute lower respiratory infection	112	227
J471	Bronchiectasis W/ exacerbation	112	227
J479	Bronchiectasis, uncomplicated	112	227
J60	Coalworker's pneumoconiosis	112	N/A
J61	Pneumoconiosis D/T asbestos & other mineral fibers	112	N/A
J620	Pneumoconiosis D/T talc dust	112	N/A
J628	Pneumoconiosis D/T other dust containing silica	112	N/A
J630	Aluminosis (of lung)	112	N/A
J631	Bauxite fibrosis (of lung)	112	N/A
J632	Berylliosis	112	N/A
J633	Graphite fibrosis (of lung)	112	N/A
J634	Siderosis	112	N/A
J635	Stannosis	112	N/A
J636	Pneumoconiosis D/T NEC inorganic dusts	112	N/A
J64	Pneumoconiosis, NOS	112	N/A
J65	Pneumoconiosis associated W/ tuberculosis	112	N/A
J660	Byssinosis	112	N/A
J661	Flax-dressers' DZ	112	N/A
J662	Cannabinosis	112	N/A
J668	Airway DZ D/T other specific organic dusts	112	N/A

Code	Code Descriptors	HCC	RXHCC
J670	Farmer's lung	112	N/A
J671	Bagassosis	112	N/A
J672	Bird fancier's lung	112	N/A
J673	Suberosis	112	N/A
J674	Maltworker's lung	112	N/A
J675	Mushroom-worker's lung	112	N/A
J676	Maple-bark-stripper's lung	112	N/A
J677	Air conditioner & humidifier lung	112	N/A
J678	Hypersensitivity pneumonitis D/T organic dust, NEC	112	N/A
J679	Hypersensitivity pneumonitis D/T organic dus, NOS	112	N/A
J680	Bronchitis & pneumonitis D/T chemicals, gases, fumes & vapors	112	N/A
J681	Pulmonary edema D/T chemicals, gases, fumes & vapors	112	N/A
J682	Upper respiratory inflammation D/T chemicals, gases, fumes & vapors, NEC	112	N/A
J683	Other acute & subacute respiratory conditions D/T chemicals, gases, fumes & vapors	112	N/A
J684	Chronic respiratory conditions D/T chemicals, gases, fumes & vapors	112	N/A
J688	Respiratory conditions D/T chemicals, gases, fumes & vapors, NEC	112	N/A
J689	Respiratory condition D/T chemicals, gases, fumes & vapors, NOS	112	N/A
J690	Pneumonitis D/T inhalation of food & vomit	114	N/A
J691	Pneumonitis D/T inhalation of oils & essences	114	N/A
J698	Pneumonitis D/T inhalation of other solids & liquids	114	N/A
J700	Acute pulmonary manifestations D/T radiation	112	227
J701	Chronic & other pulmonary manifestations D/T radiation	112	227
J702	Acute drug-induced interstitial lung disorders	112	227
J703	Chronic drug-induced interstitial lung disorders	112	227
J704	Drug-induced interstitial lung disorders, NOS	112	227
J705	Respiratory conditions D/T smoke inhalation	112	227
J708	Respiratory conditions D/T NEC external agents	112	227
J709	Respiratory conditions D/T NOS external agent	112	227
J80	Acute respiratory distress syndrome	84	N/A
J810	Acute pulmonary edema	84	N/A
J82	Pulmonary eosinophilia, NEC	112	N/A
J8401	Alveolar proteinosis	112	227
J8402	Pulmonary alveolar microlithiasis	112	227

Code	Code Descriptors	HCC	RXHCC
J8403	Idiopathic pulmonary hemosiderosis	112	227
J8409	Other alveolar & parieto-alveolar conditions	112	227
J8410	Pulmonary fibrosis, NOS	112	227
J84111	Idiopathic interstitial pneumonia, NOS	112	227
J84112	Idiopathic pulmonary fibrosis	112	227
J84113	Idiopathic non-specific interstitial pneumonitis	112	227
J84114	Acute interstitial pneumonitis	112	227
J84115	Respiratory bronchiolitis interstitial lung DZ	112	227
J84116	Cryptogenic organizing pneumonia	112	227
J84117	Desquamative interstitial pneumonia	112	227
J8417	Interstitial pulmonary DZ W/ fibrosis in DZ classified elsewhere, NEC	112	227
J842	Lymphoid interstitial pneumonia	112	227
J8481	Lymphangioleiomyomatosis	112	227
J8482	Adult pulmonary Langerhans cell histiocytosis	112	227
J8483	Surfactant mutations of lung	112	227
J84841	Neuroendocrine cell hyperplasia of infancy	112	227
J84842	Pulmonary interstitial glycogenosis	112	227
J84843	Alveolar capillary dysplasia W/ vein misalignment	112	227
J84848	Other interstitial lung DZ of childhood	112	227
J8489	Interstitial pulmonary DZ, NEC	112	227
J849	Interstitial pulmonary DZ, NOS	112	227
J850	Gangrene & necrosis of lung	115	N/A
J851	Abscess of lung W/ pneumonia	115	N/A
J852	Abscess of lung W/O pneumonia	115	N/A
J853	Abscess of mediastinum	115	N/A
J860	Pyothorax W/ fistula	115	N/A
J869	Pyothorax W/O fistula	115	N/A
J9500	Tracheostomy complication, NOS	82	N/A
J9501	Hemorrhage from tracheostomy stoma	82	N/A
J9502	Infection of tracheostomy stoma	82	N/A
J9503	Malfunction of tracheostomy stoma	82	N/A
J9504	Tracheo-esophageal fistula following tracheostomy	82	N/A
J9509	Other tracheostomy complication	82	N/A
J951	Acute pulmonary insufficiency following thoracic surgery	84	N/A
J952	Acute pulmonary insufficiency following nonthoracic surgery	84	N/A
J953	Chronic pulmonary insufficiency following surgery	84	N/A
J95821	Acute postprocedural respiratory failure	84	N/A
J95822	Acute & chronic postprocedural respiratory failure	84	N/A
J95850	Mechanical complication of respirator	82	N/A
J95851	Ventilator associated pneumonia	114	N/A

Code	Code Descriptors	HCC	RXHCC
J95859	Other complication of respirator [ventilator]	82	N/A
For codes J960- through J969-use the following 5th character: 0 NOS whether with hypoxia or hypercapnia 1 with hypoxia 2 with hypercapnia			
J960-	Acute respiratory failure	84	N/A
J961-	Chronic respiratory failure	84	N/A
J962-	Acute & chronic respiratory failure	84	N/A
J969-	Respiratory failure, NOS	84	N/A
J982	Interstitial emphysema	111	226
J983	Compensatory emphysema	111	226
J99	Respiratory disorders in DZ classified elsewhere	112	227
K200	Eosinophilic esophagitis	N/A	68
K208	Other esophagitis	N/A	68
K209	Esophagitis, NOS	N/A	68
K210	GERD W/ esophagitis	N/A	68
K219	GERD W/O esophagitis	N/A	68
K220	Achalasia of cardia	N/A	68
K222	Esophageal obstruction	N/A	68
K223	Perforation of esophagus	N/A	68
K224	Dyskinesia of esophagus	N/A	68
K225	Diverticulum of esophagus, acquired	N/A	68
K2270	Barrett's esophagus W/O dysplasia	N/A	68
K22710	Barrett's esophagus W/ low grade dysplasia	N/A	68
K22711	Barrett's esophagus W/ high grade dysplasia	N/A	68
K22719	Barrett's esophagus W/ dysplasia, NOS	N/A	68
K228	DZ of esophagus, NEC	N/A	68
K229	DZ of esophagus, NOS	N/A	68
K23	Disorders of esophagus in DZ classified elsewhere	N/A	68
K251	Acute gastric ulcer W/ perforation	33	N/A
K252	Acute gastric ulcer W/ both hemorrhage & perforation	33	N/A
K255	Chronic or NOS gastric ulcer W/ perforation	33	N/A
K256	Chronic or NOS gastric ulcer W/ both hemorrhage & perforation	33	N/A
K261	Acute duodenal ulcer W/ perforation	33	N/A
K262	Acute duodenal ulcer W/ both hemorrhage & perforation	33	N/A
K265	Chronic or NOS duodenal ulcer W/ perforation	33	N/A
K266	Chronic or NOS duodenal ulcer W/ both hemorrhage & perforation	33	N/A
K271	Acute peptic ulcer, site NOS, W/ perforation	33	N/A
K272	Acute peptic ulcer, site NOS, W/ both hemorrhage & perforation	33	N/A
K275	Chronic or NOS peptic ulcer, site NOS, W/ perforation	33	N/A

Code	Code Descriptors	HCC	RXHCC
K276	Chronic or NOS peptic ulcer, site NOS, W/ both hemorrhage & perforation	33	N/A
K281	Acute gastrojejunal ulcer W/ perforation	33	N/A
K282	Acute gastrojejunal ulcer W/ both hemorrhage & perforation	33	N/A
K285	Chronic or NOS gastrojejunal ulcer W/ perforation	33	N/A
K286	Chronic or NOS gastrojejunal ulcer W/ both hemorrhage & perforation	33	N/A
K5000	Crohn's DZ of SM intestine W/O complications	35	67
K50011	Crohn's DZ of SM intestine W/ rectal bleeding	35	67
K50012	Crohn's DZ of SM intestine W/ intestinal obstruction	33, 35	67
K50013	Crohn's DZ of SM intestine W/ fistula	35	67
K50014	Crohn's DZ of SM intestine W/ abscess	35	67
K50018	Crohn's DZ of SM intestine W/ other complication	35	67
K50019	Crohn's DZ of SM intestine W/ NOS complications	35	67
K5010	Crohn's DZ of LG intestine W/O complications	35	67
K50111	Crohn's DZ of LG intestine W/ rectal bleeding	35	67
K50112	Crohn's DZ of LG intestine W/ intestinal obstruction	33, 35	67
K50113	Crohn's DZ of LG intestine W/ fistula	35	67
K50114	Crohn's DZ of LG intestine W/ abscess	35	67
K50118	Crohn's DZ of LG intestine W/ other complication	35	67
K50119	Crohn's DZ of LG intestine W/ NOS complications	35	67
K5080	Crohn's DZ of both SM & LG intestine W/O complications	35	67
K50811	Crohn's DZ of both SM & LG intestine W/ rectal bleeding	35	67
K50812	Crohn's DZ of both SM & LG intestine W/ intestinal obstruction	33, 35	67
K50813	Crohn's DZ of both SM & LG intestine W/ fistula	35	67
K50814	Crohn's DZ of both SM & LG intestine W/ abscess	35	67
K50818	Crohn's DZ of both SM & LG intestine W/ other complication	35	67
K50819	Crohn's DZ of both SM & LG intestine W/ NOS complications	35	67
K5090	Crohn's DZ, NOS, W/O complications	35	67
K50911	Crohn's DZ, NOS, W/ rectal bleeding	35	67
K50912	Crohn's DZ, NOS, W/ intestinal obstruction	33, 35	67
K50913	Crohn's DZ, NOS, W/ fistula	35	67
K50914	Crohn's DZ, NOS, W/ abscess	35	67

Code	Code Descriptors	HCC	RXHCC
K50918	Crohn's DZ, NOS, W/ other complication	35	67
K50919	Crohn's DZ, NOS, W/ NOS complications	35	67
K5100	Ulcerative pancolitis W/O complications	35	67
K51011	Ulcerative pancolitis W/ rectal bleeding	35	67
K51012	Ulcerative pancolitis W/ intestinal obstruction	33, 35	67
K51013	Ulcerative pancolitis W/ fistula	35	67
K51014	Ulcerative pancolitis W/ abscess	35	67
K51018	Ulcerative pancolitis W/ other complication	35	67
K51019	Ulcerative pancolitis W/ NOS complications	35	67
K5120	Ulcerative proctitis W/O complications	35	67
K51211	Ulcerative proctitis W/ rectal bleeding	35	67
K51212	Ulcerative proctitis W/ intestinal obstruction	33, 35	67
K51213	Ulcerative proctitis W/ fistula	35	67
K51214	Ulcerative proctitis W/ abscess	35	67
K51218	Ulcerative proctitis W/ other complication	35	67
K51219	Ulcerative proctitis W/ NOS complications	35	67
K5130	Ulcerative rectosigmoiditis W/O complications	35	67
K51311	Ulcerative rectosigmoiditis W/ rectal bleeding	35	67
K51312	Ulcerative rectosigmoiditis W/ intestinal obstruction	33, 35	67
K51313	Ulcerative rectosigmoiditis W/ fistula	35	67
K51314	Ulcerative rectosigmoiditis W/ abscess	35	67
K51318	Ulcerative rectosigmoiditis W/ other complication	35	67
K51319	Ulcerative rectosigmoiditis W/ NOS complications	35	67
K5140	Inflammatory polyps of colon W/O complications	35	67
K51411	Inflammatory polyps of colon W/ rectal bleeding	35	67
K51412	Inflammatory polyps of colon W/ intestinal obstruction	33, 35	67
K51413	Inflammatory polyps of colon W/ fistula	35	67
K51414	Inflammatory polyps of colon W/ abscess	35	67
K51418	Inflammatory polyps of colon W/ other complication	35	67
K51419	Inflammatory polyps of colon W/ NOS complications	35	67
K5150	L sided colitis W/O complications	35	67
K51511	L sided colitis W/ rectal bleeding	35	67
K51512	L sided colitis W/ intestinal obstruction	33, 35	67
K51513	L sided colitis W/ fistula	35	67
K51514	L sided colitis W/ abscess	35	67
K51518	L sided colitis W/ other complication	35	67
K51519	L sided colitis W/ NOS complications	35	67
K5180	Ulcerative colitis W/O complications	35	67

Code	Code Descriptors	HCC	RXHCC
K51811	Ulcerative colitis NEC, W/ rectal bleeding	35	67
K51812	Ulcerative colitis NEC, W/ intestinal obstruction	33, 35	67
K51813	Ulcerative colitis NEC, W/ fistula	35	67
K51814	Ulcerative colitis NEC, W/ abscess	35	67
K51818	Ulcerative colitis NEC, W/ other complication	35	67
K51819	Ulcerative colitis NEC, W/ NOS complications	35	67
K5190	Ulcerative colitis, NOS,, W/O complications	35	67
K51911	Ulcerative colitis, NOS, W/ rectal bleeding	35	67
K51912	Ulcerative colitis, NOS, W/ intestinal obstruction	33, 35	67
K51913	Ulcerative colitis, NOS, W/ fistula	35	67
K51914	Ulcerative colitis, NOS, W/ abscess	35	67
K51918	Ulcerative colitis, NOS, W/ other complication	35	67
K51919	Ulcerative colitis, NOS, W/ NOS complications	35	67
K55011	Focal (segmental) acute (reversible) ischemia of SM intestine	107	N/A
K55012	Diffuse acute (reversible) ischemia of SM intestine	107	N/A
K55019	Acute (reversible) ischemia of SM intestine, extent NOS	107	N/A
K55021	Focal (segmental) acute infarction of SM intestine	107	N/A
K55022	Diffuse acute infarction of SM intestine	107	N/A
K55029	Acute infarction of SM intestine, extent NOS	107	N/A
K55031	Focal (segmental) acute (reversible) ischemia of LG intestine	107	N/A
K55032	Diffuse acute (reversible) ischemia of LG intestine	107	N/A
K55039	Acute (reversible) ischemia of LG intestine, extent NOS	107	N/A
K55041	Focal (segmental) acute infarction of LG intestine	107	N/A
K55042	Diffuse acute infarction of LG intestine	107	N/A
K55049	Acute infarction of LG intestine, extent NOS	107	N/A
K55051	Focal (segmental) acute (reversible) ischemia of intestine, part NOS	107	N/A
K55052	Diffuse acute (reversible) ischemia of intestine, part NOS	107	N/A
K55059	Acute (reversible) ischemia of intestine, part & extent NOS	107	N/A
K55061	Focal (segmental) acute infarction of intestine, part NOS	107	N/A
K55062	Diffuse acute infarction of intestine, part NOS	107	N/A
K55069	Acute infarction of intestine, part & extent NOS	107	N/A

Code	Code Descriptors	HCC	RXHCC
K551	Chronic vascular disorders of intestine	108	N/A
K5530	Necrotizing enterocolitis, NOS	107	N/A
K5531	Stage 1 necrotizing enterocolitis	107	N/A
K5532	Stage 2 necrotizing enterocolitis	107	N/A
K5533	Stage 3 necrotizing enterocolitis	107	N/A
K558	Vascular disorder of intestine, NEC	108	N/A
K559	Vascular disorder of intestine, NOS	108	N/A
K560	Paralytic ileus	33	N/A
K561	Intussusception	33	N/A
K562	Volvulus	33	N/A
K563	Gallstone ileus	33	N/A
K5641	Fecal impaction	33	N/A
K5649	Other impaction of intestine	33	N/A
K5650	Intestinal adhesions, NOS as to partial versus complete obstruction	33	N/A
K5651	Intestinal adhesions, with partial obstruction	33	N/A
K5652	Intestinal adhesions with complete obstruction	33	N/A
K56600	Partial intestinal obstruction, NOS as to cause	33	N/A
K56601	Complete intestinal obstruction, NOS as to cause	33	N/A
K56609	NOS intestinal obstruction, NOS as to partial vs complete obstruction	33	N/A
K56690	Partial intestinal obstruction, NEC	33	N/A
K56691	Complete intestinal obstruction, NEC	33	N/A
K56699	Intestinal obstruction unspecified as to partial vs complete obstruction, NEC	33	N/A
K567	Ileus, NOS	33	N/A
K5931	Toxic megacolon	33	N/A
K631	Perforation of intestine (nontraumatic)	33	N/A
K650	Generalized peritonitis	33	N/A
K651	Peritoneal abscess	33	N/A
K652	Spontaneous bacterial peritonitis	33	N/A
K653	Choleperitonitis	33	N/A
K654	Sclerosing mesenteritis	33	N/A
K658	Peritonitis, NEC	33	N/A
K659	Peritonitis, NOS	33	N/A
K67	Disorders of peritoneum in infectious DZ classified elsewhere	33	N/A
K6812	Psoas muscle abscess	33	N/A
K6819	Retroperitoneal abscess, NEC	33	N/A
K7030	Alcoholic cirrhosis of liver W/O ascites	28	N/A
K7031	Alcoholic cirrhosis of liver W/ ascites	28	N/A
K7040	Alcoholic hepatic failure W/O coma	28	N/A
K7041	Alcoholic hepatic failure W/ coma	27, 28	N/A
K709	Alcoholic liver DZ, NOS	28	N/A
K7111	Toxic liver DZ W/ hepatic necrosis, W/ coma	27	N/A

Code	Code Descriptors	HCC	RXHCC
K7201	Acute & subacute hepatic failure W/ coma	27	N/A
K7210	Chronic hepatic failure W/O coma	27	N/A
K7211	Chronic hepatic failure W/ coma	27	N/A
K7290	Hepatic failure, NOS W/O coma	27	N/A
K7291	Hepatic failure, NOS W/ coma	27	N/A
K730	Chronic persistent hepatitis, NEC	29	N/A
K731	Chronic lobular hepatitis, NEC	29	N/A
K732	Chronic active hepatitis, NEC	29	N/A
K738	Other chronic hepatitis, NEC	29	N/A
K739	Chronic hepatitis, NOS	29	N/A
K743	Primary biliary cirrhosis	28	N/A
K744	2ndary biliary cirrhosis	28	N/A
K745	Biliary cirrhosis, NOS	28	N/A
K7460	Cirrhosis of liver, NOS	28	N/A
K7469	Cirrhosis of liver, NEC	28	N/A
K754	Autoimmune hepatitis	29	N/A
K766	Portal hypertension	27	N/A
K767	Hepatorenal syndrome	27	N/A
K7681	Hepatopulmonary syndrome	27	N/A
K860	Alcohol-induced chronic pancreatitis	34	65
K861	Other chronic pancreatitis	34	65
K862	Cyst of pancreas	N/A	66
K863	Pseudocyst of pancreas	N/A	66
K8681	Exocrine pancreatic insufficiency	N/A	66
K8689	DZ of pancreas, NEC	N/A	66
K869	DZ of pancreas, NOS	N/A	66
K87	Disorders of gallbladder, biliary tract & pancreas in DZ classified elsewhere	N/A	66
K900	Celiac DZ	N/A	66
K901	Tropical sprue	N/A	66
K902	Blind loop syndrome, NEC	N/A	66
K903	Pancreatic steatorrhea	N/A	66
K9049	Malabsorption D/T intolerance, NEC	N/A	66
K9081	Whipple's DZ	N/A	66
K9089	Intestinal malabsorption, NEC	N/A	66
K909	Intestinal malabsorption, NOS	N/A	66
K912	Postsurgical malabsorption, NEC	N/A	66
K91850	Pouchitis	188	N/A
K91858	Complication of intestinal pouch, NEC	188	N/A
For codes K940- through K943-, use the following 5th character: 0 NOS 1 hemorrhage 2 infection 3 malfunction 9 NEC			
K940-	Colostomy complication	188	N/A
K941-	Enterostomy complication	188	N/A
K942-	Gastrostomy complication	188	N/A

Code	Code Descriptors	HCC	RXHCC
K943-	Esophagostomy complication	188	N/A
L100	Pemphigus vulgaris	N/A	314
L101	Pemphigus vegetans	N/A	314
L102	Pemphigus foliaceous	N/A	314
L103	Brazilian pemphigus [fogo selvagem]	N/A	314
L104	Pemphigus erythematosus	N/A	314
L105	Drug-induced pemphigus	N/A	314
L1081	Paraneoplastic pemphigus	N/A	314
L1089	Pemphigus, NEC	N/A	314
L109	Pemphigus, NOS	N/A	314
L1230	Acquired epidermolysis bullosa, NOS	162	N/A
L1231	Epidermolysis bullosa D/T drug	162	N/A
L1235	Acquired epidermolysis bullosa, NEC	162	N/A
L400	Psoriasis vulgaris	N/A	316
L401	Generalized pustular psoriasis	N/A	316
L402	Acrodermatitis continua	N/A	316
L403	Pustulosis palmaris et plantaris	N/A	316
L404	Guttate psoriasis	N/A	316
L4050	Arthropathic psoriasis, NOS	40	82
L4051	Distal interphalangeal psoriatic arthropathy	40	82
L4052	Psoriatic arthritis mutilans	40	82
L4053	Psoriatic spondylitis	40	82
L4054	Psoriatic juvenile arthropathy	40	82
L4059	Other psoriatic arthropathy	40	82
L408	Psoriasis, NEC	N/A	316
L409	Psoriasis, NOS	N/A	316
L410	Pityriasis lichenoides et varioliformis acuta	N/A	316
L411	Pityriasis lichenoides chronica	N/A	316
L413	SM plaque parapsoriasis	N/A	316
L414	LG plaque parapsoriasis	N/A	316
L415	Retiform parapsoriasis	N/A	316
L418	Parapsoriasis, NEC	N/A	316
L419	Parapsoriasis, NOS	N/A	316
L511	Stevens-Johnson syndrome	162	N/A
L512	Toxic epidermal necrolysis	162	N/A
L513	Stevens-Johnson syndrome-toxic epidermal necrolysis overlap syndrome	162	N/A
L89000	Pressure ulcer of NOS elbow, unstageable	158, 160	N/A
L89001	Pressure ulcer of NOS elbow, stage 1	160	N/A
L89002	Pressure ulcer of NOS elbow, stage 2	159, 160	N/A
L89003	Pressure ulcer of NOS elbow, stage 3	158, 160	N/A
L89004	Pressure ulcer of NOS elbow, stage 4	157, 160	N/A
L89009	Pressure ulcer of NOS elbow, NOS stage	160	N/A

Code	Code Descriptors	HCC	RXHCC
L89010	Pressure ulcer of R elbow, unstageable	158, 160	N/A
L89011	Pressure ulcer of R elbow, stage 1	160	N/A
L89012	Pressure ulcer of R elbow, stage 2	159, 160	N/A
L89013	Pressure ulcer of R elbow, stage 3	158, 160	N/A
L89014	Pressure ulcer of R elbow, stage 4	157, 160	N/A
L89019	Pressure ulcer of R elbow, NOS stage	160	N/A
L89020	Pressure ulcer of L elbow, unstageable	158, 160	N/A
L89021	Pressure ulcer of L elbow, stage 1	160	N/A
L89022	Pressure ulcer of L elbow, stage 2	159, 160	N/A
L89023	Pressure ulcer of L elbow, stage 3	158, 160	N/A
L89024	Pressure ulcer of L elbow, stage 4	157, 160	N/A
L89029	Pressure ulcer of L elbow, NOS stage	160	N/A
L89100	Pressure ulcer of NOS part of back, unstageable	158, 160	N/A
L89101	Pressure ulcer of NOS part of back, stage 1	160	N/A
L89102	Pressure ulcer of NOS part of back, stage 2	159, 160	N/A
L89103	Pressure ulcer of NOS part of back, stage 3	158, 160	N/A
L89104	Pressure ulcer of NOS part of back, stage 4	157, 160	N/A
L89109	Pressure ulcer of NOS part of back, NOS stage	160	N/A
L89110	Pressure ulcer of R upper back, unstageable	158, 160	N/A
L89111	Pressure ulcer of R upper back, stage 1	160	N/A
L89112	Pressure ulcer of R upper back, stage 2	159, 160	N/A
L89113	Pressure ulcer of R upper back, stage 3	158, 160	N/A
L89114	Pressure ulcer of R upper back, stage 4	157, 160	N/A
L89119	Pressure ulcer of R upper back, NOS stage	160	N/A
L89120	Pressure ulcer of L upper back, unstageable	158, 160	N/A
L89121	Pressure ulcer of L upper back, stage 1	160	N/A
L89122	Pressure ulcer of L upper back, stage 2	159, 160	N/A
L89123	Pressure ulcer of L upper back, stage 3	158, 160	N/A
L89124	Pressure ulcer of L upper back, stage 4	157, 160	N/A
L89129	Pressure ulcer of L upper back, NOS stage	160	N/A
L89130	Pressure ulcer of R lower back, unstageable	158, 160	N/A

Code	Code Descriptors	HCC	RXHCC
L89131	Pressure ulcer of R lower back, stage 1	160	N/A
L89132	Pressure ulcer of R lower back, stage 2	159, 160	N/A
L89133	Pressure ulcer of R lower back, stage 3	158, 160	N/A
L89134	Pressure ulcer of R lower back, stage 4	157, 160	N/A
L89139	Pressure ulcer of R lower back, NOS stage	160	N/A
L89140	Pressure ulcer of L lower back, unstageable	158, 160	N/A
L89141	Pressure ulcer of L lower back, stage 1	160	N/A
L89142	Pressure ulcer of L lower back, stage 2	159, 160	N/A
L89143	Pressure ulcer of L lower back, stage 3	158, 160	N/A
L89144	Pressure ulcer of L lower back, stage 4	157	N/A
L89149	Pressure ulcer of L lower back, NOS stage	160	N/A
L89150	Pressure ulcer of sacral region, unstageable	158, 160	N/A
L89151	Pressure ulcer of sacral region, stage 1	160	N/A
L89152	Pressure ulcer of sacral region, stage 2	159, 160	N/A
L89153	Pressure ulcer of sacral region, stage 3	158, 160	N/A
L89154	Pressure ulcer of sacral region, stage 4	157, 160	N/A
L89159	Pressure ulcer of sacral region, NOS stage	160	N/A
L89200	Pressure ulcer of NOS hip, unstageable	158, 160	N/A
L89201	Pressure ulcer of NOS hip, stage 1	160	N/A
L89202	Pressure ulcer of NOS hip, stage 2	159, 160	N/A
L89203	Pressure ulcer of NOS hip, stage 3	158, 160	N/A
L89204	Pressure ulcer of NOS hip, stage 4	157, 160	N/A
L89209	Pressure ulcer of NOS hip, NOS stage	160	N/A
L89210	Pressure ulcer of R hip, unstageable	158, 160	N/A
L89211	Pressure ulcer of R hip, stage 1	160	N/A
L89212	Pressure ulcer of R hip, stage 2	159, 160	N/A
L89213	Pressure ulcer of R hip, stage 3	158, 160	N/A
L89214	Pressure ulcer of R hip, stage 4	157, 160	N/A
L89219	Pressure ulcer of R hip, NOS stage	160	N/A
L89220	Pressure ulcer of L hip, unstageable	158, 160	N/A
L89221	Pressure ulcer of L hip, stage 1	160	N/A
L89222	Pressure ulcer of L hip, stage 2	159, 160	N/A

Code	Code Descriptors	HCC	RXHCC
L89223	Pressure ulcer of L hip, stage 3	158, 160	N/A
L89224	Pressure ulcer of L hip, stage 4	157, 160	N/A
L89229	Pressure ulcer of L hip, NOS stage	160	N/A
L89300	Pressure ulcer of NOS buttock, unstageable	158, 160	N/A
L89301	Pressure ulcer of NOS buttock, stage 1	160	N/A
L89302	Pressure ulcer of NOS buttock, stage 2	159, 160	N/A
L89303	Pressure ulcer of NOS buttock, stage 3	158, 160	N/A
L89304	Pressure ulcer of NOS buttock, stage 4	157, 160	N/A
L89309	Pressure ulcer of NOS buttock, NOS stage	160	N/A
L89310	Pressure ulcer of R buttock, unstageable	158, 160	N/A
L89311	Pressure ulcer of R buttock, stage 1	160	N/A
L89312	Pressure ulcer of R buttock, stage 2	159, 160	N/A
L89313	Pressure ulcer of R buttock, stage 3	158, 160	N/A
L89314	Pressure ulcer of R buttock, stage 4	157, 160	N/A
L89319	Pressure ulcer of R buttock, NOS stage	160	N/A
L89320	Pressure ulcer of L buttock, unstageable	158, 160	N/A
L89321	Pressure ulcer of L buttock, stage 1	160	N/A
L89322	Pressure ulcer of L buttock, stage 2	159, 160	N/A
L89323	Pressure ulcer of L buttock, stage 3	158, 160	N/A
L89324	Pressure ulcer of L buttock, stage 4	157, 160	N/A
L89329	Pressure ulcer of L buttock, NOS stage	160	N/A
L8940	Pressure ulcer of contiguous site of back, buttock & hip, NOS stage	160	N/A
L8941	Pressure ulcer of contiguous site of back, buttock & hip, stage 1	160	N/A
L8942	Pressure ulcer of contiguous site of back, buttock & hip, stage 2	159, 160	N/A
L8943	Pressure ulcer of contiguous site of back, buttock & hip, stage 3	158, 160	N/A
L8944	Pressure ulcer of contiguous site of back, buttock & hip, stage 4	157, 160	N/A
L8945	Pressure ulcer of contiguous site of back, buttock & hip, unstageable	158, 160	N/A
L89500	Pressure ulcer of NOS ankle, unstageable	158, 160	N/A
L89501	Pressure ulcer of NOS ankle, stage 1	160	N/A
L89502	Pressure ulcer of NOS ankle, stage 2	159, 160	N/A

Code	Code Descriptors	HCC	RXHCC
L89503	Pressure ulcer of NOS ankle, stage 3	158, 160	N/A
L89504	Pressure ulcer of NOS ankle, stage 4	157, 160	N/A
L89509	Pressure ulcer of NOS ankle, NOS stage	160	N/A
L89510	Pressure ulcer of R ankle, unstageable	158, 160	N/A
L89511	Pressure ulcer of R ankle, stage 1	160	N/A
L89512	Pressure ulcer of R ankle, stage 2	159, 160	N/A
L89513	Pressure ulcer of R ankle, stage 3	158, 160	N/A
L89514	Pressure ulcer of R ankle, stage 4	157, 160	N/A
L89519	Pressure ulcer of R ankle, NOS stage	160	N/A
L89520	Pressure ulcer of L ankle, unstageable	158, 160	N/A
L89521	Pressure ulcer of L ankle, stage 1	160	N/A
L89522	Pressure ulcer of L ankle, stage 2	159, 160	N/A
L89523	Pressure ulcer of L ankle, stage 3	158, 160	N/A
L89524	Pressure ulcer of L ankle, stage 4	157, 160	N/A
L89529	Pressure ulcer of L ankle, NOS stage	160	N/A
L89600	Pressure ulcer of NOS heel, unstageable	158, 160	N/A
L89601	Pressure ulcer of NOS heel, stage 1	160	N/A
L89602	Pressure ulcer of NOS heel, stage 2	159, 160	N/A
L89603	Pressure ulcer of NOS heel, stage 3	158, 160	N/A
L89604	Pressure ulcer of NOS heel, stage 4	157, 160	N/A
L89609	Pressure ulcer of NOS heel, NOS stage	160	N/A
L89610	Pressure ulcer of R heel, unstageable	158, 160	N/A
L89611	Pressure ulcer of R heel, stage 1	160	N/A
L89612	Pressure ulcer of R heel, stage 2	159, 160	N/A
L89613	Pressure ulcer of R heel, stage 3	158, 160	N/A
L89614	Pressure ulcer of R heel, stage 4	157, 160	N/A
L89619	Pressure ulcer of R heel, NOS stage	160	N/A
L89620	Pressure ulcer of L heel, unstageable	158, 160	N/A
L89621	Pressure ulcer of L heel, stage 1	160	N/A
L89622	Pressure ulcer of L heel, stage 2	159, 160	N/A
L89623	Pressure ulcer of L heel, stage 3	158, 160	N/A

Code	Code Descriptors	HCC	RXHCC
L89624	Pressure ulcer of L heel, stage 4	157, 160	N/A
L89629	Pressure ulcer of L heel, NOS stage	160	N/A
L89810	Pressure ulcer of head, unstageable	158, 160	N/A
L89811	Pressure ulcer of head, stage 1	160	N/A
L89812	Pressure ulcer of head, stage 2	159, 160	N/A
L89813	Pressure ulcer of head, stage 3	158, 160	N/A
L89814	Pressure ulcer of head, stage 4	157, 160	N/A
L89819	Pressure ulcer of head, NOS stage	160	N/A
L89890	Pressure ulcer of other site, unstageable	158, 160	N/A
L89891	Pressure ulcer of other site, stage 1	160	N/A
L89892	Pressure ulcer of other site, stage 2	159, 160	N/A
L89893	Pressure ulcer of other site, stage 3	158, 160	N/A
L89894	Pressure ulcer of other site, stage 4	157, 160	N/A
L89899	Pressure ulcer of other site, NOS stage	160	N/A
L8990	Pressure ulcer of NOS site, NOS stage	160	N/A
L8991	Pressure ulcer of NOS site, stage 1	160	N/A
L8992	Pressure ulcer of NOS site, stage 2	159, 160	N/A
L8993	Pressure ulcer of NOS site, stage 3	158, 160	N/A
L8994	Pressure ulcer of NOS site, stage 4	157, 160	N/A
L8995	Pressure ulcer of NOS site, unstageable	158, 160	N/A
L945	Poikiloderma vasculare atrophicans	N/A	316
For codes L9710- through L9849-, use the following 6th character: **1 limited to breakdown of skin** **2 with fat layer exposed** **3 with necrosis of muscle** **4 with necrosis of bone** **5 with muscle involvement without evidence of necrosis** **6 with bone involvement without evidence of necrosis** **8 severity NEC** **9 severity NOS**			
L9710-	Non-pressure chronic ulcer of NOS thigh	161	311
L9711-	Non-pressure chronic ulcer of R thigh	161	311
L9712-	Non-pressure chronic ulcer of L thigh	161	311
L9720-	Non-pressure chronic ulcer of NOS calf	161	311
L9721-	Non-pressure chronic ulcer of R calf	161	311
L9722-	Non-pressure chronic ulcer of L calf	161	311
L9730-	Non-pressure chronic ulcer of NOS ankle	161	311
L9731-	Non-pressure chronic ulcer of R ankle	161	311
L9732-	Non-pressure chronic ulcer of L ankle	161	311
L9740-	Non-pressure chronic ulcer of NOS heel & midfoot	161	311
L9741-	Non-pressure chronic ulcer of R heel & midfoot	161	311
L9742-	Non-pressure chronic ulcer of L heel & midfoot	161	311
L9750-	Non-pressure chronic ulcer of other part of NOS foot	161	311
L9751-	Non-pressure chronic ulcer of other part of R foot	161	311
L9752-	Non-pressure chronic ulcer of other part of L foot	161	311
L9780-	Non-pressure chronic ulcer of other part of NOS lower leg	161	311
L9781-	Non-pressure chronic ulcer of other part of R lower leg	161	311
L9782-	Non-pressure chronic ulcer of other part of L lower leg	161	311
L9790-	Non-pressure chronic ulcer of NOS part of NOS lower leg	161	311
L9791-	Non-pressure chronic ulcer of NOS part of R lower leg	161	311
L9792-	Non-pressure chronic ulcer of NOS part of L lower leg	161	311
L9841-	Non-pressure chronic ulcer of buttock	161	311
L9842-	Non-pressure chronic ulcer of back	161	311
L9849-	Non-pressure chronic ulcer of skin of other sites	161	311
M0000	Staphylococcal arthritis, NOS joint	39	N/A
For codes M0001- through M0007-, use the following 6th character: **1 right** **2 left** **9 NOS**			
M0001-	Staphylococcal arthritis, shoulder	39	N/A
M0002-	Staphylococcal arthritis, elbow	39	N/A
M0003-	Staphylococcal arthritis, wrist	39	N/A
M0004-	Staphylococcal arthritis, hand	39	N/A
M0005-	Staphylococcal arthritis, hip	39	N/A
M0006-	Staphylococcal arthritis, knee	39	N/A
M0007-	Staphylococcal arthritis, ankle & foot	39	N/A
M0008	Staphylococcal arthritis, vertebrae	39	N/A
M0009	Staphylococcal polyarthritis	39	N/A
M0010	Pneumococcal arthritis, NOS joint	39	N/A
For codes M0011- through M0017-, use the following 6th character: **1 right** **2 left** **9 NOS**			
M0011-	Pneumococcal arthritis, shoulder	39	N/A
M0012-	Pneumococcal arthritis, elbow	39	N/A
M0013-	Pneumococcal arthritis, wrist	39	N/A
M0014-	Pneumococcal arthritis, hand	39	N/A
M0015-	Pneumococcal arthritis, hip	39	N/A

Code	Code Descriptors	HCC	RXHCC
M0016-	Pneumococcal arthritis, knee	39	N/A
M0017-	Pneumococcal arthritis, ankle & foot	39	N/A
M0018	Pneumococcal arthritis, vertebrae	39	N/A
M0019	Pneumococcal polyarthritis	39	N/A
M0020	Other streptococcal arthritis, NOS joint	39	N/A
For codes M0021- through M0027-, use the following 6th character: **1 right** **2 left** **9 NOS**			
M0021-	Other streptococcal arthritis, shoulder	39	N/A
M0022-	Other streptococcal arthritis, elbow	39	N/A
M0023-	Other streptococcal arthritis, wrist	39	N/A
M0024-	Other streptococcal arthritis, hand	39	N/A
M0025-	Other streptococcal arthritis, hip	39	N/A
M0026-	Other streptococcal arthritis, knee	39	N/A
M0027-	Other streptococcal arthritis, ankle & foot	39	N/A
M0028	Other streptococcal arthritis, vertebrae	39	N/A
M0029	Other streptococcal polyarthritis	39	N/A
M0080	Arthritis D/T other bacteria, NOS joint	39	N/A
For codes M0081- through M0087-, use the following 6th character: **1 right** **2 left** **9 NOS**			
M0081-	Arthritis D/T other bacteria, shoulder	39	N/A
M0082-	Arthritis D/T other bacteria, elbow	39	N/A
M0083-	Arthritis D/T other bacteria, wrist	39	N/A
M0084-	Arthritis D/T other bacteria, hand	39	N/A
M0085-	Arthritis D/T other bacteria, hip	39	N/A
M0086-	Arthritis D/T other bacteria, knee	39	N/A
M0087-	Arthritis D/T other bacteria, ankle & foot	39	N/A
M0088	Arthritis D/T other bacteria, vertebrae	39	N/A
M0089	Polyarthritis D/T other bacteria	39	N/A
M009	Pyogenic arthritis, NOS	39	N/A
M01X0	Direct infection of NOS joint in infectious & parasitic DZ classified elsewhere	39	N/A
For codes M01X1- through M01X7-, use the following 6th character: **1 right** **2 left** **9 NOS**			
M01X1-	Direct infection of shoulder in infectious & parasitic DZ classified elsewhere	39	N/A
M01X2-	Direct infection of elbow in infectious & parasitic DZ classified elsewhere	39	N/A
M01X3-	Direct infection of wrist in infectious & parasitic DZ classified elsewhere	39	N/A
M01X4-	Direct infection of hand in infectious & parasitic DZ classified elsewhere	39	N/A
M01X5-	Direct infection of hip in infectious & parasitic DZ classified elsewhere	39	N/A
M01X6-	Direct infection of knee in infectious & parasitic DZ classified elsewhere	39	N/A

Code	Code Descriptors	HCC	RXHCC
M01X7-	Direct infection of ankle & foot in infectious & parasitic DZ classified elsewhere	39	N/A
M01X8	Direct infection of vertebrae in infectious & parasitic DZ classified elsewhere	39	N/A
M01X9	Direct infection of multiple joints in infectious & parasitic DZ classified elsewhere	39	N/A
M0210	Postdysenteric arthropathy, NOS site	39	N/A
For codes M0211- through M0217-, use the following 6th character: **1 right** **2 left** **9 NOS**			
M0211-	Postdysenteric arthropathy, shoulder	39	N/A
M0212-	Postdysenteric arthropathy, elbow	39	N/A
M0213-	Postdysenteric arthropathy, wrist	39	N/A
M0214-	Postdysenteric arthropathy, hand	39	N/A
M0215-	Postdysenteric arthropathy, hip	39	N/A
M0216-	Postdysenteric arthropathy, knee	39	N/A
M0217-	Postdysenteric arthropathy, ankle & foot	39	N/A
M0218	Postdysenteric arthropathy, vertebrae	39	N/A
M0219	Postdysenteric arthropathy, multiple sites	39	N/A
M0230	Reiter's DZ, NOS site	40	83
For codes M0231- through M0237-, use the following 6th character: **1 right** **2 left** **9 NOS**			
M0231-	Reiter's DZ, shoulder	40	83
M0232-	Reiter's DZ, elbow	40	83
M0233-	Reiter's DZ, wrist	40	83
M0234-	Reiter's DZ, hand	40	83
M0235-	Reiter's DZ, hip	40	83
M0236-	Reiter's DZ, R knee	40	83
M0237-	Reiter's DZ, R ankle & foot	40	83
M0238	Reiter's DZ, vertebrae	40	83
M0239	Reiter's DZ, multiple sites	40	83
M0280	Other reactive arthropathies, NOS site	39	N/A
For codes M0281- through M0287-, use the following 6th character: **1 right** **2 left** **9 NOS**			
M0281-	Other reactive arthropathies, shoulder	39	N/A
M0282-	Other reactive arthropathies, elbow	39	N/A
M0283-	Other reactive arthropathies, wrist	39	N/A
M0284-	Other reactive arthropathies, hand	39	N/A
M0285-	Other reactive arthropathies, hip	39	N/A
M0286-	Other reactive arthropathies, knee	39	N/A
M0287-	Other reactive arthropathies, ankle & foot	39	N/A
M0288	Other reactive arthropathies, vertebrae	39	N/A
M0289	Other reactive arthropathies, multiple sites	39	N/A
M029	Reactive arthropathy, NOS	39	N/A

Code	Code Descriptors	HCC	RXHCC
M041	Periodic fever syndromes	40	83
M042	Cryopyrin-associated periodic syndromes	40	83
M048	Autoinflammatory syndrome, NEC	40	83
M049	Autoinflammatory syndrome, NOS	40	83
M0500	Felty's syndrome, NOS site	40	83
For codes M0501- through M0507-, use the following 6th character: **1 right** **2 left** **9 NOS**			
M0501-	Felty's syndrome, shoulder	40	83
M0502-	Felty's syndrome, elbow	40	83
M0503-	Felty's syndrome, wrist	40	83
M0504-	Felty's syndrome, hand	40	83
M0505-	Felty's syndrome, hip	40	83
M0506-	Felty's syndrome, knee	40	83
M0507-	Felty's syndrome, ankle & foot	40	83
M0509	Felty's syndrome, multiple sites	40	83
M0510	Rheumatoid lung DZ W/ rheumatoid arthritis of NOS site	40	83
For codes M0511- through M0517-, use the following 6th character: **1 right** **2 left** **9 NOS**			
M0511-	Rheumatoid lung DZ W/ rheumatoid arthritis of shoulder	40	83
M0512-	Rheumatoid lung DZ W/ rheumatoid arthritis of elbow	40	83
M0513-	Rheumatoid lung DZ W/ rheumatoid arthritis of wrist	40	83
M0514-	Rheumatoid lung DZ W/ rheumatoid arthritis of hand	40	83
M0515-	Rheumatoid lung DZ W/ rheumatoid arthritis of hip	40	83
M0516-	Rheumatoid lung DZ W/ rheumatoid arthritis of knee	40	83
M0517-	Rheumatoid lung DZ W/ rheumatoid arthritis of ankle & foot	40	83
M0519	Rheumatoid lung DZ W/ rheumatoid arthritis of multiple sites	40	83
M0520	Rheumatoid vasculitis W/ rheumatoid arthritis of NOS site	40	83
For codes M0521- through M0527-, use the following 6th character: **1 right** **2 left** **9 NOS**			
M0521-	Rheumatoid vasculitis W/ rheumatoid arthritis of shoulder	40	83
M0522-	Rheumatoid vasculitis W/ rheumatoid arthritis of elbow	40	83
M0523-	Rheumatoid vasculitis W/ rheumatoid arthritis of wrist	40	83
M0524-	Rheumatoid vasculitis W/ rheumatoid arthritis of hand	40	83

Code	Code Descriptors	HCC	RXHCC
M0525-	Rheumatoid vasculitis W/ rheumatoid arthritis of hip	40	83
M0526-	Rheumatoid vasculitis W/ rheumatoid arthritis of knee	40	83
M0527-	Rheumatoid vasculitis W/ rheumatoid arthritis of ankle & foot	40	83
M0529	Rheumatoid vasculitis W/ rheumatoid arthritis of multiple sites	40	83
M0530	Rheumatoid heart DZ W/ rheumatoid arthritis of NOS site	40	83
For codes M0531- through M0537-, use the following 6th character: **1 right** **2 left** **9 NOS**			
M0531-	Rheumatoid heart DZ W/ rheumatoid arthritis of shoulder	40	83
M0532-	Rheumatoid heart DZ W/ rheumatoid arthritis of elbow	40	83
M0533-	Rheumatoid heart DZ W/ rheumatoid arthritis of wrist	40	83
M0534-	Rheumatoid heart DZ W/ rheumatoid arthritis of hand	40	83
M0535-	Rheumatoid heart DZ W/ rheumatoid arthritis of hip	40	83
M0536-	Rheumatoid heart DZ W/ rheumatoid arthritis of knee	40	83
M0537-	Rheumatoid heart DZ W/ rheumatoid arthritis of ankle & foot	40	83
M0539	Rheumatoid heart DZ W/ rheumatoid arthritis of multiple sites	40	83
M0540	Rheumatoid myopathy W/ rheumatoid arthritis of NOS site	40, 75	83
For codes M0541- through M0547-, use the following 6th character: **1 right** **2 left** **9 NOS**			
M0541-	Rheumatoid myopathy W/ rheumatoid arthritis of shoulder	40, 75	83
M0542-	Rheumatoid myopathy W/ rheumatoid arthritis of elbow	40, 75	83
M0543-	Rheumatoid myopathy W/ rheumatoid arthritis of wrist	40, 75	83
M0544-	Rheumatoid myopathy W/ rheumatoid arthritis of hand	40, 75	83
M0545-	Rheumatoid myopathy W/ rheumatoid arthritis of hip	40, 75	83
M0546-	Rheumatoid myopathy W/ rheumatoid arthritis of knee	40, 75	83
M0547-	Rheumatoid myopathy W/ rheumatoid arthritis of ankle & foot	40, 75	83
M0549	Rheumatoid myopathy W/ rheumatoid arthritis of multiple sites	40, 75	83
M0550	Rheumatoid polyneuropathy W/ rheumatoid arthritis of NOS site	40, 75	83, 159

Code	Code Descriptors	HCC	RXHCC
For codes M0551- through M0557-, use the following 6th character: **1 right** **2 left** **9 NOS**			
M0551-	Rheumatoid polyneuropathy W/ rheumatoid arthritis of shoulder	40, 75	83, 159
M0552-	Rheumatoid polyneuropathy W/ rheumatoid arthritis of elbow	40, 75	83, 159
M0553-	Rheumatoid polyneuropathy W/ rheumatoid arthritis of wrist	40, 75	83, 159
M0554-	Rheumatoid polyneuropathy W/ rheumatoid arthritis of hand	40, 75	83, 159
M0555-	Rheumatoid polyneuropathy W/ rheumatoid arthritis of hip	40, 75	83, 159
M0556-	Rheumatoid polyneuropathy W/ rheumatoid arthritis of knee	40, 75	83, 159
M0557-	Rheumatoid polyneuropathy W/ rheumatoid arthritis of ankle & foot	40, 75	83, 159
M0559	Rheumatoid polyneuropathy W/ rheumatoid arthritis of multiple sites	40, 75	83, 159
M0560	Rheumatoid arthritis of NOS site W/ involvement of organs & systems, NEC	40	83
For codes M0561- through M0567-, use the following 6th character: **1 right** **2 left** **9 NOS**			
M0561-	Rheumatoid arthritis of shoulder W/ involvement of organs & systems NEC	40	83
M0562-	Rheumatoid arthritis of elbow W/ involvement of oter organs & systems NEC	40	83
M0563-	Rheumatoid arthritis of wrist W/ involvement of organs & systems NEC	40	83
M0564-	Rheumatoid arthritis of hand W/ involvement of organs & systems NEC	40	83
M0565-	Rheumatoid arthritis of hip W/ involvement of organs & systems NEC	40	83
M0566-	Rheumatoid arthritis of knee W/ involvement of organs & systems NEC	40	83
M0567-	Rheumatoid arthritis of ankle & foot W/ involvement of organs & systems NEC	40	83
M0569	Rheumatoid arthritis of multiple sites W/ involvement of organs & systems NEC	40	83
M0570	Rheumatoid arthritis W/ RF of NOS site W/O organ or systems involvement	40	83
For codes M0571- through M0577-, use the following 6th character: **1 right** **2 left** **9 NOS**			
M0571-	Rheumatoid arthritis W/ RF of shoulder W/O organ or systems involvement	40	83
M0572-	Rheumatoid arthritis W/ RF of elbow W/O organ or systems involvement	40	83
M0573-	Rheumatoid arthritis W/ RF of wrist W/O organ or systems involvement	40	83

Code	Code Descriptors	HCC	RXHCC
M0574-	Rheumatoid arthritis W/ RF of hand W/O organ or systems involvement	40	83
M0575-	Rheumatoid arthritis W/ RF of hip W/O organ or systems involvement	40	83
M0576-	Rheumatoid arthritis W/ RF of knee W/O organ or systems involvement	40	83
M0577-	Rheumatoid arthritis W/ RF of ankle & foot W/O organ or systems involvement	40	83
M0579	Rheumatoid arthritis W/ RF of multiple sites W/O organ or systems involvement	40	83
M0580	Other rheumatoid arthritis W/ RF of NOS site	40	83
For codes M0581- through M0587-, use the following 6th character: **1 right** **2 left** **9 NOS**			
M0581-	Other rheumatoid arthritis W/ RF of shoulder	40	83
M0582-	Other rheumatoid arthritis W/ RF of elbow	40	83
M0583-	Other rheumatoid arthritis W/ RF of wrist	40	83
M0584-	Other rheumatoid arthritis W/ RF of hand	40	83
M0585-	Other rheumatoid arthritis W/ RF of hip	40	83
M0586-	Other rheumatoid arthritis W/ RF of knee	40	83
M0587-	Other rheumatoid arthritis W/ RF of ankle & foot	40	83
M0589	Other rheumatoid arthritis W/ RF of multiple sites	40	83
M059	Rheumatoid arthritis W/ RF, NOS	40	83
M0600	Rheumatoid arthritis W/O RF, NOS site	40	83
For codes M0601- through M0607-, use the following 6th character: **1 right** **2 left** **9 NOS**			
M0601-	Rheumatoid arthritis W/O RF, shoulder	40	83
M0602-	Rheumatoid arthritis W/O RF, elbow	40	83
M0603-	Rheumatoid arthritis W/O RF, wrist	40	83
M0604-	Rheumatoid arthritis W/O RF, hand	40	83
M0605-	Rheumatoid arthritis W/O RF, hip	40	83
M0606-	Rheumatoid arthritis W/O RF, knee	40	83
M0607-	Rheumatoid arthritis W/O RF, ankle & foot	40	83
M0608	Rheumatoid arthritis W/O RF, vertebrae	40	83
M0609	Rheumatoid arthritis W/O RF, multiple sites	40	83
M061	Adult-onset Still's DZ	40	83
M0620	Rheumatoid bursitis, NOS site	40	83
For codes M0621- through M0627-, use the following 6th character: **1 right** **2 left** **9 NOS**			
M0621-	Rheumatoid bursitis, shoulder	40	83
M0622-	Rheumatoid bursitis, elbow	40	83
M0623-	Rheumatoid bursitis, wrist	40	83
M0624-	Rheumatoid bursitis, hand	40	83

Code	Code Descriptors	HCC	RXHCC
M0625-	Rheumatoid bursitis, hip	40	83
M0626-	Rheumatoid bursitis, knee	40	83
M0627-	Rheumatoid bursitis, ankle & foot	40	83
M0628	Rheumatoid bursitis, vertebrae	40	83
M0629	Rheumatoid bursitis, multiple sites	40	83
M0630	Rheumatoid nodule, NOS site	40	83
For codes M0631- through M0637-, use the following 6th character: **1 right** **2 left** **9 NOS**			
M0631-	Rheumatoid nodule, shoulder	40	83
M0632-	Rheumatoid nodule, elbow	40	83
M0633-	Rheumatoid nodule, wrist	40	83
M0634-	Rheumatoid nodule, hand	40	83
M0635-	Rheumatoid nodule, hip	40	83
M0636-	Rheumatoid nodule, knee	40	83
M0637-	Rheumatoid nodule, ankle & foot	40	83
M0638	Rheumatoid nodule, vertebrae	40	83
M0639	Rheumatoid nodule, multiple sites	40	83
M064	Inflammatory polyarthropathy	40	83
M0680	NEC rheumatoid arthritis, NOS site	40	83
For codes M0681- through M0687-, use the following 6th character: **1 right** **2 left** **9 NOS**			
M0681-	NEC rheumatoid arthritis, shoulder	40	83
M0682-	NEC rheumatoid arthritis, elbow	40	83
M0683-	NEC rheumatoid arthritis, wrist	40	83
M0684-	NEC rheumatoid arthritis, hand	40	83
M0685-	NEC rheumatoid arthritis, hip	40	83
M0686-	NEC rheumatoid arthritis, knee	40	83
M0687-	NEC rheumatoid arthritis, ankle & foot	40	83
M0688	NEC rheumatoid arthritis, vertebrae	40	83
M0689	NEC rheumatoid arthritis, multiple sites	40	83
M069	Rheumatoid arthritis, NOS	40	83
M0800	NOS juvenile rheumatoid arthritis of NOS site	40	83
For codes M0801- through M0807-, use the following 6th character: **1 right** **2 left** **9 NOS**			
M0801-	NOS juvenile rheumatoid arthritis, shoulder	40	83
M0802-	NOS juvenile rheumatoid arthritis, elbow	40	83
M0803-	NOS juvenile rheumatoid arthritis, wrist	40	83
M0804-	NOS juvenile rheumatoid arthritis, hand	40	83
M0805-	NOS juvenile rheumatoid arthritis, hip	40	83
M0806-	NOS juvenile rheumatoid arthritis, knee	40	83
M0807-	NOS juvenile rheumatoid arthritis, ankle & foot	40	83
M0808	NOS juvenile rheumatoid arthritis, vertebrae	40	83

Code	Code Descriptors	HCC	RXHCC
M0809	NOS juvenile rheumatoid arthritis, multiple sites	40	83
M081	Juvenile ankylosing spondylitis	40	84
M0820	Juvenile rheumatoid arthritis W/ systemic onset, NOS site	40	83
For codes M0821- through M0827-, use the following 6th character: **1 right** **2 left** **9 NOS**			
M0821-	Juvenile rheumatoid arthritis W/ systemic onset, shoulder	40	83
M0822-	Juvenile rheumatoid arthritis W/ systemic onset, elbow	40	83
M0823-	Juvenile rheumatoid arthritis W/ systemic onset, wrist	40	83
M0824-	Juvenile rheumatoid arthritis W/ systemic onset, hand	40	83
M0825-	Juvenile rheumatoid arthritis W/ systemic onset, hip	40	83
M0826-	Juvenile rheumatoid arthritis W/ systemic onset, knee	40	83
M0827-	Juvenile rheumatoid arthritis W/ systemic onset, ankle & foot	40	83
M0828	Juvenile rheumatoid arthritis W/ systemic onset, vertebrae	40	83
M0829	Juvenile rheumatoid arthritis W/ systemic onset, multiple sites	40	83
M083	Juvenile rheumatoid polyarthritis (seronegative)	40	83
M0840	Pauciarticular juvenile rheumatoid arthritis, NOS site	40	83
For codes M0841- through M0847-, use the following 6th character: **1 right** **2 left** **9 NOS**			
M0841-	Pauciarticular juvenile rheumatoid arthritis, shoulder	40	83
M0842-	Pauciarticular juvenile rheumatoid arthritis, elbow	40	83
M0843-	Pauciarticular juvenile rheumatoid arthritis, wrist	40	83
M0844-	Pauciarticular juvenile rheumatoid arthritis, hand	40	83
M0845-	Pauciarticular juvenile rheumatoid arthritis, hip	40	83
M0846-	Pauciarticular juvenile rheumatoid arthritis, knee	40	83
M0847-	Pauciarticular juvenile rheumatoid arthritis, ankle & foot	40	83
M0848	Pauciarticular juvenile rheumatoid arthritis, vertebrae	40	83
M0880	NEC juvenile arthritis, NOS site	40	83

Code	Code Descriptors	HCC	RXHCC
For codes M0881- through M0887-, use the following 6th character: 1 right 2 left 9 NOS			
M0881-	NEC juvenile arthritis, shoulder	40	83
M0882-	NEC juvenile arthritis, elbow	40	83
M0883-	NEC juvenile arthritis, wrist	40	83
M0884-	NEC juvenile arthritis, hand	40	83
M0885-	NEC juvenile arthritis, hip	40	83
M0886-	NEC juvenile arthritis, knee	40	83
M0887-	NEC juvenile arthritis, ankle & foot	40	83
M0888	NEC juvenile arthritis, NEC site	40	83
M0889	NEC juvenile arthritis, multiple sites	40	83
M0890	Juvenile arthritis, NOS, NOS site	40	83
For codes M0891- through M0897-, use the following 6th character: 1 right 2 left 9 NOS			
M0891-	Juvenile arthritis, NOS, shoulder	40	83
M0892-	Juvenile arthritis, NOS, elbow	40	83
M0893-	Juvenile arthritis, NOS, wrist	40	83
M0894-	Juvenile arthritis, NOS, hand	40	83
M0895-	Juvenile arthritis, NOS, hip	40	83
M0896-	Juvenile arthritis, NOS, knee	40	83
M0897-	Juvenile arthritis, NOS, ankle & foot	40	83
M0898	Juvenile arthritis, NOS, vertebrae	40	83
M0899	Juvenile arthritis, NOS, multiple sites	40	83
M1200	Chronic postrheumatic arthropathy, NOS site	40	83
For codes M1201- through M1207-, use the following 6th character: 1 right 2 left 9 NOS			
M1201-	Chronic postrheumatic arthropathy, shoulder	40	83
M1202-	Chronic postrheumatic arthropathy , elbow	40	83
M1203-	Chronic postrheumatic arthropathy, wrist	40	83
M1204-	Chronic postrheumatic arthropathy, hand	40	83
M1205-	Chronic postrheumatic arthropathy, hip	40	83
M1206-	Chronic postrheumatic arthropathy, knee	40	83
M1207-	Chronic postrheumatic arthropathy, ankle & foot	40	83
M1208	Chronic postrheumatic arthropathy, NEC site	40	83
M1209	Chronic postrheumatic arthropathy, multiple sites	40	83
M300	Polyarteritis nodosa	40	84
M301	Polyarteritis W/ lung involvement [Churg-Strauss]	40	84
M302	Juvenile polyarteritis	40	84
M303	Mucocutaneous lymph node syndrome [Kawasaki]	40	84

Code	Code Descriptors	HCC	RXHCC
M308	Other conditions related to polyarteritis nodosa	40	84
M310	Hypersensitivity angiitis	40	84
M311	Thrombotic microangiopathy	40	84
M312	Lethal midline granuloma	40	84
M3130	Wegener's granulomatosis W/O renal involvement	40	84
M3131	Wegener's granulomatosis W/ renal involvement	40	84
M314	Aortic arch syndrome [Takayasu]	40	84
M315	Giant cell arteritis W/ polymyalgia rheumatica	40	84
M316	Other giant cell arteritis	40	84
M317	Microscopic polyangiitis	40	84
M318	NEC necrotizing vasculopathies	108	N/A
M319	Necrotizing vasculopathy, NOS	108	N/A
M320	Drug-induced SLE	40	84
M3210	SLE, organ or system involvement NOS	40	84
M3211	Endocarditis in SLE	40	84
M3212	Pericarditis in SLE	40	84
M3213	Lung involvement in SLE	40, 112	84, 227
M3214	Glomerular DZ in SLE	40, 141	84
M3215	Tubulo-interstitial nephropathy in SLE	40, 141	84
M3219	Other organ or system involvement in SLE	40	84
M328	Other forms of SLE	40	84
M329	SLE, NOS	40	84
M3300	Juvenile dermatomyositis, organ involvement NOS	40	84
M3301	Juvenile dermatomyositis W/ respiratory involvement	40, 112	84, 227
M3302	Juvenile dermatomyositis W/ myopathy	40, 75	84
M3303	Juvenile dermatomyositis W/O myopathy	40	84
M3309	Juvenile dermatomyositis W/ organ involvement NEC	40	84
M3310	Dermatomyositis, NEC, organ involvement NOS	40	84
M3311	Dermatomyositis, NEC, W/ respiratory involvement	40, 112	84, 227
M3312	Dermatomyositis, NEC W/ myopathy	40, 75	84
M3313	Dermatomyositis, NEC, W/O myopathy	40	84
M3319	Dermatomyositis, NEC, W/ organ involvement, NEC	40	84
M3320	Polymyositis, organ involvement NOS	40	84
M3321	Polymyositis W/ respiratory involvement	40, 112	84, 227
M3322	Polymyositis W/ myopathy	40, 75	84
M3329	Polymyositis W/ organ involvement, NEC	40	84
M3390	Dermatopolymyositis, NOS, organ involvement NOS	40	84

Code	Code Descriptors	HCC	RXHCC
M3391	Dermatopolymyositis, NOS W/ respiratory involvement	40, 112	84, 227
M3392	Dermatopolymyositis, NOS W/ myopathy	40, 75	84
M3393	Dermatopolymyositis, NOS W/O myopathy	40	84
M3399	Dermatopolymyositis, NOS W/ organ involvement NEC	40	84
M340	Progressive systemic sclerosis	40	82
M341	CR(E)ST syndrome	40	82
M342	Systemic sclerosis induced by drug & chemical	40	82
M3481	Systemic sclerosis W/ lung involvement	40, 112	82, 227
M3482	Systemic sclerosis W/ myopathy	40, 75	82
M3483	Systemic sclerosis W/ polyneuropathy	40, 75	82, 159
M3489	Systemic sclerosis, NEC	40	82
M349	Systemic sclerosis, NOS	40	82
M3500	Sicca syndrome, NOS	40	84
M3501	Sicca syndrome W/ keratoconjunctivitis	40	84
M3502	Sicca syndrome W/ lung involvement	40, 112	84, 227
M3503	Sicca syndrome W/ myopathy	40, 75	84
M3504	Sicca syndrome W/ tubulo-interstitial nephropathy	40, 141	84
M3509	Sicca syndrome W/ other organ involvement	40	84
M351	Other overlap syndromes	40	84
M352	Behcet's DZ	40	83
M353	Polymyalgia rheumatica	40	N/A
M355	Multifocal fibrosclerosis	40	84
M358	Systemic involvement of connective tissue, NEC	40	84
M359	Systemic involvement of connective tissue, NOS	40	84
M360	Dermato(poly)myositis in neoplastic DZ	40	84
M368	Systemic disorders of connective tissue in other DZ classified elsewhere	40	84
M450	Ankylosing spondylitis of multiple sites in spine	40	84
M451	Ankylosing spondylitis of occipito-atlanto-axial region	40	84
M452	Ankylosing spondylitis of cervical region	40	84
M453	Ankylosing spondylitis of cervicothoracic region	40	84
M454	Ankylosing spondylitis of thoracic region	40	84
M455	Ankylosing spondylitis of thoracolumbar region	40	84
M456	Ankylosing spondylitis lumbar region	40	84
M457	Ankylosing spondylitis of lumbosacral region	40	84
M458	Ankylosing spondylitis sacral & sacrococcygeal region	40	84
M459	Ankylosing spondylitis of NOS sites in spine	40	84

Code	Code Descriptors	HCC	RXHCC
M4600	Spinal enthesopathy, site NOS	40	84
M4601	Spinal enthesopathy, occipito-atlanto-axial region	40	84
M4602	Spinal enthesopathy, cervical region	40	84
M4603	Spinal enthesopathy, cervicothoracic region	40	84
M4604	Spinal enthesopathy, thoracic region	40	84
M4605	Spinal enthesopathy, thoracolumbar region	40	84
M4606	Spinal enthesopathy, lumbar region	40	84
M4607	Spinal enthesopathy, lumbosacral region	40	84
M4608	Spinal enthesopathy, sacral & sacrococcygeal region	40	84
M4609	Spinal enthesopathy, multiple sites in spine	40	84
M461	Sacroiliitis, NEC	40	84
M4620	Osteomyelitis of vertebra, site NOS	39	N/A
M4621	Osteomyelitis of vertebra, occipito-atlanto-axial region	39	N/A
M4622	Osteomyelitis of vertebra, cervical region	39	N/A
M4623	Osteomyelitis of vertebra, cervicothoracic region	39	N/A
M4624	Osteomyelitis of vertebra, thoracic region	39	N/A
M4625	Osteomyelitis of vertebra, thoracolumbar region	39	N/A
M4626	Osteomyelitis of vertebra, lumbar region	39	N/A
M4627	Osteomyelitis of vertebra, lumbosacral region	39	N/A
M4628	Osteomyelitis of vertebra, sacral & sacrococcygeal region	39	N/A
For codes M463- through M469-, use the following 5th character: **0 site NOS** **1 occipito-atlanto-axial region** **2 cervical region** **3 cervicothoracic region** **4 thoracic region** **5 thoracolumbar region** **6 lumbar region** **7 lumbosacral region** **8 sacral and sacrococcygeal region** **9 multiple sites in spine**			
M463-	Infection of intervertebral disc (pyogenic)	39	N/A
M465-	Other infective spondylopathies	40	84
M468-	NEC inflammatory spondylopathies	40	84
M469-	NOS inflammatory spondylopathy	40	84
M4850XA	Collapsed vertebra, NEC, site NOS, initial encounter for FX	169	87
M4851XA	Collapsed vertebra, NEC, occipito-atlanto-axial region, initial encounter for FX	169	87
M4852XA	Collapsed vertebra, NEC, cervical region, initial encounter for FX	169	87
M4853XA	Collapsed vertebra, NEC, cervicothoracic region, initial encounter for FX	169	87
M4854XA	Collapsed vertebra, NEC, thoracic region, initial encounter for FX	169	87

Code	Code Descriptors	HCC	RXHCC
M4855XA	Collapsed vertebra, NEC, thoracolumbar region, initial encounter for FX	169	87
M4856XA	Collapsed vertebra, NEC, lumbar region, initial encounter for FX	169	87
M4857XA	Collapsed vertebra, NEC, lumbosacral region, initial encounter for FX	169	87
M4858XA	Collapsed vertebra, NEC, sacral & sacrococcygeal region, initial encounter for FX	169	87
M488X1	NEC spondylopathies, occipito-atlanto-axial region	40	84
M488X2	NEC spondylopathies, cervical region	40	84
M488X3	NEC spondylopathies, cervicothoracic region	40	84
M488X4	NEC spondylopathies, thoracic region	40	84
M488X5	NEC spondylopathies, thoracolumbar region	40	84
M488X6	NEC spondylopathies, lumbar region	40	84
M488X7	NEC spondylopathies, lumbosacral region	40	84
M488X8	NEC spondylopathies, sacral & sacrococcygeal region	40	84
M488X9	NEC spondylopathies, site NOS	40	84
M4980	Spondylopathy in DZ classified elsewhere, site NOS	40	84
M4981	Spondylopathy in DZ classified elsewhere, occipito- atlanto-axial region	40	84
M4982	Spondylopathy in DZ classified elsewhere, cervical region	40	84
M4983	Spondylopathy in DZ classified elsewhere, cervicothoracic region	40	84
M4984	Spondylopathy in DZ classified elsewhere, thoracic region	40	84
M4985	Spondylopathy in DZ classified elsewhere, thoracolumbar region	40	84
M4986	Spondylopathy in DZ classified elsewhere, lumbar region	40	84
M4987	Spondylopathy in DZ classified elsewhere, lumbosacral region	40	84
M4988	Spondylopathy in DZ classified elsewhere, sacral & sacrococcygeal region	40	84
M4989	Spondylopathy in DZ classified elsewhere, multiple sites in spine	40	84
M726	Necrotizing fasciitis	39	N/A
M8000XA	Age-related osteoporosis W/ current pathological FX, NOS site, initial encounter for FX	N/A	87
M80011A	Age-related osteoporosis W/ current pathological FX, R shoulder, initial encounter for FX	N/A	87
M80012A	Age-related osteoporosis W/ current pathological FX, L shoulder, initial encounter for FX	N/A	87
M80019A	Age-related osteoporosis W/ current pathological FX, NOS shoulder, initial encounter for FX	N/A	87
M80021A	Age-related osteoporosis W/ current pathological FX, R humerus, initial encounter for FX	N/A	87
M80022A	Age-related osteoporosis W/ current pathological FX, L humerus, initial encounter for FX	N/A	87
M80029A	Age-related osteoporosis W/ current pathological FX, NOS humerus, initial encounter for FX	N/A	87
M80031A	Age-related osteoporosis W/ current pathological FX, R forearm, initial encounter for FX	N/A	87
M80032A	Age-related osteoporosis W/ current pathological FX, L forearm, initial encounter for FX	N/A	87
M80039A	Age-related osteoporosis W/ current pathological FX, NOS forearm, initial encounter for FX	N/A	87
M80041A	Age-related osteoporosis W/ current pathological FX, R hand, initial encounter for FX	N/A	87
M80042A	Age-related osteoporosis W/ current pathological FX, L hand, initial encounter for FX	N/A	87
M80049A	Age-related osteoporosis W/ current pathological FX, NOS hand, initial encounter for FX	N/A	87
M80051A	Age-related osteoporosis W/ current pathological FX, R femur, initial encounter for FX	170	87
M80052A	Age-related osteoporosis W/ current pathological FX, L femur, initial encounter for FX	170	87
M80059A	Age-related osteoporosis W/ current pathological FX, NOS femur, initial encounter for FX	170	87
M80061A	Age-related osteoporosis W/ current pathological FX, R lower leg, initial encounter for FX	N/A	87
M80062A	Age-related osteoporosis W/ current pathological FX, L lower leg, initial encounter for FX	N/A	87
M80069A	Age-related osteoporosis W/ current pathological FX, NOS lower leg, initial encounter for FX	N/A	87
M80071A	Age-related osteoporosis W/ current pathological FX, R ankle & foot, initial encounter for FX	N/A	87
M80072A	Age-related osteoporosis W/ current pathological FX, L ankle & foot, initial encounter for FX	N/A	87
M80079A	Age-related osteoporosis W/ current pathological FX, NOS ankle & foot, initial encounter for FX	N/A	87
M8008XA	Age-related osteoporosis W/ current pathological FX, vertebra(e), initial encounter for FX	169	87

Code	Code Descriptors	HCC	RXHCC
M8080XA	Other osteoporosis W/ current pathological FX, NOS site, initial encounter for FX	N/A	87
M80811A	Other osteoporosis W/ current pathological FX, R shoulder, initial encounter for FX	N/A	87
M80812A	Other osteoporosis W/ current pathological FX, L shoulder, initial encounter for FX	N/A	87
M80819A	Other osteoporosis W/ current pathological FX, NOS shoulder, initial encounter for FX	N/A	87
M80821A	Other osteoporosis W/ current pathological FX, R humerus, initial encounter for FX	N/A	87
M80822A	Other osteoporosis W/ current pathological FX, L humerus, initial encounter for FX	N/A	87
M80829A	Other osteoporosis W/ current pathological FX, NOS humerus, initial encounter for FX	N/A	87
M80831A	Other osteoporosis W/ current pathological FX, R forearm, initial encounter for FX	N/A	87
M80832A	Other osteoporosis W/ current pathological FX, L forearm, initial encounter for FX	N/A	87
M80839A	Other osteoporosis W/ current pathological FX, NOS forearm, initial encounter for FX	N/A	87
M80841A	Other osteoporosis W/ current pathological FX, R hand, initial encounter for FX	N/A	87
M80842A	Other osteoporosis W/ current pathological FX, L hand, initial encounter for FX	N/A	87
M80849A	Other osteoporosis W/ current pathological FX, NOS hand, initial encounter for FX	N/A	87
M80851A	Other osteoporosis W/ current pathological FX, R femur, initial encounter for FX	170	87
M80852A	Other osteoporosis W/ current pathological FX, L femur, initial encounter for FX	170	87
M80859A	Other osteoporosis W/ current pathological FX, NOS femur, initial encounter for FX	170	87
M80861A	Other osteoporosis W/ current pathological FX, R lower leg, initial encounter for FX	N/A	87
M80862A	Other osteoporosis W/ current pathological FX, L lower leg, initial encounter for FX	N/A	87
M80869A	Other osteoporosis W/ current pathological FX, NOS lower leg, initial encounter for FX	N/A	87
M80871A	Other osteoporosis W/ current pathological FX, R ankle & foot, initial encounter for FX	N/A	87
M80872A	Other osteoporosis W/ current pathological FX, L ankle & foot, initial encounter for FX	N/A	87
M80879A	Other osteoporosis W/ current pathological FX, NOS ankle & foot, initial encounter for FX	N/A	87
M8088XA	Other osteoporosis W/ current pathological FX, vertebra(e), initial encounter for FX	169	87
M810	Age-related osteoporosis W/O current pathological FX	N/A	87
M816	Localized osteoporosis [Lequesne]	N/A	87
M818	Other osteoporosis W/O current pathological FX	N/A	87
M830	Puerperal osteomalacia	N/A	87
M831	Senile osteomalacia	N/A	87

Code	Code Descriptors	HCC	RXHCC
M832	Adult osteomalacia D/T malabsorption	N/A	87
M833	Adult osteomalacia D/T malnutrition	N/A	87
M834	Aluminum bone DZ	N/A	87
M835	Other drug-induced osteomalacia in adults	N/A	87
M838	Other adult osteomalacia	N/A	87
M839	Adult osteomalacia, NOS	N/A	87
M8440XA	Pathological FX, NOS site, initial encounter for FX	N/A	87
M84411A	Pathological FX, R shoulder, initial encounter for FX	N/A	87
M84412A	Pathological FX, L shoulder, initial encounter for FX	N/A	87
M84419A	Pathological FX, NOS shoulder, initial encounter for FX	N/A	87
M84421A	Pathological FX, R humerus, initial encounter for FX	N/A	87
M84422A	Pathological FX, L humerus, initial encounter for FX	N/A	87
M84429A	Pathological FX, NOS humerus, initial encounter for FX	N/A	87
M84431A	Pathological FX, R ulna, initial encounter for FX	N/A	87
M84432A	Pathological FX, L ulna, initial encounter for FX	N/A	87
M84433A	Pathological FX, R radius, initial encounter for FX	N/A	87
M84434A	Pathological FX, L radius, initial encounter for FX	N/A	87
M84439A	Pathological FX, NOS ulna & radius, initial encounter for FX	N/A	87
M84441A	Pathological FX, R hand, initial encounter for FX	N/A	87
M84442A	Pathological FX, L hand, initial encounter for FX	N/A	87
M84443A	Pathological FX, NOS hand, initial encounter for FX	N/A	87
M84444A	Pathological FX, R finger(s), initial encounter for FX	N/A	87
M84445A	Pathological FX, L finger(s), initial encounter for FX	N/A	87
M84446A	Pathological FX, NOS finger(s), initial encounter for FX	N/A	87
M84451A	Pathological FX, R femur, initial encounter for FX	170	87
M84452A	Pathological FX, L femur, initial encounter for FX	170	87
M84453A	Pathological FX, NOS femur, initial encounter for FX	170	87
M84454A	Pathological FX, pelvis, initial encounter for FX	N/A	87
M84459A	Pathological FX, hip, NOS, initial encounter for FX	170	87

Code	Code Descriptors	HCC	RXHCC
M84461A	Pathological FX, R tibia, initial encounter for FX	N/A	87
M84462A	Pathological FX, L tibia, initial encounter for FX	N/A	87
M84463A	Pathological FX, R fibula, initial encounter for FX	N/A	87
M84464A	Pathological FX, L fibula, initial encounter for FX	N/A	87
M84469A	Pathological FX, NOS tibia & fibula, initial encounter for FX	N/A	87
M84471A	Pathological FX, R ankle, initial encounter for FX	N/A	87
M84472A	Pathological FX, L ankle, initial encounter for FX	N/A	87
M84473A	Pathological FX, NOS ankle, initial encounter for FX	N/A	87
M84474A	Pathological FX, R foot, initial encounter for FX	N/A	87
M84475A	Pathological FX, L foot, initial encounter for FX	N/A	87
M84476A	Pathological FX, NOS foot, initial encounter for FX	N/A	87
M84477A	Pathological FX, R toe(s), initial encounter for FX	N/A	87
M84478A	Pathological FX, L toe(s), initial encounter for FX	N/A	87
M84479A	Pathological FX, NOS toe(s), initial encounter for FX	N/A	87
M8448XA	Pathological FX, other site, initial encounter for FX	N/A	87
M8450XA	Pathological FX in neoplastic DZ, NOS site, initial encounter for FX	N/A	87
M84511A	Pathological FX in neoplastic DZ, R shoulder, initial encounter for FX	N/A	87
M84512A	Pathological FX in neoplastic DZ, L shoulder, initial encounter for FX	N/A	87
M84519A	Pathological FX in neoplastic DZ, NOS shoulder, initial encounter for FX	N/A	87
M84521A	Pathological FX in neoplastic DZ, R humerus, initial encounter for FX	N/A	87
M84522A	Pathological FX in neoplastic DZ, L humerus, initial encounter for FX	N/A	87
M84529A	Pathological FX in neoplastic DZ, NOS humerus, initial encounter for FX	N/A	87
M84531A	Pathological FX in neoplastic DZ, R ulna, initial encounter for FX	N/A	87
M84532A	Pathological FX in neoplastic DZ, L ulna, initial encounter for FX	N/A	87
M84533A	Pathological FX in neoplastic DZ, R radius, initial encounter for FX	N/A	87
M84534A	Pathological FX in neoplastic DZ, L radius, initial encounter for FX	N/A	87
M84539A	Pathological FX in neoplastic DZ, NOS ulna & radius, initial encounter for FX	N/A	87

Code	Code Descriptors	HCC	RXHCC
M84541A	Pathological FX in neoplastic DZ, R hand, initial encounter for FX	N/A	87
M84542A	Pathological FX in neoplastic DZ, L hand, initial encounter for FX	N/A	87
M84549A	Pathological FX in neoplastic DZ, NOS hand, initial encounter for FX	N/A	87
M84550A	Pathological FX in neoplastic DZ, pelvis, initial encounter for FX	N/A	87
M84551A	Pathological FX in neoplastic DZ, R femur, initial encounter for FX	170	87
M84552A	Pathological FX in neoplastic DZ, L femur, initial encounter for FX	170	87
M84553A	Pathological FX in neoplastic DZ, NOS femur, initial encounter for FX	170	87
M84559A	Pathological FX in neoplastic DZ, hip, NOS, initial encounter for FX	170	87
M84561A	Pathological FX in neoplastic DZ, R tibia, initial encounter for FX	N/A	87
M84562A	Pathological FX in neoplastic DZ, L tibia, initial encounter for FX	N/A	87
M84563A	Pathological FX in neoplastic DZ, R fibula, initial encounter for FX	N/A	87
M84564A	Pathological FX in neoplastic DZ, L fibula, initial encounter for FX	N/A	87
M84569A	Pathological FX in neoplastic DZ, NOS tibia & fibula, initial encounter for FX	N/A	87
M84571A	Pathological FX in neoplastic DZ, R ankle, initial encounter for FX	N/A	87
M84572A	Pathological FX in neoplastic DZ, L ankle, initial encounter for FX	N/A	87
M84573A	Pathological FX in neoplastic DZ, NOS ankle, initial encounter for FX	N/A	87
M84574A	Pathological FX in neoplastic DZ, R foot, initial encounter for FX	N/A	87
M84575A	Pathological FX in neoplastic DZ, L foot, initial encounter for FX	N/A	87
M84576A	Pathological FX in neoplastic DZ, NOS foot, initial encounter for FX	N/A	87
M8458XA	Pathological FX in neoplastic DZ, NEC site, initial encounter for FX	N/A	87
M8460XA	Pathological FX in other DZ, NOS site, initial encounter for FX	N/A	87
M84611A	Pathological FX in other DZ, R shoulder, initial encounter for FX	N/A	87
M84612A	Pathological FX in other DZ, L shoulder, initial encounter for FX	N/A	87
M84619A	Pathological FX in other DZ, NOS shoulder, initial encounter for FX	N/A	87
M84621A	Pathological FX in other DZ, R humerus, initial encounter for FX	N/A	87
M84622A	Pathological FX in other DZ, L humerus, initial encounter for FX	N/A	87
M84629A	Pathological FX in other DZ, NOS humerus, initial encounter for FX	N/A	87

Code	Code Descriptors	HCC	RXHCC
M84631A	Pathological FX in other DZ, R ulna, initial encounter for FX	N/A	87
M84632A	Pathological FX in other DZ, L ulna, initial encounter for FX	N/A	87
M84633A	Pathological FX in other DZ, R radius, initial encounter for FX	N/A	87
M84634A	Pathological FX in other DZ, L radius, initial encounter for FX	N/A	87
M84639A	Pathological FX in other DZ, NOS ulna & radius, initial encounter for FX	N/A	87
M84641A	Pathological FX in other DZ, R hand, initial encounter for FX	N/A	87
M84642A	Pathological FX in other DZ, L hand, initial encounter for FX	N/A	87
M84649A	Pathological FX in other DZ, NOS hand, initial encounter for FX	N/A	87
M84650A	Pathological FX in other DZ, pelvis, initial encounter for FX	N/A	87
M84651A	Pathological FX in other DZ, R femur, initial encounter for FX	170	87
M84652A	Pathological FX in other DZ, L femur, initial encounter for FX	170	87
M84653A	Pathological FX in other DZ, NOS femur, initial encounter for FX	170	87
M84659A	Pathological FX in other DZ, hip, NOS, initial encounter for FX	170	87
M84661A	Pathological FX in other DZ, R tibia, initial encounter for FX	N/A	87
M84662A	Pathological FX in other DZ, L tibia, initial encounter for FX	N/A	87
M84663A	Pathological FX in other DZ, R fibula, initial encounter for FX	N/A	87
M84664A	Pathological FX in other DZ, L fibula, initial encounter for FX	N/A	87
M84669A	Pathological FX in other DZ, NOS tibia & fibula, initial encounter for FX	N/A	87
M84671A	Pathological FX in other DZ, R ankle, initial encounter for FX	N/A	87
M84672A	Pathological FX in other DZ, L ankle, initial encounter for FX	N/A	87
M84673A	Pathological FX in other DZ, NOS ankle, initial encounter for FX	N/A	87
M84674A	Pathological FX in other DZ, R foot, initial encounter for FX	N/A	87
M84675A	Pathological FX in other DZ, L foot, initial encounter for FX	N/A	87
M84676A	Pathological FX in other DZ, NOS foot, initial encounter for FX	N/A	87
M8468XA	Pathological FX in other DZ, other site, initial encounter for FX	N/A	87
M84754A	Complete transverse atypical femoral FX, R leg, initial encounter for FX	170	N/A
M84755A	Complete transverse atypical femoral FX, L leg, initial encounter for FX	170	N/A

Code	Code Descriptors	HCC	RXHCC
M84756A	Complete transverse atypical femoral FX, NOS leg, initial encounter for FX	170	N/A
M84757A	Complete oblique atypical femoral FX, R leg, initial encounter for FX	170	N/A
M84758A	Complete oblique atypical femoral FX, L leg, initial encounter for FX	170	N/A
M84759A	Complete oblique atypical femoral FX, NOS leg, initial encounter for FX	170	N/A
M8600	Acute hematogenous osteomyelitis, NOS site	39	N/A
For codes M8601- through M8607-, use the following 6th character: **1 right** **2 left** **9 NOS**			
M8601-	Acute hematogenous osteomyelitis, shoulder	39	N/A
M8602-	Acute hematogenous osteomyelitis, humerus	39	N/A
M8603-	Acute hematogenous osteomyelitis, radius & ulna	39	N/A
M8604-	Acute hematogenous osteomyelitis, hand	39	N/A
M8605-	Acute hematogenous osteomyelitis, femur	39	N/A
M8606-	Acute hematogenous osteomyelitis, tibia & fibula	39	N/A
M8607-	Acute hematogenous osteomyelitis, ankle & foot	39	N/A
M8608	Acute hematogenous osteomyelitis, other sites	39	N/A
M8609	Acute hematogenous osteomyelitis, multiple sites	39	N/A
M8610	Other acute osteomyelitis, NOS site	39	N/A
For codes M8611- through M8617-, use the following 6th character: **1 right** **2 left** **9 NOS**			
M8611-	Other acute osteomyelitis, shoulder	39	N/A
M8612-	Other acute osteomyelitis, humerus	39	N/A
M8613-	Other acute osteomyelitis, radius & ulna	39	N/A
M8614-	Other acute osteomyelitis, hand	39	N/A
M8615-	Other acute osteomyelitis, femur	39	N/A
M8616-	Other acute osteomyelitis, tibia & fibula	39	N/A
M8617-	Other acute osteomyelitis, ankle & foot	39	N/A
M8618	Other acute osteomyelitis, other site	39	N/A
M8619	Other acute osteomyelitis, multiple sites	39	N/A
M8620	Subacute osteomyelitis, NOS site	39	N/A
For codes M8621- through M8627-, use the following 6th character: **1 right** **2 left** **9 NOS**			
M8621-	Subacute osteomyelitis, shoulder	39	N/A
M8622-	Subacute osteomyelitis, humerus	39	N/A
M8623-	Subacute osteomyelitis, radius & ulna	39	N/A

Code	Code Descriptors	HCC	RXHCC
M8624-	Subacute osteomyelitis, hand	39	N/A
M8625-	Subacute osteomyelitis, femur	39	N/A
M8626-	Subacute osteomyelitis, tibia & fibula	39	N/A
M8627-	Subacute osteomyelitis, ankle & foot	39	N/A
M8628	Subacute osteomyelitis, other site	39	N/A
M8629	Subacute osteomyelitis, multiple sites	39	N/A
M8630	Chronic multifocal osteomyelitis, NOS site	39	N/A
For codes M8631- through M8637-, use the following 6th character: **1 right** **2 left** **9 NOS**			
M8631-	Chronic multifocal osteomyelitis, shoulder	39	N/A
M8632-	Chronic multifocal osteomyelitis, humerus	39	N/A
M8633-	Chronic multifocal osteomyelitis, radius & ulna	39	N/A
M8634-	Chronic multifocal osteomyelitis, hand	39	N/A
M8635-	Chronic multifocal osteomyelitis, femur	39	N/A
M8636-	Chronic multifocal osteomyelitis, tibia & fibula	39	N/A
M8637-	Chronic multifocal osteomyelitis, ankle & foot	39	N/A
M8638	Chronic multifocal osteomyelitis, other site	39	N/A
M8639	Chronic multifocal osteomyelitis, multiple sites	39	N/A
M8640	Chronic osteomyelitis W/ draining sinus, NOS site	39	N/A
For codes M8641- through M8647-, use the following 6th character: **1 right** **2 left** **9 NOS**			
M8641-	Chronic osteomyelitis W/ draining sinus, shoulder	39	N/A
M8642-	Chronic osteomyelitis W/ draining sinus, humerus	39	N/A
M8643-	Chronic osteomyelitis W/ draining sinus, radius & ulna	39	N/A
M8644-	Chronic osteomyelitis W/ draining sinus, hand	39	N/A
M8645-	Chronic osteomyelitis W/ draining sinus, femur	39	N/A
M8646-	Chronic osteomyelitis W/ draining sinus, tibia & fibula	39	N/A
M8647-	Chronic osteomyelitis W/ draining sinus, ankle & foot	39	N/A
M8648	Chronic osteomyelitis W/ draining sinus, other site	39	N/A
M8649	Chronic osteomyelitis W/ draining sinus, multiple sites	39	N/A
M8650	Other chronic hematogenous osteomyelitis, NOS site	39	N/A

Code	Code Descriptors	HCC	RXHCC
For codes M8651- through M8657-, use the following 6th character: **1 right** **2 left** **9 NOS**			
M8651-	Other chronic hematogenous osteomyelitis, shoulder	39	N/A
M8652-	Other chronic hematogenous osteomyelitis, humerus	39	N/A
M8653-	Other chronic hematogenous osteomyelitis, radius & ulna	39	N/A
M8654-	Other chronic hematogenous osteomyelitis, hand	39	N/A
M8655-	Other chronic hematogenous osteomyelitis, femur	39	N/A
M8656-	Other chronic hematogenous osteomyelitis, tibia & fibula	39	N/A
M8657-	Other chronic hematogenous osteomyelitis, ankle & foot	39	N/A
M8658	Other chronic hematogenous osteomyelitis, other site	39	N/A
M8659	Other chronic hematogenous osteomyelitis, multiple sites	39	N/A
M8660	Other chronic osteomyelitis, NOS site	39	N/A
For codes M8661- through M8667-, use the following 6th character: **1 right** **2 left** **9 NOS**			
M8661-	Other chronic osteomyelitis, shoulder	39	N/A
M8662-	Other chronic osteomyelitis, humerus	39	N/A
M8663-	Other chronic osteomyelitis, radius & ulna	39	N/A
M8664-	Other chronic osteomyelitis, hand	39	N/A
M8665-	Other chronic osteomyelitis, thigh	39	N/A
M8666-	Other chronic osteomyelitis, tibia & fibula	39	N/A
M8667-	Other chronic osteomyelitis, ankle & foot	39	N/A
M8668	Other chronic osteomyelitis, other site	39	N/A
M8669	Other chronic osteomyelitis, multiple sites	39	N/A
M868X0	Other osteomyelitis, multiple sites	39	N/A
M868X1	Other osteomyelitis, shoulder	39	N/A
M868X2	Other osteomyelitis, upper arm	39	N/A
M868X3	Other osteomyelitis, forearm	39	N/A
M868X4	Other osteomyelitis, hand	39	N/A
M868X5	Other osteomyelitis, thigh	39	N/A
M868X6	Other osteomyelitis, lower leg	39	N/A
M868X7	Other osteomyelitis, ankle & foot	39	N/A
M868X8	Other osteomyelitis, NEC site	39	N/A
M868X9	Other osteomyelitis, NOS site	39	N/A
M869	Osteomyelitis, NOS	39	N/A
M8700	Idiopathic aseptic necrosis of NOS bone	39	80
M87011	Idiopathic aseptic necrosis of R shoulder	39	80
M87012	Idiopathic aseptic necrosis of L shoulder	39	80
M87019	Idiopathic aseptic necrosis of NOS shoulder	39	80

Code	Code Descriptors	HCC	RXHCC
M87021	Idiopathic aseptic necrosis of R humerus	39	80
M87022	Idiopathic aseptic necrosis of L humerus	39	80
M87029	Idiopathic aseptic necrosis of NOS humerus	39	80
M87031	Idiopathic aseptic necrosis of R radius	39	80
M87032	Idiopathic aseptic necrosis of L radius	39	80
M87033	Idiopathic aseptic necrosis of NOS radius	39	80
M87034	Idiopathic aseptic necrosis of R ulna	39	80
M87035	Idiopathic aseptic necrosis of L ulna	39	80
M87036	Idiopathic aseptic necrosis of NOS ulna	39	80
M87037	Idiopathic aseptic necrosis of R carpus	39	80
M87038	Idiopathic aseptic necrosis of L carpus	39	80
M87039	Idiopathic aseptic necrosis of NOS carpus	39	80
M87041	Idiopathic aseptic necrosis of R hand	39	80
M87042	Idiopathic aseptic necrosis of L hand	39	80
M87043	Idiopathic aseptic necrosis of NOS hand	39	80
M87044	Idiopathic aseptic necrosis of R finger(s)	39	80
M87045	Idiopathic aseptic necrosis of L finger(s)	39	80
M87046	Idiopathic aseptic necrosis of NOS finger(s)	39	80
M87050	Idiopathic aseptic necrosis of pelvis	39	80
M87051	Idiopathic aseptic necrosis of R femur	39	80
M87052	Idiopathic aseptic necrosis of L femur	39	80
M87059	Idiopathic aseptic necrosis of NOS femur	39	80
M87061	Idiopathic aseptic necrosis of R tibia	39	80
M87062	Idiopathic aseptic necrosis of L tibia	39	80
M87063	Idiopathic aseptic necrosis of NOS tibia	39	80
M87064	Idiopathic aseptic necrosis of R fibula	39	80
M87065	Idiopathic aseptic necrosis of L fibula	39	80
M87066	Idiopathic aseptic necrosis of NOS fibula	39	80
M87071	Idiopathic aseptic necrosis of R ankle	39	80
M87072	Idiopathic aseptic necrosis of L ankle	39	80
M87073	Idiopathic aseptic necrosis of NOS ankle	39	80
M87074	Idiopathic aseptic necrosis of R foot	39	80
M87075	Idiopathic aseptic necrosis of L foot	39	80
M87076	Idiopathic aseptic necrosis of NOS foot	39	80
M87077	Idiopathic aseptic necrosis of R toe(s)	39	80
M87078	Idiopathic aseptic necrosis of L toe(s)	39	80
M87079	Idiopathic aseptic necrosis of NOS toe(s)	39	80
M8708	Idiopathic aseptic necrosis of bone, other site	39	80
M8709	Idiopathic aseptic necrosis of bone, multiple sites	39	80
M8710	Osteonecrosis D/T drugs, NOS bone	39	80
M87111	Osteonecrosis D/T drugs, R shoulder	39	80
M87112	Osteonecrosis D/T drugs, L shoulder	39	80
M87119	Osteonecrosis D/T drugs, NOS shoulder	39	80
M87121	Osteonecrosis D/T drugs, R humerus	39	80
M87122	Osteonecrosis D/T drugs, L humerus	39	80

Code	Code Descriptors	HCC	RXHCC
M87129	Osteonecrosis D/T drugs, NOS humerus	39	80
M87131	Osteonecrosis D/T drugs of R radius	39	80
M87132	Osteonecrosis D/T drugs of L radius	39	80
M87133	Osteonecrosis D/T drugs of NOS radius	39	80
M87134	Osteonecrosis D/T drugs of R ulna	39	80
M87135	Osteonecrosis D/T drugs of L ulna	39	80
M87136	Osteonecrosis D/T drugs of NOS ulna	39	80
M87137	Osteonecrosis D/T drugs of R carpus	39	80
M87138	Osteonecrosis D/T drugs of L carpus	39	80
M87139	Osteonecrosis D/T drugs of NOS carpus	39	80
M87141	Osteonecrosis D/T drugs, R hand	39	80
M87142	Osteonecrosis D/T drugs, L hand	39	80
M87143	Osteonecrosis D/T drugs, NOS hand	39	80
M87144	Osteonecrosis D/T drugs, R finger(s)	39	80
M87145	Osteonecrosis D/T drugs, L finger(s)	39	80
M87146	Osteonecrosis D/T drugs, NOS finger(s)	39	80
M87150	Osteonecrosis D/T drugs, pelvis	39	80
M87151	Osteonecrosis D/T drugs, R femur	39	80
M87152	Osteonecrosis D/T drugs, L femur	39	80
M87159	Osteonecrosis D/T drugs, NOS femur	39	80
M87161	Osteonecrosis D/T drugs, R tibia	39	80
M87162	Osteonecrosis D/T drugs, L tibia	39	80
M87163	Osteonecrosis D/T drugs, NOS tibia	39	80
M87164	Osteonecrosis D/T drugs, R fibula	39	80
M87165	Osteonecrosis D/T drugs, L fibula	39	80
M87166	Osteonecrosis D/T drugs, NOS fibula	39	80
M87171	Osteonecrosis D/T drugs, R ankle	39	80
M87172	Osteonecrosis D/T drugs, L ankle	39	80
M87173	Osteonecrosis D/T drugs, NOS ankle	39	80
M87174	Osteonecrosis D/T drugs, R foot	39	80
M87175	Osteonecrosis D/T drugs, L foot	39	80
M87176	Osteonecrosis D/T drugs, NOS foot	39	80
M87177	Osteonecrosis D/T drugs, R toe(s)	39	80
M87178	Osteonecrosis D/T drugs, L toe(s)	39	80
M87179	Osteonecrosis D/T drugs, NOS toe(s)	39	80
M87180	Osteonecrosis D/T drugs, jaw	39	80
M87188	Osteonecrosis D/T drugs, other site	39	80
M8719	Osteonecrosis D/T drugs, multiple sites	39	80
M8720	Osteonecrosis D/T previous trauma, NOS bone	39	80
M87211	Osteonecrosis D/T previous trauma, R shoulder	39	80
M87212	Osteonecrosis D/T previous trauma, L shoulder	39	80
M87219	Osteonecrosis D/T previous trauma, NOS shoulder	39	80
M87221	Osteonecrosis D/T previous trauma, R humerus	39	80

Code	Code Descriptors	HCC	RXHCC
M87222	Osteonecrosis D/T previous trauma, L humerus	39	80
M87229	Osteonecrosis D/T previous trauma, NOS humerus	39	80
M87231	Osteonecrosis D/T previous trauma of R radius	39	80
M87232	Osteonecrosis D/T previous trauma of L radius	39	80
M87233	Osteonecrosis D/T previous trauma of NOS radius	39	80
M87234	Osteonecrosis D/T previous trauma of R ulna	39	80
M87235	Osteonecrosis D/T previous trauma of L ulna	39	80
M87236	Osteonecrosis D/T previous trauma of NOS ulna	39	80
M87237	Osteonecrosis D/T previous trauma of R carpus	39	80
M87238	Osteonecrosis D/T previous trauma of L carpus	39	80
M87239	Osteonecrosis D/T previous trauma of NOS carpus	39	80
M87241	Osteonecrosis D/T previous trauma, R hand	39	80
M87242	Osteonecrosis D/T previous trauma, L hand	39	80
M87243	Osteonecrosis D/T previous trauma, NOS hand	39	80
M87244	Osteonecrosis D/T previous trauma, R finger(s)	39	80
M87245	Osteonecrosis D/T previous trauma, L finger(s)	39	80
M87246	Osteonecrosis D/T previous trauma, NOS finger(s)	39	80
M87250	Osteonecrosis D/T previous trauma, pelvis	39	80
M87251	Osteonecrosis D/T previous trauma, R femur	39	80
M87252	Osteonecrosis D/T previous trauma, L femur	39	80
M87256	Osteonecrosis D/T previous trauma, NOS femur	39	80
M87261	Osteonecrosis D/T previous trauma, R tibia	39	80
M87262	Osteonecrosis D/T previous trauma, L tibia	39	80
M87263	Osteonecrosis D/T previous trauma, NOS tibia	39	80
M87264	Osteonecrosis D/T previous trauma, R fibula	39	80
M87265	Osteonecrosis D/T previous trauma, L fibula	39	80
M87266	Osteonecrosis D/T previous trauma, NOS fibula	39	80
M87271	Osteonecrosis D/T previous trauma, R ankle	39	80
M87272	Osteonecrosis D/T previous trauma, L ankle	39	80
M87273	Osteonecrosis D/T previous trauma, NOS ankle	39	80
M87274	Osteonecrosis D/T previous trauma, R foot	39	80
M87275	Osteonecrosis D/T previous trauma, L foot	39	80
M87276	Osteonecrosis D/T previous trauma, NOS foot	39	80

Code	Code Descriptors	HCC	RXHCC
M87277	Osteonecrosis D/T previous trauma, R toe(s)	39	80
M87278	Osteonecrosis D/T previous trauma, L toe(s)	39	80
M87279	Osteonecrosis D/T previous trauma, NOS toe(s)	39	80
M8728	Osteonecrosis D/T previous trauma, other site	39	80
M8729	Osteonecrosis D/T previous trauma, multiple sites	39	80
M8730	Other 2ndary osteonecrosis, NOS bone	39	80
M87311	Other 2ndary osteonecrosis, R shoulder	39	80
M87312	Other 2ndary osteonecrosis, L shoulder	39	80
M87319	Other 2ndary osteonecrosis, NOS shoulder	39	80
M87321	Other 2ndary osteonecrosis, R humerus	39	80
M87322	Other 2ndary osteonecrosis, L humerus	39	80
M87329	Other 2ndary osteonecrosis, NOS humerus	39	80
M87331	Other 2ndary osteonecrosis of R radius	39	80
M87332	Other 2ndary osteonecrosis of L radius	39	80
M87333	Other 2ndary osteonecrosis of NOS radius	39	80
M87334	Other 2ndary osteonecrosis of R ulna	39	80
M87335	Other 2ndary osteonecrosis of L ulna	39	80
M87336	Other 2ndary osteonecrosis of NOS ulna	39	80
M87337	Other 2ndary osteonecrosis of R carpus	39	80
M87338	Other 2ndary osteonecrosis of L carpus	39	80
M87339	Other 2ndary osteonecrosis of NOS carpus	39	80
M87341	Other 2ndary osteonecrosis, R hand	39	80
M87342	Other 2ndary osteonecrosis, L hand	39	80
M87343	Other 2ndary osteonecrosis, NOS hand	39	80
M87344	Other 2ndary osteonecrosis, R finger(s)	39	80
M87345	Other 2ndary osteonecrosis, L finger(s)	39	80
M87346	Other 2ndary osteonecrosis, NOS finger(s)	39	80
M87350	Other 2ndary osteonecrosis, pelvis	39	80
M87351	Other 2ndary osteonecrosis, R femur	39	80
M87352	Other 2ndary osteonecrosis, L femur	39	80
M87353	Other 2ndary osteonecrosis, NOS femur	39	80
M87361	Other 2ndary osteonecrosis, R tibia	39	80
M87362	Other 2ndary osteonecrosis, L tibia	39	80
M87363	Other 2ndary osteonecrosis, NOS tibia	39	80
M87364	Other 2ndary osteonecrosis, R fibula	39	80
M87365	Other 2ndary osteonecrosis, L fibula	39	80
M87366	Other 2ndary osteonecrosis, NOS fibula	39	80
M87371	Other 2ndary osteonecrosis, R ankle	39	80
M87372	Other 2ndary osteonecrosis, L ankle	39	80
M87373	Other 2ndary osteonecrosis, NOS ankle	39	80
M87374	Other 2ndary osteonecrosis, R foot	39	80
M87375	Other 2ndary osteonecrosis, L foot	39	80
M87376	Other 2ndary osteonecrosis, NOS foot	39	80
M87377	Other 2ndary osteonecrosis, R toe(s)	39	80

Code	Code Descriptors	HCC	RXHCC
M87378	Other 2ndary osteonecrosis, L toe(s)	39	80
M87379	Other 2ndary osteonecrosis, NOS toe(s)	39	80
M8738	Other 2ndary osteonecrosis, other site	39	80
M8739	Other 2ndary osteonecrosis, multiple sites	39	80
M8780	Other osteonecrosis, NOS bone	39	80
M87811	Other osteonecrosis, R shoulder	39	80
M87812	Other osteonecrosis, L shoulder	39	80
M87819	Other osteonecrosis, NOS shoulder	39	80
M87821	Other osteonecrosis, R humerus	39	80
M87822	Other osteonecrosis, L humerus	39	80
M87829	Other osteonecrosis, NOS humerus	39	80
M87831	Other osteonecrosis of R radius	39	80
M87832	Other osteonecrosis of L radius	39	80
M87833	Other osteonecrosis of NOS radius	39	80
M87834	Other osteonecrosis of R ulna	39	80
M87835	Other osteonecrosis of L ulna	39	80
M87836	Other osteonecrosis of NOS ulna	39	80
M87837	Other osteonecrosis of R carpus	39	80
M87838	Other osteonecrosis of L carpus	39	80
M87839	Other osteonecrosis of NOS carpus	39	80
M87841	Other osteonecrosis, R hand	39	80
M87842	Other osteonecrosis, L hand	39	80
M87843	Other osteonecrosis, NOS hand	39	80
M87844	Other osteonecrosis, R finger(s)	39	80
M87845	Other osteonecrosis, L finger(s)	39	80
M87849	Other osteonecrosis, NOS finger(s)	39	80
M87850	Other osteonecrosis, pelvis	39	80
M87851	Other osteonecrosis, R femur	39	80
M87852	Other osteonecrosis, L femur	39	80
M87859	Other osteonecrosis, NOS femur	39	80
M87861	Other osteonecrosis, R tibia	39	80
M87862	Other osteonecrosis, L tibia	39	80
M87863	Other osteonecrosis, NOS tibia	39	80
M87864	Other osteonecrosis, R fibula	39	80
M87865	Other osteonecrosis, L fibula	39	80
M87869	Other osteonecrosis, NOS fibula	39	80
M87871	Other osteonecrosis, R ankle	39	80
M87872	Other osteonecrosis, L ankle	39	80
M87873	Other osteonecrosis, NOS ankle	39	80
M87874	Other osteonecrosis, R foot	39	80
M87875	Other osteonecrosis, L foot	39	80
M87876	Other osteonecrosis, NOS foot	39	80
M87877	Other osteonecrosis, R toe(s)	39	80
M87878	Other osteonecrosis, L toe(s)	39	80
M87879	Other osteonecrosis, NOS toe(s)	39	80
M8788	Other osteonecrosis, other site	39	80
M8789	Other osteonecrosis, multiple sites	39	80

Code	Code Descriptors	HCC	RXHCC
M879	Osteonecrosis, NOS	39	80
M8960	Osteopathy after poliomyelitis, NOS site	39	N/A
M89611	Osteopathy after poliomyelitis, R shoulder	39	N/A
M89612	Osteopathy after poliomyelitis, L shoulder	39	N/A
M89619	Osteopathy after poliomyelitis, NOS shoulder	39	N/A
M89621	Osteopathy after poliomyelitis, R upper arm	39	N/A
M89622	Osteopathy after poliomyelitis, L upper arm	39	N/A
M89629	Osteopathy after poliomyelitis, NOS upper arm	39	N/A
M89631	Osteopathy after poliomyelitis, R forearm	39	N/A
M89632	Osteopathy after poliomyelitis, L forearm	39	N/A
M89639	Osteopathy after poliomyelitis, NOS forearm	39	N/A
M89641	Osteopathy after poliomyelitis, R hand	39	N/A
M89642	Osteopathy after poliomyelitis, L hand	39	N/A
M89649	Osteopathy after poliomyelitis, NOS hand	39	N/A
M89651	Osteopathy after poliomyelitis, R thigh	39	N/A
M89652	Osteopathy after poliomyelitis, L thigh	39	N/A
M89659	Osteopathy after poliomyelitis, NOS thigh	39	N/A
M89661	Osteopathy after poliomyelitis, R lower leg	39	N/A
M89662	Osteopathy after poliomyelitis, L lower leg	39	N/A
M89669	Osteopathy after poliomyelitis, NOS lower leg	39	N/A
M89671	Osteopathy after poliomyelitis, R ankle & foot	39	N/A
M89672	Osteopathy after poliomyelitis, L ankle & foot	39	N/A
M89679	Osteopathy after poliomyelitis, NOS ankle & foot	39	N/A
M8968	Osteopathy after poliomyelitis, other site	39	N/A
M8969	Osteopathy after poliomyelitis, multiple sites	39	N/A
M9050	Osteonecrosis in DZ classified elsewhere, NOS site	39	80
For codes M9051- through M9057-, use the following 6th character: **1 right** **2 left** **9 NOS**			
M9051-	Osteonecrosis in DZ classified elsewhere, shoulder	39	80
M9052-	Osteonecrosis in DZ classified elsewhere, upper arm	39	80
M9053-	Osteonecrosis in DZ classified elsewhere, forearm	39	80
M9054-	Osteonecrosis in DZ classified elsewhere, hand	39	80
M9055-	Osteonecrosis in DZ classified elsewhere, R thigh	39	80
M9056-	Osteonecrosis in DZ classified elsewhere, lower leg	39	80
M9057-	Osteonecrosis in DZ classified elsewhere, ankle & foot	39	80

Code	Code Descriptors	HCC	RXHCC
M9058	Osteonecrosis in DZ classified elsewhere, other site	39	80
M9059	Osteonecrosis in DZ classified elsewhere, multiple sites	39	80
M96621	FX of humerus following insertion of orthopedic implant, joint prosthesis, or bone plate, R arm	176	N/A
M96622	FX of humerus following insertion of orthopedic implant, joint prosthesis, or bone plate, L arm	176	N/A
M96629	FX of humerus following insertion of orthopedic implant, joint prosthesis, or bone plate, NOS arm	176	N/A
M96631	FX of radius or ulna following insertion of orthopedic implant, joint prosthesis, or bone plate, R arm	176	N/A
M96632	FX of radius or ulna following insertion of orthopedic implant, joint prosthesis, or bone plate, L arm	176	N/A
M96639	FX of radius or ulna following insertion of orthopedic implant, joint prosthesis, or bone plate, NOS arm	176	N/A
M9665	FX of pelvis following insertion of orthopedic implant, joint prosthesis, or bone plate	176	N/A
M96661	FX of femur following insertion of orthopedic implant, joint prosthesis, or bone plate, R leg	176	N/A
M96662	FX of femur following insertion of orthopedic implant, joint prosthesis, or bone plate, L leg	176	N/A
M96669	FX of femur following insertion of orthopedic implant, joint prosthesis, or bone plate, NOS leg	176	N/A
M96671	FX of tibia or fibula following insertion of orthopedic implant, joint prosthesis, or bone plate, R leg	176	N/A
M96672	FX of tibia or fibula following insertion of orthopedic implant, joint prosthesis, or bone plate, L leg	176	N/A
M96679	FX of tibia or fibula following insertion of orthopedic implant, joint prosthesis, or bone plate, NOS leg	176	N/A
M9669	FX of other bone following insertion of orthopedic implant, joint prosthesis, or bone plate	176	N/A
M9701XA	Periprosthetic FX around internal prosthetic R hip joint, initial encounter	170	N/A
M9702XA	Periprosthetic FX around internal prosthetic L hip joint, initial encounter	170	N/A

Code	Code Descriptors	HCC	RXHCC
For codes N00- through N07-, use the following 4th character: 0 with minor glomerular abnormality 1 with focal and segmental glomerular lesions 2 with diffuse membranous glomerulonephritis 3 with diffuse mesangial proliferative glomerulonephritis 4 with diffuse endocapillary proliferative glomerulonephritis 5 with diffuse mesangiocapillary glomerulonephritis 6 with dense deposit disease 7 with diffuse crescentic glomerulonephritis 8 with morphological changes NEC 9 with morphological changes NOS			
N00-	Acute nephritic syndrome	141	N/A
N01-	Rapidly progressive nephritic syndrome	141	N/A
N02-	Recurrent & persistent hematuria	141	N/A
N03-	Chronic nephritic syndrome	141	N/A
N04-	Nephrotic syndrome	141	N/A
N05-	Nephritic syndrome NOS	141	N/A
N06-	Isolated proteinuria	141	N/A
N07-	Hereditary nephropathy, NEC	141	N/A
N08	Glomerular disorders in DZ classified elsewhere	141	N/A
N140	Analgesic nephropathy	141	N/A
N141	Nephropathy induced by other drugs, medicaments & biological substances	141	N/A
N142	Nephropathy induced by NOS drug, medicament or biological substance	141	N/A
N143	Nephropathy induced by heavy metals	141	N/A
N144	Toxic nephropathy, NEC	141	N/A
N150	Balkan nephropathy	141	N/A
N158	NEC renal tubulo-interstitial DZ	141	N/A
N170	Acute kidney failure W/ tubular necrosis	135	N/A
N171	Acute kidney failure W/ acute cortical necrosis	135	N/A
N172	Acute kidney failure W/ medullary necrosis	135	N/A
N178	Acute kidney failure, NEC	135	N/A
N179	Acute kidney failure, NOS	135	N/A
N181	CKD, stage 1	139	N/A
N182	CKD, stage 2 (mild)	139	N/A
N183	CKD, stage 3 (moderate)	138	N/A
N184	CKD, stage 4 (severe)	137	263
N185	CKD, stage 5	136	262
N186	ESRD	136	261
N189	CKD, NOS	139	N/A
N19	Kidney failure, NOS	140	N/A
N250	Renal osteodystrophy	N/A	87
N251	Nephrogenic diabetes insipidus	23	41
N2581	2ndary hyperparathyroidism of renal origin	23	41
N262	Page kidney	N/A	187
N280	Ischemia & infarction of kidney	107	N/A
N99510	Cystostomy hemorrhage	176	N/A

Code	Code Descriptors	HCC	RXHCC
N99511	Cystostomy infection	176	N/A
N99512	Cystostomy malfunction	176	N/A
N99518	Cystostomy complication, NEC	176	N/A
N99520	Hemorrhage of incontinent external stoma of urinary tract	176	N/A
N99521	Infection of incontinent external stoma of urinary tract	176	N/A
N99522	Malfunction of incontinent external stoma of urinary tract	176	N/A
N99523	Herniation of incontinent stoma of urinary tract	176	N/A
N99524	Stenosis of incontinent stoma of urinary tract	176	N/A
N99528	Complication of incontinent external stoma of urinary tract, NEC	176	N/A
N99530	Hemorrhage of continent stoma of urinary tract	176	N/A
N99531	Infection of continent stoma of urinary tract	176	N/A
N99532	Malfunction of continent stoma of urinary tract	176	N/A
N99533	Herniation of continent stoma of urinary tract	176	N/A
N99534	Stenosis of continent stoma of urinary tract	176	N/A
N99538	Complication of continent stoma of urinary tract, NEC	176	N/A
P360	Sepsis of newborn D/T streptococcus, group B	2	N/A
P3610	Sepsis of newborn D/T NOS streptococci	2	N/A
P3619	Sepsis of newborn D/T other streptococci	2	N/A
P362	Sepsis of newborn D/T Staphylococcus aureus	2	N/A
P3630	Sepsis of newborn D/T NOS staphylococci	2	N/A
P3639	Sepsis of newborn D/T other staphylococci	2	N/A
P364	Sepsis of newborn D/T E. coli	2	N/A
P365	Sepsis of newborn D/T anaerobes	2	N/A
P368	Bacterial sepsis of newborn, NEC	2	N/A
P369	Bacterial sepsis of newborn, NOS	2	N/A
Q000	Anencephaly	72	157
Q001	Craniorachischisis	72	157
Q002	Iniencephaly	72	157
Q010	Frontal encephalocele	72	157
Q011	Nasofrontal encephalocele	72	157
Q012	Occipital encephalocele	72	157
Q018	Encephalocele, NEC	72	157
Q019	Encephalocele, NOS	72	157
Q02	Microcephaly	72	157
Q030	Malformations of aqueduct of Sylvius	72	157
Q031	Atresia of foramina of Magendie & Luschka	72	157
Q038	Congenital hydrocephalus, NEC	72	157
Q039	Congenital hydrocephalus, NOS	72	157

Code	Code Descriptors	HCC	RXHCC
Q040	Congenital malformations of corpus callosum	72	157
Q041	Arhinencephaly	72	157
Q042	Holoprosencephaly	72	157
Q043	Other reduction deformities of brain	72	157
Q044	Septo-optic dysplasia of brain	72	157
Q045	Megalencephaly	72	157
Q046	Congenital cerebral cysts	72	157
Q048	Congenital malformation of brain, NEC	72	157
Q049	Congenital malformation of brain, NOS	72	157
Q050	Cervical spina bifida W/ hydrocephalus	72	157
Q051	Thoracic spina bifida W/ hydrocephalus	72	157
Q052	Lumbar spina bifida W/ hydrocephalus	72	157
Q053	Sacral spina bifida W/ hydrocephalus	72	157
Q054	NOS spina bifida W/ hydrocephalus	72	157
Q055	Cervical spina bifida W/O hydrocephalus	72	157
Q056	Thoracic spina bifida W/O hydrocephalus	72	157
Q057	Lumbar spina bifida W/O hydrocephalus	72	157
Q058	Sacral spina bifida W/O hydrocephalus	72	157
Q059	Spina bifida, NOS	72	157
Q060	Amyelia	72	157
Q061	Hypoplasia & dysplasia of spinal cord	72	157
Q062	Diastematomyelia	72	157
Q063	Other congenital cauda equina malformations	72	157
Q064	Hydromyelia	72	157
Q068	Congenital malformation of spinal cord, NEC	72	157
Q069	Congenital malformation of spinal cord, NOS	72	157
Q0700	Arnold-Chiari syndrome W/O spina bifida or hydrocephalus	72	157
Q0701	Arnold-Chiari syndrome W/ spina bifida	72	157
Q0702	Arnold-Chiari syndrome W/ hydrocephalus	72	157
Q0703	Arnold-Chiari syndrome W/ spina bifida & hydrocephalus	72	157
Q078	Congenital malformation of nervous system, NEC	72	157
Q079	Congenital malformation of nervous system, NOS	72	157
Q245	Malformation of coronary vessels	N/A	188
Q6111	Cystic dilatation of collecting ducts	139	N/A
Q6119	Other polycystic kidney, infantile type	139	N/A
Q796	Ehlers-Danlos syndrome	N/A	84
Q8500	Neurofibromatosis, NOS	12	N/A
Q8501	Neurofibromatosis, type 1	12	N/A
Q8502	Neurofibromatosis, type 2	12	N/A
Q8503	Schwannomatosis	12	N/A
Q8509	Neurofibromatosis, NEC	12	N/A
Q851	Tuberous sclerosis	12	19

Code	Code Descriptors	HCC	RXHCC
Q858	Phakomatoses, NEC	12	19
Q859	Phakomatosis, NOS	12	19
Q8740	Marfan's syndrome, NOS	N/A	84
Q87410	Marfan's syndrome W/ aortic dilation	N/A	84
Q87418	Marfan's syndrome W/ other cardiovascular manifestations	N/A	84
Q8742	Marfan's syndrome W/ ocular manifestations	N/A	84
Q8743	Marfan's syndrome W/ skeletal manifestation	N/A	84
Q8782	Arterial tortuosity syndrome	N/A	84
Q910	Trisomy 18, nonmosaicism	N/A	148
Q911	Trisomy 18, mosaicism	N/A	148
Q912	Trisomy 18, translocation	N/A	148
Q913	Trisomy 18, NOS	N/A	148
Q914	Trisomy 13, nonmosaicism	N/A	148
Q915	Trisomy 13, mosaicism	N/A	148
Q916	Trisomy 13, translocation	N/A	148
Q917	Trisomy 13, NOS	N/A	148
Q920	Whole chromosome trisomy, nonmosaicism	N/A	148
Q921	Whole chromosome trisomy, mosaicism	N/A	148
Q922	Partial trisomy	N/A	148
Q925	Duplications W/ other complex rearrangements	N/A	148
Q9261	Marker chromosomes in normal individual	N/A	148
Q9262	Marker chromosomes in abnormal individual	N/A	148
Q927	Triploidy & polyploidy	N/A	148
Q928	NEC trisomies & partial trisomies of autosomes	N/A	148
Q929	Trisomy & partial trisomy of autosomes, NOS	N/A	148
Q930	Whole chromosome monosomy, nonmosaicism	N/A	148
Q931	Whole chromosome monosomy, mosaicism	N/A	148
Q932	Chromosome replaced W/ ring, dicentric or isochromosome	N/A	148
Q933	Deletion of short arm of chromosome 4	N/A	148
Q934	Deletion of short arm of chromosome 5	N/A	148
Q935	Other deletions of part of a chromosome	N/A	148
Q937	Deletions W/ other complex rearrangements	N/A	148
Q9381	Velo-cardio-facial syndrome	N/A	148
Q9388	Other microdeletions	N/A	148
Q9389	Deletions from autosomes, NEC	N/A	148
Q939	Deletion from autosomes, NOS	N/A	148
Q952	Balanced autosomal rearrangement in abnormal individual	N/A	148
Q953	Balanced sex/autosomal rearrangement in abnormal individual	N/A	148
Q992	Fragile X chromosome	N/A	148

Code	Code Descriptors	HCC	RXHCC
R092	Respiratory arrest	83	N/A
R4020	Coma, NOS	80	N/A
For codes R40211- through R40244-, use the following 7th character: 0 time NOS 1 in the field [EMT or ambulance] 2 at arrival to emergency department 3 at hospital admission 4 24 hours or more after hospital admission			
R40211-	Coma scale, eyes open, never	80	N/A
R40212-	Coma scale, eyes open, to pain	80	N/A
R40221-	Coma scale, best verbal response, none	80	N/A
R40222-	Coma scale, best verbal response, incomprehensible words	80	N/A
R40231-	Coma scale, best motor response, none	80	N/A
R40232-	Coma scale, best motor response, extension	80	N/A
R40234-	Coma scale, best motor response, flexion withdrawal	80	N/A
R40243-	GCS score 3-8	80	N/A
R40244-	Other coma, W/O documented GCS score, or W/ partial score reported	80	N/A
R403	Persistent vegetative state	80	N/A
R532	Functional quadriplegia	70	N/A
R5600	Simple febrile convulsions	79	165
R5601	Complex febrile convulsions	79	165
R561	Post traumatic seizures	79	165
R569	Convulsions, NOS	79	165
R570	Cardiogenic shock	84	N/A
R571	Hypovolemic shock	2	N/A
R578	Shock, NEC	2	N/A
R579	Shock, NOS	84	N/A
R64	Cachexia	21	N/A
R6510	SIRS of non-infectious origin W/O acute organ dysfunction	2	N/A
R6511	SIRS of non-infectious origin W/ acute organ dysfunction	2	N/A
R6520	Severe sepsis W/O septic shock	2	N/A
R6521	Severe sepsis W/ septic shock	2	N/A
For codes S020XX-through S0292X-, only the following 7th characters risk-adjust: A initial encounter for closed fracture B initial encounter for open fracture S sequela			
S020XX-	FX of vault of skull	167	N/A
S02101-	FX of base of skull, R side	167	N/A
S02102-	FX of base of skull, L side	167	N/A
S02109-	FX of base of skull, NOS side	167	N/A
S02110-	Type I occipital condyle FX, NOS side	167	N/A
S02111-	Type II occipital condyle FX, NOS side	167	N/A
S02112-	Type III occipital condyle FX, NOS side	167	N/A
S02113-	NOS occipital condyle FX	167	N/A

Code	Code Descriptors	HCC	RXHCC
S02118-	Other FX of occiput, NOS side	167	N/A
S02119-	NOS FX of occiput	167	N/A
S0211A-	Type I occipital condyle FX, R side	167	N/A
S0211B-	Type I occipital condyle FX, L side	167	N/A
S0211C-	Type II occipital condyle FX, R side	167	N/A
S0211D-	Type II occipital condyle FX, L side	167	N/A
S0211E-	Type III occipital condyle FX, R side	167	N/A
S0211F-	Type III occipital condyle FX, L side for closed FX	167	N/A
S0211G-	Other FX of occiput, R side	167	N/A
S0211H-	Other FX of occiput, L side	167	N/A
S0219X-	Other FX of base of skull	167	N/A
S0230X-	FX of orbital floor, NOS side	167	N/A
S0231X-	FX of orbital floor, R side	167	N/A
S0232X-	FX of orbital floor, L side	167	N/A
S02400-	Malar FX, NOS side	167	N/A
S02401-	Maxillary FX, NOS side	167	N/A
S02402-	Zygomatic FX, NOS side	167	N/A
S0240A-	Malar FX, R side	167	N/A
S0240B-	Malar FX, L side	167	N/A
S0240C-	Maxillary FX, R side	167	N/A
S0240D-	Maxillary FX, L side	167	N/A
S0240E-	Zygomatic FX, R side	167	N/A
S0240F-	Zygomatic FX, L side	167	N/A
S02411-	LeFort I FX	167	N/A
S02412-	LeFort II FX	167	N/A
S02413-	LeFort III FX	167	N/A
S0242X-	FX of alveolus of maxilla	167	N/A
S02600-	FX of NOS part of body of mandible, NOS side	167	N/A
S02601-	FX of NOS part of body of R mandible	167	N/A
S02602-	FX of NOS part of body of L mandible	167	N/A
S02609-	FX of mandible, NOS	167	N/A
S02610-	FX of condylar process of mandible, NOS side	167	N/A
S02611-	FX of condylar process of R mandible	167	N/A
S02612-	FX of condylar process of L mandible	167	N/A
S02620-	FX of subcondylar process of mandible, NOS side	167	N/A
S02621-	FX of subcondylar process of R mandible	167	N/A
S02622-	FX of subcondylar process of L mandible	167	N/A
S02630-	FX of coronoid process of mandible, NOS side	167	N/A
S02631-	FX of coronoid process of R mandible	167	N/A
S02632-	FX of coronoid process of L mandible	167	N/A
S02640-	FX of ramus of mandible, NOS side	167	N/A
S02641-	FX of ramus of R mandible	167	N/A
S02642-	FX of ramus of L mandible	167	N/A

Code	Code Descriptors	HCC	RXHCC
S02650-	FX of angle of mandible, NOS side	167	N/A
S02651-	FX of angle of R mandible	167	N/A
S02652-	FX of angle of L mandible	167	N/A
S0266X-	FX of symphysis of mandible	167	N/A
S02670-	FX of alveolus of mandible, NOS side	167	N/A
S02671-	FX of alveolus of R mandible	167	N/A
S02672-	FX of alveolus of L mandible	167	N/A
S0269X-	FX of mandible of NEC site	167	N/A
S0280X-	FX of NEC skull & facial bones, NOS side	167	N/A
S0281X-	FX of NEC skull & facial bones, R side	167	N/A
S0282X-	FX of NEC skull & facial bones, L side	167	N/A
S0291X-	NOS FX of skull	167	N/A
S0292X-	NOS FX of facial bones	167	N/A
S060X0S	Concussion W/O LOC, sequela	167	N/A
S060X1S	Concussion W/ LOC of 30 minutes or less, sequela	167	N/A
S060X9S	Concussion W/ LOC of NOS duration, sequela	167	N/A
For codes S061X0- through S061X2-, only the following 7th characters risk-adjust: A initial encounter S sequela			
S061X0-	Traumatic cerebral edema W/O LOC	167	N/A
S061X1-	Traumatic cerebral edema W/ LOC of 30 minutes or less	167	N/A
S061X2-	Traumatic cerebral edema W/ LOC of 31 minutes to 59 minutes	167	N/A
S061X3A	Traumatic cerebral edema W/ LOC of 1 HR to 5 HR 59 minutes, initial encounter	166	N/A
S061X3S	Traumatic cerebral edema W/ LOC of 1 HR to 5 HR 59 minutes, sequela	167	N/A
S061X4A	Traumatic cerebral edema W/ LOC of 6 HR to 24 HR, initial encounter	166	N/A
S061X4S	Traumatic cerebral edema W/ LOC of 6 HR to 24 HR, sequela	167	N/A
S061X5A	Traumatic cerebral edema W/ LOC greater than 24 HR W/ return to pre-existing conscious level, initial encounter	166	N/A
S061X5S	Traumatic cerebral edema W/ LOC greater than 24 HR W/ return to pre-existing conscious level, sequela	167	N/A
S061X6A	Traumatic cerebral edema W/ LOC greater than 24 HR W/O return to pre-existing conscious level W/ patient surviving, initial encounter	166	N/A
For codes S061X9- through S062X2-, only the following 7th characters risk-adjust: A initial encounter S sequela			
S061X9-	Traumatic cerebral edema W/ LOC of NOS duration	167	N/A
S062X0-	Diffuse TBI W/O LOC	167	N/A
S062X1-	Diffuse TBI W/ LOC of 30 minutes or less	167	N/A

Code	Code Descriptors	HCC	RXHCC
S062X2-	Diffuse TBI W/ LOC of 31 minutes to 59 minutes	167	N/A
S062X3A	Diffuse TBI W/ LOC of 1 HR to 5 HR 59 minutes, initial encounter	166	N/A
S062X3S	Diffuse TBI W/ LOC of 1 HR to 5 HR 59 minutes, sequela	167	N/A
S062X4A	Diffuse TBI W/ LOC of 6 HR to 24 HR, initial encounter	166	N/A
S062X4S	Diffuse TBI W/ LOC of 6 HR to 24 HR, sequela	167	N/A
S062X5A	Diffuse TBI W/ LOC greater than 24 HR W/ return to pre-existing conscious levels, initial encounter	166	N/A
S062X5S	Diffuse TBI W/ LOC greater than 24 HR W/ return to pre-existing conscious levels, sequela	167	N/A
S062X6A	Diffuse TBI W/ LOC greater than 24 HR W/O return to pre-existing conscious level W/ patient surviving, initial encounter	166	N/A
S062X6S	Diffuse TBI W/ LOC greater than 24 HR W/O return to pre-existing conscious level W/ patient surviving, sequela	167	N/A
For codes S062X9- through S06302-, only the following 7th characters risk-adjust: A initial encounter S sequela			
S062X9-	Diffuse TBI W/ LOC of NOS duration	167	N/A
S06300-	NOS focal TBI W/O LOC	167	N/A
S06301-	NOS focal TBI W/ LOC of 30 minutes or less	167	N/A
S06302-	NOS focal TBI W/ LOC of 31 minutes to 59 minutes	167	N/A
S06303A	Unspecified focal TBI W/ LOC of 1 HR to 5 HR 59 minutes, initial encounter	166	N/A
S06303S	Unspecified focal TBI W/ LOC of 1 HR to 5 HR 59 minutes, sequela	167	N/A
S06304A	Unspecified focal TBI W/ LOC of 6 HR to 24 HR, initial encounter	166	N/A
S06304S	Unspecified focal TBI W/ LOC of 6 HR to 24 HR, sequela	167	N/A
S06305A	Unspecified focal TBI W/ LOC greater than 24 HR W/ return to pre-existing conscious level, initial encounter	166	N/A
S06305S	Unspecified focal TBI W/ LOC greater than 24 HR W/ return to pre-existing conscious level, sequela	167	N/A
S06306A	Unspecified focal TBI W/ LOC greater than 24 HR W/O return to pre-existing conscious level W/ patient surviving, initial encounter	166	N/A
S06306S	Unspecified focal TBI W/ LOC greater than 24 HR W/O return to pre-existing conscious level W/ patient surviving, sequela	167	N/A
S06309-	NOS focal TBI W/ LOC of NOS duration	167	N/A
S06310-	Contusion & laceration of R cerebrum W/O LOC	167	N/A

Code	Code Descriptors	HCC	RXHCC
S06311-	Contusion & laceration of R cerebrum W/ LOC of 30 minutes or less	167	N/A
S06312-	Contusion & laceration of R cerebrum W/ LOC of 31 minutes to 59 minutes	167	N/A
For codes S06309- through S06312-, only the following 7th characters risk-adjust: A initial encounter S sequela			
S06313A	Contusion & laceration of R cerebrum W/ LOC of 1 HR to 5 HR 59 minutes, initial encounter	166	N/A
S06313S	Contusion & laceration of R cerebrum W/ LOC W/ LOC of 1 HR to 5 HR 59 minutes, sequela	167	N/A
S06314A	Contusion & laceration of R cerebrum W/ LOC of 6 HR to 24 HR, initial encounter	166	N/A
S06314S	Contusion & laceration of R cerebrum W/ LOC of 6 HR to 24 HR, sequela	167	N/A
S06315A	Contusion & laceration of R cerebrum W/ LOC W/ LOC greater than 24 HR W/ return to pre-existing conscious level, initial encounter	166	N/A
S06315S	Contusion & laceration of R cerebrum W/ LOC W/ LOC greater than 24 HR W/ return to pre-existing conscious level, sequela	167	N/A
S06316A	Contusion & laceration of R cerebrum W/ LOC greater than 24 HR W/O return to pre-existing conscious level W/ patient surviving, initial encounter	166	N/A
S06316S	Contusion & laceration of R cerebrum W/ LOC greater than 24 HR W/O return to pre-existing conscious level W/ patient surviving, sequela	167	N/A
For codes S06319- through S06322-, only the following 7th characters risk-adjust: A initial encounter S sequela			
S06319-	Contusion & laceration of R cerebrum W/ LOC of NOS duration	167	N/A
S06320-	Contusion & laceration of L cerebrum W/O LOC	167	N/A
S06321-	Contusion & laceration of L cerebrum W/ LOC of 30 minutes or less	167	N/A
S06322-	Contusion & laceration of L cerebrum W/ LOC of 31 minutes to 59 minutes	167	N/A
S06323A	Contusion & laceration of L cerebrum W/ LOC of 1 HR to 5 HR 59 minutes, initial encounter	166	N/A
S06323S	Contusion & laceration of L cerebrum W/ LOC of 1 HR to 5 HR 59 minutes, sequela	167	N/A
S06324A	Contusion & laceration of L cerebrum W/ LOC of 6 HR to 24 HR, initial encounter	166	N/A
S06324S	Contusion & laceration of L cerebrum W/ LOC of 6 HR to 24 HR, sequela	167	N/A

Code	Code Descriptors	HCC	RXHCC
S06325A	Contusion & laceration of L cerebrum W/ LOC greater than 24 HR W/ return to pre-existing conscious level, initial encounter	166	N/A
S06325S	Contusion & laceration of L cerebrum W/ LOC greater than 24 HR W/ return to pre-existing conscious level, sequela	167	N/A
S06326A	Contusion & laceration of L cerebrum W/ LOC greater than 24 HR W/O return to pre-existing conscious level W/ patient surviving, initial encounter	166	N/A
S06326S	Contusion & laceration of L cerebrum W/ LOC greater than 24 HR W/O return to pre-existing conscious level W/ patient surviving, sequela	167	N/A
For codes S06329- through S06332-, only the following 7th characters risk-adjust: A initial encounter S sequela			
S06329-	Contusion & laceration of L cerebrum W/ LOC of NOS duration	167	N/A
S06330-	Contusion & laceration of cerebrum, NOS, W/O LOC, initial encounter	167	N/A
S06331-	Contusion & laceration of cerebrum, NOS, W/ LOC of 30 minutes or less	167	N/A
S06332-	Contusion & laceration of cerebrum, NOS, W/ LOC of 31 minutes to 59 minutes	167	N/A
S06333A	Contusion & laceration of cerebrum, unspecified, W/ LOC of 1 HR to 5 HR 59 minutes, initial encounter	166	N/A
S06333S	Contusion & laceration of cerebrum, unspecified, W/ LOC of 1 HR to 5 HR 59 minutes, sequela	167	N/A
S06334A	Contusion & laceration of cerebrum, unspecified, W/ LOC of 6 HR to 24 HR, initial encounter	166	N/A
S06334S	Contusion & laceration of cerebrum, unspecified, W/ LOC of 6 HR to 24 HR, sequela	167	N/A
S06335A	Contusion & laceration of cerebrum, unspecified, W/ LOC greater than 24 HR W/ return to pre-existing conscious level, initial encounter	166	N/A
S06335S	Contusion & laceration of cerebrum, unspecified, W/ LOC greater than 24 HR W/ return to pre-existing conscious level, sequela	167	N/A
S06336A	Contusion & laceration of cerebrum, unspecified, W/ LOC greater than 24 HR W/O return to pre-existing conscious level W/ patient surviving, initial encounter	166	N/A
S06336S	Contusion & laceration of cerebrum, unspecified, W/ LOC greater than 24 HR W/O return to pre-existing conscious level W/ patient surviving, sequela	167	N/A

Code	Code Descriptors	HCC	RXHCC
For codes S06339- through S06342-, only the following 7th characters risk-adjust: A initial encounter S sequela			
S06339-	Contusion & laceration of cerebrum, NOS, W/ LOC of NOS duration	167	N/A
S06340-	Traumatic hemorrhage of R cerebrum W/O LOC	167	N/A
S06341-	Traumatic hemorrhage of R cerebrum W/ LOC of 30 minutes or less	167	N/A
S06342-	Traumatic hemorrhage of R cerebrum W/ LOC of 31 minutes to 59 minutes	167	N/A
S06343A	Traumatic hemorrhage of R cerebrum W/ LOC of 1 HR to 5 HR 59 minutes, initial encounter	166	N/A
S06343S	Traumatic hemorrhage of R cerebrum W/ LOC of 1 HR to 5 HR 59 minutes, sequela	167	N/A
S06344A	Traumatic hemorrhage of R cerebrum W/ LOC of 6 HR to 24 HR, initial encounter	166	N/A
S06344S	Traumatic hemorrhage of R cerebrum W/ LOC of 6 HR to 24 HR, sequela	167	N/A
S06345A	Traumatic hemorrhage of R cerebrum W/ LOC greater than 24 HR W/ return to pre-existing conscious level, initial encounter	166	N/A
S06345S	Traumatic hemorrhage of R cerebrum W/ LOC greater than 24 HR W/ return to pre-existing conscious level, sequela	167	N/A
S06346A	Traumatic hemorrhage of R cerebrum W/ LOC greater than 24 HR W/O return to pre-existing conscious level W/ patient surviving, initial encounter	166	N/A
S06346S	Traumatic hemorrhage of R cerebrum W/ LOC greater than 24 HR W/O return to pre-existing conscious level W/ patient surviving, sequela	167	N/A
For codes S06349- through S06352-, only the following 7th characters risk-adjust: A initial encounter S sequela			
S06349-	Traumatic hemorrhage of R cerebrum W/ LOC of NOS duration	167	N/A
S06350-	Traumatic hemorrhage of L cerebrum W/O LOC	167	N/A
S06351-	Traumatic hemorrhage of L cerebrum W/ LOC of 30 minutes or less	167	N/A
S06352-	Traumatic hemorrhage of L cerebrum W/ LOC of 31 minutes to 59 minutes	167	N/A
S06353A	Traumatic hemorrhage of L cerebrum W/ LOC of 1 HR to 5 HR 59 minutes, initial encounter	166	N/A
S06353S	Traumatic hemorrhage of L cerebrum W/ LOC of 1 HR to 5 HR 59 minutes, sequela	167	N/A
S06354A	Traumatic hemorrhage of L cerebrum W/ LOC of 6 HR to 24 HR, initial encounter	166	N/A
S06354S	Traumatic hemorrhage of L cerebrum W/ LOC of 6 HR to 24 HR, sequela	167	N/A

Code	Code Descriptors	HCC	RXHCC
S06355A	Traumatic hemorrhage of L cerebrum W/ LOC greater than 24 HR W/ return to pre-existing conscious level, initial encounter	166	N/A
S06355S	Traumatic hemorrhage of L cerebrum W/ LOC greater than 24 HR W/ return to pre-existing conscious level, sequela	167	N/A
S06356A	Traumatic hemorrhage of L cerebrum W/ LOC greater than 24 HR W/O return to pre-existing conscious level W/ patient surviving, initial encounter	166	N/A
S06356S	Traumatic hemorrhage of L cerebrum W/ LOC greater than 24 HR W/O return to pre-existing conscious level W/ patient surviving, sequela	167	N/A
For codes S06359- through S06362-, only the following 7th characters risk-adjust: **A initial encounter** **S sequela**			
S06359-	Traumatic hemorrhage of L cerebrum W/ LOC of NOS duration	167	N/A
S06360-	Traumatic hemorrhage of cerebrum, NOS, W/O LOC	167	N/A
S06361-	Traumatic hemorrhage of cerebrum, NOS, W/ LOC of 30 minutes or less	167	N/A
S06362-	Traumatic hemorrhage of cerebrum, NOS, W/ LOC of 31 minutes to 59 minutes	167	N/A
S06363A	Traumatic hemorrhage of cerebrum, unspecified, W/ LOC of 1 HR to 5 HR 59 minutes, initial encounter	166	N/A
S06363S	Traumatic hemorrhage of cerebrum, unspecified, W/ LOC of 1 HR to 5 HR 59 minutes, sequela	167	N/A
S06364A	Traumatic hemorrhage of cerebrum, unspecified, W/ LOC of 6 HR to 24 HR, initial encounter	166	N/A
S06364S	Traumatic hemorrhage of cerebrum, unspecified, W/ LOC of 6 HR to 24 HR, sequela	167	N/A
S06365A	Traumatic hemorrhage of cerebrum, unspecified, W/ LOC greater than 24 HR W/ return to pre-existing conscious level, initial encounter	166	N/A
S06365S	Traumatic hemorrhage of cerebrum, unspecified, W/ LOC greater than 24 HR W/ return to pre-existing conscious level, sequela	167	N/A
S06366A	Traumatic hemorrhage of cerebrum, unspecified, W/ LOC greater than 24 HR W/O return to pre-existing conscious level W/ patient surviving, initial encounter	166	N/A
S06366S	Traumatic hemorrhage of cerebrum, unspecified, W/ LOC greater than 24 HR W/O return to pre-existing conscious level W/ patient surviving, sequela	167	N/A

Code	Code Descriptors	HCC	RXHCC
For codes S06369- through S06372-, only the following 7th characters risk-adjust: **A initial encounter** **S sequela**			
S06369-	Traumatic hemorrhage of cerebrum, NOS, W/ LOC of NOS duration	167	N/A
S06370-	Contusion, laceration, & hemorrhage of cerebellum W/O LOC	167	N/A
S06371-	Contusion, laceration, & hemorrhage of cerebellum W/ LOC of 30 minutes or less	167	N/A
S06372-	Contusion, laceration, & hemorrhage of cerebellum W/ LOC of 31 minutes to 59 minutes	167	N/A
S06373A	Contusion, laceration, & hemorrhage of cerebellum W/ LOC of 1 HR to 5 HR 59 minutes, initial encounter	166	N/A
S06373S	Contusion, laceration, & hemorrhage of cerebellum W/ LOC of 1 HR to 5 HR 59 minutes, sequela	167	N/A
S06374A	Contusion, laceration, & hemorrhage of cerebellum W/ LOC of 6 HR to 24 HR, initial encounter	166	N/A
S06374S	Contusion, laceration, & hemorrhage of cerebellum W/ LOC of 6 HR to 24 HR, sequela	167	N/A
S06375A	Contusion, laceration, & hemorrhage of cerebellum W/ LOC greater than 24 HR W/ return to pre-existing conscious level, initial encounter	166	N/A
S06375S	Contusion, laceration, & hemorrhage of cerebellum W/ LOC greater than 24 HR W/ return to pre-existing conscious level, sequela	167	N/A
S06376A	Contusion, laceration, & hemorrhage of cerebellum W/ LOC greater than 24 HR W/O return to pre-existing conscious level W/ patient surviving, initial encounter	166	N/A
S06376S	Contusion, laceration, & hemorrhage of cerebellum W/ LOC greater than 24 HR W/O return to pre-existing conscious level W/ patient surviving, sequela	167	N/A
For codes S06379- through S06382-, only the following 7th characters risk-adjust: **A initial encounter** **S sequela**			
S06379-	Contusion, laceration, & hemorrhage of cerebellum W/ LOC of NOS duration	167	N/A
S06380-	Contusion, laceration, & hemorrhage of brainstem W/O LOC	167	N/A
S06381-	Contusion, laceration, & hemorrhage of brainstem W/ LOC of 30 minutes or less	167	N/A
S06382-	Contusion, laceration, & hemorrhage of brainstem W/ LOC of 31 minutes to 59 minutes	167	N/A
S06383A	Contusion, laceration, & hemorrhage of brainstem W/ LOC of 1 HR to 5 HR 59 minutes, initial encounter	166	N/A

Code	Code Descriptors	HCC	RXHCC
S06383S	Contusion, laceration, & hemorrhage of brainstem W/ LOC of 1 HR to 5 HR 59 minutes, sequela	167	N/A
S06384A	Contusion, laceration, & hemorrhage of brainstem W/ LOC of 6 HR to 24 HR, initial encounter	166	N/A
S06384S	Contusion, laceration, & hemorrhage of brainstem W/ LOC of 6 HR to 24 HR, sequela	167	N/A
S06385A	Contusion, laceration, & hemorrhage of brainstem W/ LOC greater than 24 HR W/ return to pre-existing conscious level, initial encounter	166	N/A
S06385S	Contusion, laceration, & hemorrhage of brainstem W/ LOC greater than 24 HR W/ return to pre-existing conscious level, sequela	167	N/A
S06386A	Contusion, laceration, & hemorrhage of brainstem W/ LOC greater than 24 HR W/O return to pre-existing conscious level W/ patient surviving, initial encounter	166	N/A
S06386S	Contusion, laceration, & hemorrhage of brainstem W/ LOC greater than 24 HR W/O return to pre-existing conscious level W/ patient surviving, sequela	167	N/A
For codes S06389- through S064X2-, only the following 7th characters risk-adjust: A initial encounter S sequela			
S06389-	Contusion, laceration, & hemorrhage of brainstem W/ LOC of NOS duration	167	N/A
S064X0-	Epidural hemorrhage W/O LOC,	167	N/A
S064X1-	Epidural hemorrhage W/ LOC of 30 minutes or less	167	N/A
S064X2-	Epidural hemorrhage W/ LOC of 31 minutes to 59 minutes	167	N/A
S064X3A	Epidural hemorrhage W/ LOC of 1 HR to 5 HR 59 minutes, initial encounter	166	N/A
S064X3S	Epidural hemorrhage W/ LOC of 1 HR to 5 HR 59 minutes, sequela	167	N/A
S064X4A	Epidural hemorrhage W/ LOC of 6 HR to 24 HR, initial encounter	166	N/A
S064X4S	Epidural hemorrhage W/ LOC of 6 HR to 24 HR, sequela	167	N/A
S064X5A	Epidural hemorrhage W/ LOC greater than 24 HR W/ return to pre-existing conscious level, initial encounter	166	N/A
S064X5S	Epidural hemorrhage W/ LOC greater than 24 HR W/ return to pre-existing conscious level, sequela	167	N/A
S064X6A	Epidural hemorrhage W/ LOC greater than 24 HR W/O return to pre-existing conscious level W/ patient surviving, initial encounter	166	N/A
S064X6S	Epidural hemorrhage W/ LOC greater than 24 HR W/O return to pre-existing conscious level W/ patient surviving, sequela	167	N/A

Code	Code Descriptors	HCC	RXHCC
For codes S064X9- through S065X2-, only the following 7th characters risk-adjust: A initial encounter S sequela			
S064X9-	Epidural hemorrhage W/ LOC of NOS duration	167	N/A
S065X0-	Traumatic subdural hemorrhage W/O LOC	167	N/A
S065X1-	Traumatic subdural hemorrhage W/ LOC of 30 minutes or less	167	N/A
S065X2-	Traumatic subdural hemorrhage W/ LOC of 31 minutes to 59 minutes	167	N/A
S065X3A	Traumatic subdural hemorrhage W/ LOC of 1 HR to 5 HR 59 minutes, initial encounter	166	N/A
S065X3S	Traumatic subdural hemorrhage W/ LOC of 1 HR to 5 HR 59 minutes, sequela	167	N/A
S065X4A	Traumatic subdural hemorrhage W/ LOC of 6 HR to 24 HR, initial encounter	166	N/A
S065X4S	Traumatic subdural hemorrhage W/ LOC of 6 HR to 24 HR, sequela	167	N/A
S065X5A	Traumatic subdural hemorrhage W/ LOC greater than 24 HR W/ return to pre-existing conscious level, initial encounter	166	N/A
S065X5S	Traumatic subdural hemorrhage W/ LOC greater than 24 HR W/ return to pre-existing conscious level, sequela	167	N/A
S065X6A	Traumatic subdural hemorrhage W/ LOC greater than 24 HR W/O return to pre-existing conscious level W/ patient surviving, initial encounter	166	N/A
S065X6S	Traumatic subdural hemorrhage W/ LOC greater than 24 HR W/O return to pre-existing conscious level W/ patient surviving, sequela	167	N/A
For codes S065X9- through S066X2-, only the following 7th characters risk-adjust: A initial encounter S sequela			
S065X9-	Traumatic subdural hemorrhage W/ LOC of NOS duration	167	N/A
S066X0-	Traumatic subarachnoid hemorrhage W/O LOC	167	N/A
S066X1-	Traumatic subarachnoid hemorrhage W/ LOC of 30 minutes or less	167	N/A
S066X2-	Traumatic subarachnoid hemorrhage W/ LOC of 31 minutes to 59 minutes	167	N/A
S066X3A	Traumatic subarachnoid hemorrhage W/ LOC of 1 HR to 5 HR 59 minutes, initial encounter	166	N/A
S066X3S	Traumatic subarachnoid hemorrhage W/ LOC of 1 HR to 5 HR 59 minutes, sequela	167	N/A
S066X4A	Traumatic subarachnoid hemorrhage W/ LOC of 6 HR to 24 HR, initial encounter	166	N/A
S066X4S	Traumatic subarachnoid hemorrhage W/ LOC of 6 HR to 24 HR, sequela	167	N/A

Code	Code Descriptors	HCC	RXHCC
S066X5A	Traumatic subarachnoid hemorrhage W/ LOC greater than 24 HR W/ return to pre-existing conscious level, initial encounter	166	N/A
S066X5S	Traumatic subarachnoid hemorrhage W/ LOC greater than 24 HR W/ return to pre-existing conscious level, sequela	167	N/A
S066X6A	Traumatic subarachnoid hemorrhage W/ LOC greater than 24 HR W/O return to pre-existing conscious level W/ patient surviving, initial encounter	166	N/A
S066X6S	Traumatic subarachnoid hemorrhage W/ LOC greater than 24 HR W/O return to pre-existing conscious level W/ patient surviving, sequela	167	N/A
For codes S066X9- through S06812-, only the following 7th characters risk-adjust: A initial encounter S sequela			
S066X9-	Traumatic subarachnoid hemorrhage W/ LOC of NOS duration	167	N/A
S06810-	Injury of R internal carotid artery, intracranial portion, NEC W/O LOC	167	N/A
S06811-	Injury of R internal carotid artery, intracranial portion, NEC W/ LOC of 30 minutes or less	167	N/A
S06812-	Injury of R internal carotid artery, intracranial portion, NEC W/ LOC of 31 minutes to 59 minutes	167	N/A
S06813A	Injury of R internal carotid artery, intracranial portion, not elsewhere classified W/ LOC of 1 HR to 5 HR 59 minutes, initial encounter	166	N/A
S06813S	Injury of R internal carotid artery, intracranial portion, not elsewhere classified W/ LOC of 1 HR to 5 HR 59 minutes, sequela	167	N/A
S06814A	Injury of R internal carotid artery, intracranial portion, not elsewhere classified W/ LOC of 6 HR to 24 HR, initial encounter	166	N/A
S06814S	Injury of R internal carotid artery, intracranial portion, not elsewhere classified W/ LOC of 6 HR to 24 HR, sequela	167	N/A
S06815A	Injury of R internal carotid artery, intracranial portion, not elsewhere classified W/ LOC greater than 24 HR W/ return to pre-existing conscious level, initial encounter	166	N/A
S06815S	Injury of R internal carotid artery, intracranial portion, not elsewhere classified W/ LOC greater than 24 HR W/ return to pre-existing conscious level, sequela	167	N/A
S06816A	Injury of R internal carotid artery, intracranial portion, not elsewhere classified W/ LOC greater than 24 HR W/O return to pre-existing conscious level W/ patient surviving, initial encounter	166	N/A
S06816S	Injury of R internal carotid artery, intracranial portion, not elsewhere classified W/ LOC greater than 24 HR W/O return to pre-existing conscious level W/ patient surviving, sequela	167	N/A
For codes S06819- through S06822-, only the following 7th characters risk-adjust: A initial encounter S sequela			
S06819-	Injury of R internal carotid artery, intracranial portion, NEC W/ LOC of NOS duration	167	N/A
S06820-	Injury of L internal carotid artery, intracranial portion, NEC W/O LOC	167	N/A
S06821-	Injury of L internal carotid artery, intracranial portion, NEC W/ LOC of 30 minutes or less	167	N/A
S06822-	Injury of L internal carotid artery, intracranial portion, NEC W/ LOC of 31 minutes to 59 minutes	167	N/A
S06823A	Injury of L internal carotid artery, intracranial portion, not elsewhere classified W/ LOC of 1 HR to 5 HR 59 minutes, initial encounter	166	N/A
S06823S	Injury of L internal carotid artery, intracranial portion, not elsewhere classified W/ LOC of 1 HR to 5 HR 59 minutes, sequela	167	N/A
S06824A	Injury of L internal carotid artery, intracranial portion, not elsewhere classified W/ LOC of 6 HR to 24 HR, initial encounter	166	N/A
S06824S	Injury of L internal carotid artery, intracranial portion, not elsewhere classified W/ LOC of 6 HR to 24 HR, sequela	167	N/A
S06825A	Injury of L internal carotid artery, intracranial portion, not elsewhere classified W/ LOC greater than 24 HR W/ return to pre-existing conscious level, initial encounter	166	N/A
S06825S	Injury of L internal carotid artery, intracranial portion, not elsewhere classified W/ LOC greater than 24 HR W/ return to pre-existing conscious level, sequela	167	N/A
S06826A	Injury of L internal carotid artery, intracranial portion, not elsewhere classified W/ LOC greater than 24 HR W/O return to pre-existing conscious level W/ patient surviving, initial encounter	166	N/A
S06826S	Injury of L internal carotid artery, intracranial portion, not elsewhere classified W/ LOC greater than 24 HR W/O return to pre-existing conscious level W/ patient surviving, sequela	167	N/A
For codes S06829- through S06892-, only the following 7th characters risk-adjust: A initial encounter S sequela			
S06829-	Injury of L internal carotid artery, intracranial portion, NEC W/ LOC of NOS duration	167	N/A

Code	Code Descriptors	HCC	RXHCC
S06890-	NEC intracranial injury W/O LOC	167	N/A
S06891-	NEC intracranial injury W/ LOC of 30 minutes or less	167	N/A
S06892-	NEC intracranial injury W/ LOC of 31 minutes to 59 minutes	167	N/A
S06893A	Other specified intracranial injury W/ LOC of 1 HR to 5 HR 59 minutes, initial encounter	166	N/A
S06893S	Other specified intracranial injury W/ LOC of 1 HR to 5 HR 59 minutes, sequela	167	N/A
S06894A	Other specified intracranial injury W/ LOC of 6 HR to 24 HR, initial encounter	166	N/A
S06894S	Other specified intracranial injury W/ LOC of 6 HR to 24 HR, sequela	167	N/A
S06895A	Other specified intracranial injury W/ LOC greater than 24 HR W/ return to pre-existing conscious level, initial encounter	166	N/A
S06895S	Other specified intracranial injury W/ LOC greater than 24 HR W/ return to pre-existing conscious level, sequela	167	N/A
S06896A	Other specified intracranial injury W/ LOC greater than 24 HR W/O return to pre-existing conscious level W/ patient surviving, initial encounter	166	N/A
S06896S	Other specified intracranial injury W/ LOC greater than 24 HR W/O return to pre-existing conscious level W/ patient surviving, sequela	167	N/A
For codes S06899- through S069X2-, only the following 7th characters risk-adjust: A initial encounter S sequela			
S06899-	NEC intracranial injury W/ LOC of NOS duration	167	N/A
S069X0-	NOS intracranial injury W/O LOC	167	N/A
S069X1-	NOS intracranial injury W/ LOC of 30 minutes or less	167	N/A
S069X2-	NOS intracranial injury W/ LOC of 31 minutes to 59 minutes	167	N/A
S069X3A	Unspecified intracranial injury W/ LOC of 1 HR to 5 HR 59 minutes, initial encounter	166	N/A
S069X3S	Unspecified intracranial injury W/ LOC of 1 HR to 5 HR 59 minutes, sequela	167	N/A
S069X4A	Unspecified intracranial injury W/ LOC of 6 HR to 24 HR, initial encounter	166	N/A
S069X4S	Unspecified intracranial injury W/ LOC of 6 HR to 24 HR, sequela	167	N/A
S069X5A	Unspecified intracranial injury W/ LOC greater than 24 HR W/ return to pre-existing conscious level, initial encounter	166	N/A
S069X5S	Unspecified intracranial injury W/ LOC greater than 24 HR W/ return to pre-existing conscious level, sequela	167	N/A
S069X6A	Unspecified intracranial injury W/ LOC greater than 24 HR W/O return to pre-existing conscious level W/ patient surviving, initial encounter	166	N/A

Code	Code Descriptors	HCC	RXHCC
S069X6S	Unspecified intracranial injury W/ LOC greater than 24 HR W/O return to pre-existing conscious level W/ patient surviving, sequela	167	N/A
S069X9A	Unspecified intracranial injury W/ LOC of unspecified duration, initial encounter	167	N/A
S069X9S	Unspecified intracranial injury W/ LOC of unspecified duration, sequela	167	N/A
For codes S069X5- through S069X9-, only the following 7th characters risk-adjust: A initial encounter S sequela			
S069X5-	NOS intracranial injury W/ LOC greater than 24 HR W/ return to pre-existing conscious level	166	N/A
S069X6-	NOS intracranial injury W/ LOC greater than 24 HR W/O return to pre-existing conscious level W/ patient surviving	166	N/A
S069X9-	NOS intracranial injury W/ LOC of NOS duration	167	N/A
For codes S12000- through S12691-, only the following 7th characters risk-adjust: A initial encounter for closed fracture B initial encounter for open fracture			
S12000-	NOS displaced FX of 1st cervical vertebra	169	N/A
S12001-	NOS nondisplaced FX of 1st cervical vertebra	169	N/A
S1201X-	Stable burst FX of 1st cervical vertebra	169	N/A
S1202X-	Unstable burst FX of 1st cervical vertebra	169	N/A
S12030-	Displaced posterior arch FX of 1st cervical vertebra	169	N/A
S12031-	Nondisplaced posterior arch FX of 1st cervical vertebra	169	N/A
S12040-	Displaced lateral mass FX of 1st cervical vertebra,	169	N/A
S12041-	Nondisplaced lateral mass FX of 1st cervical vertebra	169	N/A
S12090-	Other displaced FX of 1st cervical vertebra	169	N/A
S12091-	Other nondisplaced FX of 1st cervical vertebra	169	N/A
S12100-	NOS displaced FX of 2nd cervical vertebra	169	N/A
S12101-	NOS nondisplaced FX of 2nd cervical vertebra	169	N/A
S12110-	Anterior displaced Type II dens FX	169	N/A
S12111-	Posterior displaced Type II dens FX	169	N/A
S12112-	Nondisplaced Type II dens FX	169	N/A
S12120-	Other displaced dens FX	169	N/A
S12121-	Other nondisplaced dens FX	169	N/A
S12130-	NOS traumatic displaced spondylolisthesis of 2nd cervical vertebra	169	N/A
S12131-	NOS traumatic nondisplaced spondylolisthesis of 2nd cervical vertebra	169	N/A
S1214X-	Type III traumatic spondylolisthesis of 2nd cervical vertebra	169	N/A

Code	Code Descriptors	HCC	RXHCC
S12150-	Other traumatic displaced spondylolisthesis of 2nd cervical vertebra	169	N/A
S12151-	Other traumatic nondisplaced spondylolisthesis of 2nd cervical vertebra	169	N/A
S12190-	Other displaced FX of 2nd cervical vertebra	169	N/A
S12191-	Other nondisplaced FX of 2nd cervical vertebra	169	N/A
S12200-	NOS displaced FX of 3rd cervical vertebra	169	N/A
S12201-	NOS nondisplaced FX of 3rd cervical vertebra	169	N/A
S12230-	NOS traumatic displaced spondylolisthesis of 3rd cervical vertebra	169	N/A
S12231-	NOS traumatic nondisplaced spondylolisthesis of 3rd cervical vertebra	169	N/A
S1224X-	Type III traumatic spondylolisthesis of 3rd cervical vertebra	169	N/A
S12250-	Other traumatic displaced spondylolisthesis of 3rd cervical vertebra	169	N/A
S12251-	Other traumatic nondisplaced spondylolisthesis of 3rd cervical vertebra	169	N/A
S12290-	Other displaced FX of 3rd cervical vertebra	169	N/A
S12291-	Other nondisplaced FX of 3rd cervical vertebra	169	N/A
S12300-	NOS displaced FX of 4th cervical vertebra	169	N/A
S12301-	NOS nondisplaced FX of 4th cervical vertebra	169	N/A
S12330-	NOS traumatic displaced spondylolisthesis of 4th cervical vertebra	169	N/A
S12331-	NOS traumatic nondisplaced spondylolisthesis of 4th cervical vertebra	169	N/A
S1234X-	Type III traumatic spondylolisthesis of 4th cervical vertebra	169	N/A
S12350-	Other traumatic displaced spondylolisthesis of 4th cervical vertebra	169	N/A
S12351-	Other traumatic nondisplaced spondylolisthesis of 4th cervical vertebra	169	N/A
S12390-	Other displaced FX of 4th cervical vertebra	169	N/A
S12391-	Other nondisplaced FX of 4th cervical vertebra	169	N/A
S12400-	NOS displaced FX of 5th cervical vertebra	169	N/A
S12401-	NOS nondisplaced FX of 5th cervical vertebra	169	N/A
S12430-	NOS traumatic displaced spondylolisthesis of 5th cervical vertebra	169	N/A
S12431-	NOS traumatic nondisplaced spondylolisthesis of 5th cervical vertebra	169	N/A
S1244X-	Type III traumatic spondylolisthesis of 5th cervical vertebra	169	N/A
S12450-	Other traumatic displaced spondylolisthesis of 5th cervical vertebraX	169	N/A
S12451-	Other traumatic nondisplaced spondylolisthesis of 5th cervical vertebra	169	N/A
S12490-	Other displaced FX of 5th cervical vertebra	169	N/A

Code	Code Descriptors	HCC	RXHCC
S12491-	Other nondisplaced FX of 5th cervical vertebra,	169	N/A
S12500-	NOS displaced FX of 6th cervical vertebra	169	N/A
S12501-	NOS nondisplaced FX of 6th cervical vertebra	169	N/A
S12530-	NOS traumatic displaced spondylolisthesis of 6th cervical vertebra	169	N/A
S12531-	NOS traumatic nondisplaced spondylolisthesis of 6th cervical vertebra	169	N/A
S1254X-	Type III traumatic spondylolisthesis of 6th cervical vertebra	169	N/A
S12550-	Other traumatic displaced spondylolisthesis of 6th cervical vertebra	169	N/A
S12551-	Other traumatic nondisplaced spondylolisthesis of 6th cervical vertebra	169	N/A
S12590-	Other displaced FX of 6th cervical vertebra	169	N/A
S12591-	Other nondisplaced FX of 6th cervical vertebra	169	N/A
S12600-	NOS displaced FX of 7th cervical vertebra	169	N/A
S12601-	NOS nondisplaced FX of 7th cervical vertebra	169	N/A
S12630-	NOS traumatic displaced spondylolisthesis of 7th cervical vertebra	169	N/A
S12631-	NOS traumatic nondisplaced spondylolisthesis of 7th cervical vertebra	169	N/A
S1264X-	Type III traumatic spondylolisthesis of 7th cervical vertebra	169	N/A
S12650-	Other traumatic displaced spondylolisthesis of 7th cervical vertebra	169	N/A
S12651-	Other traumatic nondisplaced spondylolisthesis of 7th cervical vertebra	169	N/A
S12690-	Other displaced FX of 7th cervical vertebra	169	N/A
S12691-	Other nondisplaced FX of 7th cervical vertebra	169	N/A
S128XXA	FX of neck, NEC, initial encounter	169	N/A
S129XXA	FX of neck, NOS, initial encounter	169	N/A
For codes S140XX- through S14159-, only the following 7th characters risk-adjust: A initial encounter D subsequent encounter S sequela			
S140XX-	Concussion & edema of cervical spinal cord	72	N/A
S14101-	NOS injury at C1 level of cervical spinal cord	72	N/A
S14102-	NOS injury at C2 level of cervical spinal cord	72	N/A
S14103-	NOS injury at C3 level of cervical spinal cord	72	N/A
S14104-	NOS injury at C4 level of cervical spinal cord	72	N/A
S14105-	NOS injury at C5 level of cervical spinal cord	72	N/A
S14106-	NOS injury at C6 level of cervical spinal cord	72	N/A
S14107-	NOS injury at C7 level of cervical spinal cord	72	N/A
S14108-	NOS injury at C8 level of cervical spinal cord	72	N/A
S14109-	NOS injury at NOS level of cervical spinal cord	72	N/A

Code	Code Descriptors	HCC	RXHCC
S14111-	Complete lesion at C1 level of cervical spinal cord	70	N/A
S14112-	Complete lesion at C2 level of cervical spinal cord	70	N/A
S14113-	Complete lesion at C3 level of cervical spinal cord	70	N/A
S14114-	Complete lesion at C4 level of cervical spinal cord	70	N/A
S14115-	Complete lesion at C5 level of cervical spinal cord	70	N/A
S14116-	Complete lesion at C6 level of cervical spinal cord	70	N/A
S14117-	Complete lesion at C7 level of cervical spinal cord	70	N/A
S14118-	Complete lesion at C8 level of cervical spinal cord	70	N/A
S14119-	Complete lesion at NOS level of cervical spinal cord	70	N/A
S14121-	Central cord syndrome at C1 level of cervical spinal cord	72	N/A
S14122-	Central cord syndrome at C2 level of cervical spinal cord	72	N/A
S14123-	Central cord syndrome at C3 level of cervical spinal cord	72	N/A
S14124-	Central cord syndrome at C4 level of cervical spinal cord	72	N/A
S14125-	Central cord syndrome at C5 level of cervical spinal cord	72	N/A
S14126-	Central cord syndrome at C6 level of cervical spinal cord	72	N/A
S14127-	Central cord syndrome at C7 level of cervical spinal cord	72	N/A
S14128-	Central cord syndrome at C8 level of cervical spinal cord	72	N/A
S14129-	Central cord syndrome at NOS level of cervical spinal cord	72	N/A
S14131-	Anterior cord syndrome at C1 level of cervical spinal cord	72	N/A
S14132-	Anterior cord syndrome at C2 level of cervical spinal cord	72	N/A
S14133-	Anterior cord syndrome at C3 level of cervical spinal cord	72	N/A
S14134-	Anterior cord syndrome at C4 level of cervical spinal cord	72	N/A
S14135-	Anterior cord syndrome at C5 level of cervical spinal cord	72	N/A
S14136-	Anterior cord syndrome at C6 level of cervical spinal cord	72	N/A
S14137-	Anterior cord syndrome at C7 level of cervical spinal cord	72	N/A
S14138-	Anterior cord syndrome at C8 level of cervical spinal cord	72	N/A
S14139-	Anterior cord syndrome at NOS level of cervical spinal cord	72	N/A

Code	Code Descriptors	HCC	RXHCC
S14141-	Brown-Sequard syndrome at C1 level of cervical spinal cord	72	N/A
S14142-	Brown-Sequard syndrome at C2 level of cervical spinal cord	72	N/A
S14143-	Brown-Sequard syndrome at C3 level of cervical spinal cord	72	N/A
S14144-	Brown-Sequard syndrome at C4 level of cervical spinal cord	72	N/A
S14145-	Brown-Sequard syndrome at C5 level of cervical spinal cord	72	N/A
S14146-	Brown-Sequard syndrome at C6 level of cervical spinal cord	72	N/A
S14147-	Brown-Sequard syndrome at C7 level of cervical spinal cord	72	N/A
S14148-	Brown-Sequard syndrome at C8 level of cervical spinal cord	72	N/A
S14149-	Brown-Sequard syndrome at NOS level of cervical spinal cord	72	N/A
S14151-	Other incomplete lesion at C1 level of cervical spinal cord	72	N/A
S14152-	Other incomplete lesion at C2 level of cervical spinal cord	72	N/A
S14153-	Other incomplete lesion at C3 level of cervical spinal cord	72	N/A
S14154-	Other incomplete lesion at C4 level of cervical spinal cord	72	N/A
S14155-	Other incomplete lesion at C5 level of cervical spinal cord	72	N/A
S14156-	Other incomplete lesion at C6 level of cervical spinal cord	72	N/A
S14157-	Other incomplete lesion at C7 level of cervical spinal cord	72	N/A
S14158-	Other incomplete lesion at C8 level of cervical spinal cord	72	N/A
S14159-	Other incomplete lesion at NOS level of cervical spinal cord	72	N/A
For codes S22000- through S22089-, only the following 7th characters risk-adjust: A initial encounter for closed fracture B initial encounter for open fracture			
S22000-	Wedge compression FX of NOS thoracic vertebra	169	N/A
S22001-	Stable burst FX of NOS thoracic vertebra	169	N/A
S22002-	Unstable burst FX of NOS thoracic vertebra	169	N/A
S22008-	Other FX of NOS thoracic vertebra	169	N/A
S22009-	NOS FX of NOS thoracic vertebra	169	N/A
S22010-	Wedge compression FX of 1st thoracic vertebra	169	N/A
S22011-	Stable burst FX of 1st thoracic vertebra	169	N/A
S22012-	Unstable burst FX of 1st thoracic vertebra	169	N/A
S22018-	Other FX of 1st thoracic vertebra	169	N/A
S22019-	NOS FX of 1st thoracic vertebra	169	N/A

Code	Code Descriptors	HCC	RXHCC
S22020-	Wedge compression FX of 2nd thoracic vertebra	169	N/A
S22021-	Stable burst FX of 2nd thoracic vertebra	169	N/A
S22022-	Unstable burst FX of 2nd thoracic vertebra	169	N/A
S22028-	Other FX of 2nd thoracic vertebra	169	N/A
S22029-	NOS FX of 2nd thoracic vertebra	169	N/A
S22030-	Wedge compression FX of 3rd thoracic vertebra	169	N/A
S22031-	Stable burst FX of 3rd thoracic vertebra	169	N/A
S22032-	Unstable burst FX of 3rd thoracic vertebra	169	N/A
S22038-	Other FX of 3rd thoracic vertebra	169	N/A
S22039-	NOS FX of 3rd thoracic vertebra	169	N/A
S22040-	Wedge compression FX of 4th thoracic vertebra	169	N/A
S22041-	Stable burst FX of 4th thoracic vertebra	169	N/A
S22042-	Unstable burst FX of 4th thoracic vertebra	169	N/A
S22048-	Other FX of 4th thoracic vertebra	169	N/A
S22049-	NOS FX of 4th thoracic vertebra	169	N/A
S22050-	Wedge compression FX of T5-T6 vertebra	169	N/A
S22051-	Stable burst FX of T5-T6 vertebra	169	N/A
S22052-	Unstable burst FX of T5-T6 vertebra	169	N/A
S22058-	Other FX of T5-T6 vertebra	169	N/A
S22059-	NOS FX of T5-T6 vertebra	169	N/A
S22060-	Wedge compression FX of T7-T8 vertebra	169	N/A
S22061-	Stable burst FX of T7-T8 vertebra	169	N/A
S22062-	Unstable burst FX of T7-T8 vertebra	169	N/A
S22068-	Other FX of T7-T8 thoracic vertebra	169	N/A
S22069-	NOS FX of T7-T8 vertebra	169	N/A
S22070-	Wedge compression FX of T9-T10 vertebra	169	N/A
S22071-	Stable burst FX of T9-T10 vertebra	169	N/A
S22072-	Unstable burst FX of T9-T10 vertebra	169	N/A
S22078-	Other FX of T9-T10 vertebra	169	N/A
S22079-	NOS FX of T9-T10 vertebra	169	N/A
S22080-	Wedge compression FX of T11-T12 vertebra	169	N/A
S22081-	Stable burst FX of T11-T12 vertebra	169	N/A
S22082-	Unstable burst FX of T11-T12 vertebra	169	N/A
S22088-	Other FX of T11-T12 vertebra	169	N/A
S22089-	NOS FX of T11-T12 vertebra	169	N/A
For codes S240XX- through S24159-, only the following 7th characters risk-adjust: A initial encounter D subsequent encounter S sequela			
S240XX-	Concussion & edema of thoracic spinal cord	72	N/A
S24101-	NOS injury at T1 level of thoracic spinal cord	72	N/A
S24102-	NOS injury at T2-T6 level of thoracic spinal cord	72	N/A
S24103-	NOS injury at T7-T10 level of thoracic spinal cord,	72	N/A
S24104-	NOS injury at T11-T12 level of thoracic spinal cord	72	N/A
S24109-	NOS injury at NOS level of thoracic spinal cord,	72	N/A
S24111-	Complete lesion at T1 level of thoracic spinal cord,	71	N/A
S24112-	Complete lesion at T2-T6 level of thoracic spinal cord	71	N/A
S24113-	Complete lesion at T7-T10 level of thoracic spinal cord	71	N/A
S24114-	Complete lesion at T11-T12 level of thoracic spinal cord	71	N/A
S24119-	Complete lesion at NOS level of thoracic spinal cord,	71	N/A
S24131-	Anterior cord syndrome at T1 level of thoracic spinal cord	72	N/A
S24132-	Anterior cord syndrome at T2-T6 level of thoracic spinal cord	72	N/A
S24133-	Anterior cord syndrome at T7-T10 level of thoracic spinal cord	72	N/A
S24134-	Anterior cord syndrome at T11-T12 level of thoracic spinal cord	72	N/A
S24139-	Anterior cord syndrome at NOS level of thoracic spinal cord	72	N/A
S24141-	Brown-Sequard syndrome at T1 level of thoracic spinal cord	72	N/A
S24142-	Brown-Sequard syndrome at T2-T6 level of thoracic spinal cord	72	N/A
S24143-	Brown-Sequard syndrome at T7-T10 level of thoracic spinal cord	72	N/A
S24144-	Brown-Sequard syndrome at T11-T12 level of thoracic spinal cord	72	N/A
S24149-	Brown-Sequard syndrome at NOS level of thoracic spinal cord	72	N/A
S24151-	Other incomplete lesion at T1 level of thoracic spinal cord	72	N/A
S24152-	Other incomplete lesion at T2-T6 level of thoracic spinal cord	72	N/A
S24153-	Other incomplete lesion at T7-T10 level of thoracic spinal cord	72	N/A
S24154-	Other incomplete lesion at T11-T12 level of thoracic spinal cord	72	N/A
S24159-	Other incomplete lesion at NOS level of thoracic spinal cord	72	N/A
For codes S32000- through S329XX-, only the following 7th characters risk-adjust: A initial encounter for closed fracture B initial encounter for open fracture			
S32000-	Wedge compression FX of NOS lumbar vertebra	169	N/A
S32001-	Stable burst FX of NOS lumbar vertebra	169	N/A
S32002-	Unstable burst FX of NOS lumbar vertebra	169	N/A
S32008-	Other FX of NOS lumbar vertebra	169	N/A
S32009-	NOS FX of NOS lumbar vertebra	169	N/A

Code	Code Descriptors	HCC	RXHCC
S32010-	Wedge compression FX of 1st lumbar vertebra	169	N/A
S32011-	Stable burst FX of 1st lumbar vertebra	169	N/A
S32012-	Unstable burst FX of 1st lumbar vertebra	169	N/A
S32018-	Other FX of 1st lumbar vertebra	169	N/A
S32019-	NOS FX of 1st lumbar vertebra	169	N/A
S32020-	Wedge compression FX of 2nd lumbar vertebra	169	N/A
S32021-	Stable burst FX of 2nd lumbar vertebra	169	N/A
S32022-	Unstable burst FX of 2nd lumbar vertebra	169	N/A
S32028-	Other FX of 2nd lumbar vertebra	169	N/A
S32029-	NOS FX of 2nd lumbar vertebra	169	N/A
S32030-	Wedge compression FX of 3rd lumbar vertebra	169	N/A
S32031-	Stable burst FX of 3rd lumbar vertebra	169	N/A
S32032-	Unstable burst FX of 3rd lumbar vertebra	169	N/A
S32038-	Other FX of 3rd lumbar vertebra	169	N/A
S32039-	NOS FX of 3rd lumbar vertebra	169	N/A
S32040-	Wedge compression FX of 4th lumbar vertebra	169	N/A
S32041-	Stable burst FX of 4th lumbar vertebra	169	N/A
S32042-	Unstable burst FX of 4th lumbar vertebra	169	N/A
S32048-	Other FX of 4th lumbar vertebra	169	N/A
S32049-	NOS FX of 4th lumbar vertebra	169	N/A
S32050-	Wedge compression FX of 5th lumbar vertebra	169	N/A
S32051-	Stable burst FX of 5th lumbar vertebra	169	N/A
S32052-	Unstable burst FX of 5th lumbar vertebra	169	N/A
S32058-	Other FX of 5th lumbar vertebra	169	N/A
S32059-	NOS FX of 5th lumbar vertebra	169	N/A
S3210X-	NOS FX of sacrum	169	N/A
S32110-	Nondisplaced Zone I FX of sacrum	169	N/A
S32111-	Minimally displaced Zone I FX of sacrum	169	N/A
S32112-	Severely displaced Zone I FX of sacrum	169	N/A
S32119-	NOS Zone I FX of sacrum	169	N/A
S32120-	Nondisplaced Zone II FX of sacrum	169	N/A
S32121-	Minimally displaced Zone II FX of sacrum	169	N/A
S32122-	Severely displaced Zone II FX of sacrum	169	N/A
S32129-	NOS Zone II FX of sacrum	169	N/A
S32130-	Nondisplaced Zone III FX of sacrum	169	N/A
S32131-	Minimally displaced Zone III FX of sacrum	169	N/A
S32132-	Severely displaced Zone III FX of sacrum	169	N/A
S32139-	NOS Zone III FX of sacrum	169	N/A
S3214X-	Type 1 FX of sacrum	169	N/A
S3215X-	Type 2 FX of sacrum	169	N/A
S3216X-	Type 3 FX of sacrum	169	N/A
S3217X-	Type 4 FX of sacrum	169	N/A
S3219X-	Other FX of sacrum	169	N/A

Code	Code Descriptors	HCC	RXHCC
S322XX-	FX of coccyx	169	N/A
S32301-	NOS FX of R ilium	170	N/A
S32302-	NOS FX of L ilium	170	N/A
S32309-	NOS FX of NOS ilium	170	N/A
S32311-	Displaced avulsion FX of R ilium	170	N/A
S32312-	Displaced avulsion FX of L ilium	170	N/A
S32313-	Displaced avulsion FX of NOS ilium	170	N/A
S32314-	Nondisplaced avulsion FX of R ilium	170	N/A
S32315-	Nondisplaced avulsion FX of L ilium	170	N/A
S32316-	Nondisplaced avulsion FX of NOS ilium	170	N/A
S32391-	Other FX of R ilium	170	N/A
S32392-	Other FX of L ilium	170	N/A
S32399-	Other FX of NOS ilium	170	N/A
S32401-	NOS FX of R acetabulum	170	N/A
S32402-	NOS FX of L acetabulum	170	N/A
S32409-	NOS FX of NOS acetabulum	170	N/A
S32411-	Displaced FX of anterior wall of R acetabulum	170	N/A
S32412-	Displaced FX of anterior wall of L acetabulum	170	N/A
S32413-	Displaced FX of anterior wall of NOS acetabulum	170	N/A
S32414-	Nondisplaced FX of anterior wall of R acetabulum	170	N/A
S32415-	Nondisplaced FX of anterior wall of L acetabulum	170	N/A
S32416-	Nondisplaced FX of anterior wall of NOS acetabulum	170	N/A
S32421-	Displaced FX of posterior wall of R acetabulum	170	N/A
S32422-	Displaced FX of posterior wall of L acetabulum, initial encounter for closed FX	170	N/A
S32423-	Displaced FX of posterior wall of NOS acetabulum	170	N/A
S32424-	Nondisplaced FX of posterior wall of R acetabulum, initial encounter for closed FX	170	N/A
S32425-	Nondisplaced FX of posterior wall of L acetabulum	170	N/A
S32426-	Nondisplaced FX of posterior wall of NOS acetabulum	170	N/A
S32431-	Displaced FX of anterior column [iliopubic] of R acetabulum	170	N/A
S32432-	Displaced FX of anterior column [iliopubic] of L acetabulum	170	N/A
S32433-	Displaced FX of anterior column [iliopubic] of NOS acetabulum	170	N/A
S32434-	Nondisplaced FX of anterior column [iliopubic] of R acetabulum	170	N/A
S32435-	Nondisplaced FX of anterior column [iliopubic] of L acetabulum	170	N/A
S32436-	Nondisplaced FX of anterior column [iliopubic] of NOS acetabulum	170	N/A

Code	Code Descriptors	HCC	RXHCC
S32441-	Displaced FX of posterior column [ilioischial] of R acetabulum	170	N/A
S32442-	Displaced FX of posterior column [ilioischial] of L acetabulum	170	N/A
S32443-	Displaced FX of posterior column [ilioischial] of NOS acetabulum	170	N/A
S32444-	Nondisplaced FX of posterior column [ilioischial] of R acetabulum	170	N/A
S32445-	Nondisplaced FX of posterior column [ilioischial] of L acetabulum	170	N/A
S32446-	Nondisplaced FX of posterior column [ilioischial] of NOS acetabulum	170	N/A
S32451-	Displaced transverse FX of R acetabulum	170	N/A
S32452-	Displaced transverse FX of L acetabulum	170	N/A
S32453-	Displaced transverse FX of NOS acetabulum	170	N/A
S32454-	Nondisplaced transverse FX of R acetabulum	170	N/A
S32455-	Nondisplaced transverse FX of L acetabulum	170	N/A
S32456-	Nondisplaced transverse FX of NOS acetabulum	170	N/A
S32461-	Displaced associated transverse-posterior FX of R acetabulum	170	N/A
S32462-	Displaced associated transverse-posterior FX of L acetabulum	170	N/A
S32463-	Displaced associated transverse-posterior FX of NOS acetabulum	170	N/A
S32464-	Nondisplaced associated transverse-posterior FX of R acetabulum	170	N/A
S32465-	Nondisplaced associated transverse-posterior FX of L acetabulum	170	N/A
S32466-	Nondisplaced associated transverse-posterior FX of NOS acetabulum	170	N/A
S32471-	Displaced FX of medial wall of R acetabulum	170	N/A
S32472-	Displaced FX of medial wall of L acetabulum	170	N/A
S32473-	Displaced FX of medial wall of NOS acetabulum	170	N/A
S32474-	Nondisplaced FX of medial wall of R acetabulum	170	N/A
S32475-	Nondisplaced FX of medial wall of L acetabulum,	170	N/A
S32476-	Nondisplaced FX of medial wall of NOS acetabulum,	170	N/A
S32481-	Displaced dome FX of R acetabulum	170	N/A
S32482-	Displaced dome FX of L acetabulum	170	N/A
S32483-	Displaced dome FX of NOS acetabulum	170	N/A
S32484-	Nondisplaced dome FX of R acetabulum	170	N/A
S32485-	Nondisplaced dome FX of L acetabulum	170	N/A
S32486-	Nondisplaced dome FX of NOS acetabulum	170	N/A
S32491-	NEC FX of R acetabulum	170	N/A
S32492-	NEC FX of L acetabulum	170	N/A
S32499-	NEC FX of NOS acetabulum	170	N/A
S32501-	NOS FX of R pubis	170	N/A

Code	Code Descriptors	HCC	RXHCC
S32502-	NOS FX of L pubis	170	N/A
S32509-	NOS FX of NOS pubis	170	N/A
S32511-	FX of superior rim of R pubis	170	N/A
S32512-	FX of superior rim of L pubis	170	N/A
S32519-	FX of superior rim of NOS pubis	170	N/A
S32591-	NEC FX of R pubis	170	N/A
S32592-	NEC FX of L pubis	170	N/A
S32599-	NEC FX of NOS pubis	170	N/A
S32601-	NOS FX of R ischium	170	N/A
S32602-	NOS FX of L ischium	170	N/A
S32609-	NOS FX of NOS ischium	170	N/A
S32611-	Displaced avulsion FX of R ischium	170	N/A
S32612-	Displaced avulsion FX of L ischium	170	N/A
S32613-	Displaced avulsion FX of NOS ischium	170	N/A
S32614-	Nondisplaced avulsion FX of R ischium	170	N/A
S32615-	Nondisplaced avulsion FX of L ischium	170	N/A
S32616-	Nondisplaced avulsion FX of NOS ischium	170	N/A
S32691-	NEC FX of R ischium	170	N/A
S32692-	NEC FX of L ischium	170	N/A
S32699-	NEC FX of NOS ischium	170	N/A
S32810-	Multiple FXs of pelvis W/ stable disruption of pelvic ring	170	N/A
S32811-	Multiple FXs of pelvis W/ unstable disruption of pelvic ring	170	N/A
S3282X-	Multiple FXs of pelvis W/O disruption of pelvic ring	170	N/A
S3289X-	FX of other parts of pelvis	170	N/A
S329XX-	FX of NOS parts of lumbosacral spine & pelvis	170	N/A
For codes S3401X- through S34139-, use the following 7th characters: A initial encounter D subsequent encounter S sequela			
S3401X-	Concussion & edema of lumbar spinal cord	72	N/A
S3402X-	Concussion & edema of sacral spinal cord	72	N/A
S34101-	NOS injury to L1 level of lumbar spinal cord	72	N/A
S34102-	NOS injury to L2 level of lumbar spinal cord	72	N/A
S34103-	NOS injury to L3 level of lumbar spinal cord	72	N/A
S34104-	NOS injury to L4 level of lumbar spinal cord	72	N/A
S34105-	NOS injury to L5 level of lumbar spinal cord	72	N/A
S34109-	NOS injury to NOS level of lumbar spinal cord	72	N/A
S34111-	Complete lesion of L1 level of lumbar spinal cord	72	N/A
S34112-	Complete lesion of L2 level of lumbar spinal cord	72	N/A
S34113-	Complete lesion of L3 level of lumbar spinal cord	72	N/A

Code	Code Descriptors	HCC	RXHCC
S34114-	Complete lesion of L4 level of lumbar spinal cord	72	N/A
S34115-	Complete lesion of L5 level of lumbar spinal cord	72	N/A
S34119-	Complete lesion of NOS level of lumbar spinal cord	72	N/A
S34121-	Incomplete lesion of L1 level of lumbar spinal cord	72	N/A
S34122-	Incomplete lesion of L2 level of lumbar spinal cord	72	N/A
S34123-	Incomplete lesion of L3 level of lumbar spinal cord	72	N/A
S34124-	Incomplete lesion of L4 level of lumbar spinal cord	72	N/A
S34125-	Incomplete lesion of L5 level of lumbar spinal cord	72	N/A
S34129-	Incomplete lesion of NOS level of lumbar spinal cord	72	N/A
S34131-	Complete lesion of sacral spinal cord	72	N/A
S34132-	Incomplete lesion of sacral spinal cord	72	N/A
S34139-	NOS injury to sacral spinal cord	72	N/A
S343XXA	Injury of cauda equina, initial encounter	72	N/A
S48011A	Complete traumatic amputation at R shoulder joint, initial encounter	173	N/A
S48011S	Complete traumatic amputation at R shoulder joint, sequela	189	N/A
S48012A	Complete traumatic amputation at L shoulder joint, initial encounter	173	N/A
S48012S	Complete traumatic amputation at L shoulder joint, sequela	189	N/A
S48019A	Complete traumatic amputation at NOS shoulder joint, initial encounter	173	N/A
S48019S	Complete traumatic amputation at NOS shoulder joint, sequela	189	N/A
S48021A	Partial traumatic amputation at R shoulder joint, initial encounter	173	N/A
S48021S	Partial traumatic amputation at R shoulder joint, sequela	189	N/A
S48022A	Partial traumatic amputation at L shoulder joint, initial encounter	173	N/A
S48022S	Partial traumatic amputation at L shoulder joint, sequela	189	N/A
S48029A	Partial traumatic amputation at NOS shoulder joint, initial encounter	173	N/A
S48029S	Partial traumatic amputation at NOS shoulder joint, sequela	189	N/A
S48111A	Complete traumatic amputation at level between R shoulder & elbow, initial encounter	173	N/A
S48111S	Complete traumatic amputation at level between R shoulder & elbow, sequela	189	N/A
S48112A	Complete traumatic amputation at level between L shoulder & elbow, initial encounter	173	N/A
S48112S	Complete traumatic amputation at level between L shoulder & elbow, sequela	189	N/A
S48119A	Complete traumatic amputation at level between NOS shoulder & elbow, initial encounter	173	N/A
S48119S	Complete traumatic amputation at level between NOS shoulder & elbow, sequela	189	N/A
S48121A	Partial traumatic amputation at level between R shoulder & elbow, initial encounter	173	N/A
S48121S	Partial traumatic amputation at level between R shoulder & elbow, sequela	189	N/A
S48122A	Partial traumatic amputation at level between L shoulder & elbow, initial encounter	173	N/A
S48122S	Partial traumatic amputation at level between L shoulder & elbow, sequela	189	N/A
S48129A	Partial traumatic amputation at level between NOS shoulder & elbow, initial encounter	173	N/A
S48129S	Partial traumatic amputation at level between NOS shoulder & elbow, sequela	189	N/A
S48911A	Complete traumatic amputation of R shoulder & upper arm, level NOS, initial encounter	173	N/A
S48911S	Complete traumatic amputation of R shoulder & upper arm, level NOS, sequela	189	N/A
S48912A	Complete traumatic amputation of L shoulder & upper arm, level NOS, initial encounter	173	N/A
S48912S	Complete traumatic amputation of L shoulder & upper arm, level NOS, sequela	189	N/A
S48919A	Complete traumatic amputation of NOS shoulder & upper arm, level NOS, initial encounter	173	N/A
S48919S	Complete traumatic amputation of NOS shoulder & upper arm, level NOS, sequela	189	N/A
S48921A	Partial traumatic amputation of R shoulder & upper arm, level NOS, initial encounter	173	N/A
S48921S	Partial traumatic amputation of R shoulder & upper arm, level NOS, sequela	189	N/A
S48922A	Partial traumatic amputation of L shoulder & upper arm, level NOS, initial encounter	173	N/A
S48922S	Partial traumatic amputation of L shoulder & upper arm, level NOS, sequela	189	N/A
S48929A	Partial traumatic amputation of NOS shoulder & upper arm, level NOS, initial encounter	173	N/A
S48929S	Partial traumatic amputation of NOS shoulder & upper arm, level NOS, sequela	189	N/A
S58011A	Complete traumatic amputation at elbow level, R arm, initial encounter	173	N/A
S58011S	Complete traumatic amputation at elbow level, R arm, sequela	189	N/A

Code	Code Descriptors	HCC	RXHCC
S58012A	Complete traumatic amputation at elbow level, L arm, initial encounter	173	N/A
S58012S	Complete traumatic amputation at elbow level, L arm, sequela	189	N/A
S58019A	Complete traumatic amputation at elbow level, NOS arm, initial encounter	173	N/A
S58019S	Complete traumatic amputation at elbow level, NOS arm, sequela	189	N/A
S58021A	Partial traumatic amputation at elbow level, R arm, initial encounter	173	N/A
S58021S	Partial traumatic amputation at elbow level, R arm, sequela	189	N/A
S58022A	Partial traumatic amputation at elbow level, L arm, initial encounter	173	N/A
S58022S	Partial traumatic amputation at elbow level, L arm, sequela	189	N/A
S58029A	Partial traumatic amputation at elbow level, NOS arm, initial encounter	173	N/A
S58029S	Partial traumatic amputation at elbow level, NOS arm, sequela	189	N/A
S58111A	Complete traumatic amputation at level between elbow & wrist, R arm, initial encounter	173	N/A
S58111S	Complete traumatic amputation at level between elbow & wrist, R arm, sequela	189	N/A
S58112A	Complete traumatic amputation at level between elbow & wrist, L arm, initial encounter	173	N/A
S58112S	Complete traumatic amputation at level between elbow & wrist, L arm, sequela	189	N/A
S58119A	Complete traumatic amputation at level between elbow & wrist, NOS arm, initial encounter	173	N/A
S58119S	Complete traumatic amputation at level between elbow & wrist, NOS arm, sequela	189	N/A
S58121A	Partial traumatic amputation at level between elbow & wrist, R arm, initial encounter	173	N/A
S58121S	Partial traumatic amputation at level between elbow & wrist, R arm, sequela	189	N/A
S58122A	Partial traumatic amputation at level between elbow & wrist, L arm, initial encounter	173	N/A
S58122S	Partial traumatic amputation at level between elbow & wrist, L arm, sequela	189	N/A
S58129A	Partial traumatic amputation at level between elbow & wrist, NOS arm, initial encounter	173	N/A
S58129S	Partial traumatic amputation at level between elbow & wrist, NOS arm, sequela	189	N/A
S58911A	Complete traumatic amputation of R forearm, level NOS, initial encounter	173	N/A
S58911S	Complete traumatic amputation of R forearm, level NOS, sequela	189	N/A
S58912A	Complete traumatic amputation of L forearm, level NOS, initial encounter	173	N/A
S58912S	Complete traumatic amputation of L forearm, level NOS, sequela	189	N/A
S58919A	Complete traumatic amputation of NOS forearm, level NOS, initial encounter	173	N/A
S58919S	Complete traumatic amputation of NOS forearm, level NOS, sequela	189	N/A
S58921A	Partial traumatic amputation of R forearm, level NOS, initial encounter	173	N/A
S58921S	Partial traumatic amputation of R forearm, level NOS, sequela	189	N/A
S58922A	Partial traumatic amputation of L forearm, level NOS, initial encounter	173	N/A
S58922S	Partial traumatic amputation of L forearm, level NOS, sequela	189	N/A
S58929A	Partial traumatic amputation of NOS forearm, level NOS, initial encounter	173	N/A
S58929S	Partial traumatic amputation of NOS forearm, level NOS, sequela	189	N/A
S68011S	Complete traumatic metacarpophalangeal amputation of R thumb, sequela	189	N/A
S68012S	Complete traumatic metacarpophalangeal amputation of L thumb, sequela	189	N/A
S68019S	Complete traumatic metacarpophalangeal amputation of NOS thumb, sequela	189	N/A
S68021S	Partial traumatic metacarpophalangeal amputation of R thumb, sequela	189	N/A
S68022S	Partial traumatic metacarpophalangeal amputation of L thumb, sequela	189	N/A
S68029S	Partial traumatic metacarpophalangeal amputation of NOS thumb, sequela	189	N/A
S68110S	Complete traumatic metacarpophalangeal amputation of R index finger, sequela	189	N/A
S68111S	Complete traumatic metacarpophalangeal amputation of L index finger, sequela	189	N/A
S68112S	Complete traumatic metacarpophalangeal amputation of R middle finger, sequela	189	N/A
S68113S	Complete traumatic metacarpophalangeal amputation of L middle finger, sequela	189	N/A
S68114S	Complete traumatic metacarpophalangeal amputation of R ring finger, sequela	189	N/A
S68115S	Complete traumatic metacarpophalangeal amputation of L ring finger, sequela	189	N/A
S68116S	Complete traumatic metacarpophalangeal amputation of R little finger, sequela	189	N/A
S68117S	Complete traumatic metacarpophalangeal amputation of L little finger, sequela	189	N/A
S68118S	Complete traumatic metacarpophalangeal amputation of other finger, sequela	189	N/A
S68119S	Complete traumatic metacarpophalangeal amputation of NOS finger, sequela	189	N/A
S68120S	Partial traumatic metacarpophalangeal amputation of R index finger, sequela	189	N/A

Code	Code Descriptors	HCC	RXHCC
S68121S	Partial traumatic metacarpophalangeal amputation of L index finger, sequela	189	N/A
S68122S	Partial traumatic metacarpophalangeal amputation of R middle finger, sequela	189	N/A
S68123S	Partial traumatic metacarpophalangeal amputation of L middle finger, sequela	189	N/A
S68124S	Partial traumatic metacarpophalangeal amputation of R ring finger, sequela	189	N/A
S68125S	Partial traumatic metacarpophalangeal amputation of L ring finger, sequela	189	N/A
S68126S	Partial traumatic metacarpophalangeal amputation of R little finger, sequela	189	N/A
S68127S	Partial traumatic metacarpophalangeal amputation of L little finger, sequela	189	N/A
S68128S	Partial traumatic metacarpophalangeal amputation of other finger, sequela	189	N/A
S68129S	Partial traumatic metacarpophalangeal amputation of NOS finger, sequela	189	N/A
S68411A	Complete traumatic amputation of R hand at wrist level, initial encounter	173	N/A
S68411S	Complete traumatic amputation of R hand at wrist level, sequela	189	N/A
S68412A	Complete traumatic amputation of L hand at wrist level, initial encounter	173	N/A
S68412S	Complete traumatic amputation of L hand at wrist level, sequela	189	N/A
S68419A	Complete traumatic amputation of NOS hand at wrist level, initial encounter	173	N/A
S68419S	Complete traumatic amputation of NOS hand at wrist level, sequela	189	N/A
S68421A	Partial traumatic amputation of R hand at wrist level, initial encounter	173	N/A
S68421S	Partial traumatic amputation of R hand at wrist level, sequela	189	N/A
S68422A	Partial traumatic amputation of L hand at wrist level, initial encounter	173	N/A
S68422S	Partial traumatic amputation of L hand at wrist level, sequela	189	N/A
S68429A	Partial traumatic amputation of NOS hand at wrist level, initial encounter	173	N/A
S68429S	Partial traumatic amputation of NOS hand at wrist level, sequela	189	N/A
S68511S	Complete traumatic transphalangeal amputation of R thumb, sequela	189	N/A
S68512S	Complete traumatic transphalangeal amputation of L thumb, sequela	189	N/A
S68519S	Complete traumatic transphalangeal amputation of NOS thumb, sequela	189	N/A
S68521S	Partial traumatic transphalangeal amputation of R thumb, sequela	189	N/A
S68522S	Partial traumatic transphalangeal amputation of L thumb, sequela	189	N/A
S68529S	Partial traumatic transphalangeal amputation of NOS thumb, sequela	189	N/A

Code	Code Descriptors	HCC	RXHCC
S68610S	Complete traumatic transphalangeal amputation of R index finger, sequela	189	N/A
S68611S	Complete traumatic transphalangeal amputation of L index finger, sequela	189	N/A
S68612S	Complete traumatic transphalangeal amputation of R middle finger, sequela	189	N/A
S68613S	Complete traumatic transphalangeal amputation of L middle finger, sequela	189	N/A
S68614S	Complete traumatic transphalangeal amputation of R ring finger, sequela	189	N/A
S68615S	Complete traumatic transphalangeal amputation of L ring finger, sequela	189	N/A
S68616S	Complete traumatic transphalangeal amputation of R little finger, sequela	189	N/A
S68617S	Complete traumatic transphalangeal amputation of L little finger, sequela	189	N/A
S68618S	Complete traumatic transphalangeal amputation of other finger, sequela	189	N/A
S68619S	Complete traumatic transphalangeal amputation of NOS finger, sequela	189	N/A
S68620S	Partial traumatic transphalangeal amputation of R index finger, sequela	189	N/A
S68621S	Partial traumatic transphalangeal amputation of L index finger, sequela	189	N/A
S68622S	Partial traumatic transphalangeal amputation of R middle finger, sequela	189	N/A
S68623S	Partial traumatic transphalangeal amputation of L middle finger, sequela	189	N/A
S68624S	Partial traumatic transphalangeal amputation of R ring finger, sequela	189	N/A
S68625S	Partial traumatic transphalangeal amputation of L ring finger, sequela	189	N/A
S68626S	Partial traumatic transphalangeal amputation of R little finger, sequela	189	N/A
S68627S	Partial traumatic transphalangeal amputation of L little finger, sequela	189	N/A
S68628S	Partial traumatic transphalangeal amputation of other finger, sequela	189	N/A
S68629S	Partial traumatic transphalangeal amputation of NOS finger, sequela	189	N/A
S68711A	Complete traumatic transmetacarpal amputation of R hand, initial encounter	173	N/A
S68711S	Complete traumatic transmetacarpal amputation of R hand, sequela	189	N/A
S68712A	Complete traumatic transmetacarpal amputation of L hand, initial encounter	173	N/A
S68712S	Complete traumatic transmetacarpal amputation of L hand, sequela	189	N/A
S68719A	Complete traumatic transmetacarpal amputation of NOS hand, initial encounter	173	N/A
S68719S	Complete traumatic transmetacarpal amputation of NOS hand, sequela	189	N/A
S68721A	Partial traumatic transmetacarpal amputation of R hand, initial encounter	173	N/A

Code	Code Descriptors	HCC	RXHCC
S68721S	Partial traumatic transmetacarpal amputation of R hand, sequela	189	N/A
S68722A	Partial traumatic transmetacarpal amputation of L hand, initial encounter	173	N/A
S68722S	Partial traumatic transmetacarpal amputation of L hand, sequela	189	N/A
S68729A	Partial traumatic transmetacarpal amputation of NOS hand, initial encounter	173	N/A
S68729S	Partial traumatic transmetacarpal amputation of NOS hand, sequela	189	N/A
For codes S72001- through S72466-, only the following 7th characters risk-adjust: **A initial encounter for closed fracture** **B initial encounter for open FX type I or II** **C initial encounter for open FX type IIIA, IIIB, or IIIC**			
S72001-	FX of NOS part of neck of R femur	170	N/A
S72002-	FX of NOS part of neck of L femur	170	N/A
S72009-	FX of NOS part of neck of NOS femur	170	N/A
S72011-	NOS intracapsular FX of R femur	170	N/A
S72012-	NOS intracapsular FX of L femur	170	N/A
S72019-	NOS intracapsular FX of NOS femur	170	N/A
S72021-	Displaced FX of epiphysis (separation) (upper) of R femur	170	N/A
S72022-	Displaced FX of epiphysis (separation) (upper) of L femur	170	N/A
S72023-	Displaced FX of epiphysis (separation) (upper) of NOS femur	170	N/A
S72024-	Nondisplaced FX of epiphysis (separation) (upper) of R femur	170	N/A
S72025-	Nondisplaced FX of epiphysis (separation) (upper) of L femur	170	N/A
S72026-	Nondisplaced FX of epiphysis (separation) (upper) of NOS femur	170	N/A
S72031-	Displaced midcervical FX of R femur	170	N/A
S72032-	Displaced midcervical FX of L femur	170	N/A
S72033-	Displaced midcervical FX of NOS femur	170	N/A
S72034-	Nondisplaced midcervical FX of R femur	170	N/A
S72035-	Nondisplaced midcervical FX of L femur	170	N/A
S72036-	Nondisplaced midcervical FX of NOS femur	170	N/A
S72041-	Displaced FX of base of neck of R femur	170	N/A
S72042-	Displaced FX of base of neck of L femur	170	N/A
S72043-	Displaced FX of base of neck of NOS femur	170	N/A
S72044-	Nondisplaced FX of base of neck of R femur	170	N/A
S72045-	Nondisplaced FX of base of neck of L femur	170	N/A
S72046-	Nondisplaced FX of base of neck of NOS femur	170	N/A
S72051-	NOS FX of head of R femur	170	N/A
S72052-	NOS FX of head of L femur	170	N/A
S72059-	NOS FX of head of NOS femur	170	N/A
S72061-	Displaced articular FX of head of R femur	170	N/A
S72062-	Displaced articular FX of head of L femur	170	N/A

Code	Code Descriptors	HCC	RXHCC
S72063-	Displaced articular FX of head of NOS femur	170	N/A
S72064-	Nondisplaced articular FX of head of R femur	170	N/A
S72065-	Nondisplaced articular FX of head of L femur	170	N/A
S72066-	Nondisplaced articular FX of head of NOS femur,	170	N/A
S72091-	Other FX of head & neck of R femur	170	N/A
S72092-	Other FX of head & neck of L femur	170	N/A
S72099-	Other FX of head & neck of NOS femur	170	N/A
S72101-	NOS trochanteric FX of R femur	170	N/A
S72102-	NOS trochanteric FX of L femur	170	N/A
S72109-	NOS trochanteric FX of NOS femur	170	N/A
S72111-	Displaced FX of greater trochanter of R femur	170	N/A
S72112-	Displaced FX of greater trochanter of L femur	170	N/A
S72113-	Displaced FX of greater trochanter of NOS femur	170	N/A
S72114-	Nondisplaced FX of greater trochanter of R femur	170	N/A
S72115-	Nondisplaced FX of greater trochanter of L femur	170	N/A
S72116-	Nondisplaced FX of greater trochanter of NOS femur	170	N/A
S72121-	Displaced FX of lesser trochanter of R femur	170	N/A
S72122-	Displaced FX of lesser trochanter of L femur	170	N/A
S72123-	Displaced FX of lesser trochanter of NOS femur	170	N/A
S72124-	Nondisplaced FX of lesser trochanter of R femur	170	N/A
S72125-	Nondisplaced FX of lesser trochanter of L femur	170	N/A
S72126-	Nondisplaced FX of lesser trochanter of NOS femur	170	N/A
S72131-	Displaced apophyseal FX of R femur	170	N/A
S72132-	Displaced apophyseal FX of L femur	170	N/A
S72133-	Displaced apophyseal FX of NOS femur	170	N/A
S72134-	Nondisplaced apophyseal FX of R femur	170	N/A
S72135-	Nondisplaced apophyseal FX of L femur	170	N/A
S72136-	Nondisplaced apophyseal FX of NOS femur	170	N/A
S72141-	Displaced intertrochanteric FX of R femur	170	N/A
S72142-	Displaced intertrochanteric FX of L femur	170	N/A
S72143-	Displaced intertrochanteric FX of NOS femur	170	N/A
S72144-	Nondisplaced intertrochanteric FX of R femur	170	N/A
S72145-	Nondisplaced intertrochanteric FX of L femur	170	N/A
S72146-	Nondisplaced intertrochanteric FX of NOS femur	170	N/A
S7221X-	Displaced subtrochanteric FX of R femur	170	N/A
S7222X-	Displaced subtrochanteric FX of L femur	170	N/A

Code	Code Descriptors	HCC	RXHCC
S7223X-	Displaced subtrochanteric FX of NOS femur	170	N/A
S7224X-	Nondisplaced subtrochanteric FX of R femur	170	N/A
S7225X-	Nondisplaced subtrochanteric FX of L femur	170	N/A
S7226X-	Nondisplaced subtrochanteric FX of NOS femur	170	N/A
S72301-	NOS FX of shaft of R femur	170	N/A
S72302-	NOS FX of shaft of L femur	170	N/A
S72309-	NOS FX of shaft of NOS femur	170	N/A
S72321-	Displaced transverse FX of shaft of R femur	170	N/A
S72322-	Displaced transverse FX of shaft of L femur	170	N/A
S72323-	Displaced transverse FX of shaft of NOS femur	170	N/A
S72324-	Nondisplaced transverse FX of shaft of R femur	170	N/A
S72325-	Nondisplaced transverse FX of shaft of L femur	170	N/A
S72326-	Nondisplaced transverse FX of shaft of NOS femur,	170	N/A
S72331-	Displaced oblique FX of shaft of R femur	170	N/A
S72332-	Displaced oblique FX of shaft of L femur	170	N/A
S72333-	Displaced oblique FX of shaft of NOS femur	170	N/A
S72334-	Nondisplaced oblique FX of shaft of R femur	170	N/A
S72335-	Nondisplaced oblique FX of shaft of L femur	170	N/A
S72336-	Nondisplaced oblique FX of shaft of NOS femur	170	N/A
S72341-	Displaced spiral FX of shaft of R femur	170	N/A
S72342-	Displaced spiral FX of shaft of L femur	170	N/A
S72343-	Displaced spiral FX of shaft of NOS femur	170	N/A
S72344-	Nondisplaced spiral FX of shaft of R femur	170	N/A
S72345-	Nondisplaced spiral FX of shaft of L femur	170	N/A
S72346-	Nondisplaced spiral FX of shaft of NOS femur	170	N/A
S72351-	Displaced comminuted FX of shaft of R femur	170	N/A
S72352-	Displaced comminuted FX of shaft of L femur	170	N/A
S72353-	Displaced comminuted FX of shaft of NOS femur	170	N/A
S72354-	Nondisplaced comminuted FX of shaft of R femur	170	N/A
S72355-	Nondisplaced comminuted FX of shaft of L femur	170	N/A
S72356-	Nondisplaced comminuted FX of shaft of NOS femur	170	N/A
S72361-	Displaced segmental FX of shaft of R femur	170	N/A
S72362-	Displaced segmental FX of shaft of L femur	170	N/A
S72363-	Displaced segmental FX of shaft of NOS femur	170	N/A
S72364-	Nondisplaced segmental FX of shaft of R femur	170	N/A

Code	Code Descriptors	HCC	RXHCC
S72365-	Nondisplaced segmental FX of shaft of L femur	170	N/A
S72366-	Nondisplaced segmental FX of shaft of NOS femur	170	N/A
S72391-	Other FX of shaft of R femur	170	N/A
S72392-	Other FX of shaft of L femur	170	N/A
S72399-	Other FX of shaft of NOS femur	170	N/A
S72401-	NOS FX of lower end of R femur	170	N/A
S72402-	NOS FX of lower end of L femur	170	N/A
S72409-	NOS FX of lower end of NOS femur	170	N/A
S72411-	Displaced NOS condyle FX of lower end of R femur	170	N/A
S72412-	Displaced NOS condyle FX of lower end of L femur	170	N/A
S72413-	Displaced NOS condyle FX of lower end of NOS femur	170	N/A
S72414-	Nondisplaced NOS condyle FX of lower end of R femur	170	N/A
S72415-	Nondisplaced NOS condyle FX of lower end of L femur	170	N/A
S72416-	Nondisplaced NOS condyle FX of lower end of NOS femur	170	N/A
S72421-	Displaced FX of lateral condyle of R femur	170	N/A
S72422-	Displaced FX of lateral condyle of L femur	170	N/A
S72423-	Displaced FX of lateral condyle of NOS femur	170	N/A
S72424-	Nondisplaced FX of lateral condyle of R femur	170	N/A
S72425-	Nondisplaced FX of lateral condyle of L femur	170	N/A
S72426-	Nondisplaced FX of lateral condyle of NOS femur	170	N/A
S72431-	Displaced FX of medial condyle of R femur	170	N/A
S72432-	Displaced FX of medial condyle of L femur	170	N/A
S72433-	Displaced FX of medial condyle of NOS femur	170	N/A
S72434-	Nondisplaced FX of medial condyle of R femur	170	N/A
S72435-	Nondisplaced FX of medial condyle of L femur	170	N/A
S72436-	Nondisplaced FX of medial condyle of NOS femur	170	N/A
S72441-	Displaced FX of lower epiphysis (separation) of R femur	170	N/A
S72442-	Displaced FX of lower epiphysis (separation) of L femur	170	N/A
S72443-	Displaced FX of lower epiphysis (separation) of NOS femur	170	N/A
S72444-	Nondisplaced FX of lower epiphysis (separation) of R femur	170	N/A
S72445-	Nondisplaced FX of lower epiphysis (separation) of L femur	170	N/A

Code	Code Descriptors	HCC	RXHCC
S72446-	Nondisplaced FX of lower epiphysis (separation) of NOS femur	170	N/A
S72451-	Displaced supracondylar FX W/O intracondylar extension of lower end of R femur	170	N/A
S72452-	Displaced supracondylar FX W/O intracondylar extension of lower end of L femur	170	N/A
S72453-	Displaced supracondylar FX W/O intracondylar extension of lower end of NOS femur	170	N/A
S72454-	Nondisplaced supracondylar FX W/O intracondylar extension of lower end of R femur	170	N/A
S72455-	Nondisplaced supracondylar FX W/O intracondylar extension of lower end of L femur	170	N/A
S72456-	Nondisplaced supracondylar FX W/O intracondylar extension of lower end of NOS femur	170	N/A
S72461-	Displaced supracondylar FX W/ intracondylar extension of lower end of R femur	170	N/A
S72462-	Displaced supracondylar FX W/ intracondylar extension of lower end of L femur	170	N/A
S72463-	Displaced supracondylar FX W/ intracondylar extension of lower end of NOS femur	170	N/A
S72464-	Nondisplaced supracondylar FX W/ intracondylar extension of lower end of R femur	170	N/A
S72465-	Nondisplaced supracondylar FX W/ intracondylar extension of lower end of L femur	170	N/A
S72466-	Nondisplaced supracondylar FX W/ intracondylar extension of lower end of NOS femur	170	N/A
S72471A	Torus FX of lower end of R femur, initial encounter for closed FX	170	N/A
S72472A	Torus FX of lower end of L femur, initial encounter for closed FX	170	N/A
S72479A	Torus FX of lower end of NOS femur, initial encounter for closed FX	170	N/A
For codes S72491- through S7292X-, only the following 7th characters risk-adjust: **A initial encounter for closed fracture** **B initial encounter for open FX type I or II** **C initial encounter for open FX type IIIA, IIIB, or IIIC**			
S72491-	Other FX of lower end of R femur	170	N/A
S72492-	Other FX of lower end of L femur	170	N/A
S72499-	Other FX of lower end of NOS femur	170	N/A
S728X1-	Other FX of R femur	170	N/A
S728X2-	Other FX of L femur	170	N/A
S728X9-	Other FX of NOS femur	170	N/A

Code	Code Descriptors	HCC	RXHCC
S7290X-	NOS FX of NOS femur	170	N/A
S7291X-	NOS FX of R femur	170	N/A
S7292X-	NOS FX of L femur	170	N/A
S73001A	NOS subluxation of R hip, initial encounter	170	N/A
S73002A	NOS subluxation of L hip, initial encounter	170	N/A
S73003A	NOS subluxation of NOS hip, initial encounter	170	N/A
S73004A	NOS dislocation of R hip, initial encounter	170	N/A
S73005A	NOS dislocation of L hip, initial encounter	170	N/A
S73006A	NOS dislocation of NOS hip, initial encounter	170	N/A
S73011A	Posterior subluxation of R hip, initial encounter	170	N/A
S73012A	Posterior subluxation of L hip, initial encounter	170	N/A
S73013A	Posterior subluxation of NOS hip, initial encounter	170	N/A
S73014A	Posterior dislocation of R hip, initial encounter	170	N/A
S73015A	Posterior dislocation of L hip, initial encounter	170	N/A
S73016A	Posterior dislocation of NOS hip, initial encounter	170	N/A
S73021A	Obturator subluxation of R hip, initial encounter	170	N/A
S73022A	Obturator subluxation of L hip, initial encounter	170	N/A
S73023A	Obturator subluxation of NOS hip, initial encounter	170	N/A
S73024A	Obturator dislocation of R hip, initial encounter	170	N/A
S73025A	Obturator dislocation of L hip, initial encounter	170	N/A
S73026A	Obturator dislocation of NOS hip, initial encounter	170	N/A
S73031A	Other anterior subluxation of R hip, initial encounter	170	N/A
S73032A	Other anterior subluxation of L hip, initial encounter	170	N/A
S73033A	Other anterior subluxation of NOS hip, initial encounter	170	N/A
S73034A	Other anterior dislocation of R hip, initial encounter	170	N/A
S73035A	Other anterior dislocation of L hip, initial encounter	170	N/A
S73036A	Other anterior dislocation of NOS hip, initial encounter	170	N/A
S73041A	Central subluxation of R hip, initial encounter	170	N/A
S73042A	Central subluxation of L hip, initial encounter	170	N/A
S73043A	Central subluxation of NOS hip, initial encounter	170	N/A
S73044A	Central dislocation of R hip, initial encounter	170	N/A

Code	Code Descriptors	HCC	RXHCC
S73045A	Central dislocation of L hip, initial encounter	170	N/A
S73046A	Central dislocation of NOS hip, initial encounter	170	N/A
S78011A	Complete traumatic amputation at R hip joint, initial encounter	173	N/A
S78011D	Complete traumatic amputation at R hip joint, subsequent encounter	189	N/A
S78011S	Complete traumatic amputation at R hip joint, sequela	189	N/A
S78012A	Complete traumatic amputation at L hip joint, initial encounter	173	N/A
S78012D	Complete traumatic amputation at L hip joint, subsequent encounter	189	N/A
S78012S	Complete traumatic amputation at L hip joint, sequela	189	N/A
S78019A	Complete traumatic amputation at NOS hip joint, initial encounter	173	N/A
S78019D	Complete traumatic amputation at NOS hip joint, subsequent encounter	189	N/A
S78019S	Complete traumatic amputation at NOS hip joint, sequela	189	N/A
S78021A	Partial traumatic amputation at R hip joint, initial encounter	173	N/A
S78021D	Partial traumatic amputation at R hip joint, subsequent encounter	189	N/A
S78021S	Partial traumatic amputation at R hip joint, sequela	189	N/A
S78022A	Partial traumatic amputation at L hip joint, initial encounter	173	N/A
S78022D	Partial traumatic amputation at L hip joint, subsequent encounter	189	N/A
S78022S	Partial traumatic amputation at L hip joint, sequela	189	N/A
S78029A	Partial traumatic amputation at NOS hip joint, initial encounter	173	N/A
S78029D	Partial traumatic amputation at NOS hip joint, subsequent encounter	189	N/A
S78029S	Partial traumatic amputation at NOS hip joint, sequela	189	N/A
S78111A	Complete traumatic amputation at level between R hip & knee, initial encounter	173	N/A
S78111D	Complete traumatic amputation at level between R hip & knee, subsequent encounter	189	N/A
S78111S	Complete traumatic amputation at level between R hip & knee, sequela	189	N/A
S78112A	Complete traumatic amputation at level between L hip & knee, initial encounter	173	N/A
S78112D	Complete traumatic amputation at level between L hip & knee, subsequent encounter	189	N/A
S78112S	Complete traumatic amputation at level between L hip & knee, sequela	189	N/A
S78119A	Complete traumatic amputation at level between NOS hip & knee, initial encounter	173	N/A
S78119D	Complete traumatic amputation at level between NOS hip & knee, subsequent encounter	189	N/A
S78119S	Complete traumatic amputation at level between NOS hip & knee, sequela	189	N/A
S78121A	Partial traumatic amputation at level between R hip & knee, initial encounter	173	N/A
S78121D	Partial traumatic amputation at level between R hip & knee, subsequent encounter	189	N/A
S78121S	Partial traumatic amputation at level between R hip & knee, sequela	189	N/A
S78122A	Partial traumatic amputation at level between L hip & knee, initial encounter	173	N/A
S78122D	Partial traumatic amputation at level between L hip & knee, subsequent encounter	189	N/A
S78122S	Partial traumatic amputation at level between L hip & knee, sequela	189	N/A
S78129A	Partial traumatic amputation at level between NOS hip & knee, initial encounter	173	N/A
S78129D	Partial traumatic amputation at level between NOS hip & knee, subsequent encounter	189	N/A
S78129S	Partial traumatic amputation at level between NOS hip & knee, sequela	189	N/A
S78911A	Complete traumatic amputation of R hip & thigh, level NOS, initial encounter	173	N/A
S78911D	Complete traumatic amputation of R hip & thigh, level NOS, subsequent encounter	189	N/A
S78911S	Complete traumatic amputation of R hip & thigh, level NOS, sequela	189	N/A
S78912A	Complete traumatic amputation of L hip & thigh, level NOS, initial encounter	173	N/A
S78912D	Complete traumatic amputation of L hip & thigh, level NOS, subsequent encounter	189	N/A
S78912S	Complete traumatic amputation of L hip & thigh, level NOS, sequela	189	N/A
S78919A	Complete traumatic amputation of NOS hip & thigh, level NOS, initial encounter	173	N/A
S78919D	Complete traumatic amputation of NOS hip & thigh, level NOS, subsequent encounter	189	N/A
S78919S	Complete traumatic amputation of NOS hip & thigh, level NOS, sequela	189	N/A
S78921A	Partial traumatic amputation of R hip & thigh, level NOS, initial encounter	173	N/A
S78921D	Partial traumatic amputation of R hip & thigh, level NOS, subsequent encounter	189	N/A
S78921S	Partial traumatic amputation of R hip & thigh, level NOS, sequela	189	N/A
S78922A	Partial traumatic amputation of L hip & thigh, level NOS, initial encounter	173	N/A

Code	Code Descriptors	HCC	RXHCC
S78922D	Partial traumatic amputation of L hip & thigh, level NOS, subsequent encounter	189	N/A
S78922S	Partial traumatic amputation of L hip & thigh, level NOS, sequela	189	N/A
S78929A	Partial traumatic amputation of NOS hip & thigh, level NOS, initial encounter	173	N/A
S78929D	Partial traumatic amputation of NOS hip & thigh, level NOS, subsequent encounter	189	N/A
S78929S	Partial traumatic amputation of NOS hip & thigh, level NOS, sequela	189	N/A
S79001A	NOS physeal FX of upper end of R femur, initial encounter for closed FX	170	N/A
S79002A	NOS physeal FX of upper end of L femur, initial encounter for closed FX	170	N/A
S79009A	NOS physeal FX of upper end of NOS femur, initial encounter for closed FX	170	N/A
S79011A	Salter-Harris Type I physeal FX of upper end of R femur, initial encounter for closed FX	170	N/A
S79012A	Salter-Harris Type I physeal FX of upper end of L femur, initial encounter for closed FX	170	N/A
S79019A	Salter-Harris Type I physeal FX of upper end of NOS femur, initial encounter for closed FX	170	N/A
S79091A	Other physeal FX of upper end of R femur, initial encounter for closed FX	170	N/A
S79092A	Other physeal FX of upper end of L femur, initial encounter for closed FX	170	N/A
S79099A	Other physeal FX of upper end of NOS femur, initial encounter for closed FX	170	N/A
S79101A	NOS physeal FX of lower end of R femur, initial encounter for closed FX	170	N/A
S79102A	NOS physeal FX of lower end of L femur, initial encounter for closed FX	170	N/A
S79109A	NOS physeal FX of lower end of NOS femur, initial encounter for closed FX	170	N/A
S79111A	Salter-Harris Type I physeal FX of lower end of R femur, initial encounter for closed FX	170	N/A
S79112A	Salter-Harris Type I physeal FX of lower end of L femur, initial encounter for closed FX	170	N/A
S79119A	Salter-Harris Type I physeal FX of lower end of NOS femur, initial encounter for closed FX	170	N/A
S79121A	Salter-Harris Type II physeal FX of lower end of R femur, initial encounter for closed FX	170	N/A
S79122A	Salter-Harris Type II physeal FX of lower end of L femur, initial encounter for closed FX	170	N/A
S79129A	Salter-Harris Type II physeal FX of lower end of NOS femur, initial encounter for closed FX	170	N/A
S79131A	Salter-Harris Type III physeal FX of lower end of R femur, initial encounter for closed FX	170	N/A
S79132A	Salter-Harris Type III physeal FX of lower end of L femur, initial encounter for closed FX	170	N/A
S79139A	Salter-Harris Type III physeal FX of lower end of NOS femur, initial encounter for closed FX	170	N/A

Code	Code Descriptors	HCC	RXHCC
S79141A	Salter-Harris Type IV physeal FX of lower end of R femur, initial encounter for closed FX	170	N/A
S79142A	Salter-Harris Type IV physeal FX of lower end of L femur, initial encounter for closed FX	170	N/A
S79149A	Salter-Harris Type IV physeal FX of lower end of NOS femur, initial encounter for closed FX	170	N/A
S79191A	Other physeal FX of lower end of R femur, initial encounter for closed FX	170	N/A
S79192A	Other physeal FX of lower end of L femur, initial encounter for closed FX	170	N/A
S79199A	Other physeal FX of lower end of NOS femur, initial encounter for closed FX	170	N/A
S88011A	Complete traumatic amputation at knee level, R lower leg, initial encounter	173	N/A
S88011D	Complete traumatic amputation at knee level, R lower leg, subsequent encounter	189	N/A
S88011S	Complete traumatic amputation at knee level, R lower leg, sequela	189	N/A
S88012A	Complete traumatic amputation at knee level, L lower leg, initial encounter	173	N/A
S88012D	Complete traumatic amputation at knee level, L lower leg, subsequent encounter	189	N/A
S88012S	Complete traumatic amputation at knee level, L lower leg, sequela	189	N/A
S88019A	Complete traumatic amputation at knee level, NOS lower leg, initial encounter	173	N/A
S88019D	Complete traumatic amputation at knee level, NOS lower leg, subsequent encounter	189	N/A
S88019S	Complete traumatic amputation at knee level, NOS lower leg, sequela	189	N/A
S88021A	Partial traumatic amputation at knee level, R lower leg, initial encounter	173	N/A
S88021D	Partial traumatic amputation at knee level, R lower leg, subsequent encounter	189	N/A
S88021S	Partial traumatic amputation at knee level, R lower leg, sequela	189	N/A
S88022A	Partial traumatic amputation at knee level, L lower leg, initial encounter	173	N/A
S88022D	Partial traumatic amputation at knee level, L lower leg, subsequent encounter	189	N/A
S88022S	Partial traumatic amputation at knee level, L lower leg, sequela	189	N/A
S88029A	Partial traumatic amputation at knee level, NOS lower leg, initial encounter	173	N/A
S88029D	Partial traumatic amputation at knee level, NOS lower leg, subsequent encounter	189	N/A
S88029S	Partial traumatic amputation at knee level, NOS lower leg, sequela	189	N/A
S88111A	Complete traumatic BKA, R lower leg, initial encounter	173	N/A
S88111D	Complete traumatic BKA, R lower leg, subsequent encounter	189	N/A

Code	Code Descriptors	HCC	RXHCC
S88111S	Complete traumatic BKA, R lower leg, sequela	189	N/A
S88112A	Complete traumatic BKA, L lower leg, initial encounter	173	N/A
S88112D	Complete traumatic BKA, L lower leg, subsequent encounter	189	N/A
S88112S	Complete traumatic BKA, L lower leg, sequela	189	N/A
S88119A	Complete traumatic BKA, NOS lower leg, initial encounter	173	N/A
S88119D	Complete traumatic BKA, NOS lower leg, subsequent encounter	189	N/A
S88119S	Complete traumatic BKA, NOS lower leg, sequela	189	N/A
S88121A	Partial traumatic BKA, R lower leg, initial encounter	173	N/A
S88121D	Partial traumatic BKA, R lower leg, subsequent encounter	189	N/A
S88121S	Partial traumatic BKA, R lower leg, sequela	189	N/A
S88122A	Partial traumatic BKA, L lower leg, initial encounter	173	N/A
S88122D	Partial traumatic BKA, L lower leg, subsequent encounter	189	N/A
S88122S	Partial traumatic BKA, L lower leg, sequela	189	N/A
S88129A	Partial traumatic BKA, NOS lower leg, initial encounter	173	N/A
S88129D	Partial traumatic BKA, NOS lower leg, subsequent encounter	189	N/A
S88129S	Partial traumatic BKA, NOS lower leg, sequela	189	N/A
S88911A	Complete traumatic amputation of R lower leg, level NOS, initial encounter	173	N/A
S88911D	Complete traumatic amputation of R lower leg, level NOS, subsequent encounter	189	N/A
S88911S	Complete traumatic amputation of R lower leg, level NOS, sequela	189	N/A
S88912A	Complete traumatic amputation of L lower leg, level NOS, initial encounter	173	N/A
S88912D	Complete traumatic amputation of L lower leg, level NOS, subsequent encounter	189	N/A
S88912S	Complete traumatic amputation of L lower leg, level NOS, sequela	189	N/A
S88919A	Complete traumatic amputation of NOS lower leg, level NOS, initial encounter	173	N/A
S88919D	Complete traumatic amputation of NOS lower leg, level NOS, subsequent encounter	189	N/A
S88919S	Complete traumatic amputation of NOS lower leg, level NOS, sequela	189	N/A
S88921A	Partial traumatic amputation of R lower leg, level NOS, initial encounter	173	N/A
S88921D	Partial traumatic amputation of R lower leg, level NOS, subsequent encounter	189	N/A
S88921S	Partial traumatic amputation of R lower leg, level NOS, sequela	189	N/A

Code	Code Descriptors	HCC	RXHCC
S88922A	Partial traumatic amputation of L lower leg, level NOS, initial encounter	173	N/A
S88922D	Partial traumatic amputation of L lower leg, level NOS, subsequent encounter	189	N/A
S88922S	Partial traumatic amputation of L lower leg, level NOS, sequela	189	N/A
S88929A	Partial traumatic amputation of NOS lower leg, level NOS, initial encounter	173	N/A
S88929D	Partial traumatic amputation of NOS lower leg, level NOS, subsequent encounter	189	N/A
S88929S	Partial traumatic amputation of NOS lower leg, level NOS, sequela	189	N/A
S98011A	Complete traumatic amputation of R foot at ankle level, initial encounter	173	N/A
S98011D	Complete traumatic amputation of R foot at ankle level, subsequent encounter	189	N/A
S98011S	Complete traumatic amputation of R foot at ankle level, sequela	189	N/A
S98012A	Complete traumatic amputation of L foot at ankle level, initial encounter	173	N/A
S98012D	Complete traumatic amputation of L foot at ankle level, subsequent encounter	189	N/A
S98012S	Complete traumatic amputation of L foot at ankle level, sequela	189	N/A
S98019A	Complete traumatic amputation of NOS foot at ankle level, initial encounter	173	N/A
S98019D	Complete traumatic amputation of NOS foot at ankle level, subsequent encounter	189	N/A
S98019S	Complete traumatic amputation of NOS foot at ankle level, sequela	189	N/A
S98021A	Partial traumatic amputation of R foot at ankle level, initial encounter	173	N/A
S98021D	Partial traumatic amputation of R foot at ankle level, subsequent encounter	189	N/A
S98021S	Partial traumatic amputation of R foot at ankle level, sequela	189	N/A
S98022A	Partial traumatic amputation of L foot at ankle level, initial encounter	173	N/A
S98022D	Partial traumatic amputation of L foot at ankle level, subsequent encounter	189	N/A
S98022S	Partial traumatic amputation of L foot at ankle level, sequela	189	N/A
S98029A	Partial traumatic amputation of NOS foot at ankle level, initial encounter	173	N/A
S98029D	Partial traumatic amputation of NOS foot at ankle level, subsequent encounter	189	N/A
S98029S	Partial traumatic amputation of NOS foot at ankle level, sequela	189	N/A
S98111A	Complete traumatic amputation of R great toe, initial encounter	173	N/A
S98111D	Complete traumatic amputation of R great toe, subsequent encounter	189	N/A
S98111S	Complete traumatic amputation of R great toe, sequela	189	N/A

Code	Code Descriptors	HCC	RXHCC
S98112A	Complete traumatic amputation of L great toe, initial encounter	173	N/A
S98112D	Complete traumatic amputation of L great toe, subsequent encounter	189	N/A
S98112S	Complete traumatic amputation of L great toe, sequela	189	N/A
S98119A	Complete traumatic amputation of NOS great toe, initial encounter	173	N/A
S98119D	Complete traumatic amputation of NOS great toe, subsequent encounter	189	N/A
S98119S	Complete traumatic amputation of NOS great toe, sequela	189	N/A
S98121A	Partial traumatic amputation of R great toe, initial encounter	173	N/A
S98121D	Partial traumatic amputation of R great toe, subsequent encounter	189	N/A
S98121S	Partial traumatic amputation of R great toe, sequela	189	N/A
S98122A	Partial traumatic amputation of L great toe, initial encounter	173	N/A
S98122D	Partial traumatic amputation of L great toe, subsequent encounter	189	N/A
S98122S	Partial traumatic amputation of L great toe, sequela	189	N/A
S98129A	Partial traumatic amputation of NOS great toe, initial encounter	173	N/A
S98129D	Partial traumatic amputation of NOS great toe, subsequent encounter	189	N/A
S98129S	Partial traumatic amputation of NOS great toe, sequela	189	N/A
S98131A	Complete traumatic amputation of one R lesser toe, initial encounter	173	N/A
S98131D	Complete traumatic amputation of one R lesser toe, subsequent encounter	189	N/A
S98131S	Complete traumatic amputation of one R lesser toe, sequela	189	N/A
S98132A	Complete traumatic amputation of one L lesser toe, initial encounter	173	N/A
S98132D	Complete traumatic amputation of one L lesser toe, subsequent encounter	189	N/A
S98132S	Complete traumatic amputation of one L lesser toe, sequela	189	N/A
S98139A	Complete traumatic amputation of one NOS lesser toe, initial encounter	173	N/A
S98139D	Complete traumatic amputation of one NOS lesser toe, subsequent encounter	189	N/A
S98139S	Complete traumatic amputation of one NOS lesser toe, sequela	189	N/A
S98141A	Partial traumatic amputation of one R lesser toe, initial encounter	173	N/A
S98141D	Partial traumatic amputation of one R lesser toe, subsequent encounter	189	N/A
S98141S	Partial traumatic amputation of one R lesser toe, sequela	189	N/A

Code	Code Descriptors	HCC	RXHCC
S98142A	Partial traumatic amputation of one L lesser toe, initial encounter	173	N/A
S98142D	Partial traumatic amputation of one L lesser toe, subsequent encounter	189	N/A
S98142S	Partial traumatic amputation of one L lesser toe, sequela	189	N/A
S98149A	Partial traumatic amputation of one NOS lesser toe, initial encounter	173	N/A
S98149D	Partial traumatic amputation of one NOS lesser toe, subsequent encounter	189	N/A
S98149S	Partial traumatic amputation of one NOS lesser toe, sequela	189	N/A
S98211A	Complete traumatic amputation of two or more R lesser toes, initial encounter	173	N/A
S98211D	Complete traumatic amputation of two or more R lesser toes, subsequent encounter	189	N/A
S98211S	Complete traumatic amputation of two or more R lesser toes, sequela	189	N/A
S98212A	Complete traumatic amputation of two or more L lesser toes, initial encounter	173	N/A
S98212D	Complete traumatic amputation of two or more L lesser toes, subsequent encounter	189	N/A
S98212S	Complete traumatic amputation of two or more L lesser toes, sequela	189	N/A
S98219A	Complete traumatic amputation of two or more NOS lesser toes, initial encounter	173	N/A
S98219D	Complete traumatic amputation of two or more NOS lesser toes, subsequent encounter	189	N/A
S98219S	Complete traumatic amputation of two or more NOS lesser toes, sequela	189	N/A
S98221A	Partial traumatic amputation of two or more R lesser toes, initial encounter	173	N/A
S98221D	Partial traumatic amputation of two or more R lesser toes, subsequent encounter	189	N/A
S98221S	Partial traumatic amputation of two or more R lesser toes, sequela	189	N/A
S98222A	Partial traumatic amputation of two or more L lesser toes, initial encounter	173	N/A
S98222D	Partial traumatic amputation of two or more L lesser toes, subsequent encounter	189	N/A
S98222S	Partial traumatic amputation of two or more L lesser toes, sequela	189	N/A
S98229A	Partial traumatic amputation of two or more NOS lesser toes, initial encounter	173	N/A
S98229D	Partial traumatic amputation of two or more NOS lesser toes, subsequent encounter	189	N/A
S98229S	Partial traumatic amputation of two or more NOS lesser toes, sequela	189	N/A
S98311A	Complete traumatic amputation of R midfoot, initial encounter	173	N/A
S98311D	Complete traumatic amputation of R midfoot, subsequent encounter	189	N/A

Code	Code Descriptors	HCC	RXHCC
S98311S	Complete traumatic amputation of R midfoot, sequela	189	N/A
S98312A	Complete traumatic amputation of L midfoot, initial encounter	173	N/A
S98312D	Complete traumatic amputation of L midfoot, subsequent encounter	189	N/A
S98312S	Complete traumatic amputation of L midfoot, sequela	189	N/A
S98319A	Complete traumatic amputation of NOS midfoot, initial encounter	173	N/A
S98319D	Complete traumatic amputation of NOS midfoot, subsequent encounter	189	N/A
S98319S	Complete traumatic amputation of NOS midfoot, sequela	189	N/A
S98321A	Partial traumatic amputation of R midfoot, initial encounter	173	N/A
S98321D	Partial traumatic amputation of R midfoot, subsequent encounter	189	N/A
S98321S	Partial traumatic amputation of R midfoot, sequela	189	N/A
S98322A	Partial traumatic amputation of L midfoot, initial encounter	173	N/A
S98322D	Partial traumatic amputation of L midfoot, subsequent encounter	189	N/A
S98322S	Partial traumatic amputation of L midfoot, sequela	189	N/A
S98329A	Partial traumatic amputation of NOS midfoot, initial encounter	173	N/A
S98329D	Partial traumatic amputation of NOS midfoot, subsequent encounter	189	N/A
S98329S	Partial traumatic amputation of NOS midfoot, sequela	189	N/A
S98911A	Complete traumatic amputation of R foot, level NOS, initial encounter	173	N/A
S98911D	Complete traumatic amputation of R foot, level NOS, subsequent encounter	189	N/A
S98911S	Complete traumatic amputation of R foot, level NOS, sequela	189	N/A
S98912A	Complete traumatic amputation of L foot, level NOS, initial encounter	173	N/A
S98912D	Complete traumatic amputation of L foot, level NOS, subsequent encounter	189	N/A
S98912S	Complete traumatic amputation of L foot, level NOS, sequela	189	N/A
S98919A	Complete traumatic amputation of NOS foot, level NOS, initial encounter	173	N/A
S98919D	Complete traumatic amputation of NOS foot, level NOS, subsequent encounter	189	N/A
S98919S	Complete traumatic amputation of NOS foot, level NOS, sequela	189	N/A
S98921A	Partial traumatic amputation of R foot, level NOS, initial encounter	173	N/A
S98921D	Partial traumatic amputation of R foot, level NOS, subsequent encounter	189	N/A

Code	Code Descriptors	HCC	RXHCC
S98921S	Partial traumatic amputation of R foot, level NOS, sequela	189	N/A
S98922A	Partial traumatic amputation of L foot, level NOS, initial encounter	173	N/A
S98922D	Partial traumatic amputation of L foot, level NOS, subsequent encounter	189	N/A
S98922S	Partial traumatic amputation of L foot, level NOS, sequela	189	N/A
S98929A	Partial traumatic amputation of NOS foot, level NOS, initial encounter	173	N/A
S98929D	Partial traumatic amputation of NOS foot, level NOS, subsequent encounter	189	N/A
S98929S	Partial traumatic amputation of NOS foot, level NOS, sequela	189	N/A
T1491	Suicide attempt	58	N/A
T1491XA	Suicide attempt, initial encounter	58	N/A
T1491XD	Suicide attempt, subsequent encounter	58	N/A
T1491XS	Suicide attempt, sequela	58	N/A
T3111	Burns involving 10-19% of TBSA W/ 10-19% 3rd-degree burns	162	N/A
T3121	Burns involving 20-29% of TBSA W/ 10-19% 3rd-degree burns	162	N/A
T3122	Burns involving 20-29% of TBSA W/ 20-29% 3rd-degree burns	162	N/A
T3131	Burns involving 30-39% of TBSA W/ 10-19% 3rd-degree burns	162	N/A
T3132	Burns involving 30-39% of TBSA W/ 20-29% 3rd-degree burns	162	N/A
T3133	Burns involving 30-39% of TBSA W/ 30-39% 3rd-degree burns	162	N/A
T3141	Burns involving 40-49% of TBSA W/ 10-19% 3rd-degree burns	162	N/A
T3142	Burns involving 40-49% of TBSA W/ 20-29% 3rd-degree burns	162	N/A
T3143	Burns involving 40-49% of TBSA W/ 30-39% 3rd-degree burns	162	N/A
T3144	Burns involving 40-49% of TBSA W/ 40-49% 3rd-degree burns	162	N/A
T3151	Burns involving 50-59% of TBSA W/ 10-19% 3rd-degree burns	162	N/A
T3152	Burns involving 50-59% of TBSA W/ 20-29% 3rd-degree burns	162	N/A
T3153	Burns involving 50-59% of TBSA W/ 30-39% 3rd-degree burns	162	N/A
T3154	Burns involving 50-59% of TBSA W/ 40-49% 3rd-degree burns	162	N/A
T3155	Burns involving 50-59% of TBSA W/ 50-59% 3rd-degree burns	162	N/A
T3161	Burns involving 60-69% of TBSA W/ 10-19% 3rd-degree burns	162	N/A
T3162	Burns involving 60-69% of TBSA W/ 20-29% 3rd-degree burns	162	N/A

Code	Code Descriptors	HCC	RXHCC
T3163	Burns involving 60-69% of TBSA W/ 30-39% 3rd-degree burns	162	N/A
T3164	Burns involving 60-69% of TBSA W/ 40-49% 3rd-degree burns	162	N/A
T3165	Burns involving 60-69% of TBSA W/ 50-59% 3rd-degree burns	162	N/A
T3166	Burns involving 60-69% of TBSA W/ 60-69% 3rd-degree burns	162	N/A
T3171	Burns involving 70-79% of TBSA W/ 10-19% 3rd-degree burns	162	N/A
T3172	Burns involving 70-79% of TBSA W/ 20-29% 3rd-degree burns	162	N/A
T3173	Burns involving 70-79% of TBSA W/ 30-39% 3rd-degree burns	162	N/A
T3174	Burns involving 70-79% of TBSA W/ 40-49% 3rd-degree burns	162	N/A
T3175	Burns involving 70-79% of TBSA W/ 50-59% 3rd-degree burns	162	N/A
T3176	Burns involving 70-79% of TBSA W/ 60-69% 3rd-degree burns	162	N/A
T3177	Burns involving 70-79% of TBSA W/ 70-79% 3rd-degree burns	162	N/A
T3181	Burns involving 80-89% of TBSA W/ 10-19% 3rd-degree burns	162	N/A
T3182	Burns involving 80-89% of TBSA W/ 20-29% 3rd-degree burns	162	N/A
T3183	Burns involving 80-89% of TBSA W/ 30-39% 3rd-degree burns	162	N/A
T3184	Burns involving 80-89% of TBSA W/ 40-49% 3rd-degree burns	162	N/A
T3185	Burns involving 80-89% of TBSA W/ 50-59% 3rd-degree burns	162	N/A
T3186	Burns involving 80-89% of TBSA W/ 60-69% 3rd-degree burns	162	N/A
T3187	Burns involving 80-89% of TBSA W/ 70-79% 3rd-degree burns	162	N/A
T3188	Burns involving 80-89% of TBSA W/ 80-89% 3rd-degree burns	162	N/A
T3191	Burns involving 90% or more of TBSA W/ 10-19% 3rd-degree burns	162	N/A
T3192	Burns involving 90% or more of TBSA W/ 20-29% 3rd-degree burns	162	N/A
T3193	Burns involving 90% or more of TBSA W/ 30-39% 3rd-degree burns	162	N/A
T3194	Burns involving 90% or more of TBSA W/ 40-49% 3rd-degree burns	162	N/A
T3195	Burns involving 90% or more of TBSA W/ 50-59% 3rd-degree burns	162	N/A
T3196	Burns involving 90% or more of TBSA W/ 60-69% 3rd-degree burns	162	N/A
T3197	Burns involving 90% or more of TBSA W/ 70-79% 3rd-degree burns	162	N/A
T3198	Burns involving 90% or more of TBSA W/ 80-89% 3rd-degree burns	162	N/A

Code	Code Descriptors	HCC	RXHCC
T3199	Burns involving 90% or more of TBSA W/ 90% or more 3rd-degree burns	162	N/A
T3211	Corrosions involving 10-19% of TBSA W/ 10-19% 3rd-degree corrosion	162	N/A
T3221	Corrosions involving 20-29% of TBSA W/ 10-19% 3rd-degree corrosion	162	N/A
T3222	Corrosions involving 20-29% of TBSA W/ 20-29% 3rd-degree corrosion	162	N/A
T3231	Corrosions involving 30-39% of TBSA W/ 10-19% 3rd-degree corrosion	162	N/A
T3232	Corrosions involving 30-39% of TBSA W/ 20-29% 3rd-degree corrosion	162	N/A
T3233	Corrosions involving 30-39% of TBSA W/ 30-39% 3rd-degree corrosion	162	N/A
T3241	Corrosions involving 40-49% of TBSA W/ 10-19% 3rd-degree corrosion	162	N/A
T3242	Corrosions involving 40-49% of TBSA W/ 20-29% 3rd-degree corrosion	162	N/A
T3243	Corrosions involving 40-49% of TBSA W/ 30-39% 3rd-degree corrosion	162	N/A
T3244	Corrosions involving 40-49% of TBSA W/ 40-49% 3rd-degree corrosion	162	N/A
T3251	Corrosions involving 50-59% of TBSA W/ 10-19% 3rd-degree corrosion	162	N/A
T3252	Corrosions involving 50-59% of TBSA W/ 20-29% 3rd-degree corrosion	162	N/A
T3253	Corrosions involving 50-59% of TBSA W/ 30-39% 3rd-degree corrosion	162	N/A
T3254	Corrosions involving 50-59% of TBSA W/ 40-49% 3rd-degree corrosion	162	N/A
T3255	Corrosions involving 50-59% of TBSA W/ 50-59% 3rd-degree corrosion	162	N/A
T3261	Corrosions involving 60-69% of TBSA W/ 10-19% 3rd-degree corrosion	162	N/A
T3262	Corrosions involving 60-69% of TBSA W/ 20-29% 3rd-degree corrosion	162	N/A
T3263	Corrosions involving 60-69% of TBSA W/ 30-39% 3rd-degree corrosion	162	N/A
T3264	Corrosions involving 60-69% of TBSA W/ 40-49% 3rd-degree corrosion	162	N/A
T3265	Corrosions involving 60-69% of TBSA W/ 50-59% 3rd-degree corrosion	162	N/A
T3266	Corrosions involving 60-69% of TBSA W/ 60-69% 3rd-degree corrosion	162	N/A
T3271	Corrosions involving 70-79% of TBSA W/ 10-19% 3rd-degree corrosion	162	N/A
T3272	Corrosions involving 70-79% of TBSA W/ 20-29% 3rd-degree corrosion	162	N/A
T3273	Corrosions involving 70-79% of TBSA W/ 30-39% 3rd-degree corrosion	162	N/A
T3274	Corrosions involving 70-79% of TBSA W/ 40-49% 3rd-degree corrosion	162	N/A
T3275	Corrosions involving 70-79% of TBSA W/ 50-59% 3rd-degree corrosion	162	N/A

Code	Code Descriptors	HCC	RXHCC
T3276	Corrosions involving 70-79% of TBSA W/ 60-69% 3rd-degree corrosion	162	N/A
T3277	Corrosions involving 70-79% of TBSA W/ 70-79% 3rd-degree corrosion	162	N/A
T3281	Corrosions involving 80-89% of TBSA W/ 10-19% 3rd-degree corrosion	162	N/A
T3282	Corrosions involving 80-89% of TBSA W/ 20-29% 3rd-degree corrosion	162	N/A
T3283	Corrosions involving 80-89% of TBSA W/ 30-39% 3rd-degree corrosion	162	N/A
T3284	Corrosions involving 80-89% of TBSA W/ 40-49% 3rd-degree corrosion	162	N/A
T3285	Corrosions involving 80-89% of TBSA W/ 50-59% 3rd-degree corrosion	162	N/A
T3286	Corrosions involving 80-89% of TBSA W/ 60-69% 3rd-degree corrosion	162	N/A
T3287	Corrosions involving 80-89% of TBSA W/ 70-79% 3rd-degree corrosion	162	N/A
T3288	Corrosions involving 80-89% of TBSA W/ 80-89% 3rd-degree corrosion	162	N/A
T3291	Corrosions involving 90% or more of TBSA W/ 10-19% 3rd-degree corrosion	162	N/A
T3292	Corrosions involving 90% or more of TBSA W/ 20-29% 3rd-degree corrosion	162	N/A
T3293	Corrosions involving 90% or more of TBSA W/ 30-39% 3rd-degree corrosion	162	N/A
T3294	Corrosions involving 90% or more of TBSA W/ 40-49% 3rd-degree corrosion	162	N/A
T3295	Corrosions involving 90% or more of TBSA W/ 50-59% 3rd-degree corrosion	162	N/A
T3296	Corrosions involving 90% or more of TBSA W/ 60-69% 3rd-degree corrosion	162	N/A
T3297	Corrosions involving 90% or more of TBSA W/ 70-79% 3rd-degree corrosion	162	N/A
T3298	Corrosions involving 90% or more of TBSA W/ 80-89% 3rd-degree corrosion	162	N/A
T3299	Corrosions involving 90% or more of TBSA W/ 90% or more 3rd-degree corrosion	162	N/A
For codes T360X2- through T71232-, only the following 7th characters risk-adjust: A initial encounter S sequela			
T360X2-	Poisoning by penicillins, self-harm	58	N/A
T361X2-	Poisoning by cephalosporins & other beta-lactam antibiotics, self-harm	58	N/A
T362X2-	Poisoning by chloramphenicol group, self-harm	58	N/A
T363X2-	Poisoning by macrolides, self-harm	58	N/A
T364X2-	Poisoning by tetracyclines, self-harm	58	N/A
T365X2-	Poisoning by aminoglycosides, self-harm	58	N/A
T366X2-	Poisoning by rifampicins, self-harm	58	N/A
T367X2-	Poisoning by antifungal antibiotics, systemically used, self-harm	58	N/A
T368X2-	Poisoning by other systemic antibiotics, self-harm	58	N/A
T3692X-	Poisoning by NOS systemic antibiotic, self-harm	58	N/A
T370X2-	Poisoning by sulfonamides, self-harm	58	N/A
T371X2-	Poisoning by antimycobacterial drugs, self-harm	58	N/A
T372X2-	Poisoning by antimalarials & drugs acting on other blood protozoa, self-harm	58	N/A
T373X2-	Poisoning by other antiprotozoal drugs, self-harm	58	N/A
T374X2-	Poisoning by anthelminthics, self-harm	58	N/A
T375X2-	Poisoning by antiviral drugs, self-harm	58	N/A
T378X2-	Poisoning by NEC systemic anti-infectives & antiparasitics, self-harm	58	N/A
T3792X-	Poisoning by NOS systemic anti-infective & antiparasitics, self-harm	58	N/A
T380X2-	Poisoning by glucocorticoids & synthetic analogues, self-harm	58	N/A
T381X2-	Poisoning by thyroid hormones & substitutes, self-harm	58	N/A
T382X2-	Poisoning by antithyroid drugs, self-harm	58	N/A
T383X2-	Poisoning by insulin & oral hypoglycemic [antidiabetic] drugs, self-harm	58	N/A
T384X2-	Poisoning by oral contraceptives, self-harm	58	N/A
T385X2-	Poisoning by other estrogens & progestogens, self-harm	58	N/A
T386X2-	Poisoning by antigonadotrophins, antiestrogens, antiandrogens, NEC, self-harm	58	N/A
T387X2-	Poisoning by androgens & anabolic congeners, self-harm	58	N/A
T38802-	Poisoning by NOS hormones & synthetic substitutes, self-harm	58	N/A
T38812-	Poisoning by anterior pituitary [adenohypophyseal] hormones, self-harm	58	N/A
T38892-	Poisoning by other hormones & synthetic substitutes, self-harm	58	N/A
T38902-	Poisoning by NOS hormone antagonists, self-harm	58	N/A
T38992-	Poisoning by other hormone antagonists, self-harm	58	N/A
T39012-	Poisoning by aspirin, self-harm	58	N/A
T39092-	Poisoning by salicylates, self-harm	58	N/A
T391X2-	Poisoning by 4-Aminophenol derivatives, self-harm	58	N/A
T392X2-	Poisoning by pyrazolone derivatives, self-harm, initial encounter	58	N/A
T39312-	Poisoning by propionic acid derivatives, self-harm	58	N/A
T39392-	Poisoning by other nonsteroidal anti-inflammatory drugs [NSAID], self-harm	58	N/A
T394X2-	Poisoning by antirheumatics, NEC, self-harm	58	N/A

Code	Code Descriptors	HCC	RXHCC
T398X2-	Poisoning by other nonopioid analgesics & antipyretics, NEC, self-harm	58	N/A
T3992X-	Poisoning by NOS nonopioid analgesic, antipyretic & antirheumatic, self-harm	58	N/A
T400X2-	Poisoning by opium, self-harm	58	N/A
T401X2-	Poisoning by heroin, self-harm	58	N/A
T402X2-	Poisoning by other opioids, self-harm	58	N/A
T403X2-	Poisoning by methadone, self-harm,	58	N/A
T404X2-	Poisoning by other synthetic narcotics, self-harm	58	N/A
T405X2-	Poisoning by cocaine, self-harm	58	N/A
T40602-	Poisoning by NOS narcotics, self-harm	58	N/A
T40692-	Poisoning by other narcotics, self-harm	58	N/A
T407X2-	Poisoning by cannabis, self-harm	58	N/A
T408X2-	Poisoning by LSD, self-harm	58	N/A
T40902-	Poisoning by NOS psychodysleptics [hallucinogens], self-harm	58	N/A
T40992-	Poisoning by other psychodysleptics [hallucinogens], self-harm	58	N/A
T410X2-	Poisoning by inhaled anesthetics, self-harm	58	N/A
T411X2-	Poisoning by intravenous anesthetics, self-harm	58	N/A
T41202-	Poisoning by NOS general anesthetics, self-harm	58	N/A
T41292-	Poisoning by other general anesthetics, self-harm	58	N/A
T413X2-	Poisoning by local anesthetics, self-harm	58	N/A
T4142X-	Poisoning by NOS anesthetic, self-harm	58	N/A
T415X2-	Poisoning by therapeutic gases, self-harm	58	N/A
T420X2-	Poisoning by hydantoin derivatives, self-harm	58	N/A
T421X2-	Poisoning by iminostilbenes, self-harm	58	N/A
T422X2-	Poisoning by succinimides & oxazolidinediones, self-harm	58	N/A
T423X2-	Poisoning by barbiturates, self-harm	58	N/A
T424X2-	Poisoning by benzodiazepines, self-harm	58	N/A
T425X2-	Poisoning by mixed antiepileptics, self-harm	58	N/A
T426X2-	Poisoning by other antiepileptic & sedative-hypnotic drugs, self-harm	58	N/A
T4272X-	Poisoning by NOS antiepileptic & sedative-hypnotic drugs, self-harm	58	N/A
T428X2-	Poisoning by antiparkinsonism drugs & other central muscle-tone depressants, self-harm	58	N/A
T43012-	Poisoning by tricyclic antidepressants, self-harm	58	N/A
T43022-	Poisoning by tetracyclic antidepressants, self-harm	58	N/A
T431X2-	Poisoning by monoamine-oxidase-inhibitor antidepressants, self-harm	58	N/A
T43202-	Poisoning by NOS antidepressants, self-harm	58	N/A

Code	Code Descriptors	HCC	RXHCC
T43212-	Poisoning by selective serotonin & norepinephrine reuptake inhibitors, self-harm	58	N/A
T43222-	Poisoning by selective serotonin reuptake inhibitors, self-harm	58	N/A
T43292-	Poisoning by other antidepressants, self-harm	58	N/A
T433X2-	Poisoning by phenothiazine antipsychotics & neuroleptics, self-harm	58	N/A
T434X2-	Poisoning by butyrophenone & thiothixene neuroleptics, self-harm	58	N/A
T43502-	Poisoning by NOS antipsychotics & neuroleptics, self-harm	58	N/A
T43592-	Poisoning by other antipsychotics & neuroleptics, self-harm	58	N/A
T43602-	Poisoning by NOS psychostimulants, self-harm	58	N/A
T43612-	Poisoning by caffeine, self-harm	58	N/A
T43622-	Poisoning by amphetamines, self-harm	58	N/A
T43632-	Poisoning by methylphenidate, self-harm	58	N/A
T43692-	Poisoning by other psychostimulants, self-harm	58	N/A
T438X2-	Poisoning by other psychotropic drugs, self-harm	58	N/A
T4392X-	Poisoning by NOS psychotropic drug, self-harm	58	N/A
T440X2-	Poisoning by anticholinesterase agents, self-harm	58	N/A
T441X2-	Poisoning by other parasympathomimetics [cholinergics], self-harm	58	N/A
T442X2-	Poisoning by ganglionic blocking drugs, self-harm	58	N/A
T443X2-	Poisoning by other parasympatholytics [anticholinergics & antimuscarinics] & spasmolytics, self-harm	58	N/A
T444X2-	Poisoning by predominantly alpha-adrenoreceptor agonists, self-harm	58	N/A
T445X2-	Poisoning by predominantly beta-adrenoreceptor agonists, self-harm	58	N/A
T446X2-	Poisoning by alpha-adrenoreceptor antagonists, self-harm	58	N/A
T447X2-	Poisoning by beta-adrenoreceptor antagonists, self-harm	58	N/A
T448X2-	Poisoning by centrally-acting & adrenergic-neuron- blocking agents, self-harm	58	N/A
T44902-	Poisoning by NOS drugs primarily affecting autonomic nervous system, self-harm	58	N/A
T44992-	Poisoning by other drug primarily affecting autonomic nervous system, self-harm	58	N/A
T450X2-	Poisoning by antiallergic & antiemetic drugs, self-harm	58	N/A
T451X2-	Poisoning by antineoplastic & immunosuppressive drugs, self-harm	58	N/A
T452X2-	Poisoning by vitamins, self-harm	58	N/A

Code	Code Descriptors	HCC	RXHCC
T453X2-	Poisoning by enzymes, self-harm	58	N/A
T454X2-	Poisoning by iron & its compounds, self-harm	58	N/A
T45512-	Poisoning by anticoagulants, self-harm	58	N/A
T45522-	Poisoning by antithrombotic drugs, self-harm	58	N/A
T45602-	Poisoning by NOS fibrinolysis-affecting drugs, self-harm	58	N/A
T45612-	Poisoning by thrombolytic drug, self-harm	58	N/A
T45622-	Poisoning by hemostatic drug, self-harm	58	N/A
T45692-	Poisoning by other fibrinolysis-affecting drugs, self-harm	58	N/A
T457X2-	Poisoning by anticoagulant antagonists, vitamin K & other coagulants, self-harm	58	N/A
T458X2-	Poisoning by other primarily systemic & hematological agents, self-harm	58	N/A
T4592X-	Poisoning by NOS primarily systemic & hematological agent, self-harm	58	N/A
T460X2-	Poisoning by cardiac-stimulant glycosides & drugs of similar action, self-harm	58	N/A
T461X2-	Poisoning by calcium-channel blockers, self-harm	58	N/A
T462X2-	Poisoning by other antidysrhythmic drugs, self-harm	58	N/A
T463X2-	Poisoning by coronary vasodilators, self-harm, initial encounter	58	N/A
T464X2-	Poisoning by angiotensin-converting-enzyme inhibitors, self-harm	58	N/A
T465X2-	Poisoning by other antihypertensive drugs, self-harm	58	N/A
T466X2-	Poisoning by antihyperlipidemic & antiarteriosclerotic drugs, self-harm	58	N/A
T467X2-	Poisoning by peripheral vasodilators, self-harm	58	N/A
T468X2-	Poisoning by antivaricose drugs, including sclerosing agents, self-harm	58	N/A
T46902-	Poisoning by NOS agents primarily affecting cardiovascular system, self-harm	58	N/A
T46992-	Poisoning by other agents primarily affecting cardiovascular system, self-harm	58	N/A
T470X2-	Poisoning by histamine H2-receptor blockers, self-harm	58	N/A
T471X2-	Poisoning by other antacids & anti-gastric-secretion drugs, self-harm	58	N/A
T472X2-	Poisoning by stimulant laxatives, self-harm	58	N/A
T473X2-	Poisoning by saline & osmotic laxatives, self-harm	58	N/A
T474X2-	Poisoning by other laxatives, self-harm	58	N/A
T475X2-	Poisoning by digestants, self-harm	58	N/A
T476X2-	Poisoning by antidiarrheal drugs, self-harm	58	N/A
T477X2-	Poisoning by emetics, self-harm	58	N/A
T478X2-	Poisoning by other agents primarily affecting gastrointestinal system, self-harm	58	N/A

Code	Code Descriptors	HCC	RXHCC
T4792X-	Poisoning by NOS agents primarily affecting gastrointestinal system, self-harm	58	N/A
T480X2-	Poisoning by oxytocic drugs, self-harm	58	N/A
T481X2-	Poisoning by skeletal muscle relaxants, self-harm	58	N/A
T48202-	Poisoning by NOS drugs acting on muscles, self-harm	58	N/A
T48292-	Poisoning by other drugs acting on muscles, self-harm	58	N/A
T483X2-	Poisoning by antitussives, self-harm	58	N/A
T484X2-	Poisoning by expectorants, self-harm	58	N/A
T485X2-	Poisoning by other anti-common-cold drugs, self-harm	58	N/A
T486X2-	Poisoning by antiasthmatics, self-harm	58	N/A
T48902-	Poisoning by NOS agents primarily acting on respiratory system, self-harm, initial encounter	58	N/A
T48992-	Poisoning by other agents primarily acting on respiratory system, self-harm	58	N/A
T490X2-	Poisoning by local antifungal, anti-infective & anti- inflammatory drugs, self-harm	58	N/A
T491X2-	Poisoning by antipruritics, self-harm	58	N/A
T492X2-	Poisoning by local astringents & local detergents, self-harm	58	N/A
T493X2-	Poisoning by emollients, demulcents & protectants, self-harm	58	N/A
T494X2-	Poisoning by keratolytics, keratoplastics, & other hair treatment drugs & preparations, self-harm	58	N/A
T495X2-	Poisoning by ophthalmological drugs & preparations, self-harm	58	N/A
T496X2-	Poisoning by otorhinolaryngological drugs & preparations, self-harm	58	N/A
T497X2-	Poisoning by dental drugs, topically applied, self-harm	58	N/A
T498X2-	Poisoning by other topical agents, self-harm	58	N/A
T4992X-	Poisoning by NOS topical agent, self-harm	58	N/A
T500X2-	Poisoning by mineralocorticoids & their antagonists, self-harm	58	N/A
T501X2-	Poisoning by loop [high-ceiling] diuretics, self-harm	58	N/A
T502X2-	Poisoning by carbonic-anhydrase inhibitors, benzothiadiazides & other diuretics, self-harm	58	N/A
T503X2-	Poisoning by electrolytic, caloric & water-balance agents, self-harm	58	N/A
T504X2-	Poisoning by drugs affecting uric acid metabolism, self-harm	58	N/A
T505X2-	Poisoning by appetite depressants, self-harm	58	N/A
T506X2-	Poisoning by antidotes & chelating agents, self-harm	58	N/A

Code	Code Descriptors	HCC	RXHCC
T507X2-	Poisoning by analeptics & opioid receptor antagonists, self-harm	58	N/A
T508X2-	Poisoning by diagnostic agents, self-harm	58	N/A
T50902-	Poisoning by NOS drugs, medicaments & biological substances, self-harm	58	N/A
T50992-	Poisoning by other drugs, medicaments & biological substances, self-harm	58	N/A
T50A12-	Poisoning by pertussis vaccine, including combinations W/ a pertussis component, self-harm	58	N/A
T50A22-	Poisoning by mixed bacterial vaccines W/O a pertussis component, self-harm	58	N/A
T50A92-	Poisoning by other bacterial vaccines, self-harm	58	N/A
T50B12-	Poisoning by smallpox vaccines, self-harm	58	N/A
T50B92-	Poisoning by other viral vaccines, self-harm	58	N/A
T50Z12-	Poisoning by immunoglobulin, self-harm	58	N/A
T50Z92-	Poisoning by other vaccines & biological substances, self-harm	58	N/A
T510X2-	Toxic effect of ethanol, self-harm	58	N/A
T511X2-	Toxic effect of methanol, self-harm	58	N/A
T512X2-	Toxic effect of 2-Propanol, self-harm	58	N/A
T513X2-	Toxic effect of fusel oil, self-harm, initial encounter	58	N/A
T518X2-	Toxic effect of other alcohols, self-harm	58	N/A
T5192X-	Toxic effect of NOS alcohol, self-harm	58	N/A
T520X2-	Toxic effect of petroleum products, self-harm	58	N/A
T521X2-	Toxic effect of benzene, self-harm	58	N/A
T522X2-	Toxic effect of homologues of benzene, self-harm	58	N/A
T523X2-	Toxic effect of glycols, self-harm	58	N/A
T524X2-	Toxic effect of ketones, self-harm	58	N/A
T528X2-	Toxic effect of other organic solvents, self-harm	58	N/A
T5292X-	Toxic effect of NOS organic solvent, self-harm	58	N/A
T530X2-	Toxic effect of carbon tetrachloride, self-harm	58	N/A
T531X2-	Toxic effect of chloroform, self-harm	58	N/A
T532X2-	Toxic effect of trichloroethylene, self-harm	58	N/A
T533X2-	Toxic effect of tetrachloroethylene, self-harm	58	N/A
T534X2-	Toxic effect of dichloromethane, self-harm	58	N/A
T535X2-	Toxic effect of chlorofluorocarbons, self-harm	58	N/A
T536X2-	Toxic effect of other halogen derivatives of aliphatic hydrocarbons, self-harm	58	N/A
T537X2-	Toxic effect of other halogen derivatives of aromatic hydrocarbons, self-harm	58	N/A

Code	Code Descriptors	HCC	RXHCC
T5392X-	Toxic effect of NOS halogen derivatives of aliphatic & aromatic hydrocarbons, self-harm	58	N/A
T540X2-	Toxic effect of phenol & phenol homologues, self-harm	58	N/A
T541X2-	Toxic effect of other corrosive organic compounds, self-harm	58	N/A
T542X2-	Toxic effect of corrosive acids & acid-like substances, self-harm	58	N/A
T543X2-	Toxic effect of corrosive alkalis & alkali-like substances, self-harm	58	N/A
T5492X-	Toxic effect of NOS corrosive substance, self-harm	58	N/A
T550X2-	Toxic effect of soaps, self-harm	58	N/A
T551X2-	Toxic effect of detergents, self-harm	58	N/A
T560X2-	Toxic effect of lead & its compounds, self-harm	58	N/A
T561X2-	Toxic effect of mercury & its compounds, self-harm	58	N/A
T562X2-	Toxic effect of chromium & its compounds, self-harm	58	N/A
T563X2-	Toxic effect of cadmium & its compounds, self-harm	58	N/A
T564X2-	Toxic effect of copper & its compounds, self-harm	58	N/A
T565X2-	Toxic effect of zinc & its compounds, self-harm	58	N/A
T566X2-	Toxic effect of tin & its compounds, self-harm	58	N/A
T567X2-	Toxic effect of beryllium & its compounds, self-harm	58	N/A
T56812-	Toxic effect of thallium, self-harm	58	N/A
T56892-	Toxic effect of other metals, self-harm	58	N/A
T5692X-	Toxic effect of NOS metal, self-harm	58	N/A
T570X2-	Toxic effect of arsenic & its compounds, self-harm,	58	N/A
T571X2-	Toxic effect of phosphorus & its compounds, self-harm	58	N/A
T572X2-	Toxic effect of manganese & its compounds, self-harm	58	N/A
T573X2-	Toxic effect of hydrogen cyanide, self-harm	58	N/A
T578X2-	Toxic effect of NEC inorganic substances, self-harm	58	N/A
T5792X-	Toxic effect of NOS inorganic substance, self-harm	58	N/A
T5802X-	Toxic effect of carbon monoxide from motor vehicle exhaust, self-harm	58	N/A
T5812X-	Toxic effect of carbon monoxide from utility gas, self-harm	58	N/A
T582X2-	Toxic effect of carbon monoxide from incomplete combustion of other domestic fuels, self-harm	58	N/A

Code	Code Descriptors	HCC	RXHCC
T588X2-	Toxic effect of carbon monoxide from other source, self-harm	58	N/A
T5892X-	Toxic effect of carbon monoxide from NOS source, self-harm	58	N/A
T590X2-	Toxic effect of nitrogen oxides, self-harm	58	N/A
T591X2-	Toxic effect of sulfur dioxide, self-harm	58	N/A
T592X2-	Toxic effect of formaldehyde, self-harm	58	N/A
T593X2-	Toxic effect of lacrimogenic gas, self-harm	58	N/A
T594X2-	Toxic effect of chlorine gas, self-harm	58	N/A
T595X2-	Toxic effect of fluorine gas & hydrogen fluoride, self-harm	58	N/A
T596X2-	Toxic effect of hydrogen sulfide, self-harm	58	N/A
T597X2-	Toxic effect of carbon dioxide, self-harm	58	N/A
T59812-	Toxic effect of smoke, self-harm	58	N/A
T59892-	Toxic effect of NEC gases, fumes & vapors, self-harm	58	N/A
T5992X-	Toxic effect of NOS gases, fumes & vapors, self-harm	58	N/A
T600X2-	Toxic effect of organophosphate & carbamate insecticides, self-harm	58	N/A
T601X2-	Toxic effect of halogenated insecticides, self-harm	58	N/A
T602X2-	Toxic effect of other insecticides, self-harm	58	N/A
T603X2-	Toxic effect of herbicides & fungicides, self-harm	58	N/A
T604X2-	Toxic effect of rodenticides, self-harm,	58	N/A
T608X2-	Toxic effect of other pesticides, self-harm	58	N/A
T6092X-	Toxic effect of NOS pesticide, self-harm	58	N/A
T6102X-	Ciguatera fish poisoning, self-harm	58	N/A
T6112X-	Scombroid fish poisoning, self-harm	58	N/A
T61772-	Other fish poisoning, self-harm	58	N/A
T61782-	Other shellfish poisoning, self-harm	58	N/A
T618X2-	Toxic effect of other seafood, self-harm	58	N/A
T6192X-	Toxic effect of NOS seafood, self-harm	58	N/A
T620X2-	Toxic effect of ingested mushrooms, self-harm	58	N/A
T621X2-	Toxic effect of ingested berries, self-harm	58	N/A
T622X2-	Toxic effect of other ingested plant(s), self-harm	58	N/A
T628X2-	Toxic effect of NEC noxious substances eaten as food, self-harm	58	N/A
T6292X-	Toxic effect of NOS noxious substance eaten as food, self-harm	58	N/A
T63002-	Toxic effect of NOS snake venom, self-harm	58	N/A
T63012-	Toxic effect of rattlesnake venom, self-harm	58	N/A
T63022-	Toxic effect of coral snake venom, self-harm	58	N/A
T63032-	Toxic effect of taipan venom, self-harm	58	N/A
T63042-	Toxic effect of cobra venom, self-harm	58	N/A
T63062-	Toxic effect of venom of other North & South American snake, self-harm	58	N/A

Code	Code Descriptors	HCC	RXHCC
T63072-	Toxic effect of venom of other Australian snake, self-harm	58	N/A
T63082-	Toxic effect of venom of other African & Asian snake, self-harm	58	N/A
T63092-	Toxic effect of venom of other snake, self-harm	58	N/A
T63112-	Toxic effect of venom of gila monster, self-harm	58	N/A
T63122-	Toxic effect of venom of other venomous lizard, self-harm	58	N/A
T63192-	Toxic effect of venom of other reptiles, self-harm	58	N/A
T632X2-	Toxic effect of venom of scorpion, self-harm	58	N/A
T63302-	Toxic effect of NOS spider venom, self-harm	58	N/A
T63312-	Toxic effect of venom of black widow spider, self-harm	58	N/A
T63322-	Toxic effect of venom of tarantula, self-harm	58	N/A
T63332-	Toxic effect of venom of brown recluse spider, self-harm	58	N/A
T63392-	Toxic effect of venom of other spider, self-harm	58	N/A
T63412-	Toxic effect of venom of centipedes & venomous millipedes, self-harm	58	N/A
T63422-	Toxic effect of venom of ants, self-harm	58	N/A
T63432-	Toxic effect of venom of caterpillars, self-harm	58	N/A
T63442-	Toxic effect of venom of bees, self-harm	58	N/A
T63452-	Toxic effect of venom of hornets, self-harm	58	N/A
T63462-	Toxic effect of venom of wasps, self-harm	58	N/A
T63482-	Toxic effect of venom of other arthropod, self-harm	58	N/A
T63512-	Toxic effect of contact W/ stingray, self-harm	58	N/A
T63592-	Toxic effect of contact W/ other venomous fish, self-harm	58	N/A
T63612-	Toxic effect of contact W/ Portugese Man-o-war, self-harm	58	N/A
T63622-	Toxic effect of contact W/ other jellyfish, self-harmr	58	N/A
T63632-	Toxic effect of contact W/ sea anemone, self-harm	58	N/A
T63692-	Toxic effect of contact W/ other venomous marine animals, self-harm	58	N/A
T63712-	Toxic effect of contact W/ venomous marine plant, self-harm	58	N/A
T63792-	Toxic effect of contact W/ other venomous plant, self-harm	58	N/A
T63812-	Toxic effect of contact W/ venomous frog, self-harm	58	N/A
T63822-	Toxic effect of contact W/ venomous toad, self-harm	58	N/A
T63832-	Toxic effect of contact W/ NEC venomous amphibian, self-harm	58	N/A

Code	Code Descriptors	HCC	RXHCC
T63892-	Toxic effect of contact W/ NEC venomous animal, self-harm	58	N/A
T6392X-	Toxic effect of contact W/ NOS venomous animal, self-harm	58	N/A
T6402X-	Toxic effect of aflatoxin, self-harm	58	N/A
T6482X-	Toxic effect of other mycotoxin food contaminants, self-harm	58	N/A
T650X2-	Toxic effect of cyanides, self-harm	58	N/A
T651X2-	Toxic effect of strychnine & its salts, self-harm	58	N/A
T65212-	Toxic effect of chewing tobacco, self-harm	58	N/A
T65222-	Toxic effect of tobacco cigarettes, self-harm	58	N/A
T65292-	Toxic effect of other tobacco & nicotine, self-harm	58	N/A
T653X2-	Toxic effect of nitroderivatives & aminoderivatives of benzene & its homologues, self-harm	58	N/A
T654X2-	Toxic effect of carbon disulfide, self-harm	58	N/A
T655X2-	Toxic effect of nitroglycerin & other nitric acids & esters, self-harm	58	N/A
T656X2-	Toxic effect of paints & dyes, NEC, self-harm	58	N/A
T65812-	Toxic effect of latex, self-harm	58	N/A
T65822-	Toxic effect of harmful algae & algae toxins, self-harm	58	N/A
T65832-	Toxic effect of fiberglass, self-harm	58	N/A
T65892-	Toxic effect of NEC substances, self-harm	58	N/A
T6592X-	Toxic effect of NOS substance, self-harm	58	N/A
T71112-	Asphyxiation D/T smothering under pillow, self-harm	58	N/A
T71122-	Asphyxiation D/T plastic bag, self-harm	58	N/A
T71132-	Asphyxiation D/T being trapped in bed linens, self-harm	58	N/A
T71152-	Asphyxiation D/T smothering in furniture, self-harm	58	N/A
T71162-	Asphyxiation D/T hanging, self-harm	58	N/A
T71192-	Asphyxiation D/T mechanical threat to breathing D/T other causes, self-harm	58	N/A
T71222-	Asphyxiation D/T being trapped in a car trunk, self-harm	58	N/A
T71232-	Asphyxiation D/T being trapped in a refrigerator, self-harm	58	N/A
T790XXA	Air embolism (traumatic), initial encounter	173	N/A
T791XXA	Fat embolism (traumatic), initial encounter	173	N/A
T792XXA	Traumatic 2ndary & recurrent hemorrhage & seroma, initial encounter	173	N/A
T794XXA	Traumatic shock, initial encounter	173	N/A
T795XXA	Traumatic anuria, initial encounter	173	N/A
T796XXA	Traumatic ischemia of muscle, initial encounter	173	N/A
T797XXA	Traumatic subcutaneous emphysema, initial encounter	173	N/A

Code	Code Descriptors	HCC	RXHCC
T798XXA	Early complications of trauma, initial encounter, NEC	173	N/A
T799XXA	Early complication of trauma, initial encounter, NOS	173	N/A
T79A0XA	Compartment syndrome, NOS, initial encounter	173	N/A
T79A11A	Traumatic compartment syndrome of R upper extremity, initial encounter	173	N/A
T79A12A	Traumatic compartment syndrome of L upper extremity, initial encounter	173	N/A
T79A19A	Traumatic compartment syndrome of NOS upper extremity, initial encounter	173	N/A
T79A21A	Traumatic compartment syndrome of R lower extremity, initial encounter	173	N/A
T79A22A	Traumatic compartment syndrome of L lower extremity, initial encounter	173	N/A
T79A29A	Traumatic compartment syndrome of NOS lower extremity, initial encounter	173	N/A
T79A3XA	Traumatic compartment syndrome of abdomen, initial encounter	173	N/A
T79A9XA	Traumatic compartment syndrome of other sites, initial encounter	173	N/A
T8111XA	Postprocedural cardiogenic shock, initial encounter	84	N/A
T8112XA	Postprocedural septic shock, initial encounter	2	N/A
For codes T81502- through T81592-, use the following 7th characters: A initial encounter D subsequent encounter S sequela			
T81502-	Complication of foreign body accidentally L in body following kidney dialysis, NOS	134	261
T81512-	Adhesions D/T foreign body accidentally L in body following kidney dialysis	134	261
T81522-	Obstruction D/T foreign body accidentally L in body following kidney dialysis	134	261
T81532-	Perforation D/T foreign body accidentally L in body following kidney dialysis	134	261
T81592-	Other complications of foreign body accidentally L in body following kidney dialysis	134	261
T82310A	Breakdown of aortic graft , initial encounter	176	N/A
T82311A	Breakdown of carotid arterial graft, initial encounter	176	N/A
T82312A	Breakdown of femoral arterial graft, initial encounter	176	N/A
T82318A	Breakdown of other vascular grafts, initial encounter	176	N/A
T82319A	Breakdown of NOS vascular grafts, initial encounter	176	N/A
T82320A	Displacement of aortic graft , initial encounter	176	N/A
T82321A	Displacement of carotid arterial graft, initial encounter	176	N/A

Code	Code Descriptors	HCC	RXHCC
T82322A	Displacement of femoral arterial graft, initial encounter	176	N/A
T82328A	Displacement of other vascular grafts, initial encounter	176	N/A
T82329A	Displacement of NOS vascular grafts, initial encounter	176	N/A
T82330A	Leakage of aortic graft, initial encounter	176	N/A
T82331A	Leakage of carotid arterial graft, initial encounter	176	N/A
T82332A	Leakage of femoral arterial graft, initial encounter	176	N/A
T82338A	Leakage of other vascular grafts, initial encounter	176	N/A
T82339A	Leakage of NOS vascular graft, initial encounter	176	N/A
T82390A	Other mechanical complication of aortic graft , initial encounter	176	N/A
T82391A	Other mechanical complication of carotid arterial graft, initial encounter	176	N/A
T82392A	Other mechanical complication of femoral arterial graft, initial encounter	176	N/A
T82398A	Mechanical complication NEC of vascular grafts, NEC, initial encounter	176	N/A
T82399A	Mechanical complication NEC of vascular grafts, NOS, initial encounter	176	N/A
For codes T8241X- through T8249X-, use the following 7th characters: A initial encounter D subsequent encounter S sequela			
T8241X-	Breakdown of vascular dialysis catheter	134	261
T8242X-	Displacement of vascular dialysis catheter	134	261
T8243X-	Leakage of vascular dialysis catheter	134	261
T8249X-	Other complication of vascular dialysis catheter	134	261
T82510A	Breakdown of surgically created arteriovenous fistula, initial encounter	176	N/A
T82511A	Breakdown of surgically created arteriovenous shunt, initial encounter	176	N/A
T82513A	Breakdown of balloon device, initial encounter	176	N/A
T82514A	Breakdown of infusion catheter, initial encounter	176	N/A
T82515A	Breakdown of umbrella device, initial encounter	176	N/A
T82518A	Breakdown of other cardiac & vascular devices & implants, initial encounter	176	N/A
T82520A	Displacement of surgically created arteriovenous fistula, initial encounter	176	N/A
T82521A	Displacement of surgically created arteriovenous shunt, initial encounter	176	N/A
T82523A	Displacement of balloon device, initial encounter	176	N/A

Code	Code Descriptors	HCC	RXHCC
T82524A	Displacement of infusion catheter, initial encounter	176	N/A
T82525A	Displacement of umbrella device, initial encounter	176	N/A
T82528A	Displacement of other cardiac & vascular devices & implants, initial encounter	176	N/A
T82530A	Leakage of surgically created arteriovenous fistula, initial encounter	176	N/A
T82531A	Leakage of surgically created arteriovenous shunt, initial encounter	176	N/A
T82533A	Leakage of balloon device, initial encounter	176	N/A
T82534A	Leakage of infusion catheter, initial encounter	176	N/A
T82535A	Leakage of umbrella device, initial encounter	176	N/A
T82538A	Leakage of other cardiac & vascular devices & implants, initial encounter	176	N/A
T82590A	Other mechanical complication of surgically created arteriovenous fistula, initial encounter	176	N/A
T82591A	Other mechanical complication of surgically created arteriovenous shunt, initial encounter	176	N/A
T82593A	Other mechanical complication of balloon device, initial encounter	176	N/A
T82594A	Other mechanical complication of infusion catheter, initial encounter	176	N/A
T82595A	Other mechanical complication of umbrella device, initial encounter	176	N/A
T82598A	Other mechanical complication of other cardiac & vascular devices & implants, initial encounter	176	N/A
T826XXA	Infection & inflammatory reaction D/T cardiac valve prosthesis, initial encounter	176	N/A
T827XXA	Infection & inflammatory reaction D/T other cardiac & vascular devices, implants & grafts, initial encounter	176	N/A
T82818A	Embolism D/T vascular prosthetic devices, implants & grafts, initial encounter	176	N/A
T82828A	Fibrosis D/T vascular prosthetic devices, implants & grafts, initial encounter	176	N/A
T82838A	Hemorrhage D/T vascular prosthetic devices, implants & grafts, initial encounter	176	N/A
T82848A	Pain D/T vascular prosthetic devices, implants & grafts, initial encounter	176	N/A
T82856A	Stenosis of peripheral vascular stent, initial encounter	176	N/A
T82858A	Stenosis of other vascular prosthetic devices, implants & grafts, initial encounter	176	N/A
T82868A	Thrombosis D/T vascular prosthetic devices, implants & grafts, initial encounter	176	N/A
T82898A	NEC complication of vascular prosthetic devices, implants & grafts, initial encounter	176	N/A
T83010A	Breakdown of cystostomy catheter, initial encounter	176	N/A

Code	Code Descriptors	HCC	RXHCC
T83011A	Breakdown of indwelling urethral catheter, initial encounter	176	N/A
T83012A	Breakdown of nephrostomy catheter, initial encounter	176	N/A
T83018A	Breakdown of other urinary catheter, initial encounter	176	N/A
T83020A	Displacement of cystostomy catheter, initial encounter	176	N/A
T83021A	Displacement of indwelling urethral catheter, initial encounter	176	N/A
T83022A	Displacement of nephrostomy catheter, initial encounter	176	N/A
T83028A	Displacement of other urinary catheter, initial encounter	176	N/A
T83030A	Leakage of cystostomy catheter, initial encounter	176	N/A
T83031A	Leakage of indwelling urethral catheter, initial encounter	176	N/A
T83032A	Leakage of nephrostomy catheter, initial encounter	176	N/A
T83038A	Leakage of other urinary catheter, initial encounter	176	N/A
T83090A	Other mechanical complication of cystostomy catheter, initial encounter	176	N/A
T83091A	Other mechanical complication of indwelling urethral catheter, initial encounter	176	N/A
T83092A	Other mechanical complication of nephrostomy catheter, initial encounter	176	N/A
T83098A	Other mechanical complication of other urinary catheter, initial encounter	176	N/A
T83110A	Breakdown of urinary electronic stimulator device, initial encounter	176	N/A
T83111A	Breakdown of implanted urinary sphincter, initial encounter	176	N/A
T83112A	Breakdown of indwelling ureteral stent, initial encounter	176	N/A
T83113A	Breakdown of other urinary stents, initial encounter	176	N/A
T83118A	Breakdown of other urinary devices & implants, initial encounter	176	N/A
T83120A	Displacement of urinary electronic stimulator device, initial encounter	176	N/A
T83121A	Displacement of implanted urinary sphincter, initial encounter	176	N/A
T83122A	Displacement of indwelling ureteral stent, initial encounter	176	N/A
T83123A	Displacement of other urinary stents, initial encounter	176	N/A
T83128A	Displacement of other urinary devices & implants, initial encounter	176	N/A
T83190A	Other mechanical complication of urinary electronic stimulator device, initial encounter	176	N/A

Code	Code Descriptors	HCC	RXHCC
T83191A	Other mechanical complication of implanted urinary sphincter, initial encounter	176	N/A
T83192A	Other mechanical complication of indwelling ureteral stent, initial encounter	176	N/A
T83193A	Other mechanical complication of other urinary stent, initial encounter	176	N/A
T83198A	Other mechanical complication of other urinary devices & implants, initial encounter	176	N/A
T8321XA	Breakdown of graft of urinary organ, initial encounter	176	N/A
T8322XA	Displacement of graft of urinary organ, initial encounter	176	N/A
T8323XA	Leakage of graft of urinary organ, initial encounter	176	N/A
T8324XA	Erosion of graft of urinary organ, initial encounter	176	N/A
T8325XA	Exposure of graft of urinary organ, initial encounter	176	N/A
T8329XA	Other mechanical complication of graft of urinary organ, initial encounter	176	N/A
T83410A	Breakdown of implanted penile prosthesis, initial encounter	176	N/A
T83411A	Breakdown of implanted testicular prosthesis, initial encounter	176	N/A
T83418A	Breakdown of other prosthetic devices, implants & grafts of genital tract, initial encounter	176	N/A
T83420A	Displacement of implanted penile prosthesis, initial encounter	176	N/A
T83421A	Displacement of implanted testicular prosthesis, initial encounter	176	N/A
T83428A	Displacement of other prosthetic devices, implants & grafts of genital tract, initial encounter	176	N/A
T83490A	Other mechanical complication of implanted penile prosthesis, initial encounter	176	N/A
T83491A	Other mechanical complication of implanted testicular prosthesis, initial encounter	176	N/A
T83498A	Other mechanical complication of other prosthetic devices, implants & grafts of genital tract, initial encounter	176	N/A
T83510A	Infection & inflammatory reaction D/T cystostomy catheter, initial encounter	176	N/A
T83511A	Infection & inflammatory reaction D/T indwelling urethral catheter, initial encounter	176	N/A
T83512A	Infection & inflammatory reaction D/T nephrostomy catheter, initial encounter	176	N/A
T83518A	Infection & inflammatory reaction D/T other urinary catheter, initial encounter	176	N/A
T83590A	Infection & inflammatory reaction D/T implanted urinary neurostimulation device, initial encounter	176	N/A

Code	Code Descriptors	HCC	RXHCC
T83591A	Infection & inflammatory reaction D/T implanted urinary sphincter, initial encounter	176	N/A
T83592A	Infection & inflammatory reaction D/T indwelling ureteral stent, initial encounter	176	N/A
T83593A	Infection & inflammatory reaction D/T other urinary stents, initial encounter	176	N/A
T83598A	Infection & inflammatory reaction D/T other prosthetic device, implant & graft in urinary system, initial encounter	176	N/A
T8361XA	Infection & inflammatory reaction D/T implanted penile prosthesis, initial encounter	176	N/A
T8362XA	Infection & inflammatory reaction D/T implanted testicular prosthesis, initial encounter	176	N/A
T8369XA	Infection & inflammatory reaction D/T other prosthetic device, implant & graft in genital tract, initial encounter	176	N/A
T83711A	Erosion of implanted vaginal mesh to surrounding organ or tissue, initial encounter	176	N/A
T83712A	Erosion of implanted urethral mesh to surrounding organ or tissue, initial encounter	176	N/A
T83713A	Erosion of implanted urethral bulking agent to surrounding organ or tissue, initial encounter	176	N/A
T83714A	Erosion of implanted ureteral bulking agent to surrounding organ or tissue, initial encounter	176	N/A
T83718A	Erosion of other implanted mesh to organ or tissue, initial encounter	176	N/A
T83719A	Erosion of other prosthetic materials to surrounding organ or tissue, initial encounter	176	N/A
T83721A	Exposure of implanted vaginal mesh into vagina, initial encounter	176	N/A
T83722A	Exposure of implanted urethral mesh into urethra, initial encounter	176	N/A
T83723A	Exposure of implanted urethral bulking agent into urethra, initial encounter	176	N/A
T83724A	Exposure of implanted ureteral bulking agent into ureter, initial encounter	176	N/A
T83728A	Exposure of other implanted mesh into organ or tissue, initial encounter	176	N/A
T83729A	Exposure of other prosthetic materials into organ or tissue, initial encounter	176	N/A
T8379XA	NEC complications D/T other genitourinary prosthetic materials, initial encounter	176	N/A
T8381XA	Embolism D/T genitourinary prosthetic devices, implants & grafts, initial encounter	176	N/A
T8382XA	Fibrosis D/T genitourinary prosthetic devices, implants & grafts, initial encounter	176	N/A
T8383XA	Hemorrhage D/T genitourinary prosthetic devices, implants & grafts, initial encounter	176	N/A

Code	Code Descriptors	HCC	RXHCC
T8384XA	Pain D/T genitourinary prosthetic devices, implants & grafts, initial encounter	176	N/A
T8385XA	Stenosis D/T genitourinary prosthetic devices, implants & grafts, initial encounter	176	N/A
T8386XA	Thrombosis D/T genitourinary prosthetic devices, implants & grafts, initial encounter	176	N/A
T8389XA	NEC complication of genitourinary prosthetic devices, implants & grafts, initial encounter	176	N/A
T839XXA	NOS complication of genitourinary prosthetic device, implant & graft, initial encounter	176	N/A
T84010A	Broken internal R hip prosthesis, initial encounter	176	N/A
T84011A	Broken internal L hip prosthesis, initial encounter	176	N/A
T84012A	Broken internal R knee prosthesis, initial encounter	176	N/A
T84013A	Broken internal L knee prosthesis, initial encounter	176	N/A
T84018A	Broken internal joint prosthesis, other site, initial encounter	176	N/A
T84019A	Broken internal joint prosthesis, NOS site, initial encounter	176	N/A
T84020A	Dislocation of internal R hip prosthesis, initial encounter	176	N/A
T84021A	Dislocation of internal L hip prosthesis, initial encounter	176	N/A
T84022A	Instability of internal R knee prosthesis, initial encounter	176	N/A
T84023A	Instability of internal L knee prosthesis, initial encounter	176	N/A
T84028A	Dislocation of other internal joint prosthesis, initial encounter	176	N/A
T84029A	Dislocation of NOS internal joint prosthesis, initial encounter	176	N/A
T84030A	Mechanical loosening of internal R hip prosthetic joint, initial encounter	176	N/A
T84031A	Mechanical loosening of internal L hip prosthetic joint, initial encounter	176	N/A
T84032A	Mechanical loosening of internal R knee prosthetic joint, initial encounter	176	N/A
T84033A	Mechanical loosening of internal L knee prosthetic joint, initial encounter	176	N/A
T84038A	Mechanical loosening of other internal prosthetic joint, initial encounter	176	N/A
T84039A	Mechanical loosening of NOS internal prosthetic joint, initial encounter	176	N/A
T84050A	Periprosthetic osteolysis of internal prosthetic R hip joint, initial encounter	176	N/A
T84051A	Periprosthetic osteolysis of internal prosthetic L hip joint, initial encounter	176	N/A
T84052A	Periprosthetic osteolysis of internal prosthetic R knee joint, initial encounter	176	N/A

Code	Code Descriptors	HCC	RXHCC
T84053A	Periprosthetic osteolysis of internal prosthetic L knee joint, initial encounter	176	N/A
T84058A	Periprosthetic osteolysis of other internal prosthetic joint, initial encounter	176	N/A
T84059A	Periprosthetic osteolysis of NOS internal prosthetic joint, initial encounter	176	N/A
T84060A	Wear of articular bearing surface of internal prosthetic R hip joint, initial encounter	176	N/A
T84061A	Wear of articular bearing surface of internal prosthetic L hip joint, initial encounter	176	N/A
T84062A	Wear of articular bearing surface of internal prosthetic R knee joint, initial encounter	176	N/A
T84063A	Wear of articular bearing surface of internal prosthetic L knee joint, initial encounter	176	N/A
T84068A	Wear of articular bearing surface of other internal prosthetic joint, initial encounter	176	N/A
T84069A	Wear of articular bearing surface of NOS internal prosthetic joint, initial encounter	176	N/A
T84090A	Other mechanical complication of internal R hip prosthesis, initial encounter	176	N/A
T84091A	Other mechanical complication of internal L hip prosthesis, initial encounter	176	N/A
T84092A	Other mechanical complication of internal R knee prosthesis, initial encounter	176	N/A
T84093A	Other mechanical complication of internal L knee prosthesis, initial encounter	176	N/A
T84098A	Other mechanical complication of other internal joint prosthesis, initial encounter	176	N/A
T84099A	Other mechanical complication of NOS internal joint prosthesis, initial encounter	176	N/A
T84110A	Breakdown of internal fixation device of R humerus, initial encounter	176	N/A
T84111A	Breakdown of internal fixation device of L humerus, initial encounter	176	N/A
T84112A	Breakdown of internal fixation device of bone of R forearm, initial encounter	176	N/A
T84113A	Breakdown of internal fixation device of bone of L forearm, initial encounter	176	N/A
T84114A	Breakdown of internal fixation device of R femur, initial encounter	176	N/A
T84115A	Breakdown of internal fixation device of L femur, initial encounter	176	N/A
T84116A	Breakdown of internal fixation device of bone of R lower leg, initial encounter	176	N/A
T84117A	Breakdown of internal fixation device of bone of L lower leg, initial encounter	176	N/A
T84119A	Breakdown of internal fixation device of NOS bone of limb, initial encounter	176	N/A
T84120A	Displacement of internal fixation device of R humerus, initial encounter	176	N/A
T84121A	Displacement of internal fixation device of L humerus, initial encounter	176	N/A
T84122A	Displacement of internal fixation device of bone of R forearm, initial encounter	176	N/A

Code	Code Descriptors	HCC	RXHCC
T84123A	Displacement of internal fixation device of bone of L forearm, initial encounter	176	N/A
T84124A	Displacement of internal fixation device of R femur, initial encounter	176	N/A
T84125A	Displacement of internal fixation device of L femur, initial encounter	176	N/A
T84126A	Displacement of internal fixation device of bone of R lower leg, initial encounter	176	N/A
T84127A	Displacement of internal fixation device of bone of L lower leg, initial encounter	176	N/A
T84129A	Displacement of internal fixation device of NOS bone of limb, initial encounter	176	N/A
T84190A	Other mechanical complication of internal fixation device of R humerus, initial encounter	176	N/A
T84191A	Other mechanical complication of internal fixation device of L humerus, initial encounter	176	N/A
T84192A	Other mechanical complication of internal fixation device of bone of R forearm, initial encounter	176	N/A
T84193A	Other mechanical complication of internal fixation device of bone of L forearm, initial encounter	176	N/A
T84194A	Other mechanical complication of internal fixation device of R femur, initial encounter	176	N/A
T84195A	Other mechanical complication of internal fixation device of L femur, initial encounter	176	N/A
T84196A	Other mechanical complication of internal fixation device of bone of R lower leg, initial encounter	176	N/A
T84197A	Other mechanical complication of internal fixation device of bone of L lower leg, initial encounter	176	N/A
T84199A	Other mechanical complication of internal fixation device of NOS bone of limb, initial encounter	176	N/A
T84210A	Breakdown of internal fixation device of bones of hand & fingers, initial encounter	176	N/A
T84213A	Breakdown of internal fixation device of bones of foot & toes, initial encounter	176	N/A
T84216A	Breakdown of internal fixation device of vertebrae, initial encounter	176	N/A
T84218A	Breakdown of internal fixation device of other bones, initial encounter	176	N/A
T84220A	Displacement of internal fixation device of bones of hand & fingers, initial encounter	176	N/A
T84223A	Displacement of internal fixation device of bones of foot & toes, initial encounter	176	N/A
T84226A	Displacement of internal fixation device of vertebrae, initial encounter	176	N/A
T84228A	Displacement of internal fixation device of other bones, initial encounter	176	N/A

Code	Code Descriptors	HCC	RXHCC
T84290A	Other mechanical complication of internal fixation device of bones of hand & fingers, initial encounter	176	N/A
T84293A	Other mechanical complication of internal fixation device of bones of foot & toes, initial encounter	176	N/A
T84296A	Other mechanical complication of internal fixation device of vertebrae, initial encounter	176	N/A
T84298A	Other mechanical complication of internal fixation device of other bones, initial encounter	176	N/A
T84310A	Breakdown of electronic bone stimulator, initial encounter	176	N/A
T84318A	Breakdown of other bone devices, implants & grafts, initial encounter	176	N/A
T84320A	Displacement of electronic bone stimulator, initial encounter	176	N/A
T84328A	Displacement of other bone devices, implants & grafts, initial encounter	176	N/A
T84390A	Other mechanical complication of electronic bone stimulator, initial encounter	176	N/A
T84398A	Other mechanical complication of other bone devices, implants & grafts, initial encounter	176	N/A
T84410A	Breakdown of muscle & tendon graft, initial encounter	176	N/A
T84418A	Breakdown of other internal orthopedic devices, implants & grafts, initial encounter	176	N/A
T84420A	Displacement of muscle & tendon graft, initial encounter	176	N/A
T84428A	Displacement of other internal orthopedic devices, implants & grafts, initial encounter	176	N/A
T84490A	Other mechanical complication of muscle & tendon graft, initial encounter	176	N/A
T84498A	Other mechanical complication of other internal orthopedic devices, implants & grafts, initial encounter	176	N/A
T8450XA	Infection & inflammatory reaction D/T NOS internal joint prosthesis, initial encounter	176	N/A
T8451XA	Infection & inflammatory reaction D/T internal R hip prosthesis, initial encounter	176	N/A
T8452XA	Infection & inflammatory reaction D/T internal L hip prosthesis, initial encounter	176	N/A
T8453XA	Infection & inflammatory reaction D/T internal R knee prosthesis, initial encounter	176	N/A
T8454XA	Infection & inflammatory reaction D/T internal L knee prosthesis, initial encounter	176	N/A
T8459XA	Infection & inflammatory reaction D/T other internal joint prosthesis, initial encounter	176	N/A
T8460XA	Infection & inflammatory reaction D/T internal fixation device of NOS site, initial encounter	176	N/A

Code	Code Descriptors	HCC	RXHCC
T84610A	Infection & inflammatory reaction D/T internal fixation device of R humerus, initial encounter	176	N/A
T84611A	Infection & inflammatory reaction D/T internal fixation device of L humerus, initial encounter	176	N/A
T84612A	Infection & inflammatory reaction D/T internal fixation device of R radius, initial encounter	176	N/A
T84613A	Infection & inflammatory reaction D/T internal fixation device of L radius, initial encounter	176	N/A
T84614A	Infection & inflammatory reaction D/T internal fixation device of R ulna, initial encounter	176	N/A
T84615A	Infection & inflammatory reaction D/T internal fixation device of L ulna, initial encounter	176	N/A
T84619A	Infection & inflammatory reaction D/T internal fixation device of NOS bone of arm, initial encounter	176	N/A
T84620A	Infection & inflammatory reaction D/T internal fixation device of R femur, initial encounter	176	N/A
T84621A	Infection & inflammatory reaction D/T internal fixation device of L femur, initial encounter	176	N/A
T84622A	Infection & inflammatory reaction D/T internal fixation device of R tibia, initial encounter	176	N/A
T84623A	Infection & inflammatory reaction D/T internal fixation device of L tibia, initial encounter	176	N/A
T84624A	Infection & inflammatory reaction D/T internal fixation device of R fibula, initial encounter	176	N/A
T84625A	Infection & inflammatory reaction D/T internal fixation device of L fibula, initial encounter	176	N/A
T84629A	Infection & inflammatory reaction D/T internal fixation device of NOS bone of leg, initial encounter	176	N/A
T8463XA	Infection & inflammatory reaction D/T internal fixation device of spine, initial encounter	176	N/A
T8469XA	Infection & inflammatory reaction D/T internal fixation device of other site, initial encounter	176	N/A
T847XXA	Infection & inflammatory reaction D/T other internal orthopedic prosthetic devices, implants & grafts, initial encounter	176	N/A
T8481XA	Embolism D/T internal orthopedic prosthetic devices, implants & grafts, initial encounter	176	N/A
T8482XA	Fibrosis D/T internal orthopedic prosthetic devices, implants & grafts, initial encounter	176	N/A

Code	Code Descriptors	HCC	RXHCC
T8483XA	Hemorrhage D/T internal orthopedic prosthetic devices, implants & grafts, initial encounter	176	N/A
T8484XA	Pain D/T internal orthopedic prosthetic devices, implants & grafts, initial encounter	176	N/A
T8485XA	Stenosis D/T internal orthopedic prosthetic devices, implants & grafts, initial encounter	176	N/A
T8486XA	Thrombosis D/T internal orthopedic prosthetic devices, implants & grafts, initial encounter	176	N/A
T8489XA	NEC complication of internal orthopedic prosthetic devices, implants & grafts, initial encounter	176	N/A
T849XXA	NOS complication of internal orthopedic prosthetic device, implant & graft, initial encounter	176	N/A
T8501XA	Breakdown of ventricular intracranial shunt, initial encounter	176	N/A
T8502XA	Displacement of ventricular intracranial shunt, initial encounter	176	N/A
T8503XA	Leakage of ventricular intracranial shunt, initial encounter	176	N/A
T8509XA	Other mechanical complication of ventricular intracranial shunt, initial encounter	176	N/A
T85110A	Breakdown of implanted electronic neurostimulator of brain electrode, initial encounter	176	N/A
T85111A	Breakdown of implanted electronic neurostimulator of peripheral nerve electrode, initial encounter	176	N/A
T85112A	Breakdown of implanted electronic neurostimulator of spinal cord electrode, initial encounter	176	N/A
T85113A	Breakdown of implanted electronic neurostimulator, generator, initial encounter	176	N/A
T85118A	Breakdown of other implanted electronic stimulator of nervous system, initial encounter	176	N/A
T85120A	Displacement of implanted electronic neurostimulator of brain electrode, initial encounter	176	N/A
T85121A	Displacement of implanted electronic neurostimulator of peripheral nerve electrode, initial encounter	176	N/A
T85122A	Displacement of implanted electronic neurostimulator of spinal cord electrode, initial encounter	176	N/A
T85123A	Displacement of implanted electronic neurostimulator, generator, initial encounter	176	N/A
T85128A	Displacement of other implanted electronic stimulator of nervous system, initial encounter	176	N/A
T85190A	Other mechanical complication of implanted electronic neurostimulator of brain electrode, initial encounter	176	N/A

Code	Code Descriptors	HCC	RXHCC
T85191A	Other mechanical complication of implanted electronic neurostimulator of peripheral nerve electrode, initial encounter	176	N/A
T85192A	Other mechanical complication of implanted electronic neurostimulator of spinal cord electrode, initial encounter	176	N/A
T85193A	Other mechanical complication of implanted electronic neurostimulator, generator, initial encounter	176	N/A
T85199A	Other mechanical complication of other implanted electronic stimulator of nervous system, initial encounter	176	N/A
T85611A	Breakdown of intraperitoneal dialysis catheter, initial encounter	134	261
T85611D	Breakdown of intraperitoneal dialysis catheter, subsequent encounter	134	261
T85611S	Breakdown of intraperitoneal dialysis catheter, sequela	134	261
T85615A	Breakdown of other nervous system device, implant or graft, initial encounter	176	N/A
T85621A	Displacement of intraperitoneal dialysis catheter, initial encounter	134	261
T85621D	Displacement of intraperitoneal dialysis catheter, subsequent encounter	134	261
T85621S	Displacement of intraperitoneal dialysis catheter, sequela	134	261
T85625A	Displacement of other nervous system device, implant or graft, initial encounter	176	N/A
T85631A	Leakage of intraperitoneal dialysis catheter, initial encounter	134	261
T85631D	Leakage of intraperitoneal dialysis catheter, subsequent encounter	134	261
T85631S	Leakage of intraperitoneal dialysis catheter, sequela	134	261
T85635A	Leakage of other nervous system device, implant or graft, initial encounter	176	N/A
T85691A	Other mechanical complication of intraperitoneal dialysis catheter, initial encounter	134	261
T85691D	Other mechanical complication of intraperitoneal dialysis catheter, subsequent encounter	134	261
T85691S	Other mechanical complication of intraperitoneal dialysis catheter, sequela	134	261
T85695A	Other mechanical complication of other nervous system device, implant or graft, initial encounter	176	N/A
T8571XA	Infection & inflammatory reaction D/T peritoneal dialysis catheter, initial encounter	134	261
T8571XD	Infection & inflammatory reaction D/T peritoneal dialysis catheter, subsequent encounter	134	261
T8571XS	Infection & inflammatory reaction D/T peritoneal dialysis catheter, sequela	134	261

Code	Code Descriptors	HCC	RXHCC
T8572XA	Infection & inflammatory reaction D/T insulin pump, initial encounter	176	N/A
T85730A	Infection & inflammatory reaction D/T ventricular intracranial shunt, initial encounter	176	N/A
T85731A	Infection & inflammatory reaction D/T implanted electronic neurostimulator of brain, electrode, initial encounter	176	N/A
T85732A	Infection & inflammatory reaction D/T implanted electronic neurostimulator of peripheral nerve, electrode, initial encounter	176	N/A
T85733A	Infection & inflammatory reaction D/T implanted electronic neurostimulator of spinal cord, electrode, initial encounter	176	N/A
T85734A	Infection & inflammatory reaction D/T implanted electronic neurostimulator, generator, initial encounter	176	N/A
T85735A	Infection & inflammatory reaction D/T cranial or spinal infusion catheter, initial encounter	176	N/A
T85738A	Infection & inflammatory reaction D/T other nervous system device, implant or graft, initial encounter	176	N/A
T8579XA	Infection & inflammatory reaction D/T other internal prosthetic devices, implants & grafts, initial encounter	176	N/A
T85810A	Embolism D/T nervous system prosthetic devices, implants & grafts, initial encounter	176	N/A
T85820A	Fibrosis D/T nervous system prosthetic devices, implants & grafts, initial encounter	176	N/A
T85830A	Hemorrhage D/T nervous system prosthetic devices, implants & grafts, initial encounter	176	N/A
T85840A	Pain D/T nervous system prosthetic devices, implants & grafts, initial encounter	176	N/A
T85850A	Stenosis D/T nervous system prosthetic devices, implants & grafts, initial encounter	176	N/A
T85860A	Thrombosis D/T nervous system prosthetic devices, implants & grafts, initial encounter	176	N/A
T85890A	NEC complication of nervous system prosthetic devices, implants & grafts, initial encounter	176	N/A
T8600	NOS complication of bone marrow transplant	186	396
T8601	Bone marrow transplant rejection	186	396
T8602	Bone marrow transplant failure	186	396
T8603	Bone marrow transplant infection	186	396
T8609	Other complications of bone marrow transplant	186	396
T8610	Complication of kidney transplant, NOS	N/A	260
T8611	Kidney transplant rejection	N/A	260
T8612	Kidney transplant failure	N/A	260
T8613	Kidney transplant infection	N/A	260
T8619	Complication of kidney transplant, NEC	N/A	260
T8620	Complication of heart transplant, NOS	186	396

Code	Code Descriptors	HCC	RXHCC
T8621	Heart transplant rejection	186	396
T8622	Heart transplant failure	186	396
T8623	Heart transplant infection	186	396
T86290	Cardiac allograft vasculopathy	186	396
T86298	Complication of heart transplant, NEC	186	396
T8630	Complication of heart-lung transplant, NOS	186	395, 396
T8631	Heart-lung transplant rejection	186	395, 396
T8632	Heart-lung transplant failure	186	395, 396
T8633	Heart-lung transplant infection	186	395
T8633	Heart-lung transplant infection	186	396
T8639	Complications of heart-lung transplant, NEC	186	395, 396
T8640	Complication of liver transplant, NOS	186	396
T8641	Liver transplant rejection	186	396
T8642	Liver transplant failure	186	396
T8643	Liver transplant infection	186	396
T8649	Complication of liver transplant, NEC	186	396
T865	Complication of stem cell transplant	186	396
T86810	Lung transplant rejection	186	395
T86811	Lung transplant failure	186	395
T86812	Lung transplant infection	186	395
T86818	Complication of lung transplant, NEC	186	395
T86819	Complication of lung transplant, NOS	186	395
T86842	Corneal transplant infection	176	N/A
T86850	Intestine transplant rejection	186	396
T86851	Intestine transplant failure	186	396
T86852	Intestine transplant infection	186	396
T86858	Complication of intestine transplant, NEC	186	396
T86859	Complication of intestine transplant, NOS	186	396
T870X1	Complications of reattached R upper extremity	173	N/A
T870X2	Complications of reattached L upper extremity	173	N/A
T870X9	Complications of reattached NOS upper extremity	173	N/A
T871X1	Complications of reattached R lower extremity	173	N/A
T871X2	Complications of reattached L lower extremity	173	N/A
T871X9	Complications of reattached NOS lower extremity	173	N/A
T872	Complications of other reattached body part	173	N/A
T8730	Neuroma of amputation stump, NOS extremity	189	N/A
T8731	Neuroma of amputation stump, R upper extremity	189	N/A

Code	Code Descriptors	HCC	RXHCC
T8732	Neuroma of amputation stump, L upper extremity	189	N/A
T8733	Neuroma of amputation stump, R lower extremity	189	N/A
T8734	Neuroma of amputation stump, L lower extremity	189	N/A
T8740	Infection of amputation stump, NOS extremity	189	N/A
T8741	Infection of amputation stump, R upper extremity	189	N/A
T8742	Infection of amputation stump, L upper extremity	189	N/A
T8743	Infection of amputation stump, R lower extremity	189	N/A
T8744	Infection of amputation stump, L lower extremity	189	N/A
T8750	Necrosis of amputation stump, NOS extremity	189	N/A
T8751	Necrosis of amputation stump, R upper extremity	189	N/A
T8752	Necrosis of amputation stump, L upper extremity	189	N/A
T8753	Necrosis of amputation stump, R lower extremity	189	N/A
T8754	Necrosis of amputation stump, L lower extremity	189	N/A
T8781	Dehiscence of amputation stump	189	N/A
T8789	Other complications of amputation stump	189	N/A
T879	NOS complications of amputation stump	189	N/A
For codes X710XX- through X838XX-, use the following 7th characters: A initial encounter D subsequent encounter S sequela			
X710XX-	Self-harm by drowning & submersion while in bathtub	58	N/A
X711XX-	Self-harm by drowning & submersion while in swimming pool	58	N/A
X712XX-	Self-harm by drowning & submersion after jump into swimming pool	58	N/A
X713XX-	Self-harm by drowning & submersion in natural water	58	N/A
X718XX-	Self-harm by drowning & submersion, NEC	58	N/A
X719XX-	Self-harm by drowning & submersion, NOS	58	N/A
X72XXX-	Self-harm by handgun discharge	58	N/A
X730XX-	Self-harm by shotgun discharge	58	N/A
X731XX-	Self-harm by hunting rifle discharge	58	N/A
X732XX-	Self-harm by machine gun discharge	58	N/A
X738XX-	Self-harm by other larger firearm discharge	58	N/A
X739XX-	Self-harm by NOS larger firearm discharge	58	N/A
X7401X-	Self-harm by airgun	58	N/A
X7402X-	Self-harm by paintball gun	58	N/A

Code	Code Descriptors	HCC	RXHCC
X7409X-	Self-harm by other gas, air or spring-operated gun	58	N/A
X748XX-	Self-harm by other firearm discharge	58	N/A
X749XX-	Self-harm by NOS firearm discharge	58	N/A
X75XXX-	Self-harm by explosive material	58	N/A
X76XXX-	Self-harm by smoke, fire & flames	58	N/A
X770XX-	Self-harm by steam or hot vapors	58	N/A
X771XX-	Self-harm by hot tap water	58	N/A
X772XX-	Self-harm by other hot fluids	58	N/A
X773XX-	Self-harm by hot household appliances	58	N/A
X778XX-	Self-harm by other hot objects	58	N/A
X779XX-	Self-harm by NOS hot objects	58	N/A
X780XX-	Self-harm by sharp glass	58	N/A
X781XX-	Self-harm by knife	58	N/A
X782XX-	Self-harm by sword or dagger	58	N/A
X788XX-	Self-harm by NEC sharp object	58	N/A
X789XX-	Self-harm by NOS sharp object	58	N/A
X79XXX-	Self-harm by blunt object	58	N/A
X80XXX-	Self-harm by jumping from a high place	58	N/A
X810XX-	Self-harm by jumping or lying in front of motor vehicle	58	N/A
X811XX-	Self-harm by jumping or lying in front of (subway) train	58	N/A
X818XX-	Self-harm by jumping or lying in front of other moving object	58	N/A
X820XX-	Intentional collision of motor vehicle W/ other motor vehicle	58	N/A
X821XX-	Intentional collision of motor vehicle W/ train	58	N/A
X822XX-	Intentional collision of motor vehicle W/ tree	58	N/A
X828XX-	Other self-harm by crashing of motor vehicle	58	N/A
X830XX-	Intentional self-harm by crashing of aircraft	58	N/A
X831XX-	Intentional self-harm by electrocution	58	N/A
X832XX-	Intentional self-harm by exposure to extremes of cold	58	N/A
X838XX-	Intentional self-harm by NEC means	58	N/A
Y622	Failure of sterile precautions during kidney dialysis & other perfusion	134	261
Z21	HIV infection status	1	1
Z430	Encounter for attention to tracheostomy	82	N/A
Z431	Encounter for attention to gastrostomy	188	N/A
Z432	Encounter for attention to ileostomy	188	N/A
Z433	Encounter for attention to colostomy	188	N/A
Z434	Encounter for attention to other artificial openings of digestive tract	188	N/A
Z435	Encounter for attention to cystostomy	188	N/A
Z436	Encounter for attention to other artificial openings of urinary tract	188	N/A
Z438	Encounter for attention to other artificial openings	188	N/A

Appendix B: ICD-10-CM Codes Mapped to HCCs and RxHCCs

Code	Code Descriptors	HCC	RXHCC
Z439	Encounter for attention to NOS artificial opening	188	N/A
Z44101	Encounter for fitting & adjustment of NOS R artificial leg	189	N/A
Z44102	Encounter for fitting & adjustment of NOS L artificial leg	189	N/A
Z44109	Encounter for fitting & adjustment of NOS artificial leg, NOS leg	189	N/A
Z44111	Encounter for fitting & adjustment of complete R artificial leg	189	N/A
Z44112	Encounter for fitting & adjustment of complete L artificial leg	189	N/A
Z44119	Encounter for fitting & adjustment of complete artificial leg, NOS leg	189	N/A
Z44121	Encounter for fitting & adjustment of partial artificial R leg	189	N/A
Z44122	Encounter for fitting & adjustment of partial artificial L leg	189	N/A
Z44129	Encounter for fitting & adjustment of partial artificial leg, NOS leg	189	N/A
Z4821	Encounter for aftercare following heart transplant	186	396
Z4822	Encounter for aftercare following kidney transplant	N/A	260
Z4823	Encounter for aftercare following liver transplant	186	396
Z4824	Encounter for aftercare following lung transplant	186	395
Z48280	Encounter for aftercare following heart-lung transplant	186	395, 396
Z48290	Encounter for aftercare following bone marrow transplant	186	396
Z4901	Encounter for fitting & adjustment of extracorporeal dialysis catheter	134	261
Z4902	Encounter for fitting & adjustment of peritoneal dialysis catheter	134	261
Z4931	Encounter for adequacy testing for hemodialysis	134	261
Z4932	Encounter for adequacy testing for peritoneal dialysis	134	261
Z6841	BMI 40.0-44.9, adult	22	43
Z6842	BMI 45.0-49.9, adult	22	43
Z6843	BMI 50-59.9 , adult	22	43
Z6844	BMI 60.0-69.9, adult	22	43
Z6845	BMI 70 or greater, adult	22	43
Z794	Long term use of insulin	19	31
Z89411	Acquired absence of R great toe	189	N/A
Z89412	Acquired absence of L great toe	189	N/A
Z89419	Acquired absence of NOS great toe	189	N/A
Z89421	Acquired absence of other R toe(s)	189	N/A
Z89422	Acquired absence of other L toe(s)	189	N/A
Z89429	Acquired absence of other toe(s), NOS side	189	N/A

Code	Code Descriptors	HCC	RXHCC
Z89431	Acquired absence of R foot	189	N/A
Z89432	Acquired absence of L foot	189	N/A
Z89439	Acquired absence of NOS foot	189	N/A
Z89441	Acquired absence of R ankle	189	N/A
Z89442	Acquired absence of L ankle	189	N/A
Z89449	Acquired absence of NOS ankle	189	N/A
Z89511	Acquired absence of R leg below knee	189	N/A
Z89512	Acquired absence of L leg below knee	189	N/A
Z89519	Acquired absence of NOS leg below knee	189	N/A
Z89611	Acquired absence of R leg above knee	189	N/A
Z89612	Acquired absence of L leg above knee	189	N/A
Z89619	Acquired absence of NOS leg above knee	189	N/A
Z9115	Patient's noncompliance W/ renal dialysis	134	261
Z930	Tracheostomy status	82	N/A
Z931	Gastrostomy status	188	N/A
Z932	Ileostomy status	188	N/A
Z933	Colostomy status	188	N/A
Z934	NEC artificial opening of gastrointestinal tract status	188	N/A
Z9350	NOS cystostomy status	188	N/A
Z9351	Cutaneous-vesicostomy status	188	N/A
Z9352	Appendico-vesicostomy status	188	N/A
Z9359	Other cystostomy status	188	N/A
Z936	Other artificial openings of urinary tract status	188	N/A
Z938	Other artificial opening status	188	N/A
Z939	Artificial opening status, NOS	188	N/A
Z940	Kidney transplant status	N/A	260
Z941	Heart transplant status	186	396
Z942	Lung transplant status	186	395
Z943	Heart & lungs transplant status	186	395, 396
Z944	Liver transplant status	186	396
Z9481	Bone marrow transplant status	186	396
Z9482	Intestine transplant status	186	396
Z9483	Pancreas transplant status	186	397
Z9484	Stem cells transplant status	186	396
Z95811	Presence of heart assist device	186	N/A
Z95812	Presence of fully implantable artificial heart	186	N/A
Z9911	Dependence on respirator status	82	N/A
Z9912	Encounter for respirator dependence during power failure	82	N/A
Z992	Dependence on renal dialysis	134	261

Appendix C

Evaluate Your Understanding and Abstract & Code It! Answers and Rationales

CHAPTER 1

Risk Adjustment Basics

A Answer Questions

1. D. **Rationale:** Medicare Advantage organizations (MAOs) are reimbursed based on the diagnoses submitted for their enrollees. As a result, CMS holds the MAO responsible to ensure the codes submitted are accurate.
2. A. **Rationale:** Prospective payment means that diagnoses from claims for the previous year are used by CMS to calculate risk score of an enrollee for the current year for MAOs. The risk score determines the MAO's payment from CMS for each enrollee.
3. C. **Rationale:** Pay for Performance is a transactional payment system in which a value is assigned to a service, and the value is paid when the service is performed. Pay for Performance is a provider payment system. Part C and Part D represent risk-adjusted payment systems for Medicare and Medicaid beneficiaries, and the Health Insurance Marketplace risk pools provide risk-adjusted payments to non-Medicare enrollees. In risk adjustment, payment is to the insurance company. Patients with significant comorbidities cost the insurance company more in payments to providers, and this added cost is offset by risk-adjustment payment to the insurance company. The payment is financed by CMS for Medicare patients, and by the risk pool in Health Insurance Marketplace plans.
4. D. **Rationale:** Multiple variables contribute to the risk score of a patient. Age and sex are assigned values, as are any disability status and chronic or acute diagnoses that map to HCCs. The patient's housing status, whether in the community or in an institute, also contributes to the scoring.
5. B. **Rationale:** In RA, a value is assigned to a group of chronic diseases (eg, chronic diabetic complications or metastatic cancers). These like-groups of chronic diseases are divided into hierarchical condition categories (HCCs).
6. C. **Rationale:** As a department under HSS, CMS determines the risk-adjustment payments for the MAO, and pays the MAO. The MAO is responsible for paying charges for services for members of the plan. There are no risk pools in Medicare Advantage plans.
7. A. **Rationale:** Medical documentation and coding is the primary focus of a RADV audit. Charts and coding are reviewed to validate that the diagnoses reported were captured in documentation.
8. C. **Rationale:** A per-person fee, rather than a per-service fee, is paid to the MAO that has agreed to provide health insurance coverage to enrollees of a Medicare Advantage plan. Fee payment per person, rather than per service, is called capitation. In addition, patients with significant comorbidities will cause a risk-adjusted payment to the MAO.

9. D. **Rationale:** Prediabetes is not considered a chronic condition eligible for HCC assignment, likely because prediabetes symptoms are mild and it is a reversible diagnosis.

10. A. **Rationale:** All American citizens who reach the age of 65 or who have end stage renal disease (ESRD) are eligible for Medicare Part A, hospitalization coverage. There is no charge for Part A. They may opt to pay for Medicare Part B, outpatient coverage, for about $135 per month. Medicare's expansion into RA began as a result of the Balanced Budget Act of 1997, which established Part C of Medicare. Initially called Medicare+Choice, Part C opened up Medicare programs to private insurers. RA was expanded to include drugs under the Medicare Prescription Drug, Improvement, and Modernization Act of 2003, and at that time, Medicare+Choice was renamed Medicare Advantage. Medicare Advantage Organizations (MAOs) continue to grow, with one in three Medicare enrollees today choosing an MAO rather than traditional Medicare. Drug coverage, Part D of Medicare, could be purchased separately or could be bundled into a Medicare Advantage program.

B True/False Questions

1. True. **Rationale:** Hospital coding of diagnoses historically has been more specific than physician office coding of diagnoses because inpatient diagnoses contribute to MS-DRG assignment, the payment system for hospital Medicare claims. When payment is involved, the likelihood of audit and the need for accuracy increases.

2. True. **Rationale:** Patients who have multiple, chronic comorbidities historically consume more medical services than those without chronic comorbidities.

3. False. **Rationale:** Pull-down menus in EHRs often do not offer all code possibilities, do not contain guidelines or code-specific notes, and the descriptions are not always complete. Often, default codes appear first on the list of pull-down menus.

4. False. **Rationale:** NCHS is the federal agency chiefly responsible for ICD-10-CM code management and development. CMS is responsible for CMS-HCCs.

5. True. **Rationale:** Economic status, chronic disease, age, and disability are all elements that risk-adjust in Medicare Advantage. Serious acute conditions like some pneumonias, cancers, and hip fractures also risk adjust.

6. True. **Rationale:** Every diagnosis must be reported at least once a year for that diagnosis to affect payment for the care of the patient. When people enrolled in MA plans skip preventive care and do not seek out health care services for a year, lifelong chronic diseases may disappear from their risk scores, and their conditions are not monitored for prevention of complicatons.

7. False. **Rationale:** Not all risk factors are additive. For example, if a patient is diagnosed with uncomplicated diabetes in January, but diabetic nephropathy in July, only the diabetes with complication is counted. Similarly, different conditions occurring in the same patient will map to the same HCC, but the HCC will only be counted once each year for risk adjustment.

8. False. **Rationale:** Coders needn't memorize all HCCs and RAF values. Instead, coders should focus on complete and compliant ICD-10-CM code abstraction, with adherence to the AHA's *Coding Clinic*.

9. True. **Rationale:** The health exchanges created by the ACA have risk pools that use the HHS-HCC model, an HCC model that is similar to CMS-HCCs but also includes pediatric and obstetric diagnoses.

10. True. **Rationale:** Value-based payment modifiers consider the health status of the patient when determining incentive payments to the physician.

CHAPTER 2
Common Administrative Errors and Processes

A Answer Questions

1. B. **Rationale:** Every date of service requires a signature authenticating the contents of the record. There is no requirement that a copy of the radiology report be in the patient record, only that the provider discusses the results of the report in the record. Subjective findings may contribute to the use of a CPT evaluation and management code, but are not required for diagnostic coding. Coders abstract from diagnoses, not from ICD-10-CM codes.
2. C. **Rationale:** Attestations allow a provider to authenticate a medical record for which there is an unacceptable signature. Only the author of a document may sign an attestation for it.
3. D. **Rationale:** An audit log is tied directly to login information. Every line of data added to a record is time-stamped and identified by author in the audit log. This is essential for record integrity.
4. D. **Rationale:** A nurse is an unacceptable provider, but the *ICD-10-CM Guidelines* state that a nurse may document a BMI score or depth of skin ulcer, and this documentation is acceptable when accompanied by related documentation (eg, morbid obesity, decubitus ulcer of heel) from an acceptable provider.
5. C. **Rationale:** A registered nurse must always work under the direction of an acceptable provider. Both GNP-BC and CNS-BC are ACPs, advanced clinical practitioners.
6. D. **Rationale:** A problem list may identify resolved conditions from the past (eg, acute tonsillitis); chronic, ongoing conditions (eg, Alzheimer's dementia); and may be abstracted if there is support for the diagnosis elsewhere in the record (eg, in the case of Alzheimer's dementia, a discussion that the patient's cognitive decline has stabilized, according to her daughter).
7. D. **Rationale:** Pain is perceived by the patient, and would, therefore, be a subjective finding. If the subjective finding is affirmed by the provider or brought into the assessment and plan, it may be abstracted. BMI, +3 edema, and rhonchi are all elements that are observed or measured by the provider, and so would be considered objective findings.
8. B. **Rationale:** Telemedicine is considered an acceptable POS for RA if CMS has approved the circumstances for fee-for-service payment. Typically, telemedicine is approved for remote locales.
9. D. **Rationale:** Without a proper signature authenticating the discharge summary, an inpatient chart must be coded as individual encounters, for each provider visit on each day, using outpatient rules.
10. A. **Rationale:** The date a service is performed should be used as the date of service. In this case, use the date the consulting provider examined the patient.

B True/False Questions

1. True. **Rationale:** Because interventional radiologists are performing a treatment on the patient, and use radiology as support of the approach they use for surgery, they are considered acceptable providers.
2. False. **Rationale:** While facilities and local regulations may require that a scribe self-identify and sign documentation the scribe transcribed for the provider, CMS makes no such requirement. Documentation transcribed by a scribe must simply be signed and dated by the provider who authors it. The DOS of a service must always be identified, even in a dated letter from a consulting provider to the referring provider. With the DOS, the letter can be abstracted for risk adjustment. The letter's date cannot be used instead.

3. True. **Rationale:** Consultations are acceptable documents, but can be confusing in code abstraction because they may contain the date the letter was written in addition to the date of the encounter. Always use the date of the encounter as the date of service. Many coders mistakenly use the date the letter was written, which is an error.

4. True. **Rationale:** An objective observation is one that is experienced by the provider. A subjective observation is one that is shared by the patient.

5. False. **Rationale:** Psychiatric hospitals and outpatient mental health clinics are acceptable places of service.

6. False. **Rationale:** In many outpatient EHRs, the problem list self-populates from the previous medical encounter into the current one. If a new diagnosis develops, it is added to the existing list, but none of the old diagnoses drop off. Problem lists cannot be considered documentation generated for a current DOS, unless dated for the DOS, the narrative sates that the problem list is updated to reflect current diagnoses, or the diagnosis is supported elsewhere in the record.

7. False. **Rationale:** CMS expects a separate login for each person entering data into an EHR.

8. False. **Rationale:** A transfer is an inpatient administrative document and not considered appropriate for RA coding.

9. True. **Rationale:** Each DOS for each provider during the hospitalization of an inpatient record must be coded as an outpatient encounter using outpatient rules if the record does not contain an acceptable discharge summary.

10. True. **Rationale:** Axis 3 in a behavioral medicine chart lists comorbidities that may affect the patient's psychiatric condition. Diabetic patients have a higher incidence of depression, and so would be appropriate to enumerate in a listing of chronic or acute comorbidities.

CHAPTER 3
Clinical Documentation and Coding for RA

A Answer Questions

1. C. **Rationale:** A causal relationship is one that is cause and effect. Etiology describes the disease that causes symptoms or complications. These symptoms or complications are manifestations. Causal relationships can be identified through the codes in ICD-10-CM.

2. C. **Rationale:** History of present illness is the physician's description of the patient's complaint. It is acceptable for coding. Past medical history contains the patient's medical history, and the problem list is a historic list of illnesses. History is not acceptable for coding current conditions, according to guidelines. The medication list may also be pulled forward from past visits, and may not contain diagnoses.

3. D. **Rationale:** A SOAP note is a type of medical documentation that includes subjective information from the patient,objective findings by the physician, assessment of the diagnosis, and plans for treatment. "Refer to neurology clinic" would fall under the treatment plan, or P.

4. B. **Rationale:** A personal history of a foot amputation would indicate the patient has a lower-extremity amputation status, which risk-adjusts. The other conditions do not risk-adjust.

5. D. **Rationale:** The word "with" should be interpreted to mean "associated with" or "due to" when it appears in the Alphabetic Index. The classification presumes a causal relationship between the two conditions linked by these terms in the Alphabetic Index or Tabular List.

6. A. **Rationale:** "Code first" is an instruction that appears with codes that report manifestations. These manifestation codes can only be reported secondary to the underlying cause of the disease. "Use additional code" and "Code also" instruct coders to report comorbidities that are commonly, but not always, associated with a diagnosis (eg, smoking with chronic obstructive pulmonary disease [COPD]).

7. A. **Rationale:** The coder cannot seek information from other encounters in order to correctly code the current encounter. Each encounter note must stand on its own documentation merits, and the coder is required to abstract the diagnoses as documented by the physician.

8. B. **Rationale:** The physician has documented "dementia, stable," so the diagnosis has support and can be documented. The specific ICD-10-CM code must be ignored, so it cannot inform code choice for abstraction. The correct code is F03.90, *Unspecified dementia without behavioral disturbance*, which is supported by the code description, "dementia, stable."

9. C. **Rationale:** To select a code in the classification that corresponds to a diagnosis or reason for visit documented in a medical record, first locate the term in the Alphabetic Index, and then verify the code in the Tabular List. Read and be guided by instructional notations that appear in both the Alphabetic Index and the Tabular List. If the lookup involves a neoplasm, the correct method would be to first reference the Alphabetic Index, followed by the Table of Neoplasms, and then followed by the Tabular List.

10. D. **Rationale:** Physicians should spell out acronyms in the first reference (eg, diabetes mellitus [DM]), or develop a list of acceptable acronyms for the policies and procedures manual within their practice. The ICD-10-CM Alphabetic Index does have some acronyms for some conditions (eg, HIV).

C Audit Exercises

1. D. **Rationale:** Unspecified congestive heart failure and unspecified atrial fibrillation are both supported in the document's Subjective section and in the Assessment/Plan. The patient did not have an emergent stroke during this office visit, as evidenced by the continuation of physical therapy. No acute stroke code should be reported. The patient's irregular gait is caused by the stroke, so it is inappropriate to report code R00.9. A more specific code should be selected. The patient has hyperlipidemia, but the Subjective section further specifies "mixed hyperlipidemia." This should be reported with code E78.2, *Mixed hyperlipidemia*, rather than reporting an unspecified variant.

2. B. **Rationale:** The patient has sequela of the stroke, which manifests as left-sided weakness. This left-sided weakness is to be reported as hemiparesis. Without more specificity on the type of stroke the patient experienced, an unspecified type is selected.

3. C. **Rationale:** The patient's blood glucose is abnormally high but it is not addressed in the documentation. All other test results were within normal range.

4. A. **Rationale:** Vitamin A supplements are routinely prescribed to people who are at risk of or who have osteoporosis. Coding the osteoporosis would depend on the individual coding policies of the workplace.

5. C. **Rationale:** While the note is signed and dated, there is nothing in the signature that indicates Orville Hawkins is an acceptable provider.

CHAPTER 4
Clinical Documentation and Coding Integrity: Part I (A-C)

Amputation

Abstract & Code It! Patient 1

Z44.121	Encounter for fitting and adjustment of partial artificial right leg
Z89.511	Acquired absence of right leg below knee

Rationale: While the encounter code captures the lower-extremity amputation status, code Z85.511 reports the full extent of the limb loss, so it would also be reported. Report status-codes when they contribute additional information to the record, but not if they are redundant to diagnoses. For example, it is unnecessary to report colostomy status for a patient who has a diagnosis of colostomy stoma infection.

Abstract & Code It! Patient 2

I73.9	Peripheral vascular disease, unspecified
Z89.412	Acquired absence of left great toe

Rationale: Always check the physical examination portion of the medical record, because diagnoses may be discovered there. Diminished pedal pulses and bilateral ankle discoloration are associated with atherosclerosis, but only the less specific peripheral vascular disease is documented. Report the documented diagnoses.

Abstract & Code It! Patient 3

E11.52	Type 2 diabetes with diabetic peripheral angiopathy with gangrene

Rationale: Do not code amputation status, as the amputation is being performed during this surgery. Amputation status would be appropriate during a subsequent encounter in which it is documented. The default for diabetes when the type is not identified is type 2. The patient's peripheral vascular disease, gangrene, and diabetes are captured with the single code reporting diabetes and its manifestations, so a second code is not necessary. Code E11.52 maps to three different HCCs and two RxHCCs, so the risks facing this patient are sufficiently captured with the single code.

Arrest, Shock, Ventilator Status

Abstract & Code It! Patient 1

J96.21	Acute and chronic respiratory failure with hypoxia
J96.22	Acute and chronic respiratory failure with hypercapnia
J43.1	Panlobular emphysema
Z99.11	Dependence on respirator [ventilator] status
Z87.891	Personal history of nicotine dependence

Rationale: There is no single code to capture acute respiratory failure with hypoxia and hypercapnia, so two codes are required to capture the condition. The personal history of nicotine dependence is pertinent to the emphysema diagnosis, and the ICD-10-CM guidelines instructs us to also code any tobacco use or dependence for patients with respiratory disease. The key to reporting respirator dependence is documentation that mechanical ventilation was "required."

Abstract & Code It! Patient 2

A41.59	Other Gram-negative sepsis
B96.1	Klebsiella pneumoniae (K. pneumoniae) as the cause of diseases classified elsewhere
J80	Acute respiratory distress syndrome
R65.21	Severe sepsis with septic shock

Rationale: Obviously, this is a very brief description for a very sick patient. Actual documentation would be much more detailed, but enough information is provided for adequate coding. Adult respiratory distress syndrome (ARDS) and septic shock are indicators of severe sepsis in this patient. There is no specific code for *Klebsiella pneumoniae* sepsis. Therefore, a code of "other" sepsis agent is reported with a specific infection code to capture the *Klebsiella pneumoniae.*

Abstract & Code It! Patient 3

J95.821	Acute postprocedural respiratory failure
C34.32	Malignant neoplasm of lower lobe, left bronchus or lung
Z99.11	Dependence on respirator [ventilator] status

Rationale: Using the Alphabetic Index will guide the coder away from typical codes for respiratory failure found in category J96, and to the correct codes for postprocedural respiratory conditions. The procedure in question was for lung cancer. Therefore, the lung cancer would also be reported. The patient "requires" mechanical ventilation, and code Z99.11 captures the dependence.

Arthritis and Inflammatory Disorders

Abstract & Code It!

M06.041	Rheumatoid arthritis without rheumatoid factor, right hand
M06.042	Rheumatoid arthritis without rheumatoid factor, left hand

Rationale: Remember that rheumatoid-factor status must be documented by the physician in order for it to be coded. The coder may not assume that a rheumatoid factor of 54 indicates the patient has positive rheumatoid factor. Coders cannot infer diagnoses from laboratory values. The Assessment in the medical record states "seronegative," so that must be coded, despite the laboratory results. If positive or negative status of rheumatoid factor is not identified, report code M06.9, *Rheumatoid arthritis, unspecified*, unless organ involvement, rheumatoid nodule or bursitis, or juvenile rheumatoid arthritis is documented. There is no need to report the symptoms of fever, fatigue, swelling, or pain associated with rheumatoid arthritis.

Autism

Abstract & Code It! Patient 1

F84.9	Pervasive developmental disorder, unspecified
F70	Mild intellectual disabilities

Rationale: Report intellectual disabilities when they are documented. The Alphabetic Index has an entry for Autism/atypical. Do not assume that all autism is coded as autism spectrum disorder.

Abstract & Code It! Patient 2

R56.9	Unspecified convulsions
Q99.2	Fragile X syndrome
F84.0	Autistic disorder

Rationale: The patient's autism spectrum disorder is captured with code F84.0. Fragile X syndrome is pertinent to the encounter. While the coder may be tempted to report unspecified epilepsy for this patient because the seizures seem to be recurrent, the documentation does not support an epilepsy diagnosis. Instead, report unspecified convulsions until a firm diagnosis is made.

Abstract & Code It! Patient 3

F80.9	Developmental disorder of speech and language, unspecified

Rationale: Physician and outpatient facilities cannot code uncertain diagnoses (eg, rule out, suspected), whereas inpatient facilities can if it is documented by the physician at the time of discharge. In this case, the outpatient evaluation states autism is suspected. Therefore, it cannot be reported. Code F80.9 is found in the Alphabetic Index under Disorder/communication.

Behavioral Disorders

Abstract & Code It! Patient 1

Z13.89	Encounter for screening of other disorder

Rationale: There is no diagnosis of depression documented. Only the results of a screening test is noted. The physician must document depression in order for it to be coded. A screening test is a tool, not a diagnosis. Code Z13.89 is found in the Alphabetic Index under Screening/depression.

Abstract & Code It! Patient 2

F33.3	Major depressive disorder, single episode, severe with psychotic symptoms
Z91.14	Patient's other noncompliance with medication regimen

Rationale: The physician has not documented the episodic nature of the patient's depression (eg, recurrent or single episode). The default is single episode unless the coder can query the physician. Noncompliance with medication may have led to the need for hospitalization, but the cause of noncompliance is not documented. Therefore, report code Z91.14, rather than codes for intentional noncompliance.

Abstract & Code It! Patient 3

F32.9	Major depressive disorder, single episode, unspecified

Rationale: Without more information, the default code for depression is reported.

Blood Disorders

Abstract & Code It! Patient 1

I85.11	Secondary esophageal varices with bleeding
D62	Acute posthemorrhagic anemia
K70.9	Alcoholic liver disease, unspecified
F10.21	Alcohol dependence in remission
K76.6	Portal hypertension

Rationale: The patient's causal relationships in this scenario are complex: The anemia is caused by the bleeding varices, the varices are caused by the liver disease and portal hypertension, which in turn are caused by the alcoholism. All conditions should be captured.

Abstract & Code It! Patient 2

D61.2	Aplastic anemia due to other external agents
Y84.2	Radiological procedure and radiotherapy as the cause of abnormal reaction of the patient, or later complication, without mention of misadventure at the time of the procedure.
C22.0	Liver cell carcinoma

Rationale: The patient's liver cancer is active because he is still undergoing radiotherapy. The patient has anemia due to the radiotherapy. The anemia code is found in the Alphabetic Index under Anemia/aplastic/due to/radiation. A note at code D61.2 instructs the coder to "Code first, if applicable, toxic effects" and references T51-T65, which are drug codes. Locating the code for the appropriate adverse effect requires the coder to remember to review the Alphabetic Index to External Causes, where code Y84.2 can be found under Complication/radiological procedure or therapy.

Abstract & Code It! Patient 3

D62	Acute posthemorrhagic anemia
D68.32	Hemorrhagic disorder due to extrinsic circulating anticoagulants
K24.4	Chronic or unspecified duodenal ulcer with hemorrhage
T45.515A	Adverse effects of anticoagulants

Rationale: The patient has acute anemia due to hemorrhage from a duodenal ulcer. Complicating the reporting of this case is a current history of anticoagulant therapy, which led to the acute condition. We are instructed to use an additional code to report the drug responsible for the hemorrhagic disorder, therefore, code T45.515A is also reported. See Disorder/drug-induced hemorrhagic D68.32 in the Alphabetic Index for guidance on how to report the problem caused by warfarin. Code D68.32 instructs coders to "Use additional code for adverse effect, if applicable, to identify drug" and suggests code T45.515 or T45.525 as options.

Cerebral Palsy

Abstract & Code It! Patient 1

M41.47	Neuromuscular scoliosis, lumbosacral region
G80.1	Spastic diplegic cerebral palsy

Rationale: Refer to the Alphabetic Index, under Scoliosis/secondary (to)/cerebral palsy – *see* Scoliosis, neuromuscular. A note under code M41.4 *Neuromuscular scoliosis*, states that these codes should be used for scoliosis secondary to cerebral palsy, and to also code the underlying condition (eg, cerebral palsy).

Abstract & Code It! Patient 2

M80.872	Other osteoporosis with current pathological fracture, left ankle and foot
G80.0	Spastic quadriplegic cerebral palsy
T42.0X5A	Adverse effect of hydantoin derivatives, initial encounter
G40.009	Localization-related (focal) (partial) idiopathic epilepsy and epileptic syndromes with seizures of localized onset, not intractable, without status epilepticus

F70	Mild intellectual disabilities
Z79.899	Other long term (current) drug therapy
Z99.3	Dependence on wheelchair

Rationale: Often, fetal or infant brain injuries result in a complex of comorbidities, as is likely the case for this patient, who has epilepsy, cerebral palsy, and intellectual disabilities. The long-term use of epilepsy medication has caused secondary osteoporosis in this patient, resulting in the calcaneal fracture. The drug itself is captured with the T-code, but code Z79.899 captures the long-term use of the drug. Note that the dependence on wheelchair is also reported, along with the mild intellectual disabilities.

Abstract & Code It! Patient 3

G80.8	Other cerebral palsy

Rationale: There is no entry under Palsy/cerebral for triplegia, however, Triplegia/congenital classifies to code G80.8 in the Alphabetic Index. We did not report the delayed walking (R62.0, *Delayed milestone*) because although the patient was noted as not walking at age two, a diagnosis (eg, delayed walking) was not documented. Coders cannot make assumptions based on data; they should only report diagnoses documented in the medical record.

Cerebrovascular Disease

Abstract & Code It!

I69.310	Attention and concentration deficit following cerebral infarction
I69.320	Aphasia following cerebral infarction
I69.321	Dysphasia following cerebral infarction
I69.322	Dysarthria following cerebral infarction
I69.354	Hemiplegia and hemiparesis following cerebral infarction affecting left non-dominant side

Rationale: The type of stroke was documented as cerebral infarction, so the appropriate codes to report are from category I69.3-. Each type of sequela from the stroke should be captured because each may require a separate form of rehabilitative therapy.

Chromosomal Abnormalities, Intellectual Disabilities, and Other Developmental Disorders

Abstract & Code It! Patient 1

F70	Mild intellectual disabilities

Rationale: Begin the search in the Alphabetic Index under Subnormal/subnormality/mental – see Disability, intellectual. Mild intellectual disability is classified to category F70. For the purposes of coding, assume the "social worker" is a licensed clinical social worker (LCSW). LCSWs are acceptable providers for behavioral health.

Abstract & Code It! Patient 2

J18.1	Lobar pneumonia, unspecified organism
Q90.9	Down syndrome, unspecified
F70	Mild intellectual disabilities

Rationale: Capture the lobal pneumonia and any causal agent, although none is documented for Patient 2. The patient's Down syndrome complicates his care, so report the Down syndrome. Also report the level of intellectual disability, when it is documented.

Abstract & Code It! Patient 3

J20.0	Acute bronchitis due to Mycoplasma pneumoniae
F71	Moderate intellectual disabilities
G09	Sequelae of inflammatory disease of the central nervous system

Rationale: The patient's intellectual disability is the result of a childhood illness, which is captured with code G09, which is found in the Alphabetic Index under Sequela/meningitis/other or unspecified cause. Be careful to use the combination codes for bronchitis or pneumonia when they exist, and capture the patient's intellectual disability.

Complications

Abstract & Code It! Patient 1

T82.7XXA	Infection and inflammatory reaction due to other cardiac and vascular devices, implants and grafts, initial encounter

A41.02	Sepsis due to Methicillin resistant Staphylococcus aureus
E11.22	Type 2 diabetes mellitus with diabetic chronic kidney disease
N18.6	End stage renal disease
Z99.2	Dependence on renal dialysis

Rationale: Cause-and-effect relationships, when documented, should be coded. Here, diabetes caused nephropathy, causing end-stage renal disease, causing dependence on dialysis, causing a need for the dialysis catheter, which became infected. All conditions should be captured. A note at code E11.22 instructs coders to use an additional code to report the stage of chronic kidney disease. Infection of a dialysis catheter is found under Complication/catheter/dialysis/infection. Report a combination code for the sepsis because the causal agent is known and a specific code exists.

Abstract & Code It! Patient 2

T83.721A	Exposure of implanted vaginal mesh into vagina
Y73.2	Prosthetic and other implants, materials and accessory gastroenterology and urology devices associated with adverse incidents

Rationale: Pain would be considered a sign and symptom of the exposure of the implanted mesh and would not be separately reported. "Extrusion of implanted mesh" is an inclusion term under code T83.72, although there is no entry addressing vaginal mesh under Extrusion in the Alphabetic Index. If finding a code becomes difficult, perform a word search of the Alphabetic Index or Tabular List in the electronic version of the ICD-10-CM code set. Both the Alphabetic Index and Tabular List would yield results, which would lead to correct code selection if the search were for "vaginal mesh."

Abstract & Code It! Patient 3

K50.012	Crohn's disease of small intestine with intestinal obstruction
K50.011	Crohn's disease of small intestine with rectal bleeding
D62	Acute posthemorrhagic anemia

Rationale: The Alphabetic Index establishes a link between the Crohn's disease and rectal bleeding, which is indicated in the guideline in which the term "with" in the Alphabetic Index establishes a causal relationship. See Enteritis/regional/small intestine/with/complication/rectal bleeding. There is no single code that captures the bleeding and the intestinal obstruction, so two codes are required for reporting the Crohn's disease. The posthemorrhage anemia is also reported.

Congestive Heart Failure

Abstract & Code It! Patient 1

I11.0	Hypertensive heart disease with heart failure
I50.9	Heart failure, unspecified
I51.7	Cardiomegaly

Rationale: The Alphabetic Index directs the coder to Hypertrophy/cardiac and code I51.7 from Dilatation/ventricular. When hypertension appears "with" heart failure, a combination code from category I11, *Hypertensive heart disease*, is reported rather than code I10, *Essential (primary) hypertension*, even when documentation does not link the conditions, unless the physician documents another cause for the hypertension. Congestive heart failure is nonspecific, which is reported with code I50.9. An inclusion note with code I50.9 states, "Congestive heart failure, NOS."

Abstract & Code It! Patient 2

I50.82	Biventricular heart failure
I50.23	Acute on chronic systolic (congestive) heart failure

Rationale: According to the instructions under code I50.82, coders should report the specific form of heart failure in addition to the biventricular heart failure.

Abstract & Code It! Patient 3

I50.84	End stage heart failure
I50.43	Acute on chronic combined systolic (congestive) and diastolic (congestive) heart failure
J96.11	Chronic respiratory failure with hypoxia
I11.0	Hypertensive heart disease with heart failure
Z66	Do not resuscitate

Rationale: Capture the hypertensive heart disease with three codes: one for the hypertension, one for the type of heart failure, and one for end-stage heart failure. A note at code I50.84 instructs the coder to code the type of heart failure, if known. A single code captures the hypoxia and chronic respiratory failure. Coding the "do not resuscitate" status contributes to the complete clinical picture for this moribund patient.

CHAPTER 4

Clinical Documentation and Coding Integrity: Part 2 of 4 (D-M)

Dementia

Abstract & Code It! Patient 1

G30.0	Alzheimer's disease with early onset
F02.90	Dementia without behavioral disturbance

Rationale: While the patient is documented as being "pre-senile," Alzheimer's disease is coded in keeping with the conventions of ICD-10-CM, which requires two codes based on the use of bracketed codes with code G30.0 in the Alphabetic Index.

Abstract & Code It! Patient 2

I70.91	Generalized atherosclerosis
F01.50	Vascular dementia without behavioral disturbance
Z86.73	Personal history of transient ischemic attack (TIA), and cerebral infarction without residual deficits

Rationale: Coders are instructed to first code the underlying physiological condition or sequela of cerebrovascular disease for code F01, *Vascular dementia*. A code from category I69 cannot be reported to address dementia as sequela of stroke because an Excludes1 note with code Z86.73 precludes reporting codes from category I69 with the TIA code. Furthermore, the documentation does not link the TIAs to the dementia. Coders can, however, report the generalized atherosclerosis.

Abstract & Code It! Patient 3

B96.1	Klebisella pneumoniae as the cause of diseases classified elsewhere
N39.0	Urinary tract infection, site not specified
R41.0	Disorientation, unspecified

Rationale: Take care to use the physician's documented language in determining code lookups. This patient was not diagnosed with dementia, but was experiencing a transient disorientation that is common in elderly patients with urinary tract or other infections.

Diabetes Mellitus

Abstract & Code It! Patient 1

E11.9	Type 2 diabetes without complications
K05.10	Chronic gingivitis, plaque induced
F17.210	Nicotine dependence, cigarettes, uncomplicated

Rationale: Only those specific complications listed under "with" in the Alphabetic Index under Diabetes can be linked to the diabetes without documentation of a link. In this case, no such link was made for the gingivitis. Smoking status is pertinent to the diabetes as well as the gingivitis.

Abstract & Code It! Patient 2

E11.40	Type 2 diabetes mellitus with diabetic neuropathy, unspecified
E11.65	Type 2 diabetes mellitus with hyperglycemia
E66.01	Morbid (severe) obesity due to excess calories
Z68.42	Body mass index [BMI] 45.0-49.9, adult

Rationale: "Out of control" diabetes is reported as hyperglycemia in ICD-10-CM. Therefore, code E11.65 is reported in addition to code E11.40. Report as many codes for diabetes as are required to capture the patient's complications. The default for documented "diabetes" is type 2 when the type is not specified.

Abstract & Code It! Patient 3

I13.0	Hypertensive heart and chronic kidney disease with heart failure and stage 1 through stage 4 chronic kidney disease, or unspecified chronic kidney disease
I50.22	Chronic systolic (congestive) heart failure
E11.22	Type 2 diabetes mellitus with diabetic chronic kidney disease
N18.4	Chronic kidney disease, stage 4
Z79.84	Long-term (current) use of oral hypoglycemic drugs

Rationale: Unless documentation states another specific cause for the hypertension, it would be linked to both the heart failure and the kidney disease, and the kidney disease would also be linked to the diabetes. This is based on ICD-10-CM Alphabetic Index rules. Report the metformin therapy with code Z79.84.

Drug/Alcohol Use Disorders

Abstract & Code It!

F10.282	Alcohol dependence with alcohol-induced sleep disorder
F33.1	Major depressive disorder, recurrent, moderate
F42.4	Excoriation (skin-picking) disorder
G31.84	Mild cognitive impairment
I25.2	Old myocardial infarction
F17.210	Nicotine dependence, cigarettes, uncomplicated
F11.21	Opioid dependence, in remission

Rationale: This is an example of a chart that must be combed through carefully to capture all diagnoses. Many of the diagnoses are not listed in the behavioral health–axis chart. The patient's insomnia is linked to the alcohol using the Alphabetic Index convention for reporting diagnoses "with." The skin-picking condition is reported in addition to the depression. The personal history of IV opioid dependence is reported as "in remission," as directed by the Index entry, History/personal/drug dependence – see Dependence, drug, by type, in remission.

Esophageal Reflux

Abstract & Code It!

J45.909	Unspecified asthma, uncomplicated
K21.9	Gastroesophageal reflux disease without esophagitis
Z87.891	Personal history of tobacco dependence

Rationale: In the Alphabetic Index, see Rhinitis/allergic/with/asthma J45.90. No second code for the rhinitis is required. No policy has been established to allow coders to code vitamin D deficiency from the problem-list entry, even though it is supported by the problem list. But because there is no evidence the problem list was reviewed, vitamin D deficiency cannot be reported. Personal history of smoking was abstracted because it is pertinent to the asthma and reflux diagnosis, and in keeping with a "Use additional code" note at category J45, *Asthma*.

Heart Arrhythmias

Abstract & Code It! Patient 1

I49.5	Sick sinus syndrome

Rationale: Report sick sinus syndrome (SSS) because that is the reason for the procedure. In future encounters, the status code for pacemaker should be used instead.

Abstract & Code It! Patient 2

Z00.00	Encounter for general adult examination without abnormal findings
Z95.0	Presence of cardiac pacemaker

Rationale: As the patient is asymptomatic and no other treatment beyond the pacemaker is noted, only the presence of the cardiac pacemaker would be reported. An examination code identifies the reason for the encounter.

Abstract & Code It! Patient 3

I48.2	Chronic atrial fibrillation
Z95.0	Presence of cardiac pacemaker
Z79.2	Long term (current) use of antithrombotics/antiplatelets

Rationale: The patient with chronic atrial fibrillation has a pacemaker, but also requires medication to prevent blood clots. Therefore, the code for atrial fibrillation is reported in addition to the presence of the pacemaker. Report the long-term use of clopidogrel as well.

HIV and Opportunistic Infections

Abstract & Code It! Patient 1

K52.1	Toxic gastroenteritis and colitis
T37.5X5A	Adverse effect of antiviral drugs, initial encounter
Z21	Asymptomatic human immunodeficiency virus [HIV] infection status

Rationale: The colitis is HIV-associated because of the HIV medication, not because of an opportunistic infection. This patient's colitis is an adverse reaction to medication. Report the colitis, the adverse effect, and the patient's HIV-positive status.

Abstract & Code It! Patient 2

B20	Human immunodeficiency virus [HIV] disease
B59	Pneumocystosis

Rationale: "Due to HIV" is key in this documentation: It identifies that the patient has an HIV disease. Report the HIV disease and the pneumocytosis. Although the pneumocytosis is in the Infectious Disease chapter of ICD-10-CM, it is a pneumonia-specific diagnosis, so no other code is required to report the pneumonia.

Abstract & Code It! Patient 3

Z21	Asymptomatic human immunodeficiency virus [HIV] infection status

Rationale: The patient has an HIV-positive status, is on HIV medications, and has healthy laboratory results. Report code Z21.

Hyperlipidemia

Abstract & Code It! Patient 1

E78.2	Mixed hyperlipidemia

Rationale: See High/cholesterol/with high triglycerides in the Alphabetic Index. Note that high triglycerides without elevated cholesterol is reported with code E72.1 instead.

Abstract & Code It! Patient 2

E78.00	Pure hypercholesterolemia, unspecified

Rationale: See High/cholesterol in the Alphabetic Index.

Abstract & Code It! Patient 3

E78.00	Pure hypercholesterolemia, unspecified

Rationale: See Hyperlipoproteinemia/low-density-lipoprotein-type (LDL) in the Alphabetic Index.

Hypertension

Abstract & Code It! Patient 1

I16.0	Hypertensive urgency
I10	Essential (primary) hypertension
Z91.14	Patient's other noncompliance with medication regimen

Rationale: Always report the underlying hypertension code with a hypertensive crisis code. It is not stated whether the patient's noncompliance with medications was intentional, so report code Z91.14 rather than a code for intentional noncompliance.

Abstract & Code It! Patient 2

I12.0	Hypertensive chronic kidney disease with stage 5 or end stage renal disease
N18.6	End stage renal disease
Z99.2	Dependence on renal dialysis

Rationale: Alphabetic Index conventions instructs coders to link the hypertension to the chronic kidney disease. The Tabular List directs coders to report the stage of the chronic kidney disease with code I12.0. Report dialysis dependence when it is documented (eg, "dialysis three times a week").

Abstract & Code It! Patient 3

I15.2	Hypertension secondary to endocrine disorders
E05.00	Thyrotoxicosis with diffuse goiter without thyrotoxic crisis or storm

Rationale: The patient's hypertension is secondary to thyroid disease and, therefore, both conditions must be reported.

Intestinal Disorders

Abstract & Code It! Patient 1

K56.2	Volvulus
K63.1	Perforation of intestine (nontraumatic)
K55.041	Focal (segmental) acute infarction of large intestine

Rationale: There is no combination code for volvulus with complications. Each complication must be separately reported in addition to the volvulus.

Abstract & Code It! Patient 2

K25.4	Chronic or unspecified gastric ulcer with hemorrhage
D50.0	Iron deficiency anemia secondary to blood loss (chronic)

Rationale: Report the blood-loss anemia in addition to the code for gastric ulcer with hemorrhage.

Abstract & Code It! Patient 3

K50.811	Crohn's disease of both small and large intestine with rectal bleeding

Rationale: Specific codes are available for Crohn's disease that includes both the large and small intestines. Do not report Crohn's disease of the large and small intestinal separately.

Ischemic Heart Disease

Abstract & Code It! Patient 1

I20.8	Other forms of angina pectoris

Rationale: In the Alphabetic Index, see Angina/of effort – see Angina, specified NEC.

Abstract & Code It! Patient 2

E78.00	Pure hypercholesterolemia, unspecified
I25.2	Old myocardial infarction
I25.119	Atherosclerotic heart disease of native coronary artery with unspecified angina pectoris
E11.51	Type 2 diabetes mellitus with diabetic peripheral angiopathy without gangrene
I70.213	Atherosclerosis of native arteries of extremities with intermittent claudication, bilateral legs
Z79.4	Long term (current) use of insulin

Rationale: Link atherosclerosis of the extremities to the diabetes and report both conditions because code I70.213 provides much more specificity than "peripheral angiopathy without gangrene."

Abstract & Code It! Patient 3

I21.21	St elevation (STEMI) myocardial infarction involving left circumflex coronary artery

Rationale: Encounters for a myocardial infarction that occur within 28 days of the date of the infarction are reported as acute myocardial infarctions. Find oblique marginal coronary artery in the Alphabetic Index under Infarct/ST elevation/involving/oblique marginal coronary artery.

Liver Disease

Abstract & Code It! Patient 1

K70.40	Alcoholic hepatic failure without coma
F10.188	Alcohol abuse with other alcohol-induced disorder
Y90.1	Blood alcohol level of 20-39 mg/100 ml

Rationale: The alcohol abuse is reported as occurring with an alcohol-induced disorder because the physician documented "alcoholic liver failure." Encephalopathy is not synonymous with coma.

Abstract & Code It! Patient 2

K70.4	Alcoholic hepatitis failure without coma
B18.2	Chronic viral hepatitis C
F10.21	Alcohol dependence, in remission

Rationale: The patient's alcohol dependence is in remission, so report code F10.21. Ascites often occurs in liver failure and because no treatment of the ascites was documented (eg, paracentesis), the code was omitted.

Abstract & Code It! Patient 3

K70.0	Alcoholic fatty liver
F10.988	Alcohol use, unspecified, with other alcohol-induced disorder

Rationale: "Drinks regularly" cannot be reported as anything other than "use."

Malnutrition

Abstract & Code It! Patient 1

G30.9	Alzheimer's disease, unspecified
F02.80	Dementia in other diseases classified elsewhere without behavioral disturbance
R63.0	Anorexia
Z68.1	Body mass index (BMI) 19 .9 or less, adult

Rationale: Coder cannot infer early or late Alzheimer's disease based on the patient's age. Therefore, unspecified Alzheimer's disease is reported. Always report the dementia with Alzheimer's, even when not specifically documented, according to Alphabetic Index convention. While her BMI and weight loss seem to indicate malnutrition or cachexia, no diagnosis is assigned and, therefore, only the symptom anorexia and the BMI may be reported.

Abstract & Code It! Patient 2

E44.1	Mild protein-calorie malnutrition
F33.0	Major depressive disorder, recurrent, mild
Z68.1	Body mass index (BMI) 19 .9 or less, adult
Z63.4	Disappearance and death of family member

Rationale: Default for recurrent depression is code F33.0. Capture the mild malnutrition and BMI. Reporting the death of the patient's husband may be optional because the patient has underlying depression. A local policy on reporting bereavement may be appropriate.

Abstract & Code It! Patient 3

J43.9	Emphysema, unspecified

Rationale: Cachexia is a diagnosis, but cachexic is an adjective describing the patient. Cachexic is not a diagnosis. Only the emphysema is reported.

Migraine

Abstract & Code It! Patient 1

G43.A0	Cyclical vomiting, not intractable

Rationale: See Vomiting/cyclical/without refractory migraine in the Alphabetic Index.

Abstract & Code It! Patient 2

G43.109	Migraine with aura, not intractable, without status migrainosus

Rationale: Despite the severity, the migraine described for this patient is not intractable and without migrainousus.

Abstract & Code It! Patient 3

G43.019	Migraine without aura, intractable, without status migrainosus

Rationale: The patient's migraine is documented as intractable.

Motor Neuron and Myoneural Junction Disease and Inflammatory Polyneuropathies

Abstract & Code It! Patient 1

G62.0	Drug-induced polyneuropathy
T45.1X5S	Adverse effect of antineoplastic and immunosuppressive drugs
Z85.118	Personal history of other malignant neoplasm of bronchus and lung

Rationale: An instruction at code G62.0 tells coders to use additional code to identify the drug, which was antineoplastic. Report a history of lung cancer because there is no evidence that the condition is ongoing and it was treated two years ago.

Abstract & Code It! Patient 2

G12.21	Amyotrophic lateral sclerosis
E44.0	Moderate protein-calorie malnutrition
R13.19	Other dysphagia
Z68.1	Body mass index (BMI) of 19.9 or less

Rationale: The patient's amyotrophic lateral sclerosis has led to swallowing difficulties and the resultant malnutrition. Capture all conditions so that the entire clinical picture is reported.

Abstract & Code It! Patient 3

G61.0 Guillain-Barre syndrome

J96.00 Acute respiratory failure, unspecified whether with hypoxia or hypercapnia

N31.8 Other neuromuscular dysfunction of bladder

N17.9 Acute kidney failure, unspecified

R33.8 Other retention of urine

Z99.11 Dependence on respirator [ventilator] status

Rationale: Because the tracheostomy was performed during this inpatient encounter, code Z93.0, *Tracheostomy status*, would not be reported. AIDP is a form of Guillain-Barre syndrome, and the bladder dysfunction is neurogenic in origin. Report unspecified acute kidney failure, as the specific damage caused by the urinary retention was not identified.

Multiple Sclerosis

Abstract & Code It! Patient 1

G37.5 Concentric sclerosis [Balo] of central nervous system

G81.91 Hemiplegia, unspecified, affecting right dominant side

Rationale: Note that entries under Encephalitis/periaxialis and Encephalitis/periaxial classify to different codes. Assume that the right side is the dominant side when the dominant side is not documented.

Abstract & Code It! Patient 2

G37.9 Demyelinating disease of central nervous system, unspecified

Rationale: Do not report "probable" diagnoses, except when they appear on an inpatient discharge summary that is properly authenticated by a physician. Report the unspecified demyelinating disease, which risk-adjusts.

Abstract & Code It! Patient 3

G35 Multiple sclerosis

Rationale: Only the multiple sclerosis may be reported because no specific symptoms are documented.

Muscular Dystrophy

Abstract & Code It! Patient 1

H90.0 Conductive hearing loss, bilateral

G71.0 Muscular dystrophy

Rationale: Without more information, this patient's hearing loss is reported as conductive, according to the Alphabetic Index conventions for default coding, even though facioscapulohumeral muscular dystrophy is known to cause sensorineural hearing loss. Query the physician for more specificity, if possible.

Abstract & Code It! Patient 2

G71.0 Muscular dystrophy

Rationale: Code the muscular dystrophy and any manifestations, when present. None was identified here.

Abstract & Code It! Patient 3

G71.11 Myotonic muscular dystrophy

M21.41 Flat foot [pes planus] [acquired], right foot

M21.42 Flat foot [pes planus] [acquired], left foot

Rationale: For the bilateral planovalgus deformity, two codes are required: one for each side. The only mention of "planovalgus" in the Alphabetic Index is for a congenital condition (Q66.6-), but the note says "acquired." Planovalgus is another term for flat foot, also called pes plan valgus. Acquired flat foot is reported with codes from subategory M21.4, *Flat foot* [pes planus] (acquired).

CHAPTER 4
Clinical Documentation and Coding Integrity Part 3 (N-P)

Narcolepsy

Abstract & Code It! Patient 1

I69.398	Other sequelae of cerebral infarction
G47.411	Narcolepsy in conditions classified elsewhere with cataplexy

Rationale: The narcolepsy is a late effect of the cerebral infarction that the patient had previously experienced. The sequela is captured in addition to the code for narcolepsy in conditions classified elsewhere.

Abstract & Code It! Patient 2

G47.421	Narcolepsy with cataplexy

Rationale: The first sentence cites "symptoms of" narcolepsy. We cannot code "symptoms of," but only the actual diagnosis. The diagnosis comes further in the note, with a discussion of "narcolepsy and cataplexy" responding to medication.

Abstract & Code It! Patient 3

G47.419	Narcolepsy without cataplexy

Rationale: There are types of narcolepsy that are hereditary. Code the narcolepsy, without mention of cataplexy.

Neoplasms

Abstract & Code It! Patient 1

K56.699	Other intestinal obstruction unspecified as to partial versus complete obstruction
C78.6	Secondary malignant neoplasm of retroperitoneum and peritoneum
C56.1	Malignant neoplasm of right ovary

Rationale: Exclusion notes under K56.60- and K56.69- instruct the coder to omit the code for intestinal obstruction when it is due to specified conditions, but this note is referencing digestive disorders with obstruction noted in the code (eg, K56.52, *Intestinal adhesions [bands] with complete obstruction*). The obstruction is the reason for the encounter. Report code K56.699 as there is no further description of the obstruction. Peritoneal carcinomatosis is found in the Alphabetic Index under Carcinomatosis/peritonei. It is a secondary malignancy. A right ovarian malignancy is also documented. The default for an ovarian malignancy is primary.

Abstract & Code It! Patient 2

C61	Malignant neoplasm of prostate

Rationale: A leuprolide injection is for the treatment of patient's prostate cancer only, and no increase in the size of tumor was noted in physical examination. Code the cancer as active even though it is documented as history of, as the evidence is strong.

Abstract & Code It! Patient 3

C79.51	Secondary malignant neoplasm of bone
R32	Unspecified urinary incontinence
M54.31	Sciatica, right side
Z85.118	Personal history of other malignant neoplasm of bronchus and lung

Rationale: The incontinence is reported because it is not integral to the diagnosis. This is in keeping with ICD-10-CM Guideline Section I(B.5). The sciatica is also reported. The Alphabetic Index entries for sciatica are not complete, however, using the Alphabetical Index will still lead to the correct answer. In the Alphabetic Index, locate Sciatica/due to intervertebral disc disorder – see Disorder/disc/with/radiculopathy, which will take the coder to code M51.1-. A note at code M51.1 states Excludes1 sciatica NOS (M54.3). Report code M54.3- because the extradural spine metastasis is not specifically an intervertebral disc disorder.

Neuralgia

Abstract & Code It!

B02.29	Other postherpetic nervous system involvement
E11.40	Type 2 diabetes mellitus with diabetic neuropathy, unspecified

Rationale: The herpes infection has resolved, as evidenced by documentation of "healed, with pink scarring." The assessment is postherpetic neuralgia. The diabetes is noted in the past medical history (PMH), however, there is no note that the PMH was reviewed in this encounter. Discussion of how the physician will increase the patient's medication for diabetic neuropathy to treat the neuralgia salvages the diabetes diagnosis and allows the reporting of code E11.40. Type 2 is the default when the type of diabetes in not documented.

Obesity

Abstract & Code It! Patient 1

E65	Localized adiposity

Rationale: Abdominal fat can be clinically important, ie, when it interferes with diagnostic tests.

Abstract & Code It! Patient 2

E66.01	Morbid (severe) obesity due to excess calories
I10	Benign (essential) hypertension
J44.9	Chronic obstructive pulmonary disease, unspecified
Z68.41	Body mass index (BMI) 40.0-44.9

Rationale: The COPD appears in the active record and may be reported without meeting the MEAT criteria, depending on local coding policy. The blood-pressure reading and the description "controlled" meets the MEAT criteria for the hypertension. Report the morbid obesity and supporting BMI.

Abstract & Code It! Patient 3

Z71.3	Dietary counseling and surveillance
E66.01	Morbid (severe) obesity due to excess calories
E11.9	Type 2 diabetes mellitus without complication
I10	Benign (essential) hypertension
G47.33	Obstructive sleep apnea (adult) (pediatric)
Z68.36	Body mass index (BMI) 36.0-36.9

Rationale: Although the physician's diagnosis of morbid obesity seems to conflict with the BMI of 36 (usually associated with obesity, not morbid obesity), it is the coder's responsibility to query the physician regarding the conflicting diagnoses if possible, and if not, to abstract the diagnoses as documented.

Ophthalmic Disorders

Abstract & Code It!

H35.3221	Exudative age-related macular degeneration, left eye, with active choroidal neovascularization
H35.3210	Exudative age-related macular degeneration, right eye, stage unspecified
H35.363	Drusen (degenerative) of macula, bilateral

Rationale: The right eye (OD) is documented with drusen (dilated fundus exam) and wet, age-related macular degeneration. The left eye (OS) has drusen and choroidal neovascularization in macular degeneration. Symptoms are consistent with macular degeneration and would not be reported separately.

Osteomyelitis

Abstract & Code It!

E10.621	Type 1 diabetes mellitus with foot ulcer
E10.69	Type 1 diabetes mellitus with other specified complication
E10.40	Type 1 diabetes mellitus with diabetic neuropathy, unspecified
E10.52	Type 1 diabetes mellitus with diabetic peripheral angiopathy with gangrene
M86.671	Other chronic osteomyelitis, right ankle and foot
L97.514	Non-pressure chronic ulcer of other part of right foot with necrosis of bone
B95.61	Methicillin susceptible Staphylococcus aureus infection as the cause of diseases classified elsewhere
Z89.411	Acquired absence of right great toe

Rationale: Report diabetes with as many codes as necessary to completely report the patient's condition. This patient has angiopathy, neuropathy (LOPS), a foot ulcer, and osteomyelitis ("Staphylococcus aureus invading his second phalangeal shaft"). The osteomyelitis is reported with code E10.69, and a code from the Musculoskeletal System chapter to identify the specific complication. An instruction with code E10.69 states, "Use additional code to identify complication," and a note with code E10.621 states, "Use additional code to identify site of ulcer." Report the infective agent, when documented.

Osteoporosis, Vertebral, and Pathological Fractures

Abstract & Code It! Patient 1

M80.08XA Age-related osteoporosis with current pathological fracture, vertebrae, initial encounter

Z87.310 Personal history of (healed) osteoporosis fracture

Rationale: The ICD-10-CM guidelines instruct coders to assume a fracture is pathological in a patient with osteoporosis when the fracture occurs under circumstances during which a fracture would not normally occur. Such is the case here, and so a pathological fracture due to osteoporosis is reported. The default for osteoporosis is age-related osteoporosis, unless otherwise documented. The patient has an "old" compression fracture at T-7 and T-8. Further documentation would be required to code this as a chronic, ongoing condition; it could be a healed fracture. Report code Z87.310.

Abstract & Code It! Patient 2

M40.14 Other secondary kyphosis, thoracic region

M80.08XS Age-related osteoporosis with current pathological vertebral fracture, sequela

M54.89 Other dorsalgia

Rationale: The kyphosis is sequela of collapsed vertebra and due to osteoporosis. The brace is to help with the back pain, so that should be reported separately.

Abstract & Code It! Patient 3

S22.031A Stable burst fracture of third thoracic vertebra, initial encounter for closed fracture

Rationale: This fracture is not stated as pathological and, therefore, it would be reported as an injury.

Pancreatic Disorders

Abstract & Code It! Patient 1

K85.30 Drug induced acute pancreatitis without necrosis or infection

T38.3X5A Adverse effect of insulin and oral hypoglycemic [antidiabetic] drugs

Rationale: A note at code K85.3 instructs coders to use an additional code to report the adverse effect. A quick search for "sitagliptin" online reveals it as an antidiabetic medication for type 2 diabetics. The coder may want to query the physician if possible because diabetes is not documented.

Abstract & Code It! Patient 2

K86.0 Alcohol-induced chronic pancreatitis

F10.21 Alcohol dependence, in remission

Rationale: Report the pancreatitis and the alcohol dependence to the highest level of specificity.

Abstract & Code It! Patient 3

K85.11 Biliary acute pancreatitis with uninfected necrosis

K86.1 Other chronic pancreatitis

E84.8 Cystic fibrosis with other manifestations

K86.81 Exocrine pancreatic insufficiency

Rationale: Cystic fibrosis can damage the pancreas and block the biliary ducts, as is seen here. Report the cystic fibrosis with other manifestations, the exocrine pancreatic insufficiency, and codes for both the chronic and acute pancreatitis.

Paralysis, Malformation of Brain/Spinal Cord

Abstract & Code It! Patient 1

K94.02	Colostomy infection
B37.89	Other sites of candidiasis
G82.21	Paraplegia, complete
S24.113S	Complete lesion at T7-T10 level of thoracic spinal cord, sequela

Rationale: The colostomy infection is the reason for the encounter, and the causal agent was documented and reported as well. An injury code with a seventh character "S" reports sequela of the injury. The patient has complete paraplegia, as evidenced by the complete lesion injury.

Abstract & Code It! Patient 2

R53.2	Functional quadriplegia
G35	Multiple sclerosis

Rationale: There is one code for multiple sclerosis, regardless of severity. Reporting functional quadriplegia further explains the patient's requirements for care.

Abstract & Code It! Patient 3

I69.331	Monoplegia of upper limb following cerebral infarction affecting right dominant side

Rationale: Unilateral weakness related to a cerebrovascular accident is considered monoplegia.

Parkinson's and Huntington's Disease

Abstract & Code It!

G10	Huntington's disease
E44.0	Moderate protein-calorie malnutrition
Z68.1	Body mass index (BMI) 19.9 or less

Rationale: Do not code a gastrostomy-status code for this encounter, as the reason for the encounter was to place the gastrostomy tube. Going forward, the gastrostomy can be reported when it is documented.

Pemphigus

Abstract & Code It!

L10.0	Pemphigus vulgaris
K05.11	Chronic gingivitis, non-plaque induced

Rationale: Report the acute gingivitis to capture the inflammation of gingiva due to pemphigus vulgaris. Find code K05.11 by searching the Alphabetic Index under Inflammation/gum.

Pulmonary Disorders: Acute

Abstract & Code It! Patient 1

J86.9	Pyothorax without fistula
B95.5	Unspecified streptococcus as the cause of diseases classified elsewhere

Rationale: While an empyema can occur in numerous anatomical locations, the default is pulmonary, category J86.9. Report the infectious agent, if known.

Abstract & Code It! Patient 2

J15.5	Pneumonia due to Escherichia coli

Rationale: A single code captures both the pneumonia and the causal agent. Short-term use of oxygen is not reported. A note under code Z99.81, *Dependence on supplemental oxygen*, states, "Dependence on long-term oxygen."

Abstract & Code It! Patient 3

J15.1	Pneumonia due to Pseudomonas
J44.0	Chronic obstructive pulmonary disease with acute lower respiratory infection
J44.1	Chronic obstructive pulmonary disease with (acute) exacerbation
R09.02	Hypoxemia

Rationale: The patient's pneumonia has caused hypoxemia, which is reported. Do not assume respiratory failure because the patient has COPD. The patient is documented as having an exacerbation of the COPD in addition to the pneumonia, and both conditions should be reported. Short-term use of oxygen is not reported. A note under code Z99.81, *Dependence on supplemental oxygen*, states, "Dependence on long-term oxygen."

Pulmonary Disorders: Chronic

Abstract & Code It! Patient 1

J43.2 Centrilobular emphysema

Z87.891 Personal history of tobacco dependence

Rationale: Emphysema may be asymptomatic in early stages, but it is still reported. A note with chronic pulmonary diseases in the Tabular List instructs coders to report any current or past exposure to tobacco.

Abstract & Code It! Patient 2

J44.1 Chronic obstructive pulmonary disease with (acute) exacerbation

J96.22 Acute and chronic respiratory failure with hypercapnia

Z99.81 Dependence on supplemental oxygen

Rationale: There is no specific code for end-stage or acute chronic obstructive pulmonary disease. This patient is on continuous home oxygen, so reporting a code for dependence on supplemental oxygen is warranted.

Abstract & Code It! Patient 3

J45.41 Moderate persistent asthma with (acute) exacerbation

Rationale: The documentation for Patient 3 tells the coder everything that is pertinent to code selection in the nomenclature of ICD-10-CM.

CHAPTER 4 Clinical Documentation and Coding Integrity: Part 4 (Topics R–Z)

Renal Disorders

Abstract & Code It! Patient 1

E10.9 Type 1 diabetes mellitus without complications

R80.1 Persistent proteinuria, unspecified

Rationale: A diagnosis of nephropathy would be required in order to link the persistent proteinuria to a complication of diabetes.

Abstract & Code It! Patient 2

N18.3 Chronic kidney disease, stage 3

Rationale: While this is listed as "history of," the referral to a nephrologist and the patient's GFR provide the context and support to code an active condition. The GFR is significant for stage 4 CKD, however, do not code from laboratory results. Query the physician, if possible.

Abstract & Code It! Patient 3

N18.4 Chronic kidney disease, stage 4

Rationale: The patient's CKD trend is well documented, and code N18.4 is easily abstracted.

Seizure and Epilepsy

Abstract & Code It! Patient 1

G40.909 Epilepsy, unspecified, not intractable, without status epilepticus

Rationale: Seizure does not classify in the Alphabetic Index to epilepsy, but recurrent seizure does.

Abstract & Code It! Patient 2

Z02.4 Encounter for examination for driving license

G40.A09 Absence epileptic syndrome, not intractable, without status epilepticus

Rationale: The reason for the encounter is to obtain clearance for a driving license, which should be coded in addition to the epileptic syndrome.

Abstract & Code It! Patient 3

G80.1 Spastic diplegic cerebral palsy

G40.209 Localization-related (focal) (partial) symptomatic epilepsy and epileptic syndromes with complex partial seizures, not intractable, without status epilepticus

Rationale: Seizure disorders are not uncommon with cerebral palsy. Report both conditions. For the epilepsy code, look up Seizure/partial/complex – see Epilepsy, localization-related, symptomatic, with complex partial seizures in the Alphabetic Index. Depending on local policies, code Z99.3, *Dependence on wheelchair*, could also be reported.

Septicemia and SIRS

Abstract & Code It! Patient 1

T82.7XXA Infection and inflammatory reaction due to cardiac and vascular devices, implants and grafts, initial encounter

R78.81 Bacteremia

B95.2 Enterococcus as the cause of diseases classified elsewhere

C50.919 Malignant neoplasm of unspecified site of unspecified female breast

Rationale: The infection due to the vascular device is reported with code T82.7XXA. A note with code T82.7 instructs coders to "use additional code to identify infection." The bacteremia is reported, as well as the infective agent. The PICC line is used for chemotherapy for breast cancer; therefore, breast cancer is also reported.

Abstract & Code It! Patient 2

A41.02 Sepsis due to methicillin resistant Staphylococcus aureus

R65.20 Severe sepsis without septic shock

J96.00 Acute respiratory failure, unspecified whether with hypoxia or hypercapnia

L03.115 Cellulitis of right lower limb

Z93.0 Tracheostomy status

Z99.11 Dependence on respirator [ventilator] status

Rationale: Report severe sepsis when a patient has sepsis-related organ failure. Always drill down to the origin of the sepsis: in this case, cellulitis of the ankle. A combination code reports both the sepsis and infective agent. Report the tracheostomy status and ventilator status, so stated.

Abstract & Code It! Patient 3

Omit code.

Rationale: "Urosepsis" does not communicate a specific disorder. The Alphabetic Index instructs coders to "Code to condition" for urosepsis, but this is not possible if no other diagnosis is documented.

Skin Ulcers

Abstract & Code It!

E10.51 Type 1 diabetes mellitus with diabetic peripheral angiopathy without gangrene

E10.621 Type 1 diabetes mellitus with foot ulcer

L97.429 Non-pressure chronic ulcer of left heel and midfoot with unspecified severity

F33.9 Major depressive disorder, recurrent, unspecified

I10 Essential (primary) hypertension

E78.00 Pure hypercholesterolemia

E55.9 Vitamin D deficiency, unspecified

Z89.412 Acquired absence of left great toe

Z89.422 Acquired absence of other left toe(s)

Z87.891 Personal history of nicotine dependence

Rationale: Many diagnoses in this patient's record were not addressed during this encounter. These conditions were captured: diabetes and foot ulcer; hypercholesterolemia; recurrent depression; vitamin D deficiency; hypertension; smoking history; and amputation status. The status of the patient's right foot is unclear, as there is a note under the problem list of an "amputated foot." The documentation states that only the toes of the left foot were amputated. This illustrates the problem with coding from the problem list: The information may not be recent, or accurate. Other documentation errors affecting risk-adjusting diagnoses that would contribute to the patient's risk score are listed below:

Prostate cancer: Prostate cancer is listed in the past medical history and the patient is experiencing hyperglycemia due to Lupron. From this, we can infer the prostate cancer is still being actively treated with Lupron. Based on risk-adjustment rules from CMS, we cannot code from past medical history (PMH); therefore, query the physician.

Chronic kidney disease: The patient is noted to have CKD Stage 4 in the problem list but there is no other mention of renal disease in the note. CKD Stage 4 risk-adjusts and changes the HCC for the hypertension diagnosis, increasing its value.

Abdominal aortic aneurysm: Abdominal aortic aneurysm (AAA) appears in PMH and risk-adjusts when codeable. However, there is no evidence that this was addressed in this encounter.

Diabetic retinopathy, diabetic neuropathy, diabetic nephropathy: All three of these complications of diabetes have additional HCCs/RxHCCs beyond those for diabetes with complication, and should be reported for their additive value. Because they are not supported in the record or if they only shows up in the PMH, they are omitted. Capturing one diabetes HCC is not the equivalent of capturing all HCCs available because many of the diabetic complications have multiple, different HCCs and RxHCCs. Coding from a flawed problem list is always risky, and this problem list had issues.

Skin Burns and Severe Conditions

Abstract & Code It! Patient1

T20.32XA	Burn of third degree of lip(s), initial encounter
T31.0	Burns involving less than 10% of body surface
W86.0XXA	Exposure to domestic wiring and appliances, initial encounter

Rationale: A full-thickness burn is a third-degree burn. Report the percentage of third-degree burn secondary to the code for the burn site. An external-cause code captures the circumstances of the burn.

Abstract & Code It! Patient 2

T22.391A	Burn of third degree of multiple sites of right shoulder and upper limb, except wrist and hand, initial encounter
T21.20XA	Burn of second degree of trunk, unspecified site, initial encounter
T31.21	Burns involving 20-29% of body surface with 10-19% third degree burns
W40.1XXA	Explosion of explosive gases, initial encounter
Y92.099	Unspecified place in other non-institutional residence as the place of occurrence of the external cause

Rationale: Separate codes are required to capture the different burn degrees, and another code captures the percentage of third-degree burn. The circumstances of the accident should be reported with an external-cause code, and in some cases, reporting the place of occurrence will expedite assignment of benefits for insurance. The use of Y-codes and external-cause codes could be the subject of a policy for risk-adjustment auditing firms.

Abstract & Code It! Patient 3

T27.5XXD	Corrosion involving larynx and trachea with lung, subsequent encounter
T54.3X1D	Toxic effect of corrosive alkalis and alkali-like substances, accidental (unintentional), subsequent encounter

Rationale: The patient is no longer in the acute phase of her injury. She no longer has respiratory failure and is no longer on a ventilator, so these codes are omitted. The external-cause code can be coded, even in subsequent encounters.

Vascular Disease

Abstract & Code It!

Z01.818	Encounter for other preprocedural examination
I70.244	Atherosclerosis of native arteries of left leg with ulceration of heel and midfoot
L97.425	Non-pressure chronic ulcer of left heel and midfoot with muscle involvement without evidence of necrosis

E11.51	Type 2 diabetes mellitus with peripheral angiopathy without gangrene
E11.261	Type 2 diabetes mellitus with foot ulcer
I25.10	Atherosclerotic heart disease of native coronary artery without angina pectoris
Z79.84	Long term (current) use of oral antidiabetic drugs
Z87.891	Personal history of tobacco dependence

Rationale: This is an encounter for surgery clearance. Do not assume that the "assessment" provides the most detailed information on the diagnosis. The coder must pull together elements from several places in this record to obtain that diagnosis, but all the information is there. "Atherosclerotic" is mentioned in the Assessment/Plan under preoperative clearance and the severity of the ulcer is addressed in the musculoskeletal physical examination. Laterality is documented in the history of present illness. The Alphabetic Index conventions instruct coders to link the atherosclerosis of the extremities to the diabetes and the atherosclerosis to the ulcer. Instructions at category I70 direct coders to code use additional code to identify history of tobacco dependence, and instructions with the diabetes codes direct coders to report the long-term use of oral antidiabetic agents. Documentation errors affecting risk-adjusting diagnoses that would contribute to the patient's risk score are highlighted below:

Ostomy status: The patient has a surgical history of total colectomy and ileostomy. This should have been noted in the physical examination so that the ostomy status could be abstracted. With a colectomy, it is possible the ostomy was reversed, so coders cannot make assumptions about the surgical history of stoma.

Hypertension and polyneuropathy: The patient has a PMH of hypertension and polyneuropathy. Both of these conditions were pertinent to this examination and both risk-adjust, but neither can be reported from the PMH.

Evaluate Your Understanding

A Answer Questions

1. C. **Rationale:** A diagnosis must be captured at least once yearly for risk adjustment related to that diagnosis to occur. That said, each condition should be reported as often as the condition is assessed, given that HCCs may influence other methodologies (eg, Medicare spending per beneficiary calculation) using a shorter timeframe (eg, 6 months).
2. D. **Rationale:** Cachexia describes a condition in which a patient with an underlying pathology (eg, cancer, AIDS, or dementia) is wasting away due to resistance to nutrition. It is not determined by BMI, although most patients with cachexia will have low BMIs.
3. C. **Rationale:** Code R06.03, *Acute respiratory distress*, is new for 2018. This code may be reported for a child or an adult.
4. B. **Rationale:** ICD-10-CM Guideline Section I(C.1.a.2.f) states, "Patients with any known prior diagnosis of an HIV-related illness should be coded to B20, Human immunodeficiency virus [HIV] disease. Once a patient has developed an HIV-related illness, the patient should always be assigned code B20 on every subsequent admission/encounter. Patients previously diagnosed with any HIV illness (B20) should never be assigned to R75, Inconclusive laboratory evidence of human immunodeficiency virus [HIV], or Z21, Asymptomatic human immunodeficiency virus [HIV] infection status."
5. D. **Rationale:** All of the terms are classified to code K21.9, *Gastro-esophageal reflux disease without esophagitis*, in the Alphabetical Index.

B True/False Questions

1. True. **Rationale:** Alzheimer's disease includes an inherent diagnosis of dementia in ICD-10-CM conventions, therefore, one code is reported for the Alzheimer's disease, and a second code is required to report the dementia with or without behavioral disturbance.

2. False. **Rationale:** A coder cannot abstract codes from laboratory values. The coder should instead query the physician, or report code J96.10, *Chronic respiratory failure, unspecified whether with hypoxia or hypercapnia.*

3. False. **Rationale:** There is no code for reporting bilateral rheumatoid arthritis of any joint. If the condition is bilateral, report two codes.

4. True. **Rationale:** A diagnosis of autism spectrum disorder usually comes from a clinician qualified under the plan for behavioral health care, and that usually includes licensed clinical social workers, psychologists, or physicians specializing in autism spectrum disorder.

5. False. **Rationale:** Codes in category I69, *Sequelae of cerebrovascular disease*, should be used to indicate sequelae from codes in categories I60-I67, reported after the initial encounter for the cerebrovascular event. The initial event is reported with codes from categories I60-I69.

6. False. **Rationale:** With the exception of nicotine, uncomplicated use of a psychoactive substance is not reported if there is no link between the substance use and a complication. Omit the code.

7. True. **Rationale:** The Alphabetic Index directs readers from Disease/Crohn's to Enteritis/regional, and at that entry, regional enteritis is linked to the rectal bleeding with the word, "with." According to ICD-10-CM guidelines, this establishes a causal link between regional enteritis (Crohn's disease) and the rectal bleeding.

8. False. **Rationale:** Acute kidney injury is often the language used when an acute kidney disease has been diagnosed. Query the physician to specify the type of glomerular disease or renal tubule-interstitial disease, if circumstances regarding a traumatic injury are not documented. Encourage physicians who use the terminology "acute kidney injury" to describe a nontraumatic disorder to add "nontraumatic" to documentation to prevent abstraction errors. Acute kidney injury can occur in patients who are not experiencing acute renal failure, so identify acute renal failure when it occurs.

9. False. **Rationale:** Atherosclerosis and intermittent claudication has a causal relationship, according to the Alphabetical Index conventions as found under atherosclerosis. Instead, report a code from code I70.21, *Atherosclerosis of native arteries of extremities with intermittent claudication.* The same holds true for causal relationships between atherosclerosis and rest pain, ulceration, or gangrene.

10. False. **Rationale:** It is not enough to assign a code in an effort to document the diagnosis. Codes cannot be abstracted from codes, according to CMS. It is a physician's responsibility to describe the diagnosis and its etiology, acuity, and manifestations. The physician's language, in combination with the Alphabetic Index, should take the coder to the correct code.

CHAPTER 5

Developing Risk-Adjustment Policies

A Answer Questions

1. C. **Rationale:** In risk adjustment, the accepted standard for IRR is 95%, ie, coders abstracting the same chart should achieve the same results 95% of the time.

2. A. **Rationale:** Because CMS would be responsible for any audit of Medicare Advantage coding, direction and instructions directly from CMS would build the strongest argument for coding decisions.

3. D. **Rationale:** Policies require time and effort to research, write, maintain, and communicate. Only when a diagnosis occurs frequently enough to disrupt workflow or has a significant impact on risk payments should a policy be drafted, and then, only if a thorough research of the ICD-10-CM code set and its guidelines and the AHA's *Coding Clinic* do not answer the coding question.

4. B. **Rationale:** The first line of defense for a coder who encounters ambiguous documentation is to query the physician. In many RA coding organizations, querying the physician is not possible. In these cases, each organization must provide the coder with its expectations for the next step(s) in the coding process.

5. D. **Rationale:** A main term is usually the root defect of a diagnosis, which in this case is a block. In some cases, more than one main term may exist in a diagnosis (eg, diabetic retinopathy is classified in the Alphabetical Index under diabetes or retinopathy).

6. A. **Rationale:** COPD is described as one of the "chronic eight" in the *2008 Risk Adjustment Technical Assistance for Medicare Advantage Organizations (MAOs) Participant Guide*: "It is likely that these diagnoses would be part of a general overview of the patient's health when treating co-existing conditions for all but the most minor of medical encounters." Pneumonia and appendicitis are acute conditions and gestational diabetes resolves when the baby is delivered. COPD is a chronic, incurable disease managed throughout the life of the patient, and some risk adjustment organizations have policies that allow for the abstraction of chronic, incurable conditions from "Past Medical History" when they are accompanied by support in the body of the medical record (eg, "The patient is maintaining a PO2 level of 92% on room air during the day, but is using supplemental oxygen at night").

7. A. **Rationale:** While citations from CMS, the AHA's *Coding Clinic*, and federal resources do not guarantee a coding policy will be accepted by CMS, citations do help build a case for how a coding decision is made and may protect the organization from punitive fines should CMS disagree with the coding policy during an appeal.

8. D. **Rationale:** Organizations will obviously want to communicate coding policy with coders, but the risk-adjustment management team should also be informed so that its members are aware of the risks and benefits of the policies. Similarly, MAOs or other payer clients will need to review the policies because they carry ultimate responsibility in a CMS audit.

9. D. **Rationale:** There is no difference in risk adjustment based on the type of diabetes mellitus assigned to the patient. The difference in payment is determined by whether the patient has complications of diabetes or uncomplicated diabetes. The policy on type 1.5 diabetes may be considered by some organizations to ensure all cases of type 1.5 diabetes mellitus are reported with the same diabetes category. This aligns internal coding of type 1.5 diabetes mellitus, which in turn boosts IRR scores and improves productivity.

10. B. **Rationale:** *ICD-10-CM Guidelines* define past medical history as a "medical condition that no longer exists and is not receiving any treatment but that has the potential for recurrence, and therefore, may require continued monitoring."

C Audit Exercises

1. **Answer/Rationale:** The physician's note documents both hyperthyroidism and hypothyroidism. One of these diagnoses is in error, as the two contradict each other. Either the fatigue and mental dullness of hypothyroidism, or the anxiety and insomnia of hyperthyroidism could have contributed to her depressive symptoms. If the physician cannot be queried, what should be coded? A new policy on "Conflicts in Documentation" may be useful.

2. **Answer/Rationale:** Documentation states that the patient has prostate cancer; however, it is not being treated. Should prostate cancer be reported for this patient? A new policy on "Non-Treatment of Malignancy" would clarify for coders how to approach this scenario.

3. **Answer/Rationale:** "Metformin" supports the diabetes, but the anti-inflammatory action of prednisone could support either the COPD or the rheumatoid arthritis. There is no other support or mention of these two conditions in the note. Can a single medication that has multiple uses support multiple comorbidities in a record when there is no other support? A new policy on "Ambiguous MEAT" could answer that question.

4. **Answer/Rationale:** A Chopart disarticulation is an amputation of the foot at the midtarsal joint, with the retention of the calcaneus and talus. Can an amputation status be reported from past surgical history, and can it be reported without support? A new policy could be entitled "Amputation Status."

5. **Answer/Rationale:** The patient's BMI of 32 conflicts with the diagnosis of morbid obesity. While there are some circumstances in which the national guidelines allow physicians to document morbid obesity in a patient with a BMI under 40, those guidelines require a BMI of at least 35. Because morbid obesity risk-adjusts, how should the coder handle this? Is a physician diagnosis sufficient even when BMI evidence contradicts it? A policy entitled "Morbid Obesity Exceptions" could answer this question for coders.

Appendix D

Training/Teaching Tools

Physicians and coders are always looking for ways to improve their documentation/coding accuracy and productivity, and the training/teaching tools in Appendix D are created with both of these goals in mind. Designed to be two-sided documentation and coding sheets: 11 tools provide guidance regarding documentation and coding errors associated with common risk-adjustment diagnoses and one provides general advice that falls into the category of "best practices" for documentation and coding.

For best results, these tools are laid out as two-sided tools by topic (eg, Diabetes Mellitus Physician Documentation on one side and Diabetes Mellitus Coder Abstraction on the other side). Often, it can be helpful to provide coding information to the physicians who code and/or clinical documentation guidance to the coders who work with physicians on coding. These pages are available as downloadable two-sided PDFs and they may be distributed to the physicians and/or coders in your practice or organizations. To download these PDFs, visit amaproductupdates.org.

ARTHRITIS

Physician Documentation

Etiology of arthritis is a critical element to physician documentation. The default for arthritis not further specified is unspecified osteoarthritis, unspecified site.

Documentation Tips

- **Do not skimp on details in documentation.** Laterality and joint(s) affected by arthritis must be documented with etiology. Crucial elements for documentation of etiology are catalogued here:

Type of Arthritis	Code Category(ies)
Pyogenic: identify infective agent and whether a direct or indirect infection, and whether post-infective or reactive	**M00-M02**
Rheumatoid arthritis: note any rheumatoid factor, juvenile type, Felty's syndrome, specific organ or system involvement, bursitis, nodules, myopathy	**M05-M06, M08**
Gout: note etiology (renal, drug, lead, idiopathic, other secondary), chronic or acute, with or without tophus	**M1A, M10**
Other crystal arthropathies: specify type as hydroxyapatite deposition disease, familial chondrocalcinosis, or other	**M11**
Other: post-rheumatic and chronic, Kaschin-Beck, villonodular synovitis, palindromic rheumatism, intermittent hydrarthrosis, traumatic arthropathy, transient, allergic, monoarthritis NOS [not otherwise specified]	**M12, M13**
Arthritis in disease classified elsewhere: specify underlying disease	**M14**
Osteoarthritis: multiple sites, bilateral of single joint, primary, secondary, post-traumatic (also identify the type of trauma that led to the late effect arthritis)	**M15-M19**

- **Document the results of rheumatoid factor tests in the record.** A coder cannot infer positive or negative rheumatoid arthritis with rheumatoid factor from a test value.
- **For a patient requiring joint replacement,** documentation must include:
  - History of pain (onset, duration, character, aggravating and relieving factors)
  - Specific limitations in activities of daily living and safety issues (eg, falls)
  - Contraindications to nonsurgical solutions
  - List of failed nonsurgical treatments (ie, weight loss, medication, braces, injections, physical therapy [PT])
  - Physical exam identifying deformity, range of motion (ROM), gait, effusion, crepitus, etc
  - Results of diagnostic tests and specific type of arthritis
  - Comorbidities affecting mobility and care
- **Document any history of joint replacement.**
- **Do not rely on the medication list** to capture long-term (current) use of medications. Document current use of aspirin, NSAIDs, opioids, steroids, or immunosuppressive drugs.
- **If a patient has joint pain, stiffness, or effusion,** document the specific joint and laterality.

ARTHRITIS

Coder Abstraction

"Arthritis" defaults in ICD-10-CM to unspecified osteoarthritis of an unspecified site. Read all **Includes** and **Excludes** notes carefully to capture codes correctly and use additional codes to fully report the etiology of conditions.

Coding Tips

- **Osteoarthritis of the spine** is reported with a code from category M47, *Spondylosis,* rather than a code from category M15-M19. Spondylosis is a general term for arthritis or spinal degeneration affecting the spine and sacroiliac joints. Degenerative joint disease (DJD) is a common term describing osteoarthritis of a joint or the spine.
- **Start with the Alphabetic Index.** Although most types of arthritis are reported with codes from the ICD-10-CM musculoskeletal chapter, some forms of arthritis are reported with codes from other chapters.

Multiple Sites vs Bilateral Sites

In ICD-10-CM, polyosteoarthrtis (M15.-) is reported when multiple sites are affected by osteoarthritis, excluding the spine. Most definitions use a threshold requiring five or more sites, although ICD-10-CM does not define the term. Osteoarthritis (M16-M19) is reported when one site is arthritic, or when one bilateral site is arthritic, up to four sites for osteoarthritis.

- **Juvenile idiopathic arthritis (JIA) describes** a form of rheumatoid arthritis with onset in childhood. If RA is documented in a patient under 18 years of age, query the physician about the patient's rheumatoid arthritis type. A patient diagnosed with JIA in childhood may continue to have JIA in adulthood.

Positive and Negative Rheumatoid Factor

The Alphabetic Index to ICD-10-CM classifies rheumatoid arthritis as juvenile, seronegative, or seropositive, or with organ involvement. The lack of documentation of rheumatoid factor does not constitute "seronegative" rheumatoid arthritis.

- **Charcot's arthropathy in diabetes** is reported with code E--.610, *Diabetes with diabetic neuropathic arthropathy,* rather than a code from category M14.6-, *Charcot's joint.*
- **Gout always requires a 7th character** to report with or without tophus. All forms of secondary gout require more than one code to completely describe the condition (ie, toxic effects, renal condition, etc).

Symptom Codes or Code Categories	
M25.4--	Effusion of joint (fluid in joint)
M25.5--	Pain in joint (arthralgia)
M25.6--	Stiffness in joint
R26.2	Difficulty in walking, NOS
R29.890	Loss of height

NEOPLASMS

Physician Documentation

Neoplasms are classified in ICD-10-CM by anatomical location and histology. Essential to proper coding and documentation is noting the specific site including any laterality, and whether the neoplasm is benign, primary malignant, secondary malignant, in situ, uncertain, or unspecified.

Documentation Tips

- **Avoid words like *mass, lump, tumor, lesion,* or *growth*** if more specific language is available.
  According to ICD-10-CM nomenclature:
  - An uncertain neoplasm has been examined microscopically. Its nature cannot be predicted.
  - An unspecified neoplasm is unknown and no microscopic examination has occurred.

Active Disease, Remission, and History

Use language that allows the coder to abstract the appropriate diagnosis for the patient. In ICD-10-CM, the only malignant conditions that can be categorized as "in remission" are multiple myeloma and leukemia. Documentation of "minimal residual disease" is insufficient for coders to determine whether remission has been achieved.

Other types of cancers are identified as active disease, meaning the condition is still present or still being treated, or history of disease, meaning the condition has been eradicated and all treatment completed.

- **Do not document "history of malignant neoplasm" or "NED"** if the neoplasm is still being treated. Instead, document the continuum of care with what has been done and what is left to do. "History of" and "no evidence of disease" indicate an eradicated condition, according to coding rules.
- **If a selective estrogen receptor modulator (SERM) such as tamoxifen is being administered,** indicate whether the medication is treatment for active cancer or prophylaxis against cancer.

Metastatic Disease

Documentation of metastatic disease requires special care, as "metastatic" and "metastasis" can be ambiguous in describing the primary and secondary sites. Use of the words "to" and "from" in notes will clarify the origin of neoplasms (eg, "breast cancer with metastases to the lung" or "metastatic lung cancer from the breast"). Or, simply use the terms "secondary" and "primary."

- **Connect the dots.** For example, document anemia as caused by cancer or by cancer treatment. Document diabetes due to pancreatic carcinoma, or pathologic fracture due to breast cancer metastasizing to bone. Always document etiology and manifestation of cancer and its complications.
- **If the staging of the malignancy is known,** document this in the medical record. This helps the coder understand the severity of the patient's condition.
- **Leukemia and multiple myeloma** are the only types of cancers classified in ICD-10-CM with "remission." For other types of cancers, state "active" or "history of." For example, do not report "colon cancer in remission."
- **Differentiate in documentation** between a malignant neoplasm growing within a certain site and one that is advancing to adjacent sites (metastasizing).

NEOPLASMS

Coder Abstraction

Neoplasms can be documented in many ways. Do not make assumptions about coding "mass," "growth," "tumor," "polyp," or other terms documented. Be sure to start in the Alphabetic Index and use the exact words from the documentation. For example, a "polyp" may be indexed to a benign neoplasm, a neoplasm of uncertain behavior, an "other or unspecified disorder," and for some sites, a unique polyp code. From the Alphabetic Index, go to the Table of Neoplasms if so directed, and then to the Tabular Section of ICD-10-CM.

Coding Tips

- **Do not confuse uncertain and unspecified neoplasms.** An uncertain neoplasm has been examined microscopically, but its nature cannot be predicted. An unspecified neoplasm has an unknown etiology because no microscopic examination has been documented.
- **A cancer-staging form** is an acceptable form of documentation if authenticated by the physician.

> **History vs Active Cancer**
>
> **A cancer becomes "history of cancer"** when treatment is completed (ie, excision, radiotherapy, chemotherapy), for coding purposes. For example, following mastectomy and chemotherapy, a patient is diagnosed with secondary bone cancer, originating in the breast. The patient is reported with secondary bone cancer, and history of breast cancer.

- **"Metastatic from . . ."** indicates a primary malignancy: the original site of the cancer. "Metastatic to . . ." indicates a secondary malignancy: a new site for cancer that has grown from seeds from the original site. Query the physician if the documentation is unclear whether a site is primary or secondary. When a growing malignancy advances beyond the boundaries of its anatomic site, it is metastatic (eg, when a cancer in the ascending colon extends into the cecum).
- **Only leukemia and multiple myeloma have "remission" codes** in ICD-10-CM cancer coding. If the physician documents another form of cancer as "in remission," query to see if the patient has a history of malignancy or active disease.
- **Comorbidities are sometimes caused by the neoplasm.** Look for linking language in documentation and report related conditions when they are associated with the neoplasm.
- **Melanoma and Merkel cell carcinoma** have unique codes, as do squamous cell and basal cell carcinomas. Do not use other malignant skin neoplasm codes to report these conditions. Melanoma and Merkel cell carcinoma risk-adjust; other skin cancers do not.
- **Prostate-cancer patients and breast-cancer patients** may be treated with long-term selective estrogen receptor modulators (SERMs). These medications may be prescribed to treat an existing cancer, or to prevent cancer in a patient at risk for cancer. Read documentation carefully before assuming that a "history of cancer" is active for a patient being treated with SERMs, and query the physician if the status of the patient's cancer is unclear.

COPD AND ASTHMA

Physician Documentation

Chronic obstructive pulmonary disease (COPD) has a tremendous effect on the quality of life and activities of daily living for patients. Ensure all aspects of COPD and asthma are tracked in the medical record.

Documentation Tips

- **Always specify bronchitis as acute or chronic,** when known.
- **Document results of pulmonary function tests (PFTs)** to show airway limitations, as well as any chest computed tomography (CT) results.
- **For chronic bronchitis, document if obstructive.**
- **ICD-10-CM differentiates between COPD with acute exacerbation and COPD with acute lower respiratory infection.** Document if an exacerbation of COPD is due to infection. Be specific in the documentation, and include the infective agent when known.

COPD Codes	Descriptions
J41.0	Simple chronic bronchitis
J41.1	Mucopurulent chronic bronchitis
J41.8	Simple and mucopurulent bronchitis
J42	Unspecified chronic bronchitis
J43.0	Unilateral pulmonary emphysema
J43.1	Panlobular emphysema
J43.2	Centrilobular emphysema
J43.8	Other emphysema
J43.9	Emphysema, unspecified
J44.0	COPD with acute lower respiratory infection
J44.1	COPD with exacerbation
J44.9	COPD, unspecified

- **For COPD, document severity** (mild, moderate, severe, end-stage).
- **For asthma, document from the following choices:** severity of mild, moderate, severe, or unspecified; with type as intermittent or persistent; and episode as uncomplicated, with acute exacerbation, or with status asthmaticus; or as exercise-induced bronchospasm, cough variant asthma, or other asthma.
- **Document acute respiratory failure** when it occurs, even when it does not require intubation. Document chronic respiratory failure for any encounter in which it exists and the respiratory system is evaluated. COPD can occur with or without respiratory failure, so it should be separately noted. Document hypoxia or hypercapnia in respiratory failure, as appropriate.
- **Document any dependence on ventilator and any tracheostomy.**
- **Tobacco use or dependence, history of tobacco use, or exposure to secondary smoke** (workplace, environment, perinatal), is relevant to all respiratory conditions and should be noted. Document the type of tobacco in current use (chewing tobacco, e-cigarette, cigarettes, etc).
- **Document any tobacco counseling, treatment, or intervention.**
- **Document the patient's dependence on supplemental oxygen.**

COPD AND ASTHMA

Coder Abstraction

COPD and asthma represent clinically discrete conditions that are sometimes difficult to code accurately. Most important for bronchitis is whether it is chronic and whether it is obstructive. Both of those conditions are required for COPD.

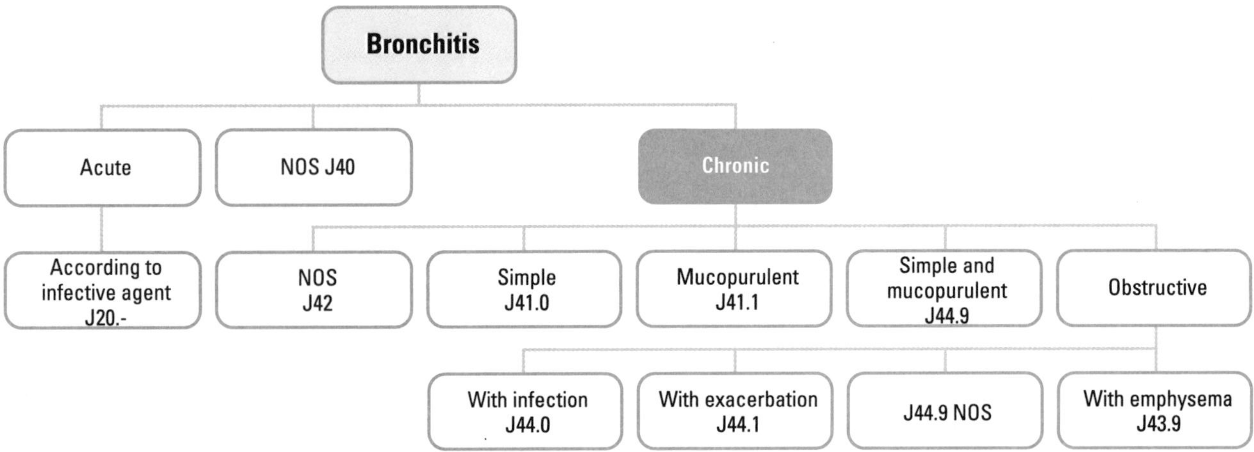

Coding Tips

- **When a patient has both COPD and emphysema,** report only the emphysema in ICD-10-CM, as COPD is included in the emphysema. See the Alphabetic Index under Disease/pulmonary/obstructive/with/emphysema J43.9. This is new for 2018.
- **When a patient is documented with both COPD and asthma,** report both conditions.
- **Code the patient's smoking status, if noted.** Do not link a current or past history of tobacco dependence with COPD, asthma, or emphysema, unless the documentation states a causal relationship between smoking and COPD. If a causal relationship is documented, report code F17.218, *Nicotine dependence, cigarettes, with other nicotine-induced disorders.*
- **Any hypoxia, hypercapnia, hypoxemia, polycythemia, or respiratory failure** in the patient with COPD or asthma should be reported.
- **If the patient's pulse oximetry reading is charted below 90** and no diagnosis of hypoxia or hypoxemia has been noted, query the physician (eg, "Is the pulseOx of XX significant for any additional diagnoses?").
- **Code Z99.11 for any dependence on a respirator,** including dependence on a continuous positive airway pressure (CPAP) or bi-level positive airway pressure (BiPAP) device when oxygen is delivered through tracheostomy.
- **Aspiration pneumonia and influenza** are excluded from code J44.0, *Chronic obstructive pulmonary disease with acute lower respiratory infection,* as the cause of the infection, according to the AHA's *Coding Clinic.*

Common Tobacco Use and History Codes	
F17.210	Nicotine dependence, cigarettes, uncomplicated
F17.211	Nicotine dependence, cigarettes, in remission
F17.218	Nicotine dependence, cigarettes, with other nicotine-induced disorders
Z72.0	Tobacco use
Z77.22	Contact with and (suspected) exposure to environmental tobacco smoke (acute)(chronic)
Z87.891	Personal history of nicotine dependence

DEMENTIA

Physician Documentation

Dementia is a progressive decline in cognition along with short- and long-term memory loss due to brain damage or disease. It is always going to affect the health of the patient and should be documented for all encounters, as it affects care planning.

Documentation Tips

- **Documentation of mental health and decline** is an important concept in senior care. Note all counseling provided for driving alternatives, safety issues, neuropsychiatric referrals or interventions, end-of-life decisions, and medication changes. Note if the patient is accompanied by a caregiver.
- **Be as specific as possible** in describing the patient's mental capabilities, symptoms, or diagnosis. Document any violent or disruptive behavior, wandering, or sundowning. The chart below provides the language of ICD-10-CM for patients at risk for dementia.

Code(s)	Symptoms
G31.84	Mild cognitive impairment
I69.-	Cognitive deficit following stroke, specify deficit; note intracerebral/subarachnoid bleed vs infarct
R41.81	Age-related cognitive decline
R41.82	Altered mental status, unspecified
R41.841	Cognitive communication deficit
R41.844	Frontal lobe and executive function deficit
R90.82	White matter disease, diagnostic imaging, NOS
Z87.820	Personal history of traumatic brain injury

- **Dementia should be linked to any known etiology** with causal language (eg, "Dementia due to Parkinson's disease"). Often, two codes are required to capture the etiology and the dementia.

Code(s)	Dementia Etiology
E--. with .49	Diabetes
E75.-	Cerebral lipidoses
F01.5-	Vascular dementia
F03.9-	Unspecified dementia
F03.9-	Senile dementia, not otherwise specified
F10.97, F10.27	Alcoholic dementia, state dependence, abuse
G10	Huntington's disease
G20	Parkinson's disease
G30.-	Alzheimer's disease, state early or late onset
G31.01	Pick's disease
G31.09	Frontotemporal dementia
G31.83	Lewy body disease
G35	Multiple sclerosis
G40.-	Epilepsy

- **Document violent, combative, or aggressive behavior** to capture the extra work required in serving a patient with behavioral disorders in dementia. Document all related comorbidities, including any depression, malnutrition, or functional quadriplegia.
- **The age of onset of Alzheimer's disease** is pertinent to outcomes. Younger patients have a greater impairment in neocortical temporal function, affecting practical application of knowledge. Later onset results in greater impairment in limbic disorders affecting visual memory and orientation. Document the patient's Alzheimer's disease as early onset (before age 65) or late onset (after age 65).

DEMENTIA

Coder Abstraction

A patient with dementia is going to have memory deficits. Over time, the patient typically becomes progressively confused. A caregiver or family member will usually accompany dementia patients to medical encounters and provide the patient's history and chief complaint.

Coding Tips

- **Report behavioral status for any patient with dementia.** The patient who is violent, aggressive, or uncooperative should be coded with behavioral disturbance. DSM-V states significant psychotic symptoms include mood disturbances, agitation, and apathy, which qualify as "behavioral disturbance." Query the physician if there are questions regarding a symptom.
- **In some cases, the behavioral disturbance, dementia, and etiology are captured with one code.** In other instances, it requires two codes to capture both.

Parkinsonism vs Parkinson's Disease

Parkinsonism is defined as tremor and abnormalities in movement. Patients with Parkinson's disease, a specific neurological disorder, have Parkinsonism, but not all patients with Parkinsonism have Parkinson's disease. Code these conditions as follows:

- **Dementia due to Parkinson's disease** G20, F02.80
- **Dementia with Parkinsonism** G31.83, F20.80

- **Wandering** is reported in addition to dementia with code Z91.83.
- **Sundowning** is reported in addition to dementia with code F05. Sundowning is not in the Alphabetic Index, but can be found as an inclusion term at code F05, *Delirium due to known physiological condition*.
- **Do not report Alzheimer's dementia** when the patient is elderly and the physician has documented only "dementia." Coders cannot assume etiology. Without a documented cause of the dementia, query the physician or report code F03.90, *Unspecified dementia without behavioral disturbance*.

Dementia due to Alcohol Dependence

ICD-10-CM assumes a link between dementia and alcohol dependence. Therefore, report code F10.27 whenever documentation states persistent dementia in a patient who is also noted to be alcohol dependent, unless the physician states otherwise.

- **Dementia is inherent to Alzheimer's, Lewy body, and Pick's disease.** If Alzheimer's is documented, report the Alzheimer's and report dementia in diseases classified elsewhere. In the Alphabetic Index, see Disease/Alzheimer's G30.9 *[F02.80]*, an indication that two codes are required, according to the ICD-10-CM guideline's etiology/manifestation convention. The Alphabetic Index also provides two codes for Disease/Lewy body G31.83 *[F02.80]*, and Disease/Pick's, G31.01 *[F02.80]*.
- **There is no time limit on when a late effect code** can be used to report a cognitive deficit from a stroke. Once the patient has been released from the hospital following an acute infarct or hemorrhage, the codes from category I69 may be used to report any cognitive deficits.
- **Delirium and other symptoms similar to dementia** may be present in an elderly patient who has a urinary tract infection or other malady. Do not make assumptions regarding the diagnosis; query the physician to answer any questions.
- **Code also any noted comorbidities** for dementia (eg, cachexia [R64], depression [F32.9], or frailty [R54]).

DIABETES MELLITUS (DM)

Physician Documentation

Diabetes is a chronic, lifelong metabolic disorder affecting uptake and storage of carbohydrate, protein, and fat. Sustained high blood glucose levels lead to the diagnosis. Diabetes should be addressed in every encounter with the diabetic patient, as it will always affect outcomes and care.

Documentation Tips

- **Document the type of diabetes as:**
  - Type 1 (autoimmune; no insulin production)
  - Type 2 (insulin resistance or low production; most common form)
  - Secondary, due to underlying condition
    - Document underlying condition (eg, cystic fibrosis, cancer, pancreatitis, Cushing's)
  - Secondary, due to drugs/chemicals
    - Document drug or chemical causing the adverse effect (eg, corticosteroids, streptozotocin, alloxan, rodenticide Vacor)
  - Other specified form of diabetes
    - Document as genetic defect, postpancreatectomy, etc
- **Do not document diabetes using these outdated terms:**
  - IDDM, NIDDM (from the 1970s; replaced with type 1 and type 2)
  - Juvenile onset, adult onset (type 1 can occur in adults; type 2 can occur in children)
  - Brittle diabetes (outdated terminology; classifies to type 1 diabetes)
- **Document when a comorbidity is *not* due to diabetes.** Coders will link the diabetes to most other conditions, as this is guidance from CMS. If the patient's CKD has another cause, be sure to document it using clear language (eg, "CKD stage 4 due to polycystic kidney disease").
- **Provide qualitative information regarding diabetic control** (eg, "Diabetes is in good control despite pneumonia. Blood glucose today is 105." "Patient's A1C is 7.6, and his goal is 6.5.").
- **Identify treatment method.** Document whether diabetes is controlled by diet and exercise, antidiabetic medications, or insulin. Note if the patient has an insulin pump.
- **Address all complications of diabetes,** with qualitative language that documents the extent or severity of the complication (eg, "10-year diabetic neuropathy has progressed to LOPS").
- **State the obvious.** Do not document "BG of 495." Instead, document, "Patient's blood glucose indicates hyperglycemia at 495." Coders cannot connect the dots or code from laboratory values.
- **Document hyperglycemia as appropriate.** High blood sugar was considered a sign and symptom of diabetes in ICD-9-CM; in ICD-10-CM, it is considered a complication of diabetes and is reported.
- **Document any status resulting from diabetes.** Ensure that the patient's vision loss, amputation, or dialysis status is discussed during the encounter, as appropriate.
- **Remember to address status of annual examinations.** Has the patient had a retinal eye examination? Foot examination? Are elevated A1Cs being addressed with changes to diet/medication? Has macroalbuminuria, hyperlipidemia, or hypertension been assessed?
- **Document all referrals** for dietetic counseling, foot care, or other therapies:

Pregnancy and Diabetes: What to Document
TYPE: Gestational, type 1, type 2, unknown diabetes, abnormal GTT
TREATMENT: Insulin, antidiabetic oral medication, diet and exercise
COMORBIDITIES: Existing complications of diabetes in pregnant patient

DIABETES MELLITUS (DM)

Coder Abstraction

Coding complications of diabetes changed with the 2017 ICD-10-CM guidelines. Now, most comorbidities found under "Diabetes/with" are considered a complication of diabetes. No linkage language from the physician is specifically required, as identified by the "with" rule in the guidelines.

Coding Tips

- **If the type of diabetes is not stated,** the guidelines tell us to report DM, type 2, unless the patient has diabetic ketoacidosis (DKA), in which case, according to the AHA's *Coding Clinic*, the default is type 1.

Types of Diabetes	
E08 Secondary diabetes	due to Cushing's, CF, cancer, pancreatitis, malnutrition
E09 Secondary diabetes	due to drugs or chemicals (code also with T36-T65)
E10 Type 1 diabetes	due to autoimmune process
E11 Type 2 diabetes	due to shortage of insulin or poor insulin transport
E13 Other specified DM	due to genetic defect, pancreatectomy, NEC

- **Don't stop with one code.** Use as many codes as required to describe all the complications of diabetes documented for the patient. However, all codes for a patient encounter should be in the same diabetes category (eg, do not report code E11.65 with code E10.43).
- **Report treatment with insulin** (Z79.4) or antidiabetic drugs (Z79.84). If patient is on insulin and oral drugs, report only the insulin.
- **Insulin may be given temporarily** for hyperglycemia therapy. This is not "long-term use." "Long- term use" describes daily injection of prescribed insulin. Code presence of an insulin pump (Z96.41).

Type 1 Diabetes and Insulin

Because type 1 DM requires insulin injections multiple times daily for survival, there is no need to code Z79.4 with type 1 diabetes.

- **Type 1.5 diabetes** does not have a separate category in ICD-10-CM, and there is no guidance. Query physicians on their preferences or refer to internal coding policies.
- **Do not overlook documented hyperglycemia or hypoglycemia.** While these conditions were once considered incidental to diabetes, if they are documented and treated, they should be reported.
- **Diabetic gastroparesis** is reported as autonomic polyneuropathy (E--.43). Because there are other forms of autonomic polyneuropathy, also report code K31.84, *Gastroparesis.*

Pregnant Patients with DM

For patients with gestational diabetes, report a code from category O24.4-, plus code Z79.84 for use of oral antidiabetic medications, if appropriate. For other forms of diabetes in pregnancy, report a code from category O24, as well as an "E" code to describe the type of diabetes. Except for type 1, also report a code for insulin or oral medication.

- **Causal links are required** for comorbidities not specifically identified in the Alphabetic Index entries under "Diabetes/with." However, a "with/other specified" comorbidity must be clearly linked in documentation. "Diabetes" documented in the same encounter as "candidiasis infection of skin of groin" does not represent a causal relationship because "Diabetes/with/other specified disorder of skin" is not specific to candidal skin infection. "Diabetic candidiasis of skin" shows a causal link.
- **Poorly controlled/out-of-control diabetes** is reported as hyperglycemia, according to the ICD-10-CM Alphabetic Index.

HEART DISEASE

Physician Documentation

Heart health is critical to overall health, and treatments may include pharmacologic, nonpharmacologic, and surgical approaches. Details are important when documenting cardiac conditions, as treatment approaches vary, depending on the exact etiology, and because ICD-10-CM heart disease specificity has increased in recent years.

Documentation Tips

- **Identify chest pain as:** during respiration, precordal, intercostal, anterior chest wall, or pleurodynia.
- **Heart failure** is documented as arteriosclerotic, left ventricular, systolic, diastolic, or combined; right heart, high output, or end-stage heart failure. Note whether acute, chronic, or acute on chronic. Congestive heart failure is a nonspecific diagnosis.
- **ICD-10-CM assumes a causal link** between heart failure and hypertension. If the heart failure is not due to hypertension, document its cause.
- **Myocardial infarct** (MI) should be noted as having occurred within the past 28 days, or as being an old MI. A subsequent MI within 28 days of another MI should be so noted by date. Identify STEMI or NSTEMI and site as left main, left anterior descending, right coronary, left circumflex, or inferior/anterior wall.
- **Document any history of** coronary artery bypass surgery, cardiac pacemaker, or heart valve replacement. Document heart transplant status or if the patient is awaiting transplant.

Atrial Fibrillation: Document Type	
I48.0	**Paroxysmal**—intermittent, stopping, starting by itself
I48.1	**Persistent**—can be stopped with treatment
I48.2	**Chronic**—cannot be stopped with treatment
I48.91	**Unspecified**—type is not documented or known

- **In coronary artery disease (CAD),** document any lipid-rich plaque or chronic total occlusion. Note if the vessels involved are native vessels or grafts, and whether the CAD is accompanied by angina pectoris, with or without spasm, or instability.
- **Document the valve associated with any heart murmur,** if known.
- **In valve disease, specify insufficiency or stenosis,** and specify which valve(s) is involved.
- **Do not rely on electronic medication lists to capture long-term use** of medications. Actively document long-term use of anticoagulants, antithrombolitics, antiplatelets, NSAIDs, aspirin, or any other pertinent pharmaceuticals in the medical record for the current encounter.
- **Link cardiac arrest** to underlying conditions, as appropriate.
- **Document pertinent symptoms** (eg, nonexertional dyspnea, fatigue, edema, or weight gain).
- **Document any current use or history of use** of tobacco for patients with heart disease.

Common Tobacco Use and History Codes	
F17.210	Nicotine dependence, cigarettes, uncomplicated
F17.211	Nicotine dependence, cigarettes, in remission
F17.218	Nicotine dependence, cigarettes, with nicotine-induced disorders
Z72.0	Tobacco use
Z77.22	Contact with and (suspected) exposure to environmental tobacco smoke (acute)(chronic)
Z87.891	Personal history of tobacco dependence

HEART DISEASE

Coder Abstraction

Cardiology is a complex specialty with its own nomenclature. Often, more than one code is required to capture the nature of the patient's condition. Refer to anatomy references or search online to understand unfamiliar diagnoses.

Coding Tips

- **If the site of an MI or the type of heart failure is not noted in the physician documentation,** seek out supporting diagnostic documents from radiology or other departments. It is acceptable for diagnostic information from other sources to support a more detailed diagnosis for the physician, so long as it is generated and signed by an acceptable risk-adjustment provider and does not contradict the treating physician's diagnosis.

Evolving Myocardial Infarctions

If an NSTEMI evolves into a STEMI, report only the STEMI. If STEMI converts to NSTEMI due to thrombolytic therapy, code only the STEMI.

- **Any acute MI that is identified as subendocardial** or nontransmural is reported as an NSTEMI (I21.4), regardless of the documented site of the MI.

Common Heart-associated Symptom Codes

Code	Symptom
R01.0	Benign murmur
R01.1	Murmur, NOS
R06.01	Orthopnea
R06.02	Shortness of breath
R42	Dizziness
R60.0	Localized edema
R94.31	Abnormal ECG

Code	Symptom
R00.0	Tachycardia, NOS
R00.1	Bradycardia, NOS
R00.2	Palpitations
R07.2	Precordal pain
R07.9	Chest pain, NOS
R53.83	Fatigue NOS
R68.84	Jaw pain

- **An encounter for a patient who experiences a second acute MI within 28 days** of a previous MI requires two codes to capture the condition: a code from I21-, *ST-elevation (STEMI) and non-ST elevation (NSTEMI) myocardial infarction,* for the initial MI, and a code from I22-, *Subsequent ST elevation (STEMI) and non-ST elevation (NSTEMI) myocardial infarction*, for the subsequent MI.
- **If a patient has a subsequent MI more than 28 days following a previous** MI, the new infarction is reported as an initial MI with a code from category I21.
- **Report any documented old MI (I25.2),** heart transplant status (Z94.1), heart valve replacement status, and any long-term use of blood-thinners, antithrombolitics, or aspirin.
- **Autogolous graft** is a graft using a vessel removed from the patient for a bypass. Nonautologous biological graft is usually composed of processed vessels from cadavers (allografts [same species]) or animals (xenografts [different species, ie, pigs or cows]).
- **In coronary artery disease,** assume the patient has native arteries if not otherwise documented. Use additional codes to report calcified coronary lesion (I25.84), lipid-rich plaque (I25.83), or chronic total occlusion (I25.82).
- **If a patient's heart arrhythmia is resolved** by placement of a pacemaker, report the pacemaker status rather than the arrhythmia. If a patient continues to take medication for the arrhythmia in addition to having a pacemaker, report the arrhythmia in addition to the pacemaker status.

HYPERTENSION

Physician Documentation

Hypertension (HTN) is a major risk factor for myocardial infarction, vascular disease, chronic kidney disease (CKD), and stroke. Blood pressure (BP) and efficacy of pharmacologic therapy should be assessed and documented at every patient encounter.

Documentation Tips

- **High BP may be incidental;** HTN is a chronic condition. Document hypertension when it exists to avoid ambiguity.
- **An isolated instance of elevated BP** should be documented and reported with code R03.0, *Elevated blood-pressure reading, without diagnosis of hypertension*. Also report code R03.0 for borderline HTN and "white coat disease."
- **A patient on medication for HTN who has normal BP readings** still has HTN, not "history of" HTN. Ensure the diagnosis is captured by noting it in documentation. Coders cannot abstract diagnoses from past medical history (PMH) notes.
- **ICD-10-CM guidelines state that a causal relationship can be assumed** for HTN when it occurs with heart failure, cardiomyopathy, or CKD. Be sure to document when these conditions coexist and are **not** related to HTN.

Hypertensive Crisis

A hypertensive crisis occurs when BP rises fast enough and high enough that it has the potential to damage organs. The American Heart Association defines **hypertensive urgency** as a systolic BP exceeding 180, or diastolic exceeding 110, without progressive organ dysfunction. **Hypertensive emergency** occurs when levels exceed 180 systolic or 120 diastolic, with impending or progressive organ damage. **Hypertensive crisis** is reported when neither urgency nor emergency is specified.

Accelerated, malignant, and uncontrolled are not terms associated with hypertensive crisis in ICD-10-CM. Rather, they are associated with code I10, *Essential (primary) hypertension*.

Also document any consequences of the uncontrolled BP.

I16.0	Hypertensive urgency
I16.1	Hypertensive emergency
I16.9	Hypertensive crisis, unspecified

- **Coders cannot abstract diagnoses from numbers.** Documentation must support the diagnosis coded. A BP reading of 180/110 cannot be coded at all. Coders can only abstract the physician's diagnoses.
- **If a patient has secondary HTN,** identify the source (eg, renovascular, other renal, or endocrine), and link the specific underlying condition to the HTN in documentation.
- **Specify a pregnant patient with HTN** as experiencing a pre-existing, gestational, pre-eclampsic, or eclampsic HTN.
- **Document the smoking status of a patient with HTN** as current smoker, history of tobacco dependence, tobacco use, or exposure to environmental tobacco smoke.
- **When a patient has HTN,** identify the etiology (eg, drug-induced [also document medication], idiopathic, orthostatic, or other cause).

HYPERTENSION

Coder Abstraction

Hypertension (HTN) is always going to affect the health of the patient and should be reported as often as documented and addressed. HTN occurring with chronic kidney disease (CKD) or congestive heart failure (CHF) requires a HTN code other than I10.

Coding Tips

- **For hypertensive cerebrovascular disease,** report a code from categories I60-I69 and the appropriate HTN code.
- **Report two codes, at a minimum, for hypertensive crisis.** Report the crisis and the underlying hypertension.

ICD-10-CM Guideline Section I(C.9.a)

The classification presumes a causal relationship between hypertension and heart involvement and between hypertension and kidney involvement, as the two conditions are linked by the term "with" in the Alphabetic Index. These conditions should be coded as related even in the absence of physician documentation explicitly linking them, unless the documentation clearly states the conditions are unrelated.

For hypertension and conditions not specifically linked by relational terms, such as "with," "associated with," or "due to" in the classification, physician documentation must link the conditions in order to be coded as related.

The causal link is established for HTN for these conditions/codes:

I50.1	Left ventricular HF	**I50.814**	Right HF due to left HF
I50.20	Systolic HF, NOS	**I50.83**	High output heart failure
I50.21	Acute systolic HF	**I50.84**	End stage heart failure
I50.22	Chronic systolic HF	**I50.89**	Other heart failure
I50.23	Acute on chronic systolic HF	**I50.9**	Congestive heart failure NOS
I50.30	Diastolic HF, NOS	**I51.4**	Myocarditis, unspecified
I50.31	Acute diastolic HF	**I51.5**	Myocardial degeneration
I50.32	Chronic diastolic HF	**I51.7**	Cardiomegaly
I50.33	Acute on chronic diastolic HF	**I51.81**	Takotsubo syndrome
I50.40	Combined (diastolic/systolic) HF, NOS	**I51.89**	Other ill-defined heart disease
I50.41	Combined (diastolic/systolic) HF, acute	**I51.9**	Heart disease, unspecified
I50.42	Combined (diastolic/systolic) HF, chronic	**N18.1**	CKD, stage 1
I50.43	Combined (diastolic/systolic) HF, acute on chronic	**N18.2**	CKD, stage 2 (mild)
I50.810	Right heart failure NOS	**N18.3**	CKD, stage 3 (moderate)
I50.811	Acute right heart failure	**N18.4**	CKD, stage 4 (severe)
I50.812	Chronic right heart failure	**N18.5**	CKD, stage 5
I50.813	Acute on chronic right heart failure	**N18.6**	End stage renal disease

Note: Do not link the CKD or heart disease to the HTN, if the physician documents another cause for the CKD or heart disease.

KIDNEY DISEASE

Physician Documentation

Renal insufficiency is a generic term that covers a broad spectrum of illness. It is often found in the medical record, and ICD-10-CM classifies it as an unspecified disorder of the kidney and ureter. Rather than simply documenting "renal insufficiency," describe the patient's condition as chronic or acute, document any known etiology, and note if the patient requires dialysis.

Documentation Tips

- **For hematuria, document whether gross,** benign essential microscopic, or asymptomatic microscopic.
- **Document microalbuminuria when it exists** in patients who have not been diagnosed with chronic kidney disease (CKD). Document nephropathy when it is diagnosed in diabetic patients with a history of more than 90 days of microalbuminuria.
- **Identify the specific stage in chronic kidney disease** as stage 1-5 or end-stage renal disease (ESRD). A coder cannot abstract based on CKD noted as "mild" or "moderate," and cannot abstract a stage from a glomerular filtration rate (GFR) result. Diagnoses must be assigned by the clinician.
- **Document the underlying cause of CKD.** ICD-10 assumes a causal relationship between CKD and hypertension and between CKD and diabetes, unless the physician documents otherwise.
- **Specify the type of glomerular disease or renal tubule-interstitial disease,** if known.
- **"Acute kidney injury"** may be confused with a traumatic injury. Add "nontraumatic" to the documentation of "acute kidney injury" to prevent misinterpretation.
- **Dependence on dialysis is not a stand-alone condition.** Document the etiology and manifestations for the kidney disorder and the stage of CKD or the acute kidney failure and its cause. Document any presence of arteriovenous shunt for dialysis. Document any noncompliance.
- **Always link a complication of dialysis** (eg, infection, hypotension, catheter break, etc) to dialysis.

Common Renal Failure Codes	
N17.0	Acute kidney failure with tubular necrosis
N17.1	Acute kidney failure with cortical necrosis
N17.2	Acute kidney failure with medullary necrosis
N17.9	Acute kidney failure, unspecified
N18.-	Add a number corresponding to stage of CKD for stages 1 through 5
N18.6	ESRD (Also code dialysis status Z99.2)
N18.9	Chronic kidney failure, unspecified
N19	Kidney failure, unspecified whether acute or chronic
P96.0	Congenital kidney failure

- **The etiology of anemia in the kidney patient** should be noted in the medical record.
- **When a patient has a transplant complication,** identify the type of complication (eg, failure, infection, or rejection).
- **Specifically document a complication of a transplant as a complication of a transplant.** For example, a patient may have CKD and a transplanted kidney, and the CKD may be a complication of the transplant, but unless it is documented as such, the transplant status and CKD are reported as two unrelated conditions.
- **ARF is an acronym for acute renal failure or acute respiratory failure.** Spell out first reference.
- **Note if a patient is awaiting a kidney transplant,** or has a status as a transplant recipient.

KIDNEY DISEASE

Coder Abstraction

Chronic kidney disease (CKD) or chronic renal failure (CRF) covers all degrees of chronic, decreased, and irreversible renal function, representing conditions that range from mild to end-stage. CKD is reported based on the renal function of the patient, as determined by the patient's GFR, albuminuria, and other factors. In contrast, acute renal failure comes on rapidly, and may be reversible. It is usually due to an interruption of the blood supply to the kidney, ureteral blockage, or kidney infection/damage.

Coding Tips

- **If both ESRD and stage 5 CKD are documented**, code only the ESRD.
- **Do not assign a CKD code based on GFR** or on a notation of mild, moderate, severe disease. Query the physician to assign the stage of CKD if it is not documented, or report unspecified.
- **The presence of CKD in a patient with a transplanted kidney** is not necessarily a complication of the transplant. The condition must be so stated to be coded as a complication.
- **Documentation of persistent microalbuminuria in a diabetic patient** may be indicative of CKD. Query the physician to determine how this should be reported

Do Not Assign Code I10 in a Patient with CKD

Choose a hypertension code from category I12, *Hypertensive chronic kidney disease,* or I13, *Hypertensive heart and chronic kidney disease,* for patients with hypertension and CKD, unless the physician states otherwise.

- **ARF is an acronym with several meanings.** If acute renal failure is not stated or obvious from context, query the physician regarding the acronym.
- **Assume a causal link between CKD** and diabetes or hypertension, unless documentation states otherwise. If the patient has diabetes, hypertension, and CKD, query the physician to determine if both conditions are responsible for the CKD, or only one should be linked to the hypertension. If the physician cannot be queried, report both links.
- **Always code documented kidney transplant status and dialysis status,** or any of the status codes listed below, when they are documented.

Status Codes Associated with Kidneys	
Z76.82	Awaiting kidney transplant
Z90.5	Nephrectomy status
Z91.15	Noncompliance with renal dialysis
Z94.0	Presence of transplanted kidney
Z97.8	Presence of artificial kidney
Z98.85	Transplanted kidney removed
Z99.2	Dependence on dialysis
Z99.2	Dialysis status

- **For a patient with EPO-resistant anemia (D63.1),** code also the underlying CKD.
- **Documented cardiorenal syndrome usually describes** acute decompensated congestive heart failure resulting in acute kidney failure. There is no code for this syndrome, which the Alphabetic Index classifies to hypertension. Be sure to capture all elements of the syndrome by querying the physician if the elements are not documented completely.

OBESITY/MALNUTRITION

Physician Documentation

Excess weight or malnutrition is always going to affect the health of the patient and should be documented for any encounter in which the condition is observed. **Body mass index (BMI)** is a valuable screening tool for weight and nutrition status.

Documentation Tips

- **Ensure the patient's BMI** is calculated at least once annually.
- **Document a weight-related diagnosis** for any patient with an abnormal BMI as follows:

BMI	Associated Condition
less than 16.0	severe malnutrition
16.00-16.99	moderate malnutrition
17.00-18.49	mild malnutrition
18.5-24.99	normal
25.00-29.00	overweight
30 to less than 39.9	obese (Classes 1 and 2)
40 or greater	morbidly obese (extreme, severe, Class 3)

- **If a patient's weight is causing other health issues,** document the health issues and link them to the weight diagnosis. Similarly, if the weight issue is caused by an underlying cause (eg, hypothyroidism, Cushing's syndrome, AIDS), document the underlying cause.
- **Document malnutrition, obesity, or morbid obesity in pregnant patient** during each encounter that addresses the patient's weight.
- **Document a treatment plan** for each patient's weight problem.
- **Cachexia** is weight loss despite caloric intake, seen in some end-stage diseases. Always document cachexia when it is observed. "Cachexic" describes a patient, but is not a diagnosis of cachexia.
- **Report any sequelae** of hyperalimentation in a patient who remains obese, or who has successfully undergone bariatric surgery (eg, bilateral osteoarthritis of the knees, as sequelae of morbid obesity).

Associated ICD-10-CM Diagnosis		Directive
E40	Kwashiorkor	Caution: Very rarely seen in US
E41	Nutritional marasmus	Caution: Very rarely seen in US
E42	Marasmic kwashiorkor	Caution: Very rarely seen in US
E43	Severe protein-calorie malnutrition NOS	Document also BMI
E44.0	Moderate protein-calorie malnutrition	Document also BMI
E44.1	Mild protein-calorie malnutrition	Document also BMI
E45	Retarded growth following malnutrition	Document also BMI
E46	Unspecified protein calorie malnutrition	Document also BMI
E66.01	Morbid (severe) obesity due to excess calories	Document also BMI
E66.09	Other obesity due to excess calories	Document also BMI
E66.1	Drug-induced obesity	Document also drug and BMI
E66.2	Morbid (severe) obesity with alveolar hypoventilation	Document also BMI
E66.3	Overweight	Document also BMI
E66.9	Obesity, unspecified	More specificity desired. Document BMI
E68	Sequelae of hyperalimentation	Document also condition
R64	Cachexia	Document also BMI

OBESITY/MALNUTRITION

Coder Abstraction

Excess weight or malnutrition is always going to affect the health of the patient and should be reported as often as it is documented and addressed by the physician. **BMI** is an important quality measure tool, and is coded whenever documented.

Coding Tips

- **Code BMI with any encounter in which it is documented along with a weight-related diagnosis.** There are HCPCS Level II codes for reporting compliance with BMI quality measures and these can be reported in physician offices when a weight diagnosis is not present. Some EHRs automatically generate the HCPCS Level II BMI codes; in other systems, coders abstract them.
- **A pregnant patient being treated or assessed for a weight diagnosis** (ie, morbid obesity, malnutrition) has a complication of pregnancy, even if the physician does not state it is a complication of pregnancy. Two codes are reported: one for the complication of pregnancy and one for the condition.

ICD-10-CM Guideline Section I(C.15.a.1)

It is the provider's responsibility to state that the condition being treated is not affecting the pregnancy.

- **If a BMI seems inappropriate to the diagnosis,** query the physician. If a query is not possible, code the two conditions, even if they conflict (eg, report an overweight diagnosis with BMI reflecting morbid obesity).
- **Obese abdomen or abdominal obesity** describes localized fat, not obesity. A person with a normal BMI may have abdominal obesity. It is clinically significant because it impairs the physical examination.
- **"Cachexic" is not a diagnosis;** "cachexia" is. Cachexia occurs when the patient's metabolism resists nutrition in late stages of AIDS, COPD, dementia, and other diseases.
- **Use caution in reporting kwashiorkor,** as this disease is usually limited to newly weaned children in impoverished countries. Query the physician if kwashiorkor appears in the chart of an elderly patient.
- **Use the Alphabetic Index** to find the exact language of the documentation (eg, abnormal weight loss, underweight).

Adult BMI Code	BMI Description
Z68.1	19 or less, adult
Z68.- -	Append first two digits of BMI to Z68 to create codes for all adult BMIs from 20.0 through 39.9. For example, a BMI of 34.5 would be reported as Z68.34.
Z68.41	40.9-44.9, adult
Z68.42	45.0-49.9, adult
Z68.43	50.0-59.9, adult
Z68.44	60.0-69.9, adult
Z68.45	70.0 or greater, adult

- **Report localized adiposity** for any "apron of fat" documented by the physician. These conditions can lead to integumentary complications.

STROKE AND INFARCTION

Physician Documentation

Do not document cardiovascular accident (CVA). Classification of stroke in ICD-10-CM requires more information than many physicians have traditionally documented, and coding of sequelae of stroke and infarction also demands a level of detail often missing in medical records. Etiology and site of stroke or infarction impact outcomes, so document as thoroughly as possible during emergent and ongoing care.

Documentation Tips

- **Identify the etiology of an acute stroke, infarction, or transient ischemic attack (TIA)** by category as shown below:

Codes	Stroke Type
I60.-	Spontaneous subarachnoid hemorrhage
I61.-	Spontaneous intracerebral hemorrhage
I62.-	Spontaneous subdural hemorrhage
I63.0-I63.2	Thrombosis/embolus precerebral arteries
I63.3-I63.5	Thrombosis/embolus cerebral arteries
I63.6	Venous thrombosis
I63.8	Other specified cerebral infarction
I63.9	Unspecified cerebral infarction
G45.9	Transient cerebral ischemic attack, unspecified (TIA)

- **In addition to the stroke or infarction type,** the vessel and laterality should be documented.
- **Once a patient has been released from the acute-care facility** following the initial stroke or infarction, the stroke or infarction is classified by its late effects. Therefore, document an encounter as an acute event or sequelae. The site and type of stroke impact long-term care coding, so identify whether the initial event was hemorrhagic or ischemic, and document affected site.
- **Document specific symptoms** of cognitive deficit following stroke (eg, attention, memory, executive function, psychomotor, visuospatial, social, emotional). Document other symptoms, including aphasia, dysphasia, dysarthria, apraxia, dysphagia, facial weakness, ataxia, or fluency disorder, or paralyses, including monoplegia or paraplegia.
- **For patients experiencing hemiplegia from stroke or infarction,** document which side is dominant, and which is affected. Document a link between the hemiplegia and the CVA as appropriate.

Etiology of Sequelae

Document in each encounter for sequelae of stroke, if the original stroke was due to subarachnoid hemorrhage, intracerebral hemorrhage, intracranial hemorrhage, or cerebral infarction.

- **Clearly identify the cause-and-effect relationship** of any cerebrovascular accident that occurs due to a surgical intervention. Specify whether the event occurred intraoperatively or postprocedurally, and whether infarction or hemorrhage. For cerebral hemorrhage, the type of surgery that was being performed must also be documented.
- **Document any tissue plasminogen activator (tPa) administration** and time started. If the stroke was aborted, document that fact.
- **Identify tobacco use** history, as appropriate. Document any coexisting hypertension, atrial fibrillation, coronary artery disease (CAD), or hypertension.

STROKE AND INFARCTION

Coder Abstraction

Seek answers to these questions when coding a stroke, infarction, or hemorrhage. First, ask if the cerebral event is acute and emergent or a previous event. Second, look for documentation of the site, laterality, and type of stroke or infarction.

Coding Tips

- **Documentation of unilateral weakness due to a stroke** is considered by ICD-10-CM to be hemiparesis/hemiplegia due to the stroke, and should be reported separately. Hemiparesis is not considered a normal sign or symptom of stroke and is always reported separately.
- **If the patient's dominant side is not documented,** assume the right side is dominant, except for ambidextrous patients. In ambidextrous patients, assume the affected side is dominant.
- **Report any and all neurological deficits** of a cerebrovascular accident that are exhibited anytime during a hospitalization, even if the deficits resolve before the patient is released from the hospital.
- **Once the patient has completed the initial treatment** for stroke and is released from acute care, report deficits with codes from category I69, *Sequelae of cerebral infarction*. Neurologic deficits may be present at the time of the acute event, or may arise at any time after the condition, reported with codes from categories I60-I67.
- **If the physician is not specific in recording the site of a stroke or infarction,** it is permissible for coders to use the accompanying CT scans or other radiological reports to report the specific anatomic site, so long as the diagnoses are documented and authenticated by a radiologist.
- **Codes from categories I60-I69 should never be used** to report traumatic intracranial injuries.

ICD-10-CM Guideline Section I(C.9.c)

Medical record documentation should clearly specify the cause-and-effect relationship between the medical intervention and the cerebrovascular accident, in order to assign a code for an intraoperative or postprocedural cerebrovascular accident.

- **Normally, do not report codes from categories I60-I67 with codes from category I69.** However, if the patient has deficits from an old cerebrovascular event and is currently having a new cerebrovascular event, both categories may be reported.
- **If a patient has a history of a past cerebrovascular event** and has no residual sequelae, report code Z86.73, *Personal history of transient ischemic attack (TIA), and cerebral infarction without residual deficits.*
- **If a patient is diagnosed with bilateral nontraumatic intracerebral hemorrhages,** report code I61.6, *Nontraumatic intracerebral hemorrhage, multiple localized.* For bilateral subarachnoid hemorrhage, assign a code for each site. Categories I65 and I66 classify bilateral conditions with unique codes.
- **Also code any documented atrial fibrillation,** coronary artery disease, diabetes mellitus, or hypertension, as these comorbidities are stroke risk factors.

Term	Definition
Stenosis	Narrowing of lumen
Thrombus	Stationary blood clot lodged in vessel
Occlusion	Complete/partial obstruction of lumen
Embolism	Blood clot or other clot carried through vessel to new location, usually lodging in a smaller vessel

SUBSTANCE USE/MENTAL DISORDERS

Physician Documentation

Psychiatric conditions can affect the health and wellness of the patient, and determine how well the patient will comply with any treatment plan. The trend today is a more holistic approach toward the patient, and psychiatric conditions are being diagnosed or treated by primary care physicians in increasing numbers. Prevention and screening and coordination of care with behavioral health specialists help provide opportunities for earlier intervention and improved outcomes.

Documentation Tips

- **Document the recurring nature of a disorder in each encounter.** The medical record for each date of service must stand on its own. A diagnosis in the patient's problem list or past medical history can't be abstracted unless it is addressed in the record for the current encounter.
- **Clearly state the status of substance or alcohol** as use, abuse, or dependence. Link any complication to the substance (eg, alcoholic psychosis or opioid-related constipation). Similarly, document if the conditions are not linked because the classification presumes some relationship.
- **In major depressive disorder,** note the severity as mild, moderate, severe, severe with psychosis, or in partial or full remission.
- **In bipolar disorder,** note whether the current episode is manic or depressive, and whether mild, moderate, severe, severe and psychotic, or in remission (ie, full or partial with a description of the most recent episode as hypomanic, manic, depressed, or mixed).
- **A drug or alcohol "use disorder"** is insufficient for code abstraction. Describe the manifestations of the drug or alcohol use requiring intervention, or specify mild, moderate, or severe use disorder.
- **Intellectual disability affects** a patient's ability to provide a medical history or follow a treatment plan. Document it at every encounter with the disabled patient.
- **Make a note regarding the administration** and results of a depression screening, and if suicide risk was assessed. Document any suicidal ideation.
- **ICD-10-CM provides codes for behaviors** that have not yet been classified to behavioral disorders, but that may contribute to the need for further treatment or study. Among those codes:

Psychosocial Circumstances and Encounters	
R41.0	Disorientation, unspecified
R41.82	Altered mental status, unspecified
R41.840	Attention and concentration deficit
R44.3	Hallucinations, unspecified
R45.83	Excessive crying
R45.84	Anhedonia
R45.86	Emotional lability
R45.87	Impulsiveness
R46.0	Very low level of personal hygiene
R46.2	Strange and inexplicable behavior
R46.81	Obsessive-compulsive behavior

- **Identify post-traumatic stress disorder (PTSD)** as acute or chronic.
- **In obsessive-compulsive disorder,** note any hoarding, skin-picking, obsessive acts, or neuroses.
- **ICD-10-CM assumes a link between alcoholism and any of the following:** persisting amnestic disorder; anxiety disorder; mood disorder; psychotic disorder; sexual dysfunction; or sleep disorder. Document if the conditions should not be linked.
- **Document time** when it is invested in counseling and coordination of care.

SUBSTANCE USE/MENTAL DISORDERS

Coder Abstraction

Drug and alcohol problems and behavioral disorders are increasingly diagnosed and treated by the patient's primary care physician, and should be reported as often as they are documented and assessed or treated.

Coding Tips

- **Documentation of "traits" is not documentation of a disorder.** For example, if a patient is said to have "borderline personality traits," the physician has not documented borderline personality disorder.
- **If documented drug use is not treated or noted as affecting the patient's health, *do not* code it.** A patient's incidental use of drugs is only reported when the use affects treatment or care of a patient (eg, other psychiatric conditions exacerbated by drug use or liver disease documented as affected by the use of recreational drugs).

Use, Abuse, and Dependence

When the physician refers to use or abuse with dependence of the same substance, report only the dependence. If the physician reports use and abuse of the same substance, report only abuse.

- **Diagnoses for children** are at times found in what seems to be an "adult" area of diagnoses in ICD-10-CM, and diagnoses for adults in the "children's" section. For example, the diagnosis for an adult with new onset attention deficit disorder is reported with a code from category F90, in a section entitled "Behavioral and emotional disorders with onset usually occurring in childhood and adolescence." Confidently code behavioral disorders from the Alphabetic Index.
- **Always code intellectual disability when it is documented.** Intellectual disability always affects a patient's ability to follow a treatment plan or to provide a pertinent medical history.
- **Report postpartum depression** with code F53, *Puerperal psychosis,* rather than a code from the pregnancy chapter of ICD-10-CM. Report other behavioral disorders with codes from category O99.34, *Other mental disorders complicating pregnancy, childbirth, and the puerperium.* ICD-10-CM guidelines say that any comorbidity affects pregnancy, so any pre-existing or newly diagnosed behavioral disorder would be reported as a complication of pregnancy, unless the physician specifically states the disorder does not affect the pregnancy.

Assume Causal Relationship for Alcohol Dependence and These Diagnoses	
F10.24	Alcohol dependence with alcohol-induced mood disorder
F10.250	Alcohol dependence with alcohol-induced psychotic disorder with delusions
F10.251	Alcohol dependence with alcohol-induced psychotic disorder with hallucinations
F10.26	Alcohol dependence with alcohol-induced persisting amnestic disorder
F10.280	Alcohol dependence with alcohol-induced anxiety disorder
F10.281	Alcohol dependence with alcohol-induced sexual dysfunction
F10.282	Alcohol dependence with alcohol-induced sleep disorder

- **Do not make assumptions regarding the language** physicians use in describing patient conditions. Use the Alphabetic Index to look up the exact terminology from the medical record to properly abstract the diagnosis code. Never report a more complex condition than what is documented and indexed.

BEST PRACTICES

Physician Documentation

This teaching tool addresses common coding and compliance shortcomings. Minor changes to documentation habits can lead to greater accuracy in abstraction, better compliance, and more appropriate risk scores, quality ratings, and reimbursement.

Documentation Tips

- **Do not use "history of"** to describe a known, active condition. In ICD-10-CM, "history of" always describes a condition that is resolved. Instead of saying "history of," quantify the continuum of care (eg, "Mr. Doe is being seen today for his Parkinson's disease, first diagnosed 7 years ago.").
- **Do not use "history of"** to describe a condition in remission. Instead, document "in remission."
- **Consider each encounter** as a stand-alone account of the patient's health and document accordingly. Coders are not permitted to seek clarity from previous encounter notes.
- **Use an Assessment/Plan format** that clearly aligns each diagnosis to a treatment plan. Example:

Assessment	Plan
1. Type 2 diabetes mellitus	1. Metformin, 500 mg bid; draw A1C in 3 months
2. CKD, stage 3	2. Staff set up appointment with nephrology clinic
3. Bilateral osteoarthritis, knees	3. Patient to continue naproxen as directed

- **Think in ink.** Chronic conditions affect the chief complaint in almost all cases, and physicians think about them, but may not write about them. Document how each chronic condition is affected (eg, "Diabetes is in good control despite pneumonia. Blood glucose today is 105.").
- **Use linking language for related conditions:** "Aphagia due to CVA" rather than "Aphagia and CVA."
- **Specifically identify any complication** and clearly document what caused the complication.
- **State the obvious.** Do not document "GFR of 48." Instead, document, "Chronic kidney disease (CKD) stage 3, GFR of 48." Coders are not permitted to connect the dots or code from laboratory values.
- **Ensure documentation is unique to the encounter.** Use cut-and-paste function with caution!
- **Be specific.** Is the condition acute or chronic? What is the cause? Where is the bleeding? Drug "abuse" or "dependence"? Details yield different diagnostic codes and affect risk scores.
- **Acknowledge pertinent laboratory or radiology results** in the body of the documentation.
- **Document status conditions** at least annually and whenever they affect care and/or are evaluated:

Document These Status Conditions	
Amputation	Asymptomatic HIV status
Dependence on respirator	Dialysis
Ostomy	Transplant
Intellectual disability	History of myocardial infarction

- **Do not say "All systems negative."** Name specific systems reviewed.
- **Document time** when more than 10 minutes have been spent face-to-face with the patient.
- **Tell the whole story.** If physicians do not record what they did, they cannot be paid for it.
- **Review and update problem lists and medication lists** and document having done so.
- **Check administrative details.** Electronic signatures require name, credentials, and date. Written signatures must be legible with credentials.
- **Review and update problem lists** and address each chronic condition at least yearly.

BEST PRACTICES

Coder Abstraction

Proper code look-up affects code selection, which can affect the physician's compliance and reimbursement. The patients are affected too, as the codes assigned become part of their permanent health record.

Coding Tips

- **Follow the instructions** in coding references, including guidelines, chapter-level instructions, and code-specific instructions. Follow the AHA's *Coding Clinic* for guidance.
- **Don't stop at the Alphabetic Index.** The Index points to the correct direction, but it does not always give the exact code. Look up the code in the Tabular Section after finding it in the Index.
- **Pay attention to who is "talking."** Do not code patients' self-diagnoses. Do not code diagnoses written by medical assistant or nurse. Code only diagnoses documented by the physician or other acceptable provider.
- **Watch out for "cloning."** Be aware of what is unique to the current encounter and what is copied from previous encounters. Some electronic health records (EHRs) pull information forward automatically. Do not code from information that has not been referenced or updated by the physician during the current encounter.

Chronic Diseases Rule

Chronic diseases treated on an ongoing basis may be coded and reported as many times as the patient receives treatment and care of the condition(s).

- **Check physician coding.** If a physician assigns codes in documentation, check them. The physician is the expert clinician, while coders are the experts at coding. The physician's words matter more than the codes they select or document. Documented codes without language describing the diagnosis cannot be abstracted.
- **Never make assumptions** about what the note means. A blood glucose reading of 900 cannot be reported as hyperglycemia, unless the physician documents it as such. Query the physician, and the physician can amend the note to reflect the condition, if appropriate; only then can it be coded.

Uncertain or Differential Diagnoses

In the outpatient environment, do not code diagnoses documented as "probable," "suspected," "questionable," "rule-out," or "working" diagnoses. Do not code "differential" diagnoses.

- **Link related conditions** when they are documented as related. Use the Alphabetic Index to determine which conditions are automatically linked by the "with" convention in the ICD-10-CM guidelines.
- **Search and research the Internet** often to understand medications and conditions referenced in documentation. Medscape, National Institutes of Health, and MedlinePlus are dependable resources.
- **Use language** found in the documentation when searching the Alphabetic Index.
- **Read the entire note.** Often, diagnoses are buried within the operative or physical examination notes. Do not rely solely on the assessment.
- **Do not depend completely on software code-lookup programs.** These are not always complete.
- **Always code these status conditions** when present: ostomy, dialysis, HIV positive, transplant, amputation, dependence on respirator.
- **Update codebooks,** resources, and software for ICD-10-CM effective October 1 of each year.
- **A rule of thumb for coding:** If a patient is on medication for a condition, and the condition would return if medication were stopped, code the condition.
- **Never code from superbills.**

Code Index

Note: Page numbers indicated by f, t, and ce refer to figure, table, and clinical examples.

Code Index

HCCs

RxHCCs

Subject Index

Note: Page numbers indicated by f, t, and ce refer to figure, table, and clinical examples.

Subject Index